Nuclear Medicine Imaging:
A Teaching File
Second Edition

Nuclear Medicine Imaging:
A Teaching File
Second Edition

Edited by

M. Reza Habibian, MD
Associate Professor
Department of Radiology and Radiological Sciences
Vanderbilt University Medical Center
Chief, Nuclear Medicine/Ultrasound Service
Tennessee Valley Healthcare System
Nashville, Tennessee

Dominique Delbeke, MD, PhD
Professor
Department of Radiology and Radiological Sciences
Director of Division of Nuclear Medicine/PET
Vanderbilt University Medical Center
Nashville, Tennessee

William H. Martin, MD
Associate Professor of Radiology and Medicine
Co-Director of Nuclear Cardiology
Department of Radiology and Radiological Sciences
Vanderbilt University Medical Center
Nashville, Tennessee

João V. Vitola, MD
Associate Professor
Department of Medicine, Federal University of Paraná Medical School
Director, Quanta Medicina Nuclear
Curitiba, Paraná, Brazil

Martin P. Sandler, MD
Professor of Radiology and Medicine
Associate Vice-Chancellor for Hospital Affairs
Vanderbilt University Medical Center
Nashville, Tennessee

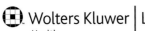

Wolters Kluwer | Lippincott Williams & Wilkins
Health
Philadelphia · Baltimore · New York · London
Buenos Aires · Hong Kong · Sydney · Tokyo

Acquisitions Editor: Lisa McAllister
Managing Editor: Kerry Barrett
Project Manager: Nicole Walz
Manufacturing Manager: Kathleen Brown
Senior Marketing Manager: Angela Panetta
Design Coordinator: Stephen Druding
Cover Designer: Larry Didona
Production Services: Aptara®

Second Edition
© 2009 by Lippincott Williams & Wilkins, a Wolters Kluwer business
© 1999 by Lippincott Williams & Wilkins

Printed in China

Library of Congress Cataloging-in-Publication Data

Nuclear medicine imaging : a teaching file / edited by M. Reza Habibian . . . [et al.]. – 2nd ed.
     p. ; cm.
   Includes bibliographical references and index.
   ISBN 978-0-7817-6988-4
1. Radioisotope scanning—Case studies.   I. Habibian M. Reza.
   [DNLM: 1. Radionuclide Imaging—methods.   2. Nuclear Medicine.   WN 203 N964 2009]
   RC78.7.R4N755 2009
   616.07'575—dc22   2008019362

Care has been taken to confirm the accuracy of the information presented and to describe generally accepted practices. However, the authors, editors, and publisher are not responsible for errors or omissions or for any consequences from application of the information in this book and make no warranty, expressed or implied, with respect to the currency, completeness, or accuracy of the contents of the publication. Application of this information in a particular situation remains the professional responsibility of the practitioner; the clinical treatments described and recommended may not be considered absolute and universal recommendations.

The authors, editors, and publisher have exerted every effort to ensure that drug selection and dosage set forth in this text are in accordance with current recommendations and practice at the time of publication. However, in view of ongoing research, changes in government regulations, and the constant flow of information relating to drug therapy and drug reactions, the reader is urged to check the package insert for each drug for any change in indications and dosage and for added warnings and precautions. This is particularly important when the recommended agent is a new or infrequently employed drug.

Some drugs and medical devices presented in this publication have Food and Drug Administration (FDA) clearance for limited use in restricted research settings. It is the responsibility of health care providers to ascertain the FDA status of each drug or device planned for use in their clinical practice.

The publishers have made every effort to trace copyright holders for borrowed material. If they have inadvertently overlooked any, they will be pleased to make the necessary arrangements at the first opportunity.

To purchase additional copies of this book, call our customer service department at (800) 638-3030 or fax orders to (301) 223-2320. International customers should call (301) 223-2300. Visit Lippincott Williams & Wilkins on the Internet at: LWW.com. Lippincott Williams & Wilkins customer service representatives are available from 8:30 am to 6 pm, EST.

10 9 8 7 6 5 4 3 2 1

DEDICATION

This book is dedicated to the nuclear medicine and radiology residents who have provided us the stimulus to produce *Nuclear Medicine Imaging: A Teaching File*. We hope they will enjoy reading these cases even more than we did writing them.

CONTRIBUTORS

Carlos Cunha Pereira Neto, MD
Co-Director, Quanta Medicina Nuclear
Curitiba, Paraná, Brazil

Dominique Delbeke, MD, PhD
Professor
Department of Radiology and Radiological Sciences
Director of Division of Nuclear Medicine/PET
Vanderbilt University Medical Center
Nashville, Tennessee

M. Reza Habibian, MD
Associate Professor
Department of Radiology and Radiological Sciences
Vanderbilt University Medical Center
Chief, Nuclear Medicine/Ultrasound Service
Tennessee Valley Healthcare System
Nashville, Tennessee

William H. Martin, MD
Associate Professor of Radiology and Medicine
Co-Director of Nuclear Cardiology
Department of Radiology and Radiological Sciences
Vanderbilt University Medical Center
Nashville, Tennessee

James A. Patton, PhD
Professor of Radiology and Physics
Department of Radiology and Radiological Sciences
Vanderbilt University Medical Center
Nashville, Tennessee

Martin P. Sandler, MD
Professor of Radiology and Medicine
Associate Vice-Chancellor for Hospital Affairs
Vanderbilt University Medical Center
Nashville, Tennessee

Chirayu Shah, MD
Division of Nuclear Medicine
Department of Radiology and Radiological Sciences
Vanderbilt University Medical Center
Nashville, Tennessee

João V. Vitola, MD
Associate Professor
Department of Medicine, Federal University of Paraná
    Medical School
Director, Quanta Medicina Nuclear
Curitiba, Paraná, Brazil

PUBLISHER'S FOREWORD

Teaching Files are one of the hallmarks of education in radiology. There has long been a need for a comprehensive series of books, using the Teaching File format, which would provide the kind of personal "consultation with the experts" normally found only in the setting of a teaching hospital. Lippincott Williams & Wilkins is proud to have created such a series; our goal is to provide the resident and practicing radiologist with a useful resource that answers this need.

Actual cases have been culled from extensive teaching files in a major medical center. The discussions presented mimic those performed on a daily basis between residents and faculty members customary in many radiology teaching programs.

The format of the books is designed so that each case can be studied as an unknown, if so desired. A consistent format is used to present each case. A brief clinical history is given, followed by several images. Then, relevant findings, followed by a discussion of the case, differential diagnosis, and final diagnosis are given. The authors thereby guide the reader through the interpretation of each case.

We hope that this series will become a valuable and trusted teaching tool for radiologists at any stage of training or practice, and that it will also be a benefit to clinicians whose patients undergo these imaging studies.

The Publisher

FOREWORD

Participating in education is a major reason that physicians enjoy being in an academic environment. Academic physicians provide education to several audiences including medical students, residents, and practicing physicians in several formats, including didactic lectures, case presentations, textbooks, and teaching files. The various formats are appropriate for certain audiences. The teaching file approach is particularly applicable to specialties such as radiology and nuclear medicine, in which we are asked to make diagnoses based on findings on images. The teaching file approach is particularly applicable to nuclear medicine because of the new imaging studies that continue to be developed and because of the need to have examples for medical students, residents, and practicing physicians. *Nuclear Medicine Imaging: A Teaching File*, edited by Drs. M. Reza Habibian, Dominique Delbeke, William H. Martin, João V. Vitola, and Martin P. Sandler, provides an excellent overview of nuclear medicine through the case presentation (teaching file) format.

Nuclear medicine encompasses a wide variety of topics. In its infancy, nuclear medicine consisted primarily of imaging of the thyroid, lung perfusion, liver–spleen, bone, kidney, and blood–brain permeability. The applications of nuclear medicine have grown tremendously, particularly in the area of cardiovascular and oncologic diseases. The importance of myocardial perfusion imaging is demonstrated by its rapid and continued growth. The growth in oncology has been hastened by the use of gallium 67 citrate and more recently by the use of fluorine-18 2-2-fluoro-deoxyglucose (^{18}F-FDG) and PET imaging. Oncology imaging agents, such as radiolabeled antibodies, Octreoscan, and MIBG, also contribute to the growth of nuclear medicine imaging in oncology.

Nuclear Medicine Imaging: A Teaching File covers the gamut of procedures performed in most departments. The book is composed of chapters that are based on organ systems. A brief overview of each topic is presented, and the bulk of the teaching is in the case presentations. This book focuses on the clinical information that is available from nuclear medicine imaging studies. The presentation of the images with a brief history permits readers to determine the findings and come to a diagnosis before the findings and diagnoses are described in the text. Thus, the readers can compare their interpretation of the images with those of the authors, if they wish to test themselves. Otherwise, the chapters can be read like a textbook to educate the readers in the various uses of nuclear medicine imaging.

Each chapter integrates the imaging studies that have been routinely available with the newer imaging studies that are only now becoming available. In Chapter 1 the use of thyroid imaging is demonstrated in addition to the use of radionuclide imaging in evaluation of hyperparathyroidism and neuroendocrine tumors. In Chapter 4 the use of brain perfusion imaging and radionuclide cisternography is included with cases using cerebral perfusion imaging with acetazolamide challenge and with metabolic imaging using ^{18}F-FDG.

The use of case presentation is an effective method of learning and reviewing nuclear medicine imaging. The authors and editors have provided excellent clinical material for portraying the clinical applications of nuclear medicine, *Nuclear Medicine Imaging: A Teaching File* is an up-to-date resource of nuclear medicine imaging studies.

Physicians practicing nuclear medicine will find this book to be an excellent review of the current status of nuclear medicine. Medical students and residents will find that this book provides an excellent in-depth overview of nuclear medicine. The editors are to be congratulated on their development of these cases, outlined in an enjoyable format for learning, that provide such contemporary information in this rapidly changing specialty of nuclear medicine.

R. Edward Coleman, MD
Professor of Radiology and Director of Nuclear Medicine
Department of Radiology
Duke University Medical Center
Durham, North Carolina

PREFACE

Since the publication of the first edition of *Nuclear Medicine Imaging: A Teaching File,* in 1999, dramatic technological advancements have occurred in the field of nuclear medicine, necessitating the publication of the second edition.

The second edition is a complete revision of the text. Many new cases and illustrations have been introduced to add to or replace the old cases; however, a remnant of several of the original cases has been preserved. In spite of these changes, the impetus for producing *Nuclear Medicine: A Teaching File,* has not changed. The second edition has been designed to provide an updated single reference source of nuclear medicine cases, including positron emission tomography, that may be used as a comprehensive teaching reference. The book is designed to be used within the private practice milieu, by residents in nuclear medicine or radiology, by medical students, and by specialists whose fields overlap with nuclear imaging.

This edition is divided into nine chapters. The first eight of these are devoted to clinical nuclear medicine, each chapter covering a variety of cases ranging from the simple to the more complex. The subjects of the thyroid nodule, hyperthyroidism, and thyroid cancer have been reviewed in depth, along with current available clinical guidelines. Similarly, the practical approach in the selection of lung ventilation/perfusion imaging versus pulmonary CT angiography in the diagnosis of pulmonary embolism has been presented. Chapters 3 and 8 have extensive references that will allow the interested reader to research in greater depth the rapidly expanding and changing fields of nuclear cardiology and oncology imaging using both short- and long-lived radioisotopes. Chapter 9 has been devoted to a series of case presentations of imaging artifacts that continue to be important and often confusing in the daily practice of nuclear medicine.

In order to keep the price of this text as low as possible, most of the figures are presented in black and white, although, when necessary, the liberal use of color images was not avoided.

We sincerely hope that this text will provide nuclear medicine physicians, radiologists, trainees, and others interested in nuclear imaging with a reference text of teaching files that will enhance their practice of clinical nuclear medicine as well as provide a valuable resource for those preparing for board certification or maintenance of certification examinations.

M. Reza Habibian, MD
Dominique Delbeke, MD, PhD
William H. Martin, MD
João V. Vitola, MD, PhD
Martin P. Sandler, MD

ACKNOWLEDGMENTS

We would like to thank all contributors, including the authors and publishers who have granted us permission to reproduce their tables and illustrations. We are indebted to Jaime Branch for her editorial assistance, as well as to John Bobbitt of Vanderbilt University Medical Center and Brandon Lunday of the Nashville Veterans Affairs Medical Center for their production of the illustrations. Special thanks to David Burkett, the Radiation Safety Officer at the Nashville Veterans Affairs Medical Center for assistance in reorganizing the illustrations and figures. We are also grateful to Dr. Ronald Walker for his review, advice, and critique in preparation of this edition. We wish to acknowledge the work of all the technologists at both institutions, without whom this work could not have been produced.

CONTENTS

CHAPTER FOUR NEUROLOGIC IMAGING 155

Dominique Delbeke and Carlos Cunha Pereira Neto

CHAPTER FIVE GASTROINTESTINAL AND CORRELATIVE ABDOMINAL NUCLEAR MEDICINE IMAGING 202

M. Reza Habibian and Chirayu Shah

CHAPTER SIX RENAL SCINTIGRAPHY 259

Carlos Cunha Pereira Neto and Dominique Delbeke

CHAPTER SEVEN MUSCULOSKELETAL SCINTIGRAPHY 306

M. Reza Habibian and Carlos Cunha Pereira Neto

CHAPTER EIGHT ONCOLOGIC IMAGING 423

Dominique Delbeke and William H. Martin

CHAPTER NINE ARTIFACTS 512

James A. Patton

CHAPTER ONE

ENDOCRINE IMAGING

William H. Martin, Martin P. Sandler,
and M. Reza Habibian

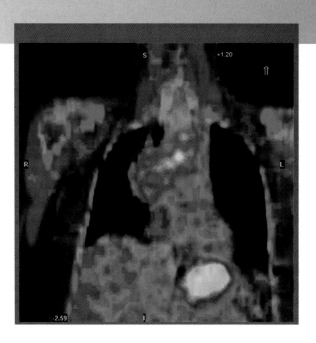

This chapter includes a series of scintigraphic case presentations with correlative imaging of the thyroid, parathyroid, and adrenal glands. Imaging of neuroendocrine tumors is addressed in Chapter 8.

THYROID GLAND

The shield-shaped thyroid gland is normally positioned anterior and lateral to the cricoid cartilage, although it may be located more superiorly anterior to the thyroid cartilage or more inferiorly anterior to the trachea. The thyroid contains two lobes, each with superior and inferior poles, an isthmus, and often a pyramidal lobe that originates from the isthmus or the medial aspect of either lobe. The pyramidal lobe develops along the distal thyroglossal duct, thus its location. Similarly, thyroid tissue may be ectopically located anywhere along its embryonic migration track—i.e., as a lingual thyroid at the base of the tongue, within a vestigial midline thyroglossal duct cyst, or further caudally within the mediastinum. The normal thyroid weighs 15 to 20 g; a mildly enlarged 30-g gland is barely palpable, whereas a 40-g gland is easily palpable and often visible with deglutition if the neck is extended. Goiters as large as 60 g or more are easily visible in the unextended neck.

Within the regulation of the hypothalamic–pituitary axis, the functions of the thyroid gland include the trapping of iodine, the synthesis and storage of hormones, and the release of these hormones into the circulation (Fig. 1.A). This ability to trap iodine is not unique to the thyroid gland, because trapping also occurs in the salivary glands, gastric mucosa, and breast, but none of these other tissues is able to organify the trapped iodine to synthesize thyroid hormones.

Thyroid Gland Scintigraphy

Technetium 99m- (^{99m}Tc) pertechnetate or iodine 123 (^{123}I) may be used to image the thyroid gland. The advantage of using ^{123}I as compared with ^{99m}Tc is that ^{123}I is not only trapped, as is pertechnetate, but is also organified, thus providing a more accurate representation of thyroid function. Owing to its low cost and ready availability, ^{99m}Tc-pertechnetate is more frequently used and, in most instances, provides comparable diagnostic information. To obtain the maximum image quality and spatial resolution, a pinhole collimator is used to acquire anterior and oblique images. Oblique imaging may sometimes demonstrate a small posterior nodule (Fig. 1.B, lower) not seen on the anterior images (Fig. 1.B, upper).

^{131}I is used primarily for the determination of thyroid uptake. Although ^{131}I is used routinely to detect recurrent and metastatic thyroid cancer, the high radiation dose from its

HYPOTHALAMIC-PITUITARY-THYROID AXIS

Figure 1.A

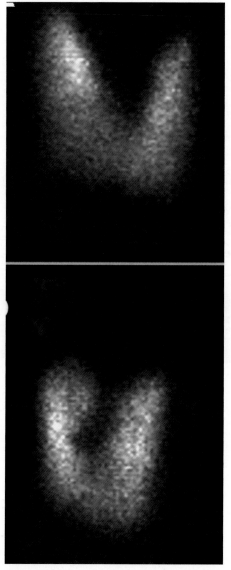

Figure 1.B

beta emissions as well as its high-energy gamma emission (364 keV) precludes its use in routine thyroid imaging.

Thyroid hormone therapy with either thyroxine (T_4, Synthroid®) or tri-iodothyronine (T_3, Cytomel®) will suppress the hypothalamic–pituitary–thyroid axis and markedly diminish the uptake of radionuclides used for thyroid imaging. Flooding the vascular pool with iodine by administering exogenous iodine, as with iodinated contrast agents, saturates the thyroid with iodine and similarly suppresses thyroidal uptake of radioiodine.

PARATHYROID GLANDS

The parathyroid glands are usually situated along the posterior aspect of the lateral thyroid lobes. They normally measure about 6 × 3 mm in width and weigh approximately 35 mg each. There are usually four parathyroid glands, two upper and two lower. Supernumerary glands have been reported in 2% to 6% of adults and may occur anywhere from the level of the submandibular glands to the arch of the aorta.

Parathyroid Gland Scintigraphy

Although technetium 99m/thallium 201 (^{99m}Tc/^{201}Tl) subtraction imaging has been used to effectively identify parathyroid pathology, ^{99m}Tc-sestamibi (^{99m}Tc-MIBI), a lipophilic cation used for both myocardial and tumor imaging, is now used. Distribution of ^{99m}Tc-MIBI is proportional to blood flow, and once intracellular, it is sequestered primarily within the mitochondria in response to the electrical potential generated across the membrane bilayers of both the cell and mitochondria. The large number of mitochondria present in the cells of parathyroid adenomas may be responsible for the avid uptake and slow release of ^{99m}Tc-MIBI in parathyroid adenomas compared with surrounding thyroid tissue. Detection and localization of parathyroid adenomas with ^{99m}Tc-MIBI can be performed by either a single radiopharmaceutical injection or a dual-isotope procedure using a low-energy high-resolution collimator with immediate and 2- to 3-hour delayed anterior (and sometimes oblique) imaging.

ADRENAL GLANDS

Each adrenal gland lies in the retroperitoneal perinephric space, near the upper poles of the kidneys. Although CT and MRI are used as the primary imaging modalities for adrenal pathology, scintigraphic techniques are important in several specific instances.

Adrenal Medulla Scintigraphy

The adrenal medulla produces and secretes the principal catecholamine epinephrine. Metaiodobenzylguanidine (MIBG) is a guanethidine analog that localizes via the norepinephrine reuptake mechanism into catecholamine storage vesicles of adrenergic nerve endings and cells of the adrenal medulla. MIBG localizes in other organs with rich adrenergic innervation, including the heart, spleen, and salivary glands. Both ^{131}I-MIBG and ^{123}I-MIBG are commercially available for imaging of neuroendocrine tumors, but ^{123}I-MIBG is not FDA-approved in the United States. ^{123}I-MIBG has more favorable dosimetry and imaging characteristics, permitting the acquisition of single photon emission computed tomography (SPECT) and SPECT-CT images.

With ^{123}I-MIBG, activity within normal adrenals as well as the uterus and prostate can be seen. Owing to radiolysis, activity within the bowel and bladder is physiologic.

Patients are pretreated with inorganic iodine (Lugol's solution or potassium iodide), 1 to 2 mg/kg per day, beginning 1 to 2 days prior and continuing for 1 week following the administration of ^{131}I-MIBG and for 3 days after ^{123}I-MIBG injection. After administration of ^{131}I-MIBG, imaging is delayed to 48 and 72 hours, whereas imaging with ^{123}I-MIBG is performed at 24 hours.

CASE 1.1

History: A 43-year-old female was noted to have a palpable nodule in the right lobe of her thyroid. Her thyroid function tests were entirely normal, and she was referred for thyroid scintigraphy (Fig. 1.1 A).

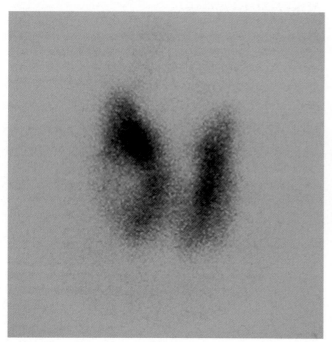

Figure 1.1 A

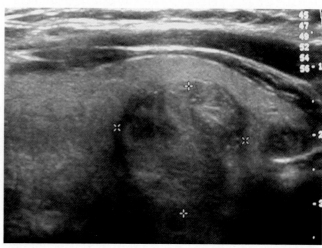

Figure 1.1 B

Findings: A scintigram of the neck following IV injection 10 mCi ^{99m}Tc-pertechnetate showed an area of markedly reduced uptake in the lower pole of the right lobe, corresponding to the palpable mass and representing a hypofunctioning nodule.

Discussion: Some 85% to 90% of thyroid nodules are hypofunctioning, but only 10% of cold nodules are malignant. The remaining hypofunctioning nodules represent degenerative nodules, nodular hemorrhage, cysts, focal thyroiditis, infiltrative disorders such as amyloid, and nonthyroid neoplasms.

A subsequent ultrasound (Fig. 1.1 B) demonstrated a 1.9-cm solid mass in the lower pole of the right lobe of the thyroid without sonographic findings suspicious of malignancy. A fine-needle-aspiration (FNA) biopsy was benign; annual sonographic surveillance was planned.

Palpable thyroid nodules occur in 5% of women and 1% of men and are detectable in 40% of people by ultrasound, more often in women and in the elderly. Approximately 5% to 10% of these nodules are malignant, depending on age, gender, family history, and prior radiation exposure. In the United States, approximately 24,000 cases of differentiated thyroid cancer are diagnosed annually. The incidence is rising, probably related to increased detectability using ultrasound. Imaging is used in an effort to aid in the differentiation of malignant from benign lesions.

Current guidelines recommend a history and physical exam followed by a serum TSH determination and an ultrasound procedure. Generally the presence of a firm nodule, rapid growth, fixation to the adjacent structures, vocal cord paralysis, ipsilateral cervical adenopathy, male gender, age younger than 20 years or older than 70 years, history of head and neck radiation, and family history of thyroid cancer are significant risk factors suggestive of increased malignant potential.

If the serum TSH is suppressed, a ^{99m}Tc-pertechnetate scan is recommended to exclude the presence of a functioning nodule, for which biopsy and ultrasound are unnecessary (see discussion of Case 1.2). If the TSH is normal or elevated, an ultrasound is recommended to document number, size, location, and specific sonographic characteristics of the nodule(s). FNA biopsy is the most accurate and cost-effective tool for evaluating thyroid nodules. Nonpalpable nodules have the same risk of malignancy as palpable nodules of similar size, so nodules identified incidentally on ultrasound or CT require evaluation similar to clinically evident nodules. Figure 1.1 C and Figure 1.1 D demonstrate an incidental hypofunctioning nodule within the medial aspect of the left lobe and isthmus. Nodules smaller than 10 mm need not be biopsied unless suspicious ultrasound characteristics are found or there is a family history of thyroid cancer or a history of radiation exposure of the head or neck. Otherwise, nodules larger than 10 mm are biopsied by FNA using ultrasound guidance, even if they are partially necrotic. Recommendations regarding multinodular goiter are reviewed in Case 1.3. FNA biopsy produces false

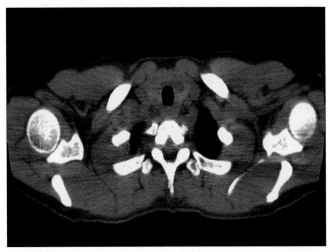

Figure 1.1 C

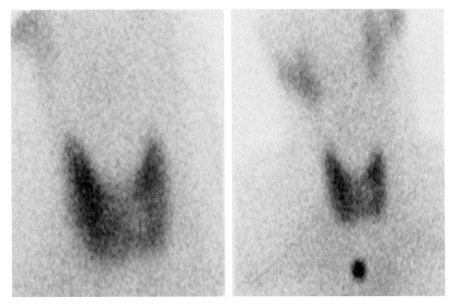

Figure 1.1 D

negatives in 1% to 3% of cases, so annual ultrasound surveillance is recommended; nodule growth of >20% in diameter is an indication for repeat biopsy.

None of the ultrasound findings can be used to either diagnose or exclude malignancy with a high degree of accuracy, but the combination of a solid hypoechoic mass with an irregular border, microcalcifications, and/or increased intranodular vascularity increase the potential for malignancy, mandating biopsy.

Diagnosis: Benign follicular neoplasm.

CASE 1.2

History: A 32-year-old female is referred for scintigraphy and ^{131}I uptake (radioactive iodine uptake, or RAIU) owing to the finding of a left neck mass and a suppressed serum TSH value.

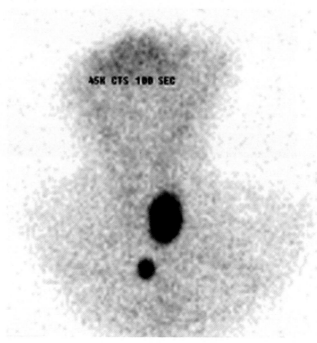

Figure 1.2 A

Findings: On the ^{99m}Tc-pertechnetate scan (Fig. 1.2 A) there is intense uptake in the palpable left thyroid nodule with complete suppression of all extranodular activity. The RAIU is elevated to 38% at 24 hours.

Discussion: These findings are consistent with an autonomously functioning follicular adenoma. The suppression of all extranodular activity is seen in patients with overt hyperthyroidism. In the context of hyperthyroidism, the solitary hyperfunctioning nodule is virtually always benign; no additional imaging or biopsy is required. Definitive treatment with ^{131}I or surgical resection is indicated to relieve the patient of her hyperthyroidism.

According to the recent American Thyroid Association guidelines for patients with thyroid nodules, scintigraphy for a nodule or multinodular goiter (MNG) is indicated only (1) in patients who have a serum TSH below the lower limit of the normal range, (2) if ectopic thyroid tissue or a retrosternal nodule is suspected, or (3) if an indeterminate FNA biopsy result is suggestive of a follicular neoplasm. If an autonomously hyperfunctioning nodule is not seen on scintigraphy in the patient with an indeterminate biopsy, thyroidectomy is recommended. A recent report of 42 consecutive nodule patients with indeterminate cytologic results found that fluorodeoxyglucose positron emission tomography (FDG-PET) had a sensitivity of 100% and a specificity of 39%, concluding that the use of FDG-PET would reduce unnecessary thyroidectomies by 39% in patients with benign disease. Other authors have reported a high negative predictive value and high sensitivity in the pre-operative evaluation of thyroid nodules. Similarly, ^{201}Tl and ^{99m}Tc sestamibi are useful adjuncts to FNA cytology in the evaluation of solitary thyroid nodules when the latter is inconclusive (see discussion of Case 1.8).

In a prospective report of 78 patients with solitary hypofunctioning thyroid nodules undergoing thallium scintigraphy preoperatively, 86% of the 65 benign lesions showed less than or equal uptake as compared with normal thyroid tissue at 3 hours, and 85% of the malignant lesions were "hot" on delayed imaging; however, 14% of the benign lesions also showed increased activity on the delayed images. In a report of 71 patients undergoing preoperative ^{99m}Tc-MIBI scintigraphy, 91% of the 23 carcinomas were positive with ^{99m}Tc-MIBI, and only 11% of the benign lesions were positive. Therefore both ^{99m}Tc-MIBI and ^{201}Tl imaging are useful adjuncts to FNA cytology in the evaluation of solitary thyroid nodules, especially when the latter is inconclusive.

Although a functioning thyroid nodule in the euthyroid patient may represent hyperplastic (sensitive to TSH stimulation) tissue, most are autonomously functioning adenomas (AFTNs) arising independently of TSH stimulation. Biochemical hyperthyroidism, often subclinical, is present in 74% of patients at presentation, although overt hyperthyroidism is less common. Over a period of 3 years after detection, 33% of AFTNs enlarge in patients not receiving definitive therapy, and 24% of euthyroid patients develop hyperthyroidism. If overt hyperthyroidism exists, the surrounding normal thyroid tissue will be suppressed, and the TSH level will be undetectable (Fig. 1.2 A).

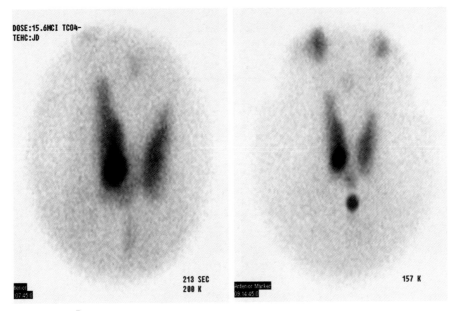

Figure 1.2 B

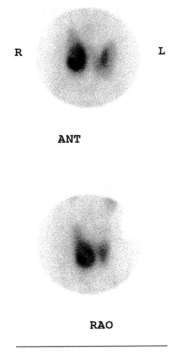

ANT

RAO

Figure 1.2 C

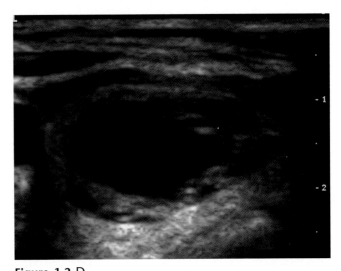

Figure 1.2 D

In euthyroid patients, surrounding extranodular thyroid tissue will be visible (Fig. 1.4B) and thyroid function studies will be normal; these patients can be followed on an annual basis. Spontaneous cystic degeneration occurs in 27%, manifested by central photopenia; there is little concern for malignancy (Figs. 1.2 C, D). Radioiodine therapy with a dose of 10 to 20 mCi is a simple, safe, and cost-effective mode of therapy, but late hypothyroidism may develop in as many as 25% of such patients. Surgery may be advisable for larger AFTNs, especially if compressive symptoms exist. As an alternative to surgery or ^{131}I treatment, percutaneous ethanol injection (PEI) is successful in alleviating hyperthyroidism in approximately 67% of patients

with toxic AFTNs, but this usually requires repeated injections under sonographic guidance; current guidelines recommend PEI only for small AFTNs (volume <5 mL) not yet completely suppressing the surrounding thyroid parenchyma, and then only if such patients are concerned about the occurrence of late hypothyroidism.

In the evaluation of a nodule appearing hyperfunctioning on ^{99m}Tc imaging, one should be aware of the occasional existence of a discordant nodule. Discordant thyroid imaging is dissociation between trapping and organification, measured respectively with ^{99m}Tc-pertechnetate and [123]I. It occurs in only 2% to 8% of thyroid nodules and is not specific for

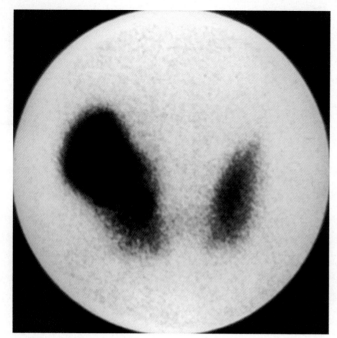

Figure 1.2 E

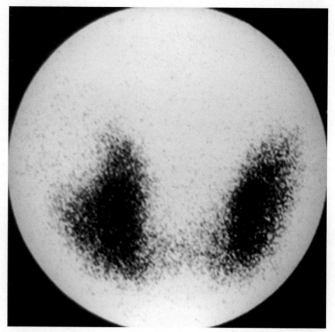

Figure 1.2 F

malignant disease. A nodule that traps ^{99m}Tc (hot) (Fig. 1.2 E) but is unable to organify iodine (cold) (Fig. 1.4F) is much more likely to be benign than malignant. This ability to trap small anions accompanied by a loss of the ability to organify iodine has been observed in adenomatous goiters, focal thyroiditis, and follicular adenomas, most often seen in multinodular goiters. If it is assumed that 8% of hot nodules with ^{99m}Tc are cold with ^{123}I and 10% of those are malignant, then less than 1% of hot nodules seen with ^{99m}Tc imaging are malignant. Additional

radioiodine imaging of hot nodules identified on a ^{99m}Tc scan should probably be reserved for patients deemed at higher risk for malignancy, and initial scintigraphy with ^{123}I rather than ^{99m}Tc-pertechnetate should be reserved for patients deemed at high risk for carcinoma, such as children, males, and patients with a prior history of radiation exposure or a family history of thyroid cancer.

Diagnosis: Toxic autonomously functioning follicular adenoma.

CASE 1.3

History: A 60-year-old woman with a history of endometrial sarcoma was referred for ^{99m}Tc-pertechnetate scintigraphy (Fig. 1.3 A) when a goiter was noted incidentally on CT imaging.

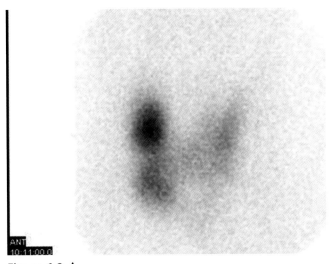

Figure 1.3 A

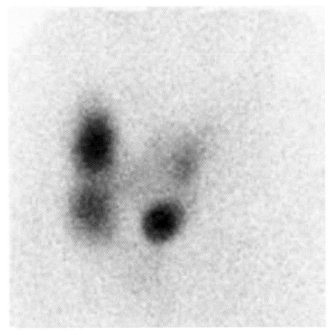

Figure 1.3 B

Findings: There is heterogeneous uptake throughout the gland with two hyperfunctioning nodules within the right lobe and a large hypofunctioning nodule within the lower pole of the left lobe. A cobalt 57 (^{57}Co) marker (Fig. 1.3 B) has been placed on a palpable nodule on the left and found to be congruent with the dominant left-lower-lobe cold nodule.

Discussion: The findings are most consistent with a typical MNG, but the left-lower-pole hypofunctioning nodule must be considered worrisome for neoplasm. In view of the history of endometrial sarcoma, the patient underwent thyroidectomy. Histopathology was consistent with MNG with no evidence of thyroid carcinoma or metastatic sarcoma.

Current guidelines affirm that patients with multiple thyroid nodules have the same risk of malignancy as those with solitary nodules, approximately 5% to 10%, depending on age, gender, radiation exposure history, family history, and other factors. If the patient has a low or low-normal serum TSH concentration, a radioiodine scan is recommended to determine the functionality of each nodule larger than 1 to 1.5 cm in diameter. FNA biopsy is recommended only for those isofunctioning or nonfunctioning nodules that demonstrate suspicious sonographic features, such as hypoechogenicity, irregular borders, microcalcifications, and/or intranodular vascularity. If none of the nodules has a suspicious sonographic appearance and multiple sonographically similar coalescent nodules are present, the likelihood of malignancy is low enough that only the largest nodule should be biopsied. If nodular growth of more than 20% in diameter and more than 2 mm occurs at serial follow-up ultrasound, repeat ultrasound-guided biopsy is recommended owing to the 1% to 3% rate of false-negative cytology results at initial FNA.

The development of MNG is related to cycling periods of stimulation followed by involution; it may be idiopathic or occur as a result of endemic iodine deficiency. Over time, the gland enlarges and evolves into an admixture of fibrosis, functional nodules, and nonfunctioning involuted nodules. Scintigraphically, the MNG is a heterogeneously appearing, asymmetrically enlarged gland with multiple cold, warm, and hot areas of various sizes (Figure 1.3 A). The differential diagnosis includes autoimmune Hashimoto's thyroiditis, multiple adenomata, and multifocal carcinoma.

In the patients with hyperthyroidism, the 24-hour RAIU in toxic nodular goiter may be elevated, but more frequently it is within the high-normal range. Treatment of toxic MNG can be accomplished with ^{131}I administration or by thyroidectomy with similarly good outcomes. Nontoxic MNG requires treatment if compressive symptoms are bothersome. In the patient with comorbidities, ^{131}I therapy, 30 mCi, often with rhTSH stimulation, can effect a 40% decrease in gland volume over the first year and 60% by the end of the second year with alleviation of compressive symptomatology.

Diagnosis: Multinodular goiter with benign dominant cold nodule.

CASE 1.4

History: A 24-year-old female patient presented with a history of recent weight loss, palpitations, anxiety, and heat intolerance. The clinical exam revealed tremulousness, moist palms, tachycardia, and a 60-g nontender goiter with no apparent nodularity by palpation. An ^{131}I uptake (RAIU) and ^{99m}Tc thyroid scan were performed (Fig. 1.4 A). Four-hour and 24-hour RAIU values were 46% (normal = 10% to 15%) and 62% (normal = 15% to 25%), respectively.

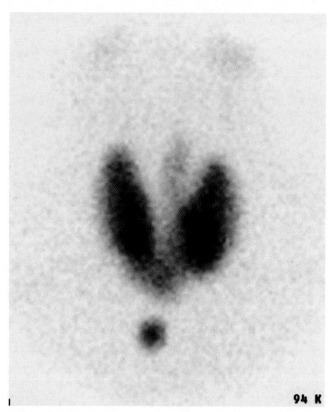

Figure 1.4 A

TABLE 1.1 Classification of hyperthyroidism

Thyroid gland (±95%)
    Diffuse toxic goiter (Graves' disease)
    Toxic nodular goiter
        Multinodular (Plummer's disease)
        Solitary nodule
    Thyroiditis (subacute)
Exogenous thyroid hormone/iodine (±4%)
    Iatrogenic
    Factitious
    Iodine-induced (Jod-Basedow)
Rarely encountered causes (±1%)
    Hypothalamic-pituitary neoplasms
    Struma ovarii
    Excessive human chorionic gonadotropin
      production by trophoblastic tissue
    Metastatic thyroid carcinoma

Reproduced from Sandler MP, Patton JA, Sacks GA, Shaff MI, Partain CL, Baxter J. Scintigraphy thyroid imaging. In: Sandler MP, Patton JA, Partain CL, eds. Thyroid and parathyroid imaging. Norwalk, CT: Appleton & Lange, 1986: 113, with permission.

Findings: There is homogenous uptake of ^{99m}Tc by the thyroid gland (250,000 counts in 60 sec) with a convex contour to the gland (Fig. 1.4 A). No nodularity is present. Mild linear activity originates from the medial aspect of the left thyroid lobe. Note the relative absence of background and salivary gland activity secondary to increased thyroidal uptake. A ^{57}Co marker has been placed on the suprasternal notch.

Discussion: The scintigraphic finding of diffuse toxic goiter and an elevated RAIU in a young woman with hyperthyroidism is diagnostic of Graves' disease. The pyramidal lobe, a remnant of the distal thyroglossal duct, is identified in less than 10% of euthyroid patients but is visualized in as many as 43% of patients with Graves' disease (Fig. 1.4 A). The hyperthyroidism of Graves' disease is often accompanied by exophthalmos and sometimes pretibial myxedema.

Hyperthyroidism is a clinical syndrome that results from supraphysiologic levels of thyroid hormones and may occur as a consequence of numerous disease processes (Table 1.1). Clinical history and physical examination combined with serum hormone and antithyroid autoantibody levels, thyroid scintigraphy, and RAIU measurement usually allow identification and differentiation of the various etiologies.

The presence of thyroid stimulatory antibodies (TSIg) in patients with Graves' disease results in both increased trapping and organification by the thyroid gland. Scintigraphic imaging of patients with Graves' disease using ^{99m}Tc or ^{123}I reveals diffusely increased thyroidal activity with minimal background and salivary gland activity (Fig. 1.4 A). The gland size will frequently but not always appear enlarged, sometimes asymmetrically. It occurs primarily in young women but also in children and in the elderly.

Patients with diffuse toxic goiter will, in most cases, have an increased RAIU at 4 and 24 hours. Occasionally, patients with Graves' disease may have a normal 24-hour RAIU but an elevated 4-hour RAIU due to rapid ^{131}I turnover (4hr/24hr RAIU >1). The low RAIU (usually ≤5%) of hyperthyroid patients with subacute or autoimmune thyroiditis is easily differentiated from the high-normal (20% to 30%) uptake seen in some patients with Graves' disease or those with toxic nodular goiters.

The thyroid scan aids in the differentiation of toxic nodular goiter from Graves' disease. In a series of 178 patients with hyperthyroidism and no suspicion of thyroid nodularity, 152 patients (85%) had typical Graves' disease but 9% had

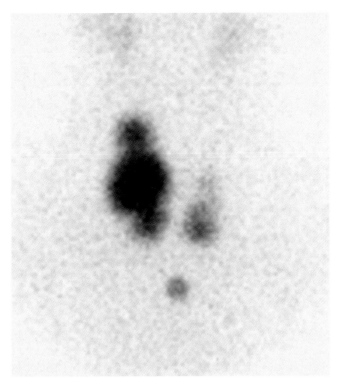

Figure 1.4 B

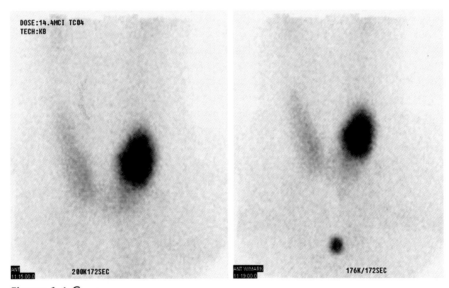

Figure 1.4 C

functioning or nonfunctioning nodules, 3% had unexpected subacute thyroiditis, and 3% had AFTNs. Although a cold nodule in a diffuse toxic goiter may represent a functioning but TSH-dependent adenoma (Marine-Lenhart syndrome), malignancy should be excluded by biopsy or thyroidectomy. Therefore scintigraphy is important in the management of patients with Graves' disease, since 15% of those patients may have associated nodularity or another diagnosis such as AFTN or subacute thyroiditis.

Figure 1.4 B is the scan of a 66-year-old female presenting with a history of fatigue, weakness, palpitations, and dyspnea on exertion. Clinical exam revealed an irregularly, irregular

rhythm, bibasilar rales, and a 40-g nodular, firm goiter. Her 24-hour RAIU was 23%. Note the heterogeneous activity throughout the thyroid gland, with several large nodules demonstrating intense trapping. A ^{57}Co marker is at the suprasternal notch. In the context of hyperthyroidism, these findings would be consistent with toxic MNG, probably complicated by atrial fibrillation and mild high-output congestive heart failure. Toxic nodular goiter may be due to multiple nodules (Fig. 1.4 B) or a solitary hyperfunctioning nodule (Fig. 1.4 C).

Patients with toxic nodular goiter are typically between the fourth and fifth decades of life and are more likely to have cardiac complications. On the other hand, patients with solitary toxic nodules are often younger, varying in age from adolescence to adulthood. Uninodular autonomously functioning adenomas are monoclonal neoplasms, but the pathogenesis of toxic MNG is less certain (see discussion of Case 1.3).

Scintigraphically, toxic MNG (Fig. 1.4 B) appears as focal areas of increased and decreased radionuclide activity scattered throughout the gland. The areas of increased activity represent islands of autonomously hyperfunctioning tissue, whereas the areas of decreased activity are areas suppressed by excessive thyroid hormone levels. Background and salivary activity are often more prominent than that seen in patients with Graves' disease, and the RAIU is often within the high-normal range rather than elevated.

Hyperthyroidism due to Graves' disease or toxic nodular goiter may be treated with ^{131}I administration. Antithyroid drug therapy achieves a permanent remission in only 10% to 14% of Graves' patients and is not a logical long-term option in toxic nodular goiter. Although thyroidectomy is effective and complications are infrequent, surgery is performed only occasionally at present, usually in patients who are unable to accept alternative therapies or who have extremely large goiters with compressive symptoms. Radioiodine therapy is effective, practical, inexpensive, and available on an outpatient basis.

[131]I should not be administered in the absence of an elevated or high-normal RAIU and confirmation of biomedical hyperthyroidism. An elevated RAIU aids in excluding other etiologies of hyperthyroidism, such as thyroiditis, iodine-induced hyperthyroidism, and factitious hyperthyroidism, all of which are associated with a low RAIU. Rarely, hyperthyroidism with diffuse goiter and elevated RAIU may be caused by excessive secretion of human chorionic gonadotropin by a trophoblastic tumor or by inappropriate secretion of TSH by a functioning pituitary adenoma.

The patient must be counseled prior to therapy regarding the advantages and disadvantages of alternative therapies. Antithyroid drug therapy requires frequent outpatient visits for monitoring and dosage adjustment and may rarely be associated with life-threatening agranulocytosis. Minor toxicity, such as skin rash, fever, hepatitis, and arthalgias, occurs in up to 5% of patients. In addition to the morbidity and rare mortality associated with thyroidectomy, there is a 25% to 50% incidence of postsurgical hypothyroidism as well as a 5% to 20% relapse rate. Because iodide readily crosses the placenta, a pregnancy test is mandatory prior to administration of ^{131}I therapy. Exposure of the fetus to ^{131}I after the 10th week of gestation may result in severe fetal hypothyroidism.

The effectiveness of radioiodine treatment for hyperthyroidism is due to radiation-induced cellular damage resulting from high-energy beta emissions, the magnitude of which is directly proportional to the radiation dose received by the thyroid gland. Some practitioners have adopted a fixed-dose administration of 10 to 15 mCi for all patients. Other physicians calculate a dose of 120 to 150 μCi/g of thyroid tissue for the usual patient with Graves' disease. Even higher dosages of 150 to 200 μCi/g may be used to produce a more rapid response in patients with severe hyperthyroidism or in typically more radioresistant cohorts such as children/adolescents, recent exposure to propylthiouracil (PTU), prior failed therapy, and those with high iodine turnover. Although estimation of thyroid size by palpation is relatively accurate for glands weighing 60 g or less, the degree of inaccuracy increases in larger glands. Ultrasound can provide a more accurate estimation of size. The calculation is made as follows: administered μCi = μCi/g desired × gland weight (g) ×100 ÷ RAIU (24 hours).

Our patient with Graves' disease, a 60-g goiter, and a 62% RAIU treated with 130 μCi/g would be prescribed a dose of 13 mCi. A higher dose is typically prescribed for patients with toxic nodular goiter. Our patient with toxic MNG complicated by atrial fibrillation and high-output heart failure would be prescribed a dose of 30 mCi based on a dose of 170 μCi/g; beta blockade should be prescribed prior to treatment.

The complications of radioiodine therapy include transient exacerbation of hyperthyroidism, possible exacerbation of existing Graves' orbitopathy, and posttherapeutic hypothyroidism (an expected consequence of treatment). It is estimated that less than 10% of patients require retreatment, and this is rarely undertaken before 3 to 4 months following therapy. Pretreatment with antithyroid medication is advisable in elderly patients, in patients with known cardiac disease, and in patients with large goiters. These medications should be discontinued 48 to 72 hours prior to administration of [131]I. The administration of beta-blocking medications before and after therapy serves to ameliorate the manifestations of hyperthyroidism but will not affect therapeutic efficacy of radioiodine.

At ^{131}I doses used in the treatment of hyperthyroidism, no increased incidence of subsequent thyroid or nonthyroid neoplasia has been reported. Although the desire for subsequent pregnancy is not a contraindication to radioiodine therapy, patients are usually advised to avoid conception for 6 months in case retreatment is required. In the context of ALARA, written radiation precautions are given to the patient regarding the need to remain a prudent distance from others for several days and to use standard hygienic measures. Long-term follow-up of thyroid status is mandatory in all patients.

Diagnosis: (1) Hyperthyroidism due to Graves' disease. (2) Hyperthyroidism due to toxic MNG.

CASE 1.5

History: A lactating 24-year-old woman presents for thyroid uptake (RAIU) and scan (Fig. 1.5) owing to a suppressed TSH accompanied by anxiety and palpitations. Her gland is nontender and only mildly enlarged, without palpable nodularity.

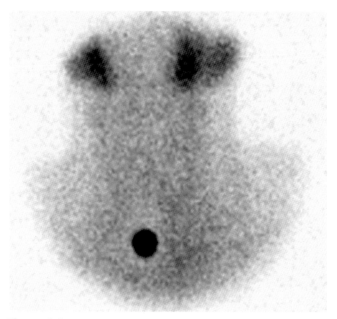

Figure 1.5

Findings: Four- and 24-hour RAIU values were markedly decreased, and ^{99m}Tc thyroid scintigraphy demonstrated diffusely diminished ^{99m}Tc trapping. No nodularity can be demonstrated and there is markedly increased background activity related to the poor thyroid uptake. There is a ^{57}Co marker on the suprasternal notch.

Discussion: In the patient with hyperthyroidism but a low RAIU, a destruction-induced hyperthyroidism is present if exogenous sources of iodine, such as iodinated contrast administration and thyroid hormone, are excluded. Subacute, presumably viral, thyroiditis is the most common cause, but this is almost always accompanied by a tender goiter. Silent autoimmune thyroiditis is also a relatively common cause of low-uptake hyperthyroidism, often occurring postpartum, and thought to be related to an exacerbation of underlying autoimmune thyroid disease. The hyperthyroidism resolves spontaneously over several months but tends to recur following subsequent pregnancies. Many of these women eventually become permanently hypothyroid.

Subacute thyroiditis, also known as de Quervain's thyroiditis, is a benign, self-limited, transient inflammatory disease of the thyroid gland presenting with a destruction-induced hyperthyroidism accompanied by a viral-like prodrome, an exquisitely tender goiter, an elevated sedimentation rate, and circulating thyroglobulin levels.

Scintigraphy may show diffusely decreased radionuclide uptake or isolated areas of impaired uptake within the gland. The RAIU by the thyroid gland is decreased, usually to < 5%. Ultrasound during the acute thyrotoxic phase demonstrates diffuse hypoechogenicity similar to that of Graves' disease, but color-flow Doppler imaging shows no increased vascularity, thus differentiating it from Graves' disease. During recovery, RAIU may rise to elevated levels before returning to normal as the process resolves. Most patients are eventually left with a normal thyroid gland, both histologically and functionally. Symptoms respond to nonsteroidal or steroidal anti-inflammatory agents and beta blockade.

Differentiation from Graves' disease is easily made because of the association of elevated thyroid hormone levels with increased radionuclide uptake in patients with Graves' disease. The other causes of low-uptake hyperthyroidism are not typically accompanied by tenderness of the thyroid gland. In addition to autoimmune (postpartum) thyroiditis, administration of amiodarone and of interferon can be associated with a destruction-induced hyperthyroidism that is indistinguishable scintigraphically from subacute thyroiditis.

Amiodarone is an antiarrhythmic pharmaceutical containing 75 mg of iodine per tablet with a half-life of over 3 months. Approximately 6% of patients treated with amiodarone develop iodine-induced hypothyroidism, but 3% develop thyrotoxicosis. Two varieties of amiodarone-induced thyrotoxicosis occur. Type I is due to iodide-induced hyperthyroidism (Jod-Basedow disease) in patients with preexisting nodular goiter or subclinical Graves' disease; owing to the prolonged half-life of amiodarone, the hyperthyroidism may be refractory to medical therapy, thus prompting thyroidectomy. Type II is amiodarone-induced destructive thyroiditis; this more common variety occurs in patients without preexisting thyroid disease. The thyrotoxicosis persists for 1 to 3 months but resolves more rapidly with glucocorticoid administration. The RAIU of type II amiodarone-induced thyrotoxicosis is near zero, but it may also be very low in type I. If the RAIU is >5%, the type I variety is likely. Of more use in the differentiation of these two types is color-flow Doppler sonography. Type I has normal or increased flow, whereas type II has decreased flow and patchy echogenicity. A mixed pattern of types I and II is common in the United States.

Approximately 9% of patients receiving interferon for hepatitis C and other disease processes develop thyroid dysfunction. Over half of these develop hyperthyroidism, with a destruction-induced hyperthyroidism appearing in many. The disease process often remits if interferon therapy is withdrawn.

The RAIU may be normal, elevated, or suppressed in patients with chronic lymphocytic Hashimoto's thyroiditis, depending on the stage of the disease. Scintigraphy reveals non-homogeneous activity throughout the gland in 50%; a pattern suggestive of either "hot" or "cold" nodules; a combination of both occurs in 30% of patients. Twenty percent of patients with lymphocytic thyroiditis have normal scintigraphic imaging. Markedly elevated thyroid autoantibody titers are typically seen in patients with chronic autoimmune thyroiditis. Hyper- or hypothyroidism associated with chronic thyroiditis does not exclude concurrent thyroid malignancy in patients with focal abnormalities.

Diagnosis: Hyperthyroidism due to postpartum autoimmune thyroiditis.

CASE 1.6

History: A 60-year-old woman with a history of dysphagia and remote left hemithyroidectomy underwent a chest x-ray (Fig. 1.6 A) followed by a CT scan of the thorax (Fig. 1.6 B). ^{123}I scintigraphy of the neck (Fig. 1.6 C) and chest with SPECT/CT fusion imaging (Fig. 1.6 D, E) was performed concurrently.

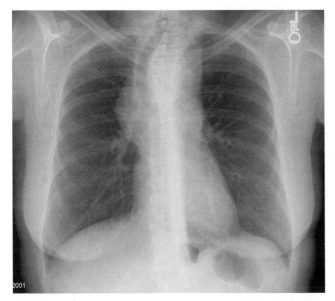

Figure 1.6 A

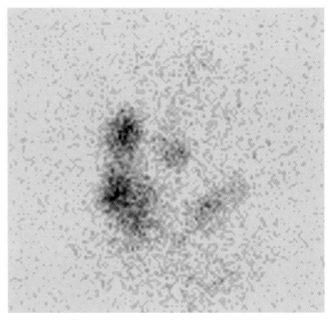

Figure 1.6 C

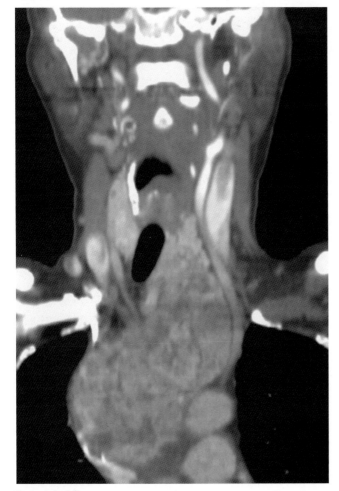

Figure 1.6 B

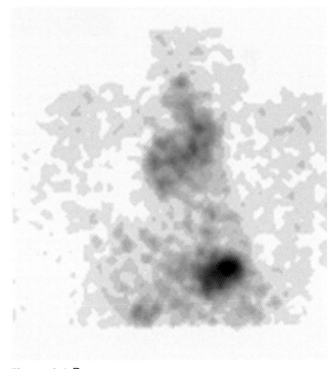

Figure 1.6 D

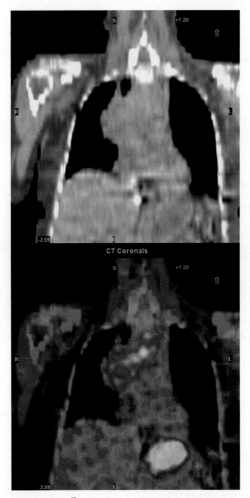

CT Coronals

Figure 1.6 E

Findings: The chest x-ray demonstrates a large anterior mediastinal and right paratracheal mass displacing the trachea to the right; this heterogeneous mass measures 7 by 9 by 12 cm on the coronal CT scan (Fig. 1.6 B), descending to the level of the right main pulmonary artery and abutting the left thyroid lobe remnant. [123]I scintigraphy shows heterogeneous uptake in the neck (Fig. 1.6 C), more on the right than on the left, extending into the thorax. Uptake is relatively poor, but the SPECT/CT fusion imaging (Figs. 1.6 D, E) clearly demonstrates that the mediastinal mass is radioiodine-avid. Physiologic gastric activity is present.

Discussion: These findings indicate that the large mediastinal mass seen on CT is a substernal goiter. In addition to mediastinal goiter, the most common anterior mediastinal masses are thymomas, lymphomas, and germ cell tumors. Although substernal aberrant thyroid accounts for only 7% to 10% of all mediastinal masses, the noninvasive demonstration of radioiodine uptake within a mediastinal mass is important, because otherwise definitive tissue diagnosis is imperative prior to initiating treatment, be it surgery, radiation, or chemotherapy. Substernal thyroid tissue is usually the result of inferior extension of a cervical goiter, but it may rarely be related to enlargement of ectopic mediastinal thyroid tissue. Continuity between the cervical and intrathoracic components of a mediastinal goiter may consist of only a narrow fibrous band not demonstrable by CT or ultrasound.

[123]I is the radionuclide of choice for imaging retrosternal thyroid masses. [123]I scintigraphy yields high-quality images of thoracic goiters even when uptake is relatively decreased. ^{99m}Tc-pertechnetate images are more difficult to interpret owing to the surrounding blood pool activity in the chest. The most common cause of false-negative scans is recent exposure of the patient to exogenous iodine, usually from a preceding contrast-enhanced CT. Rarely, a scan may be falsely positive in mediastinal teratoma, similar to the positive uptake seen with struma ovarii tumor.

CT findings of intrathoracic goiter include continuity with the cervical gland, focal calcification, high attenuation values on noncontrasted images, and marked enhancement after intravenous contrast administration. Despite the fact that clinically significant thyroid cancer occurs in only 4% of mediastinal goiters, the majority of patients with significant mediastinal goiters eventually undergo surgical resection. However, ^{131}I treatment, sometimes augmented by administration of rhTSH, can be used to reduce the size of the mass and alleviate tracheal compression in appropriate patients.

Diagnosis: Mediastinal goiter.

CASE 1.7

History: Two months following a near-total thyroidectomy for follicular carcinoma of the thyroid, 2 weeks after withdrawal of tri-iodothyronine (Cytomel®) treatment, and 48 hours after the oral administration of 2.5 mCi of ^{131}I sodium iodide, a whole-body ^{131}I radioiodine scan (RIS) was acquired on this 47-year-old man (Fig. 1.7 A). Serum TSH at the time of ^{131}I administration was appropriately elevated to 92 mIU/L.

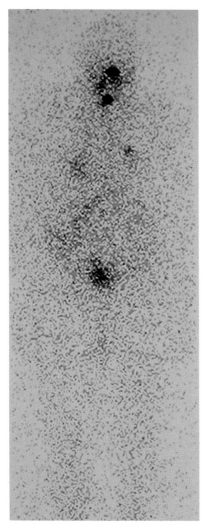

Figure 1.7 A

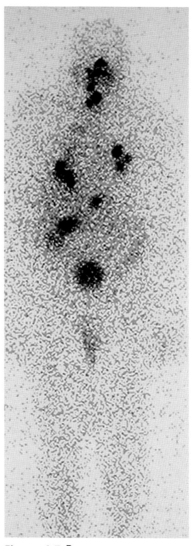

Figure 1.7 B

Findings: The anterior whole-body RIS scan (Fig. 1.7 A) is remarkable for a focus of activity in the thyroid bed as well as foci in both lungs. Physiologic activity is present in the nasopharynx, GI tract, and urinary bladder.

Discussion: This initial low-dose postthyroidectomy diagnostic RIS scan shows a postsurgical thyroid remnant as well as bilateral pulmonary metastases not recognized on a prior chest x-ray; more importantly, ^{131}I avidity is established. Owing to the presence of the pulmonary metastases, the patient received a large 232-mCi treatment dose of ^{131}I. As compared with the pretreatment RIS, a posttreatment RIS scan (Fig. 1.7 B) acquired a week later shows better delineation of the previously seen lesions as well as the identification of additional cervical and pulmonary metastases.

The ideal dose of ^{131}I to be administered for a diagnostic RIS scan to assess a patient for metastatic thyroid cancer is controversial (see discussion of Case 8.6). Most centers use 2 to 5 mCi, although the sensitivity for detection of metastases increases in direct proportion to the size of the diagnostic dose utilized. A follow up RIS scan routinely acquired 5 to 8 days following a 100- to 200-mCi therapeutic dose of ^{131}I will identify additional sites of metastatic disease in 10% to 26% of patients, resulting in an alteration in staging and/or clinical management in 10% to 15%.

Most patients with differentiated thyroid carcinoma (papillary and follicular) are treated with a 30- to 100-mCi ablative dose of ^{131}I following near-complete thyroidectomy in order to reduce the rate of recurrence and mortality and to facilitate

Chapter 1: Endocrine Imaging   17

TABLE 1.2 False-positive iodine scans

Head	**Abdomen**
Meningioma	Gallbladder
Chronic sinusitis	Gastric carcinoma
Dacryocystitis	Renal cyst
Artificial eye	Meckel's diverticulum
Neck	Cystic neurilemoma
Sialadenitis	Ectopic kidney
Carotid ectasia	Gastrointestinal tract (stool)
Saliva in esophagus[a]	**Pelvis**
Zenker's diverticulum	Scrotal hydrocele
Chest	**General[b]**
Hiatal hernia	Skin/clothes contamination
Achalasia	
Barrett's esophagus	
Mega-esophagus	
Pericardial effusion	
Pericardial cyst	
Thymus	
Lactating breasts	
Tracheostomy	
Inflammatory disease (lung)	
Fungal infection (lung)	
Lung cancer	

[a]Most mimic lung or mediastinal lesions.
[b]Many are reported on chest area mimicking lung metastases, but they could be anywhere.
Reproduced from Galloway RJ, Smallridge RC. Imaging in thyroid cancer. Endocrinol Metab Clin North AM 1996;25:93–113, with permission.

surveillance. Current recommendations do not support treating patients with stage I disease in the absence of multifocality, invasion, nodal metastases, or aggressive histopathology. As in this patient, doses of 150 to 250 mCi of ^{131}I are empirically used in patients with known or suspected residual disease.

RIS scans performed for surveillance of patients with known or suspected metastases require proper patient preparation with a low-iodine diet for 2 weeks, avoidance of exogenous sources of iodine, and TSH stimulation. Similar preparation is required for patients undergoing ^{131}I treatment. Endogenous stimulation of serum TSH to a concentration of >30 mIU/L occurs upon withdrawal of thyroxine (T_4) for 3 to 4 weeks or tri-iodothyronine (T_3)(Cytomel®) for 2 weeks. Injection of recombinant human TSH (rhTSH) (Thyrogen®) for 2 days prior to radioiodine administration while the patient continues thyroxine therapy provides scintigraphic results similar to that of withdrawal imaging and has recently been approved in the United States for initial ^{131}I ablation. For patients with concurrent hypopituitarism or with comorbid conditions potentially exacerbated by hypothyroidism, rhTSH has been used successfully for ^{131}I treatment.

In this patient, the pretreatment RIS scan provided a diagnosis of stage IV disease with distant metastases, resulting in an augmentation of the prescribed initial treatment dose. Current guidelines recommend pretreatment RIS with 1 to 3 mCi ^{131}I or use of ^{123}I only when the extent of the thyroid remnant is in question or when the results would alter the prescribed dose.

For patients with low-risk stage I and II disease, pretreatment RIS is often omitted. Stunning is the phenomenon in which the initial diagnostic dose of ^{131}I (2 to 5 mCi) reduces trapping of the subsequently administered treatment dose. The frequency of this effect and its clinical impact is controversial, but quantitative uptake studies estimate a 30% to 50% reduction of therapeutic radioiodine uptake as compared to the uptake of the diagnostic dose. Many investigators now advocate utilizing ^{123}I RIS with 1 to 5 mCi partly to avoid ^{131}I-induced stunning but also because of the superior image quality. In most reports, there is little if any difference in the sensitivity for the detection of postsurgical thyroid remnants and metastases using ^{123}I versus posttherapy high-dose ^{131}I RIS; SPECT acquisitions with or without CT fusion can be performed with diagnostic ^{123}I RIS when deemed appropriate. The lack of beta emissions and the lower gamma energy (159 keV) account for the advantages of ^{123}I over ^{131}I for scintigraphic surveillance.

Patients with differentiated thyroid cancer require long-term surveillance for recurrence utilizing periodic RIS in concert with serum Tg measurement and cervical ultrasound. The sensitivity of radioiodine imaging is approximately 50% to 70% but the specificity is over 95%. However, there are numerous causes of false positive findings with which every interpreter must be familiar (Table 1.2). The use of ^{123}I, 3 to 5 mCi, allows SPECT/CT imaging with improved differentiation of artifacts versus metastases; SPECT is also feasible with posttreatment RIS. Posttreatment ^{131}I images with SPECT-CT fusion of two

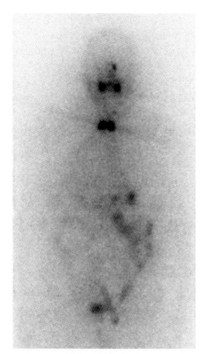

Figure 1.7 C

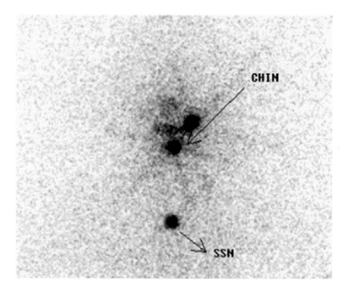

Figure 1.7 E

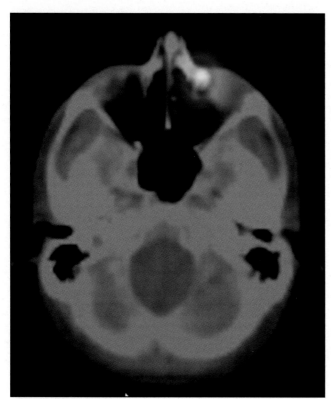

Figure 1.7 D

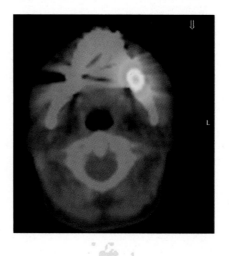

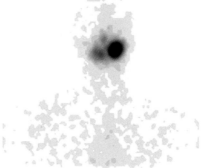

Figure 1.7 F

patients with confusing abnormal foci in the head and neck region demonstrate the utility of these techniques. Figures 1.7 C and 1.7 D demonstrate physiologic activity within the lacrimal gland and Figures 1.7 E and 1.7 F demonstrate activity within an inflammatory mandibular focus following a recent dental extraction.

Patients with persistent/recurrent disease confined to the neck should undergo complete ipsilateral or central compartmental dissection of involved compartments followed by ^{131}I therapy; up to half of these patients may become free of disease if distant metastases are absent. Whereas many practitioners use fixed doses of 150 to 200 mCi for locoregional disease and 200 to 250 mCi for the treatment of distant metastases, there is no consensus as to when more complicated dosimetric methods should be used. For iodine-avid pulmonary and skeletal metastases, current recommendations are for ^{131}I therapy every 6 to 12 months, empirically with 150 to 300 mCi or estimated by dosimetry. For lung metastases, the use of dosimetry to limit whole body retention to 80 mCi at 48 hours is advisable to reduce the risk of pulmonary fibrosis. Under current Nuclear Regulatory Commission (NRC) guidelines, most patients can be treated as outpatients if appropriate counseling and written radiation precautions are provided.

The principal side effects of ^{131}I treatment for thyroid cancer are (1) sialadenitis with usually transient change in taste, (2) lacrimal duct obstruction (Figs. 1.7 C, D) with epiphora, (3) transient gonadal dysfunction with oligomenorrhea, and (4) secondary malignancies. The risk of secondary malignancies (colon, bladder, leukemia, bone, soft tissue, breast, and salivary gland) is very low and is dose-related. Myelosuppression occurring with increasing cumulative dosages is usually mild, but a complete blood and platelet count prior to each treatment is recommended. Owing to an increased miscarriage rate over the first 6 to 12 months after treatment and the possible need for retreatment, women should avoid pregnancy for 6 to 12 months after treatment. Gonadal radiation exposure can be reduced by hydration, frequent emptying of the bladder, and the avoidance of constipation.

For patients with elevated serum Tg (above 10 ng/mL after thyroid hormone withdrawal or 5 ng/mL after rhTSH administration) and negative RIS, the current recommendation is to consider empiric ^{131}I treatment with up to 200 mCi if imaging has failed to identify the responsible tumor site(s). Up to 50% of such patients will have a positive posttreatment scan. If the posttreatment scan is negative, TSH-stimulated [18]FDG PET-CT and/or other imaging modalities is recommended, especially in patients with unstimulated serum Tg levels above 10 to 20 ng/mL (see discussion of Case 8.6).

Diagnosis: Follicular carcinoma of thyroid with metastases treated with high-dose radioactive iodine.

CASE 1.8

History: A 41-year-old man with newly diagnosed pancreatic adenocarcinoma underwent whole-body FDG-PET CT for staging.

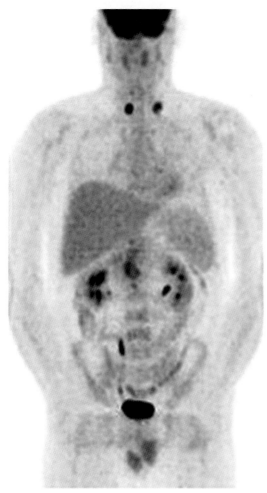

Figure 1.8 A

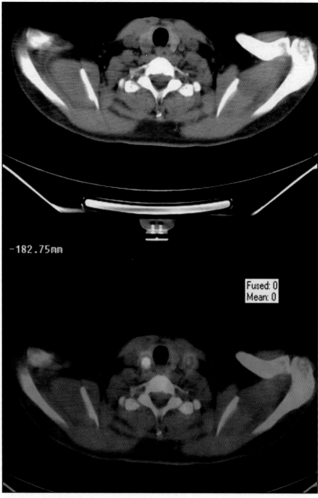

Figure 1.8 B

Findings: The MIP image (Fig. 1.8 A) demonstrates uptake within the pancreatic mass as well as a left cervical node suggestive of nodal metastasis. Incidentally, focal FDG uptake is seen within the right lobe of the thyroid, congruent with a low-attenuation mass seen on the noncontrasted CT (Fig. 1.8 B), which was performed for attenuation correction. A subsequent ultrasound demonstrates a hypoechoic mass with intranodular microcalcifications (Fig. 1.8 C) and intranodular hypervascularity (Fig. 1.8 D).

Discussion: The FDG-avid thyroid nodule discovered incidentally has ultrasound characteristics strongly suggestive of papillary thyroid carcinoma, namely microcalcifications, hypoechogenicity, and intranodular (rather than perinodular) vascularity. FNA biopsy was consistent with papillary carcinoma, but the lesion was not resected because of the patient's stage IV pancreatic carcinoma.

The evaluation of thyroid nodules identified incidentally on CT or ultrasound is reviewed in the discussion of Case 1.1. Focal FDG uptake discovered incidentally within the thyroid

on a PET-CT performed in patients without known thyroid disease is seen in approximately 1% to 2% of cases. Since many of these are not biopsied in the reported series, the actual incidence of malignant neoplasia in these nodules is not known, but it is thought to be in the range of 14% to 30%. Although metastatic disease to the thyroid from known nonthyroidal cancers does occur, most of the biopsied cases have been primary differentiated papillary or follicular carcinomas with a few medullary carcinomas. The remainder have been benign lesions such as follicular adenomas, focal thyroiditis, or multinodular goiters. Diffuse FDG uptake within the thyroid is typically related to the presence of autoimmune thyroid disease, either Hashimoto's disease or Graves' disease. Since some of these patients may be hypo- or hyperthyroid, clinical assessment should be recommended. Physiologic laryngeal uptake should not be confused with diffuse thyroidal uptake (Fig 1.8 E).

^{99m}Tc-sestamibi, ^{99m}Tc-tetrofosmin, and ^{201}Tl, utilized primarily for myocardial perfusion scintigraphy (MPS), are all

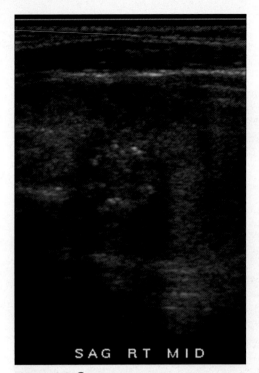

SAG RT MID

Figure 1.8 C

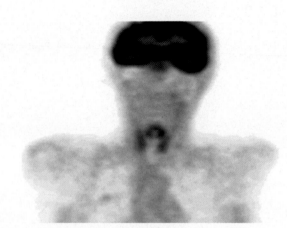

Figure 1.8 E

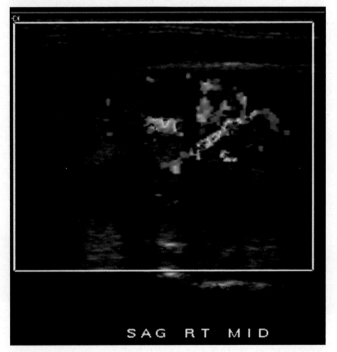

SAG RT MID

Figure 1.8 D

nonspecific tumor imaging agents. For this reason, focal or diffuse thyroid uptake identified on the rotating cine images of MPS studies must be further evaluated. Whereas diffuse uptake is generally related to the presence of goiters, multinodular or diffuse, focal uptake is typically related to the presence of benign or malignant neoplasms and should be evaluated appropriately using ^{99m}Tc-pertechnetate or ^{123}I scintigraphy and biopsied if demonstrated to be hypofunctioning. The focal thyroid uptake seen on the MPS displayed in Figure 1.8 F was hypofunctioning on ^{99m}Tc-pertechnetate imaging (Fig. 1.8 G); the biopsy was diagnostic of papillary carcinoma.

If a thyroid nodule is actually photopenic with MIBI imaging, there is a very low risk of malignancy, whereas the risk of malignancy increases eightfold if the nodule is MIBI-avid (hot). Warm or isointense findings are nonspecific. Approximately 80% of cold nodules by pertechnetate imaging that are subsequently noted to be MIBI-positive will be malignant.

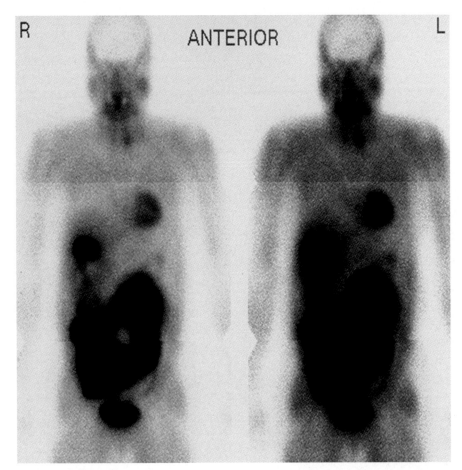

Figure 1.8 F

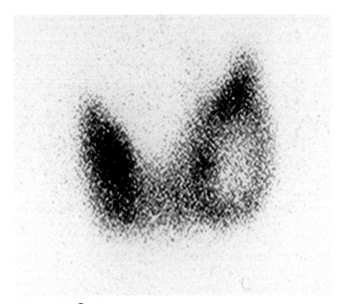

Figure 1.8 G

Similarly, 85% of malignant nodules are thallium-avid, but 14% of benign nodules are also thallium-avid.

In summary, thyroid nodules discovered incidentally by FDG-PET or on MPS performed with MIBI, tetrofosmin, or thallium should be appropriately evaluated by traditional thyroid scintigraphy and then biopsied if the nodule is hypofunctioning.

Diagnosis: (1) Papillary carcinoma of the thyroid, incidental detection with FDG-PET CT. (2) Papillary carcinoma of the thyroid, incidental detection with ^{99m}Tc-sestamibi.

History: A neonate is referred for ^{99m}Tc thyroid scintigraphy (Figs. 1.9 A, B) with confirmed primary neonatal hypothyroidism.

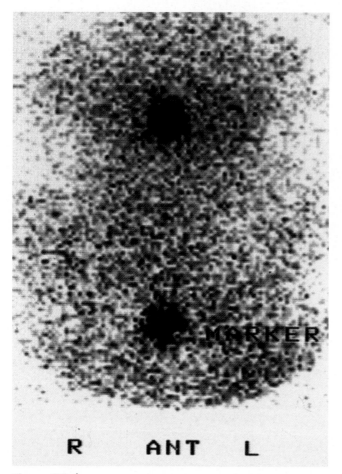

Figure 1.9 A

Figure 1.9 B

Findings: Anterior and lateral images demonstrate a focus of increased activity at the base of the tongue with no eutopic activity identified. Background activity is high, suggestive of low thyroidal uptake. A ^{57}Co marker has been placed at the suprasternal notch.

Discussion: These findings are indicative of neonatal hypothyroidism due to thyroid dysgenesis related to an ectopic lingual thyroid. No additional functioning thyroid tissue is identified.

Congenital hypothyroidism (CHT) has an incidence of 1 per 2,500 to 5,000 births, and most infants do not exhibit signs or symptoms of hypothyroidism at birth. A delay in the institution of thyroxine therapy beyond 6 to 8 weeks of life is likely to result in measurable impairment of intellectual function. Since the institution of newborn screening programs for CHT by measuring serum TSH and/or T_4 levels, the mental retardation of CHT has been eradicated in developed countries.

Thyroid dysgenesis (agenesis, hypoplasia, ectopia) is the most common (70%) cause of CHT in the United States. ^{99m}Tc-pertechnetate thyroid scintigraphy is performed immediately after CHT is confirmed. It can easily detect eutopic and ectopic thyroid tissue as well as assess the degree of thyroidal uptake. Using a pinhole collimator, multiple views are acquired 20 minutes after administration of <1 mCi of ^{99m}Tc-pertechnetate. Ectopic thyroid tissue is rarely accompanied by normally functioning eutopic tissue and is indicative of the need for lifelong thyroxine therapy (Figs. 1.9 A, B). A eutopic, often enlarged gland with increased uptake (Fig. 1.9 C) is most consistent with dyshormonogenesis; a small proportion of such cases are due to transient immaturity of the iodine organification process and will be normal at reassessment after age 3 years. Nonvisualization of the thyroid on scintigraphy is due to agenesis in over 90% of cases, the remainder being due to the presence of maternal transmission of TSH-receptor-blocking antibodies; similarly, poor uptake in a eutopic gland (Fig. 1.11D) is seen with maternal transmission of blocking antibodies. These latter patients will be euthyroid at reassessment, when the maternal antibodies have cleared the child's system. Patients with a poorly visualized eutopic gland or a nonvisualized gland or patients with images suggesting

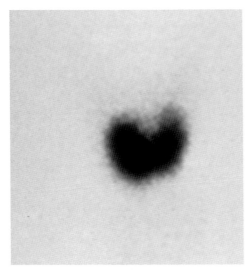

Figure 1.9 C

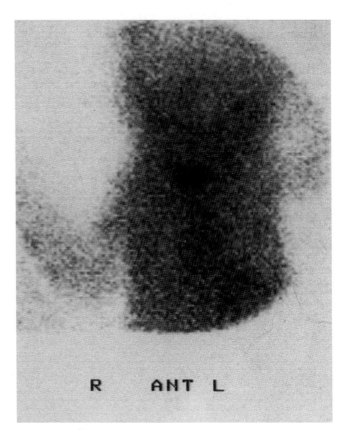

Figure 1.9 D

dyshormonogenesis are all reevaluated at age 3 to 4 years to exclude transient CHT; patients with ectopia are not reassessed.

Therefore thyroid scintigraphy in the neonate is indispensable in the proper diagnostic workup of congenital hypothyroidism because it (1) provides a more specific diagnosis,

(2) is cost-effective for selecting patients for subsequent reassessment to uncover transient CHT and discontinue thyroid hormone replacement therapy, and (3) defines dyshormonogenesis, which is familial and requires genetic counseling.

Diagnosis: Neonatal hypothyroidism due to lingual thyroid.

CASE 1.10

History: A 60-year-old euthyroid woman found to have an abnormal thyroid gland incidentally at the time of carotid sonography underwent ^{99m}Tc-pertechnetate thyroid scintigraphy (Fig. 1.10 A). The ultrasound was described as consistent with MNG versus autoimmune thyroiditis. Circulating antiperoxidase antibodies were markedly elevated.

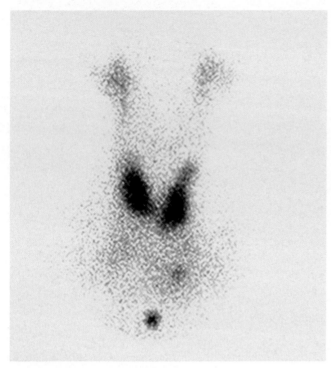

Figure 1.10 A

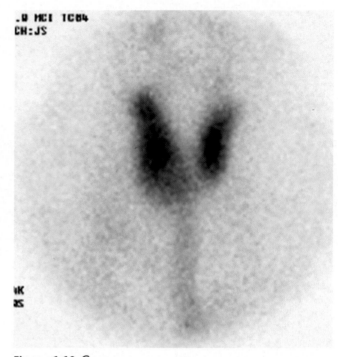

Figure 1.10 C

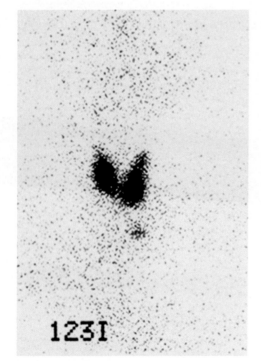

Figure 1.10 B

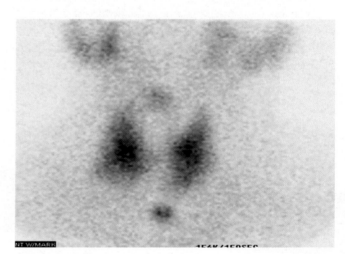

Figure 1.10 D

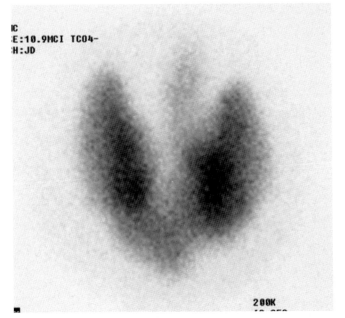

Figure 1.10 E

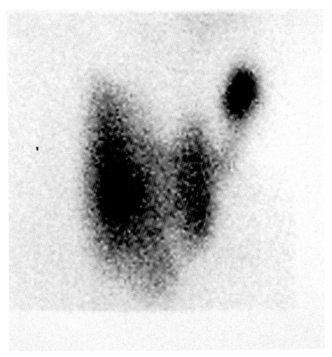

Figure 1.10 F

Findings: Anterior imaging of the thyroid (Fig. 1.10 A) demonstrates heterogeneous thyroidal uptake bilaterally, but there is a small extrathyroidal focus of activity to the left and inferior to the thyroid. This same abnormality is confirmed with a subsequent ^{123}I scan (Fig 1.10 B).

Discussion: In view of the elevated antithyroid autoantibodies, the presence of heterogeneous thyroid uptake and the heterogeneous echogenicity are most consistent with a diagnosis of Hashimoto's thyroiditis. The laterally lying focus of ^{99m}Tc uptake is of thyroid origin since it is iodine-avid. Lateral aberrant thyroid activity rarely represents an ectopic thyroid rest; it usually is due to ectopic thyroid tissue or metastatic thyroid carcinoma provided that gastroesophageal and salivary gland activity can be excluded.

At thyroidectomy, this patient had a papillary microcarcinoma in the left lobe in a background of Hashimoto's thyroiditis; the ^{123}I-avid lower cervical mass was a metastatic lymph node.

Although inflammatory nodes and nonthyroidal metastatic adenopathy can be pertechnetate-avid on occasion, they will not be iodine-avid. Physiologic salivary and esophageal activity (Fig. 1.10 C), especially within an esophageal diverticulum or with achalasia, should not be mistaken for ectopic thyroid tissue or metastatic disease. The most common ectopic thyroid tissue is midline activity within the thyroglossal duct remnant and even occasionally within a thyroglossal duct cyst, as seen in Figure 1.10 D. A pyramidal lobe, when seen, usually emanates from the medial right or left lobe and is most often visualized in association with the diffuse hyperplasia of Graves' disease (Fig. 1.10 E).

Distinction should be made between the usually metastatic aberrant lateral thyroid activity and "sequesterent nodular goiter," in which a piece of thyroid tissue appears to be completely separated from the remainder of the gland but is actually connected to the thyroid, sometimes by only a fibrous bridge (Fig. 1.10 F). The nodule is freely movable in all directions and histology shows no evidence of lymph node tissue.

Diagnosis: (1) Metastatic thyroid carcinoma appearing as lateral aberrant thyroid. (2) Sequesterent nodular goiter.

History: A 63-year-old woman with nephrolithiasis was found to have an elevated serum calcium of 11.6 mg/dL (normal 8.5 to 10.3) accompanied by an elevated serum parathyroid hormone (PTH) level of 136 pg/mL (normal 10 to 65). She had no prior history of thyroid disease.

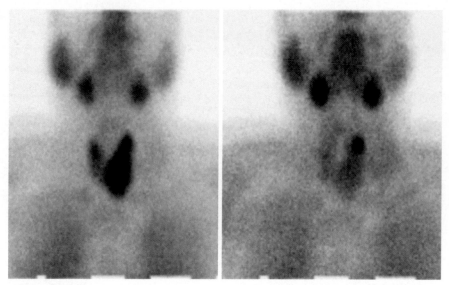

Figure 1.11 A

Findings: An immediate anterior image of the neck and upper thorax acquired after injection of 24 mCi of ^{99m}Tc-sestamibi (MIBI) (Fig. 1.11 A) demonstrates goitrous enlargement of the left lobe of the thyroid and a photopenic abnormality of the lower pole of the right lobe. On the delayed image, there is washout of the physiologic thyroid activity, with a persistent focal abnormality at the superior pole of the left thyroid lobe. Looking back, this focus is evident on the immediate images.

Discussion: The immediate image (thyroid phase) is typical of multinodular goiter. The solitary focus at the superior pole of the left lobe on the delayed image (parathyroid phase) is consistent with a parathyroid adenoma. Surprisingly, the abnormal physiologic thyroid activity washed out very well on the delayed imaging; goitrous activity often persists on 2- to 3-hour delayed imaging but will usually dissipate gradually over the ensuing 1 to 2 hours. Sensitivity for detection of a causative solitary parathyroid adenoma is 85% to 90% with dual-phase MIBI imaging, whereas multiglandular disease is identified less often (63%). Although the parathyroid pathology is usually best visualized on the delayed images, an adenoma is often detectable on the initial images (as in this case) and occasionally is seen only on the initial images owing to rapid washout from the adenoma (atypical adenoma). Although thyroid pathology and lymphadenopathy may result in false-positive findings with ^{99m}Tc-MIBI imaging, specificity is about 95%. Certainly the possibility of a false-positive finding is higher in this patient with a goiter, and the MIBI scan should be correlated with an ^{123}I thyroid image to improve specificity. In the patient with known thyroid pathology, a dual ra-

dioisotope technique is preferable; ^{99m}Tc-pertechnetate or ^{123}I-subtraction has been used with reported sensitivities of 80% to 100% and improved specificity. At surgery, this patient had a solitary superior left parathyroid adenoma and a multinodular goiter.

The diagnosis of hyperparathyroidism is made biochemically by the presence of hypercalcemia and elevated serum PTH levels, easily differentiating it from other etiologies of hypercalcemia. Since 80% of patients with primary hyperparathyroidism are asymptomatic, most are detected incidentally on routine chemistry analyses. Seventeen percent have nephrolithiasis and 10% peptic ulcer disease. Primary hyperparathyroidism results from a solitary adenoma in over 80% of cases, with multiple adenomas, diffuse hyperplasia, or rarely carcinoma accounting for the remainder. Ten percent of patients have supernumerary glands, and as many as 40% of glands may be ectopically located away from the poles of the thyroid lobes. Although the success rate of parathyroidectomy is 90% to 95% without preoperative localizing procedures, recurrent and persistent hyperparathyroidism is usually related to aberrant or ectopically located glands or recurrent hyperplasia. Reexploration is technically difficult, with a higher morbidity and poorer success rate than initial surgery. Preoperative noninvasive localization improves the cure rate of second surgery from 50% to 60% up to 90%. For these reasons and for the possibility of easier and faster surgery with unilateral neck exploration, preoperative imaging is now used routinely for localization of the offending gland or glands.

Dual-phase ^{99m}Tc-MIBI is now the universally preferred nuclear medicine technique for localization of parathyroid

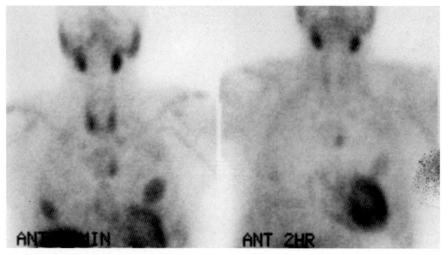

Figure 1.11 B

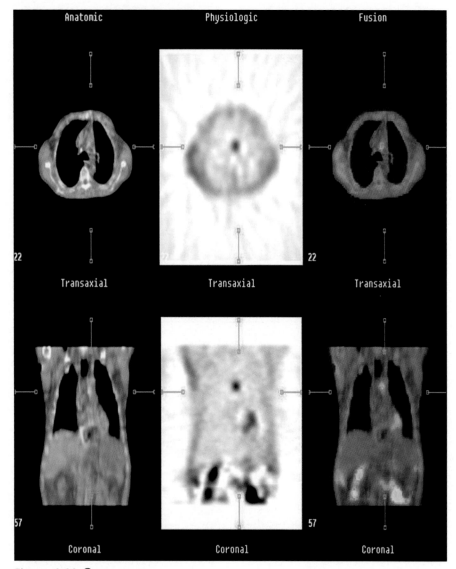

Figure 1.11 C

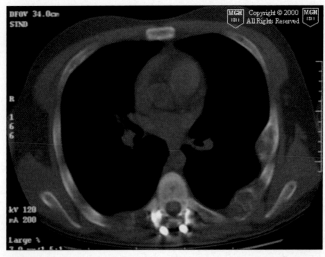

Figure 1.11 D

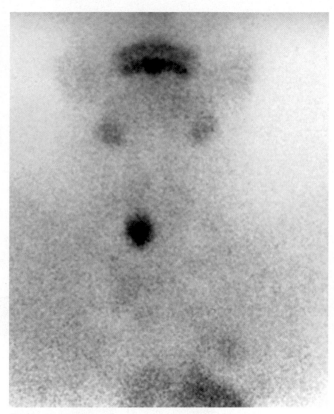

Figure 1.11 E

pathology. Anterior and sometimes oblique images of the neck and superior mediastinum are acquired 15 to 20 minutes after injection of 20 mCi of MIBI, followed by delayed imaging 2 to 3 hours later. Physiologic thyroid ^{99m}Tc-MIBI activity gradually washes out with a $T_{1/2}$ of 60 minutes, whereas parathyroid activity is stable over 2 hours, thus explaining the better visualization of parathyroid adenomas at 2 to 3 hours postinjection. Ultrasound is efficacious for cervical adenoma detection, whereas MIBI imaging is highly sensitive in the mediastinum as well as the neck.

SPECT may sometimes detect abnormalities not seen on the planar views, and SPECT/CT fusion imaging improves localization especially for ectopic glands. Parathyroid imaging has been used successfully to determine whether recurrent hyperparathyroidism following total parathyroidectomy with autotransplantation into the muscles of the neck or forearm is graft-dependent or not.

An elderly man with renal insufficiency was found to have persistent hyperparathyroidism despite the resection of $3^{1}/_{2}$ hyperplastic cervical parathyroid glands. His immediate and delayed MIBI images, displayed in Fig. 1.11 B, are diagnostic of an ectopic mediastinal parathyroid adenoma as the cause of his persistent hyperparathyroidism. SPECT-CT fusion imaging (Fig. 1.11 C) provides accurate localization for the surgeons.

The bilateral foci of thoracic activity, seen best on the immediate planar images, are brown tumors of the ribs (Fig. 1.11 D) related to osteitis fibrosa cystica from longstanding severe hyperparathyroidism and chronic renal disease. MIBI activity in the chest can also be related to primary lung or breast neoplasms, lymphoma, or metastatic pulmonary or skeletal lesions. Sestamibi is a nonspecific tumor imaging agent likely related to enhanced binding to the abundant mitochondria seen in neoplasms. Figure 1.11 E demonstrates multiple pulmonary metastases in a patient with multiple endocrine neoplasia type I (MEN I) with known metastatic gastrinoma; the lower cervical intense focus is an ectopic right inferior parathyroid adenoma. MEN I is an inherited disorder characterized by multigland parathyroid hyperplasia, pituitary adenoma, and pancreatic islet cell neoplasms. MIBI uptake within pulmonary carcinoid metastases has also been reported. Somatostatin receptor imaging is a preferred modality for this purpose (see discussion of Case 8.30).

Diagnosis: (1) Hyperparathyroidism due to a parathyroid adenoma with coexisting multinodular goiter. (2) Persistent postparathyroidectomy hyperparathyroidism due to a mediastinal parathyroid adenoma complicated by brown tumors. (3) Ectopic parathyroid adenoma in MEN I with metastatic MIBI-avid pulmonary metastases from gastrinoma.

CASE 1.12

History: A 36-year-old woman with a history of previously resected bilateral pheochromocytomas and medullary carcinoma of the thyroid presented with recurrent hyperadrenergic symptoms and elevated urinary catecholamines. A posterior view of a whole body ^{131}I-MIBG scan (Fig. 1.12 A) and concordant axial slices of subsequent CT (Fig. 1.12 B) and MR (Fig. 1.12 C) imaging are displayed.

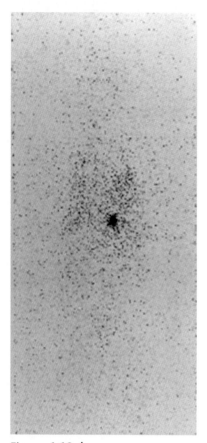

Figure 1.12 A

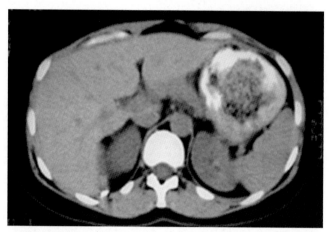

Figure 1.12 B

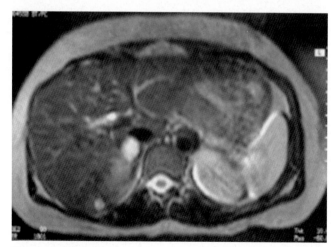

Figure 1.12 C

Findings: The MIBG image (Fig. 1.12 A) demonstrates a focus of intense activity in the upper abdomen immediately to the right of midline unaccompanied by any additional pathologic abnormalities. The nonenhanced CT image (Fig. 1.12 B) demonstrates an indeterminate contour abnormality in the region of the vena cava at the level of the caudate lobe. The MRI scan (Fig. 1.12 C) identifies a 2-cm enhancing mass with increased T2-weighted signal located just posterior to the intrahepatic inferior vena cava arising from the right adrenal bed.

Discussion: The abnormal MIBG-avid focus represents a recurrence in the right adrenal bed in this patient with MEN II and prior bilateral adrenalectomy for pheochromocytoma. This image, moreover, is similar to what one would see in a patient with a solitary right adrenal pheochromocytoma. Surgical resection of the recurrence required partial hepatectomy and partial resection of the inferior vena cava, confirming the radiologic impression of malignancy in this patient. There is

no scintigraphic evidence of recurrent MIBG-avid medullary thyroid carcinoma. Pheochromocytomas are catecholamine-secreting neoplasms arising from chromaffin cells. Approximately 10% are malignant, 10% are bilateral, 10% occur in children, and 10% to 20% are extra-adrenal in origin (paragangliomas), usually in the abdomen or pelvis but occasionally in the neck or mediastinum. Bilaterality, extra-adrenal sites and malignancy are more common in children. Because anatomic imaging studies are nonspecific and may not be sensitive for the presence of extra-adrenal foci, bilaterality, or metastatic disease, adrenal medullary scintigraphy using radioiodinated MIBG may play a pivotal role in the management of patients with pheochromocytoma, paraganglioma, and neuroblastoma (see discussion of Case 8.28). The sensitivity of ^{131}I-MIBG for the detection of primary pheochromocytoma, paraganglioma, and metastases is approximately 86%, but it is higher (95%) for ^{123}I-MIBG. Specificity is 95% to 100%. MIBG imaging is

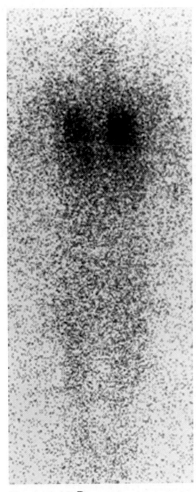

Figure 1.12 D

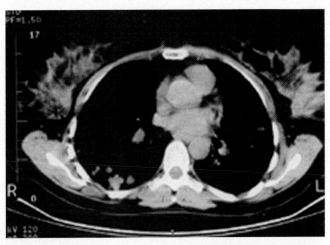

Figure 1.12 E

especially useful in differentiating postsurgical scarring from recurrence, as in this patient, as well as differentiating pheochromocytoma from neurofibroma in patients with neurofibromatosis.

The diagnosis of malignant pheochromocytoma can be made only in retrospect when local or distant spread is detected. Owing to whole-body imaging and its high degree of specificity, MIBG scintigraphy is uniquely suited to the detection of metastatic or recurrent disease, as demonstrated in this patient. Although the incidence of malignancy is reported to be 10%, the proportion of patients subsequently found to have metastatic disease has increased to levels approaching 50% with longer periods of follow-up. The most frequent sites of spread are bone (44%), liver and lymph nodes (37%), and lungs (27%). Extra-adrenal paragangliomas are metastatic at initial presentation in approximately 45% of patients.

In this patient, recurrent symptoms accompanied by progressive elevation of catecholamines prompted a repeat ^{131}I-MIBG scan (Fig. 1.12 D) 2 years after her hepatic resection. The diffuse bilateral lung activity corresponded to innumerable metastatic nodules subsequently observed on chest CT (Fig. 1.12 E). As is seen with posttherapeutic ^{131}I imaging in patients with metastatic thyroid carcinoma, sensitivity for detection of metastases is dose-dependent, and additional lesions may be identified on images obtained 7 to 10 days following a treatment dose of ^{131}I-MIBG. Partial tumor and/or biochemical responses occur in approximately 30% to 50% of patients treated with high-dose ^{131}I-MIBG. This patient has experienced stable disease over the ensuing years following three therapeutic doses of ^{131}I-MIBG.

The diagnosis of pheochromocytoma is made by the laboratory demonstration of elevated catecholamines in the plasma and/or urine in the appropriate clinical scenario. Since most primary adrenal pheochromocytomas are larger than 2 cm in diameter, they are readily identified using CT or MR imaging; contrast-enhanced CT yields a sensitivity of 98% and a specificity of 92%. The characteristic low T1 and hyperintense T2 signal with MRI is seen in virtually all pheochromocytomas and only occasionally in patients with metastatic adrenal lesions. Since adrenal masses occur in approximately 3% of the population, functional imaging with MIBG has been recommended to confirm that the mass is a pheochromocytoma and to exclude multiple tumors and metastatic disease preoperatively. However, some have not advocated the use of functional imaging in the preoperative assessment of patients with a solitary adrenal mass in the context of proven catecholamine excess, owing to the low (2%) yield of unsuspected findings. However, in patients with suspected pheochromocytoma who have nondiagnostic imaging findings with CT and MRI, MIBG

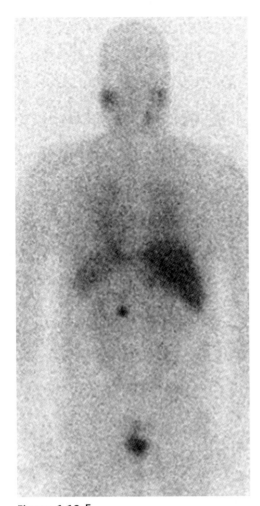

Figure 1.12 F

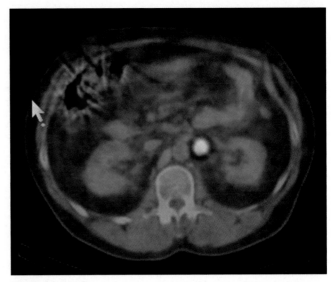

Figure 1.12 G

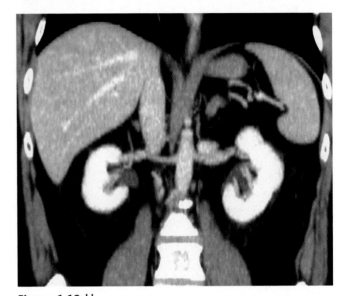

Figure 1.12 H

scintigraphy can be very useful, especially in view of its high negative predictive value.

The value of SPECT-CT fusion imaging has been demonstrated in oncology for numerous applications, improving sensitivity, specificity, and localization. The utility of SPECT-CT imaging is demonstrated in a patient who was initially thought to have a primary adrenal pheochromocytoma, by whole-body ^{123}I MIBG imaging (Fig 1.12 F) but was subsequently found to have a paraganglioma of the left renal pelvis (Figs. 1.12 G, H), as confirmed at surgery.

The sensitivity of indium 111 (^{111}In) octreotide scintigraphy for the detection of benign adrenal pheochromocytoma is only 25% as compared with over 90% for ^{123}I-MIBG scintigraphy, but the two modalities have similar efficacy in determining extent of disease in patients with malignant pheochromocytoma. Some metastases that are MIBG-negative may be somatostatin-receptor scan–positive and vice versa. Similarly, FDG-PET can be used successfully to determine the extent of disease in patients with malignant pheochromocytoma

(Fig 1.12 I). In a series of 29 pheochromocytoma patients, 58% of those with benign pheochromocytoma and 88% with malignant pheochromocytoma demonstrated FDG avidity. In the 4 patients whose pheochromocytomas were not MIBG-avid, tumor uptake of FDG was intense. Therefore most pheochromocytomas accumulate FDG, although this occurs more often with malignant pheochromocytoma. Dopamine is a better substrate for the norepinephrine transporter than other amines, and the use of ^{18}F-fluorodopamine PET is promising for the determination of metastatic disease extent, especially in patients whose tumor is not MIBG-avid.

^{123}I-MIBG imaging may be especially useful in children, who more frequently have hereditary syndromes (MEN II, von Hippel–Lindau, neurofibromatosis, familial pheochromocytoma, and Carney's triad) and are at higher risk for multifocality, extra-adrenal disease, and malignant disease. Bilateral uptake due to medullary hyperplasia may be demonstrated by MIBG scintigraphy, but its sensitivity is insufficient

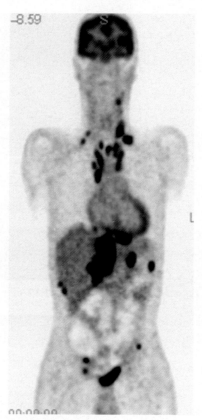

Figure 1.12 |

to exclude contralateral disease. It must be remembered that MIBG imaging, somatostatin receptor scintigraphy, and FDG-PET may detect other neuroendocrine tumors, such as medullary thyroid carcinoma, carcinoid, and islet cell tumors as well as neuroblastoma and small cell lung carcinoma (Chapter 8). This is especially important in patients with hereditary syndromes.

Diagnosis: (1) Metastatic pheochromocytoma in a patient with MEN II. (2) Paraganglioma, renal pelvis. (3) FDG-avid metastatic pheochromocytoma.

SOURCES AND SUGGESTED READING

1. Lacey NA, Jones A, Clarke SEM. Role of radionuclide imaging in hyperthyroid patients with no clinical suspicion of nodules. *Br J Radiol* 2001;74:486–489.
2. Burch HB, Shakir F, Fitzsimmons TR, et al. Diagnosis and management of the autonomously functioning thyroid nodule: the Walter Reed Army Medical Center experience, 1975–1996. *Thyroid* 1998;8: 871–880.
3. Reschini E, Ferrari C, Castellani M, et al. The trapping-only nodules of the thyroid gland: prevalence study. *Thyroid* 2006;16:757–762.
4. Sfakianakis GN, Ezuddin SH, Sanchez JE, et al. Pertechnetate scintigraphy in primary congenital hypothyroidism. *J Nucl Med* 1999;40:799–804.
5. AACE/SME Task Force. Medical guidelines for clinical practice for the diagnosis and management of thyroid nodules. *Endocr Pract* 2006;12:63–102.
6. Cooper DS, Doherty GM, Haugen BR, et al. Management guidelines for patients with thyroid nodules and differentiated thyroid cancer. *Thyroid* 2006;16:109–141.
7. Pellegriti G, Scollo C, Lumera G, et al. Clinical behavior and outcome of papillary thyroid cancers smaller than 1.5 cm in diameter: study of 299 cases. *J Clin Endocrinol Metab* 2004;89:3713–3720.
8. Alzahrani AS, Bakheet S, Mandil MA, et al. [123]I isotope as a diagnostic agent in the follow-up of patients with differentiated thyroid cancer: comparison with post ^{131}I therapy whole body scanning. *J Clin Endocrinol Metab* 2001;86:5294–5300.
9. Frates MC, Benson CB, Charboneau JW, et al and the Society of Radiologists in Ultrasound. Management of thyroid nodules detected at US: Society of Radiologists in Ultrasound consensus conference statement. *Radiology* 2005;237:794–800.
10. Sebastianes FM, Cerci JJ, Zanoni PH, et al. Role of F-18-FDG PET in preoperative assessment of cytologically indeterminate thyroid nodules. *J Clin Endocrinol Metab* 2007;92:4485–4488.
11. Kang KW, Kim SK, Kang HS, et al. Prevalence and risk of cancer of focal thyroid incidentaloma identified by 18F-fluorodeoxyglucose positron emission tomography for metastasis evaluation and cancer screening in healthy subjects. *J Clin Endocrinol Metab* 2003;88:4100–4104.
12. Siegel A, Mancuso M, Seltzer M. The spectrum of positive scan patterns in parathyroid scintigraphy. *Clin Nucl Med* 2007;32:770–774.
13. Miyakoshi M, Kamoi K, Takano T, et al. Multiple brown tumors in primary hyperparathyroidism caused by an adenoma mimicking metastatic bone disease with false positive results on computed tomography and Tc-99m sestamibi imaging: MR findings. *Endocr J* 2007;54:205–210.
14. Lavely WC, Goetze S, Friedman KP, et al. Comparison of SPECT/CT, SPECT, and planar imaging with single- and dual-phase (99m)Tc-sestamibi parathyroid scintigraphy. *J Nucl Med* 2007;48:1084–1089.
15. Ilias I, Pacak K. Current approaches and recommended algorithm for the diagnostic localization of pheochromocytoma. *J Clin Endocrinol Metab* 2004; 89:479–491.
16. van der Harst E, de Herder WW, Bruining HA, et al. [(123)I]metaiodo-benzylguanidine and [(111)In]octreotide uptake in benign and malignant pheochromocytomas. *J Clin Endocrinol Metab* 2001;86:685–693.
17. Lumachi F, Tregnaghi A, Zucchetta P, et al. Sensitivity and positive predictive value of CT, MRI and ^{123}I-MIBG scintigraphy in localizing pheochromocytomas: a prospective study. *Nucl Med Commun* 2006;27:583–587.

CHAPTER TWO

RADIONUCLIDE PULMONARY IMAGING

M. Reza Habibian
and Chirayu Shah

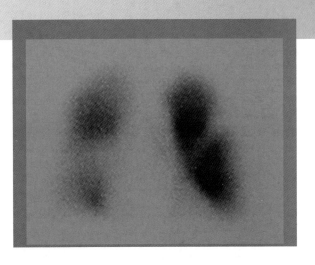

CLINICAL INDICATION

Ventilation/Perfusion Scintigraphy for Diagnosis of Pulmonary Emboli

Despite the increasing use of spiral CT angiography, the ventilation/perfusion lung scan continues to play an important role as a noninvasive procedure for the diagnosis of pulmonary emboli (1).

Pulmonary Imaging for Non-embolic Disease

Perfusion lung scan continues to be the functional image used for the estimation of regional pulmonary perfusion in order to predict postoperative pulmonary function after lobectomy or pneumonectomy (2). It is also useful in identifying the target area for resection in surgery for lung volume reduction and provides modest prognostic information (3).

The use of gallium-67 (^{67}Ga) scanning for the evaluation of pulmonary disease has diminished significantly in favor of positron emission tomography (PET). However, the gallium scan is useful in the evaluation of pulmonary sarcoidosis, HIV-positive patients with suspected *Pneumocystis carinii* pneumonia, drug- and radiation-induced pneumonitis, lung diseases associated with pneumoconiosis, and in monitoring response to therapy in patients with lymphoma (4).

PET is a noninvasive imaging modality that can differentiate benign from malignant nodules and thus replace some of the more invasive procedures. PET imaging with fluoride 18 (^{18}F) FDG is used more frequently for the characterization of solitary pulmonary nodules.

VENTILATION/PERFUSION SCINTIGRAPHY FOR DIAGNOSIS OF PULMONARY EMBOLI

As a result of the development of advanced multislice spiral CT technology as well as increased availability and acceptance of pulmonary CT angiography, the role of ventilation/perfusion lung scanning in the diagnosis of pulmonary emboli (PE) must be redefined (5,6).

1. If the chest radiograph is normal and there is no history of significant cardiopulmonary disease, the V/Q lung scan is an effective noninvasive initial study for the diagnosis of acute PE. A normal scan excludes PE and a high-probability scan can make the diagnosis.
2. When the chest x-ray finding makes it likely that the lung scan will not provide a clear diagnosis, CT angiography appears to be the first choice for many clinicians. The PIOPED II investigators also prefer CT angiography over V/Q scanning for diagnosing pulmonary embolism in many situations. However, a negative pulmonary CT angiogram does not have the same negative predictive value as a normal V/Q scan (1).

METHODOLOGY

Perfusion Scan

Perfusion lung scintigraphy is performed after the intravenous injection of technetium 99m (^{99m}Tc) macroaggregated albumin (MAA) with the patient in the supine position to avoid preferential lower lobe distribution. The injected particles are distributed in the lung in proportion to the regional pulmonary perfusion and are trapped in the pulmonary capillary and precapillary arterial beds. The usual dose of 3 to 5 mCi contains approximately 300,000 particles approximately 30 μm in size (10 to 90 μm). Blocking 1 out of 1,000 of a total 300 million precapillary arterial beds leaves a wide margin of safety, and no adverse hemodynamic effect is to be expected. However, in patients with severe pulmonary arterial hypertension as well as known or suspected right-to-left shunt, the number of particles should be reduced. A diagnostic scan still can be obtained using as few as 70,000 to 100,000 particles.

After entrapment in the pulmonary vascular bed, the particles undergo degradation and clear from the lung with a biologic half-time of 3 to 12 hours, eventually being phagocytized by the hepatic Kupffer cells. Demonstration of minimal activity in the liver on the day after lung scan should not be considered abnormal, but activity seen in other tissues, such as kidneys or brain, may signify the presence of an intra- or extracardiac shunt.

Pregnancy is a relative contraindication for radionuclide imaging, including pulmonary scintigraphy. The total dose and its appropriate number of particles should be kept to a minimum that still provides diagnostic information. A dose of 1 to 2 mCi containing 100,000 particles can be used for diagnostic purposes. However, from the standpoint of risk-to-benefit analysis, one should not be deterred from performing the scan after obtaining written informed consent. Interruption of breast-feeding following a perfusion lung scan is debatable but may not be necessary with the low dose of 1 to 2 mCi.

Ventilation Scan

The addition of ventilation images permits the determination of the regional airway abnormality and improves the specificity of a lung scan for diagnosis of PE. A positive predictive value of a perfusion scan as compared with combined V/Q images can be improved from 59% to 92% excluding a significant number of nondiagnostic scans.

Of the current radiopharmaceuticals available for ventilation scanning, xenon 133 (^{133}Xe) and ^{99m}Tc diethylenetriamine pentaacetic acid (DTPA) aerosol are the two most commonly used.

^{133}Xe is a radioactive gas with a half-life of 5.3 days. It decays by beta and gamma radiation. The photon energy is 81 keV.

The ^{133}Xe ventilation scan consists of three consecutive phases of single breath holding, equilibrium, and a washout phase. The washout phase is the most sensitive phase of the ventilation scan for the detection of airway disease.

Despite its sensitivity in detecting airway disease, ^{133}Xe is not an ideal agent. There are several disadvantages to its use: notably poor spatial resolution of the image due to its low-energy photon, relatively high radiation dose to the lung, and complexity of its disposal. Another significant disadvantage is the inability to acquire images in multiple projections.

As an alternative to ^{133}Xe, a diagnostically equal scan can be obtained with radioaerosol inhalation, which also has the advantage of providing images in multiple projections. This is very helpful for direct comparison with the perfusion images that best identify the defect.

The radioaerosol in current use is ^{99m}Tc-DTPA. A dose of approximately 30 to 40 mCi of ^{99m}Tc-DTPA is introduced into the commercially available nebulizer, which generates submicronic particles ranging from 0.1 to 0.5 μm. Through the closed system, the patient breathes a mixture of oxygen and radioaerosol for 3 to 5 minutes. This process deposits the radioaerosol into the bronchoalveolar space, thus mapping the distribution of ventilation.

Approximately 500 to 700 μCi of radioactivity reaches the lung, which is sufficient to obtain multiple images within a few minutes. The ventilation scan is usually obtained before the perfusion scan. Residual ^{99m}Tc activity from the ventilation scan will be easily overridden by a higher dose of ^{99m}Tc macroaggregated albumin (MAA) used for perfusion images.

The distribution of the aerosolized particles is affected not only by particle size but also by the presence of airway disease, which results in excessive central deposition due to turbulent airflow and poor alveolar penetration of inhaled particles. This may decrease the quality of the image, thus lowering its diagnostic validity.

Once deposited in the lungs, the ^{99m}Tc-DTPA clears from the lung across the alveolar capillary membrane into the bloodstream, with a biologic half-time of 1 to 1.5 hours; it is excreted by the kidneys. Significantly increased renal activity after ventilation scan may signify an epithelial injury state, such as damage from cigarette smoking or interstitial pulmonary fibrosis (Fig. 2.A).

Imaging Technique

Standard projections for both aerosol and perfusion scans are anterior, posterior, right posterior oblique (RPO), left posterior oblique (LPO), right lateral, left lateral, and preferably right anterior oblique (RAO) and left anterior oblique (LAO).

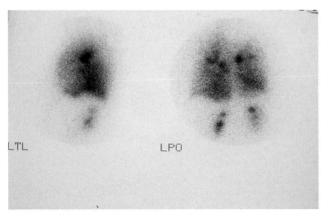

Figure 2.A ^{99m}Tc DTPA ventilation scan of a patient with interstitial pulmonary fibrosis showing increased renal activity.

After the completion of ventilation imaging, the patient is injected for perfusion scan. Injection is done in the supine position, which allows more uniform distribution of blood flow to the upper and lower lung fields. Images of perfusion are obtained in the same order, same projection, and same patient position as for ventilation, preferably with the patient in a sitting position. This reduces the ambiguity and differentiation in scan appearance due to different position and variability related to the position of the heart, diaphragm, and mediastinum.

Lateral and oblique views are important projections that only may fully demonstrate the segmental nature of the perfusion defect. The lateral segments of the lower lobe are better appreciated in the posterior oblique projection, as the lingula and middle lobe are best seen in anterior oblique projection. Oblique views also have the advantage of avoiding shine-through activity, which degrades the quality of lateral projections. The contribution of shine-through activity could be as high as 30%.

Normal Scan

The normal aerosol inhalation scan shows a uniform distribution of radioactivity outlining the lung fields. Minimal deposits of aerosol may be seen in the central airway (airway hot spot) as well as in the stomach and bowel, representing swallowed radioactive aerosol.

The normal perfusion scan also shows uniform distribution of radioactivity outlining the lung fields. The silhouette of the heart, mediastinum, hilum, aortic knob, diaphragm, and spine are readily identifiable.

Variation from normal in the pulmonary perfusion pattern is not common. Segmental defects rarely represent a normal variation; however, the presence of a subsegmental, subapical defect is not uncommon among normal subjects. To avoid overcall of the perfusion defect, attention should be given to the chest wall configuration as well as technical details during imaging. A chest wall deformity such as scoliosis or pectus excavatum may cause an apparent defect. Attenuation caused by interposition of the patient's arm on the lateral projection should not be confused as a defect. In the majority of these patients, the defect disappears by changing the patient's position slightly.

INTERPRETATION OF VENTILATION/ PERFUSION LUNG SCANS

Several schemes for interpretation of ventilation-perfusion scintigram have been developed over the years. These included the Bilo, original PIOPED, and the revised PIOPED (Table 2.1) criteria. Currently, another set of categories has been suggested by the PIOPED II study. PIOPED II is a prospective multicenter study designed to objectively evaluate the new scan categories to include a very low probability category and also to evaluate the efficacy of CT in the diagnosis of PE.

In PIOPED II, the revised PIOPED criteria for high probability have been maintained, the intermediate and low probabilities have been revised, and a very low probability criterion has been established (7,8).

TABLE 2.1 Revised PIOPED criteria for V/Q scan interpretation

High probability

≥2 large (>75% of a segment) segmental perfusion defects without corresponding ventilation or CXR abnormalities

1 large segmental perfusion defect and ≥2 moderate (25%–75% of a segment) segmental perfusion defects without corresponding ventilation or CXR abnormalities

≥4 moderate segmental perfusion defects without corresponding ventilation or CXR abnormalities

Intermediate probability

1 moderate to <2 large segmental perfusion defects without corresponding ventilation or CXR abnormalities

Corresponding V/Q defects and CXR parenchymal opacity in lower lung zone

Corresponding V/Q defects and small pleural effusion

Single moderate matched V/Q defects with normal CXR findings

Difficult to categorize as normal, low, or high probability

Low probability

Multiple matched V/Q defects, regardless of size, with normal CXR findings

Corresponding V/Q defects and CXR parenchymal opacity in upper or middle lung zone

Corresponding V/Q defects and large pleural effusion

Any perfusion defects with substantially larger CXR abnormality

Defects surrounded by normally perfused lung (stripe sign)

Single or multiple small (<25% of a segment) segmental perfusion defects with a normal CXR

Nonsegmental perfusion defects (cardiomegaly, aortic impression, enlarged hila)

Normal

No perfusion defects and perfusion outlines the shape of the lung seen on CXR

CXR = chest radiograph; V/Q = ventilation/perfusion.

Source: Reproduced from Worsley DF, Alavi A, Palevsky HI. Role of radionuclide imaging in patients with suspected pulmonary embolism. *Radiol Clin North Am* 1993;31:853, with permission.

The very low probability criteria in PIOPED II are as follows:*

a. Nonsegmental perfusion abnormalities (enlargement of the heart or hilum, elevated hemidiaphragm, linear atelectasis,

* Reprinted by permission of the Society of Nuclear Medicine, from Gottschalk A, Stein PD, Sostman HD, et al. Very low probability interpretation of V/Q lung scans in combination with low probability objective clinical assessment reliably excludes pulmonary embolism: data from PIOPED II. *J Nucl Med* 2007;48(9):1411–1415.

or costophrenic angle effusion with no other perfusion defect in either lung).

b. Perfusion defect smaller than corresponding radiographic lesion.

c. ≥2 matched V/Q defects with regionally normal chest radiograph and some areas of normal perfusion elsewhere in the lungs.

d. 1 to 3 small segmental perfusion defects (<25% of a segment).

e. Solitary triple matched defect (defined as a matched V/Q defect with associated matching chest radiographic opacification) in the middle or upper lung zone confined to a single segment.

f. Stripe sign, which consists of a stripe of perfused lung tissue between a perfusion defect and the adjacent pleural surface (best seen on a tangential view).

g. Pleural effusion equal to one third or more of the pleural cavity with no other perfusion defect in either lung.

A very low probability interpretation, according to these authors, has a positive predictive value (PPV) of 8.2%. However, a very low probability scan combined with a low clinical probability has a PPV of 3.1%, and when these data were applied only to a female patient aged <40 years, it was only 2%. Based on these findings, the authors conclude the combination of a low clinical probability and very low probability interpretation reliably excludes acute pulmonary embolus and can be used in patients whose computed tomography angiography (CTA) may be disadvantageous (women of reproductive age, compromised renal function, allergic risk).

Regardless of what criteria are being used, the classification of lung scans as normal, high probability, or very low probability is easier and the results are more reliable. However, distinguishing between low probability and intermediate probability may be difficult and some degree of uncertainty is unavoidable. In addition, an interobserver variability as much as 30% is not uncommon. Therefore adhering to the strict diagnostic criteria of lung scan interpretation may not be practical for all patients all the time. It appears that using the criteria combined with interpretative experience (gestalt), clinical evaluation, and consideration of the total situation is the best approach for the diagnosis of PE. The combination of clinical assessment and V/Q interpretation improves the chances of making the correct diagnosis when compared with either scan or clinical assessment alone (Table 2.2). It is important to note that the scintigraphic findings and clinical impression of PE are more commonly concordant than discordant.

The basic concept in formulating a rational approach to the diagnosis of PE is to observe all the clinical data—pretest probability factors and stratification of the patient with respect to underlying cardiopulmonary disease as well as ancillary scintigraphic finding and radiographs that either favor or disfavor the presence of embolic disease (9).

1. Consideration should be given to the conditions that affect the clinical probability of PE. Objective clinical probability is assessed according to the Wells test and are as follows[†]:

† Reproduced from *J Nucl Med* 2007;48:1411–1415, with permission.

TABLE 2.2   Percent probability of acute pulmonary embolus using combinations of clinical and scan findings

Clinical probability	Scan probability			
	High	**Intermediate**	**Low**	**Normal**
High	96	66	40	0
Intermediate	84	25	12	4
Low	56	16	4	2

a. Clinical signs and symptoms of deep venous thrombosis (DVT) (3 points)
b. Heart rate >100 beats/minute (1.5 points)
c. Immobilization ≥3 consecutive days or surgery in previous 4 weeks (1.5 points)
d. Previous objectively diagnosed PE or DVT (1.5 points)
e. Hemoptysis (1 point)
f. Malignancy (cancer patient receiving treatment within 6 months or receiving palliative treatment) (1 point)
g. PE as likely as or more likely than alternative diagnosis (based on history, physical examination, chest radiograph, ECG and blood test) (3 points)

A score of less than 2 considered as clinically low probability.

A score of 2 to 6 is intermediate, and a score of greater than 6 accounts for high clinical probability.

Although the history of DVT constitutes a moderate clinical risk for pulmonary emboli (20% to 70%), the presence of concurrent DVT is a high risk (70% to 80%) factor. Sonographic evidence of DVT may be seen in up to 30% of patients who have a PE and only in 15% of patients with an intermediate probability scan. Therefore a negative Doppler examination, as seen in 85% of intermediate scans, should not deter attention from the diagnosis of PE. Negative Doppler examinations in the majority of patients with angiographically confirmed PE do suggest that the thrombus has already migrated to the lung.

2. Pulmonary emboli tend to be multiple, thus producing more than two perfusion defects accompanied by a normal ventilation scan and clear chest x-ray. The wedge defect that occupies the lower and lateral border of the lower lobe seen in the anterior and lateral projections represents impaired perfusion of the two nearby segments (anterior and lateral-basilar segments). The perfusion defect of pulmonary embolism is wedge-shaped and pleural-based; therefore a centrally located defect is evidence against PE. The segmental nature of perfusion defect is also an important characteristic of PE. Bronchopulmonary segments of the lung have a rather defined boundary that can be appreciated on the surface map of the lung (Fig. 2.B). Defects that are irregular in shape and do not respect segmental boundaries are unlikely to be due to PE.

3. Perfusion defect along the fissures (fissure sign), although originally thought to be due to microembolism along the fissure, is usually related to the pleural effusion in the fissure or is caused by chronic lung disease and is not in favor of PE (Fig. 2.C).

4. Unilateral absence or near absence of perfusion in association with ventilatory abnormality strongly suggests airway disease and is not in favor of PE. In addition to the malignant and benign bronchogenic mass, stenosis of the pulmonary artery, or presence of a foreign body must be considered.

5. Multiple small serrated defects along the contour of the lung, known as a contour pattern, are usually associated with tumor microembolization and lymphatic spread of carcinoma and should not be mistaken for pulmonary embolism secondary to thrombus.

6. Although 75% of perfusion defects resolve within 3 months, the remaining 25% of defects may persist for years and thus lead to a false-positive interpretation lung scan. In patients

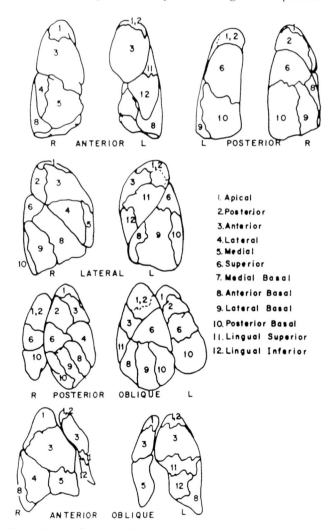

1. Apical
2. Posterior
3. Anterior
4. Lateral
5. Medial
6. Superior
7. Medial Basal
8. Anterior Basal
9. Lateral Basal
10. Posterior Basal
11. Lingual Superior
12. Lingual Inferior

Figure 2.B Surface map of the lung depicting bronchopulmonary segments.

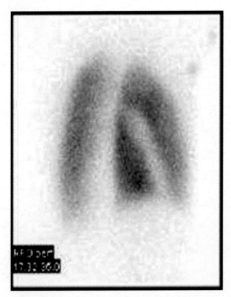

Figure 2.C An LAO perfusion scan showing a linear area of hypoperfusion consistent with fissure sign.

with documented previous PE, the positive predictive value of a high-probability scan is lower (74%) than in those without previous PE (96%). Comparison with a prior scan in such a patient is extremely important.

ROLE OF THE V/Q SCAN AND CT ANGIOGRAM IN THE MANAGEMENT OF PATIENTS WITH SUSPECTED PE

1. As mentioned earlier, the PIOPED II clinical trial investigators prefer CT pulmonary angiography over ventilation perfusion lung scanning for diagnosing PE in many situations (10). However, pulmonary CT angiography will be more diagnostic if it is combined with CT venography of the popliteal and femoral veins and the overall result are evaluated in the proper context of pretest probability. In absence of clinical assessment and CT venography, the pulmonary CT angiogram has a sensitivity of only 83%, which is not adequate for the management of PE.

2. Considering the risk of iodinated contrast, particularly in patients with impaired renal function, and the risk of radiation to the breast in women of reproductive age, pulmonary CT angiography may not be the first-line test for the diagnosis of PE in these patients. Alternatives such as the combination of venous ultrasound and V/Q lung scan may be more appropriate, as the use of the V/Q scan minimizes radiation to the breast.

3. One of the recommended approaches in the selection of V/Q scanning versus pulmonary CT angiography for providing the most favorable outcome (considering cost, risks, and availability) is based on the pretest probability of PE (11).

   a. In patients with high pretest probability, the presence of PE can be confirmed by either V/Q scanning or CT angiography. Both have the same discriminatory power in confirming PE.

   b. In patients with low pretest probability, PE can be excluded by CT angiography; if this is not available, however, a normal or near normal V/Q scan is an alternative.

   c. In excluding PE in patients with moderate pretest probability or in confirming PE in patients with low pretest probability, the V/Q scan should be avoided, as the CT angiogram has higher discriminatory power for these categories.

CASE 2.1

History: A healthy 36-year-old male with a family history of thrombophilia (not known at the time) presents with chest pain, dyspnea, and apprehension. His chest x-ray is normal. He receives a V/Q scan for evaluation of probable pulmonary emboli (Figs. 2.1 A, B).

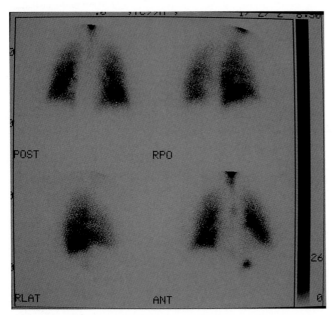

Figure 2.1 A

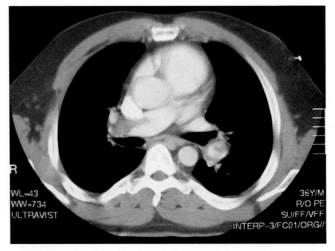

Figure 2.1 C

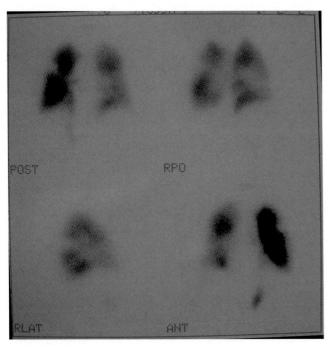

Figure 2.1 B

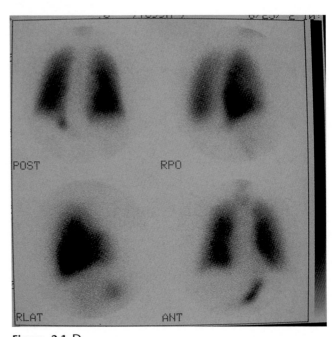

Figure 2.1 D

Findings: There are multiple large, wedge-shaped, pleural-based, mismatched defects in both lung fields. In addition, there is generalized reduced perfusion of the right lung as compared with the left. The lung scan findings indicate a high probability of acute pulmonary emboli, which were also visu-alized on CT angiography (Fig. 2.1 C) done on the same day. Multiple filling defects within the lumen of contrast-filled pulmonary arteries are seen on both sides. A follow-up perfusion scan (Fig. 2.1 D) after completion of anticoagulation therapy shows complete resolution of the perfusion abnormalities.

Discussion: Multiple large, segmental, mismatched perfusion defects are important characteristics for pulmonary emboli which, in patients with high clinical probability, have a positive predictive value of 96%.

Other causes of V/Q mismatch are previous PE, bronchogenic carcinoma, previous radiation therapy to the lung, pneumonia, tuberculosis, collagen vascular disease, intravenous drug abuse, tumor emboli, etc.; however, most of these can be excluded by clinical and other diagnostic tests.

Perfusion defects due to acute pulmonary emboli gradually regress with time and following therapy; the majority resolve within 3 months. Resolution is quicker in patients with no previous cardiovascular disease (3 to 7 days).

Obtaining a perfusion lung scan at the completion of anticoagulant therapy and at discharge is of clinical value in future management of the patient. This scan will serve as a baseline for the diagnosis of recurrent PE, which is seen as the development of a new defect.

Most patients with high-probability lung scans and a high clinical likelihood of PE require treatment and need no further diagnostic test to confirm diagnosis. Utilization of CT angiography in the workup of patients suspicious for PE is increasing. However, in patients with a high probability for PE, the discriminatory power of V/Q and CT angiography is similar and concordant positive results have been reported in 86% of interpretations.

In evaluating patients with PE, attention should be given to the risk factors for the development of DVT and PE, the most notable of which are use of estrogen, history of previous DVT or PE, and presence of concurrent DVT. Genetic disorder of thrombus formation (thrombophilia) should be kept in mind when PE occurs in young patients with no other predisposing factors. These patients are characteristically younger than the average patient with thrombosis.

Diagnosis: Acute pulmonary embolism with complete resolution.

CASE 2.2

History: A 55-year-old male who had undergone renal transplantation and now has declining renal function was flown from a long distance to the Medical Center for further evaluation and possible renal biopsy.

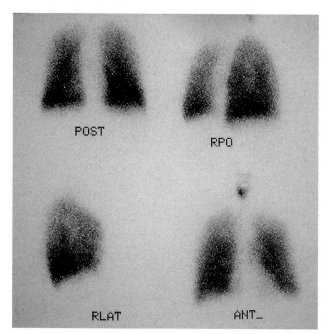

Figure 2.2 A

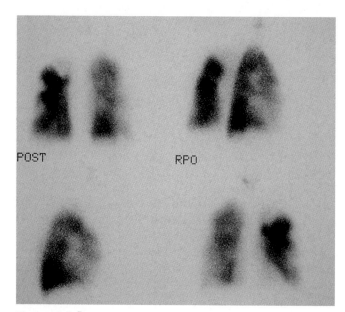

Figure 2.2 B

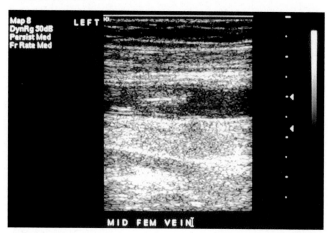

Figure 2.2 C

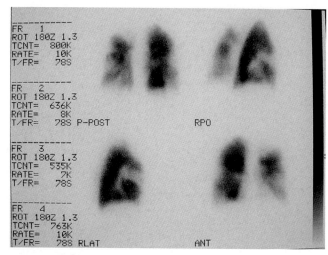

Figure 2.2 D

Shortly following his admission, the patient developed a sudden onset of right-sided chest pain and dyspnea. Cardiac enzyme, ECG, and chest radiographs were not contributory and the patient received a V/Q scan for the evaluation of probable pulmonary emboli.

Findings: V/Q lung scans (Figs. 2.2 A, B) show multiple large and moderate sized wedge-shaped, pleural-based, mismatched defects in both lungs.

Immediately following the lung scan, a lower extremity venous Doppler examination (Fig. 2.2 C) was performed. The duplex study shows large segmental venous thromboses involving the midportion of the superficial femoral vein and extending through the left popliteal vein.

The patient was managed appropriately for thromboembolic disease. A lung scan at 3-month follow-up (Fig. 2.2 D) shows persistence of multiple defects with no significant interval change.

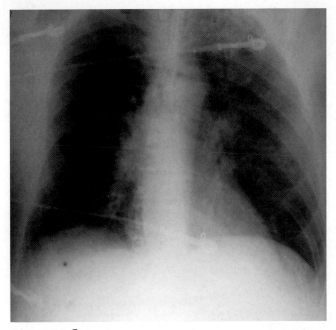

Figure 2.2 E

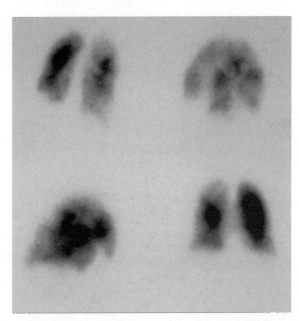

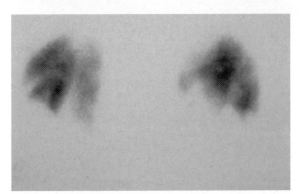

Figure 2.2 F

Discussion: In the proper clinical context and in a patient with no history of previous pulmonary emboli and a clear chest radiograph, the presence of multiple large mismatched segmental defects represents a high-probability study with a positive predictive value of 96%.

In the diagnosis of PE, regardless of the scan category, attention should be paid to the clinical presentation as well as risk factors contributing to the formation of DVT and subsequent PE. Genetic factors, use of oral contraceptives, pregnancy, puerperium, malignancy, immobilization, trauma, recent surgery, central line placement, and long airplane flight (traveler's thrombosis) are among the most important risk factors to consider.

Coexistence of PE and DVT is not unusual. The majority of PE arise from the proximal vein of the lower extremity. About one-third of patients who have PE also have detectable DVT, but more than half of the patients with PE do not demonstrate thrombosis, suggesting that the thrombus has already migrated to the lung.

Silent emboli are also not uncommon and suspected perfusion defects consistent with PE may be seen in up to 30% of patients with a positive venous duplex scan. Although these patients normally receive anticoagulant therapy, obtaining a

baseline perfusion lung scan would be helpful for evaluation of future episodes of PE.

Perfusion defects resulting from pulmonary emboli may begin to resolve within 3 to 4 days. Resolution of perfusion defect is quicker in patients with no previous cardiopulmonary disease but slower when a large defect occurs in a patient with preexisting cardiopulmonary disease. A defect not resolving by 2 to 3 months may persist for many years, and some of these patients may develop chronic changes of pulmonary emboli. It is to be noted that the most common cause of a false-positive high-probability interpretation of a lung scan is the history of PE in the past.

Pulmonary emboli are responsible for a substantial number of patients suffering from a secondary pulmonary arterial hypertension. The process is initiated by single or recurrent episodes of PE. The unresolved thrombosis proceeds to the organization stage and fibrosis, which results in stenosis or complete obstruction of the pulmonary artery; this is demonstrable by CT or conventional pulmonary angiography. On lung scan, these patients would have segmental defects in both lung fields that remain unchanged over time. These patients may benefit from the surgical procedure of pulmonary endarterectomy. It is to be noted that although CT angiography appears to be the first-line imaging procedure for the evaluation of patients suspected of having PE, V/Q pulmonary scintigraphy has a higher sensitivity and specificity for distinguishing pulmonary arterial hypertension of chronic thromboembolic disease from other causes of pulmonary arterial hypertension (idiopathic, emphysema, pulmonary fibrosis, pulmonary venous occlusive disease, sarcoidosis, and congenital heart disease such as atrial septal defect). A normal scan practically excludes chronic PE as the cause of the patient's pulmonary arterial hypertension. The patient with a chronic inflammatory disorder of the lungs and those with splenectomy are at especially high risk for developing chronic embolic pulmonary arterial hypertension.

Figures 2.2 E and 2.2 F shows a chest radiograph and perfusion scan of a 60-year-old patient with pulmonary arterial hypertension secondary to PE. On perfusion scan (Fig. 2.2 F), in addition to the presence of a segmental perfusion defect, there is generalized reduced perfusion of the right lung as compared with the left, correlating with increased lucency and reduced vascularity of the right lung seen on the radiograph (Fig. 2.2 E); this suggests a previous embolus in the right pulmonary artery. Reduced perfusion is more pronounced peripherally, consistent with diminished peripheral flow due to attenuation and pruning of the peripheral vascular branches, a known feature of pulmonary arterial hypertension.

A patient with primary pulmonary arterial hypertension may present with clinical and radiographic findings similar to those of secondary pulmonary artery hypertension; however, the perfusion lung scan in the former is normal; therefore a perfusion lung scan can be used to differentiate the two entities.

Diagnosis: Pulmonary emboli coexistent with venous thrombosis of lower extremity; unresolved perfusion defects.

CASE 2.3

History: A 63-year-old alcoholic with hepatic cirrhosis and multifocal atrial tachycardia was referred for V/Q scintigraphy to rule out PE (Figs. 2.3 A, B).

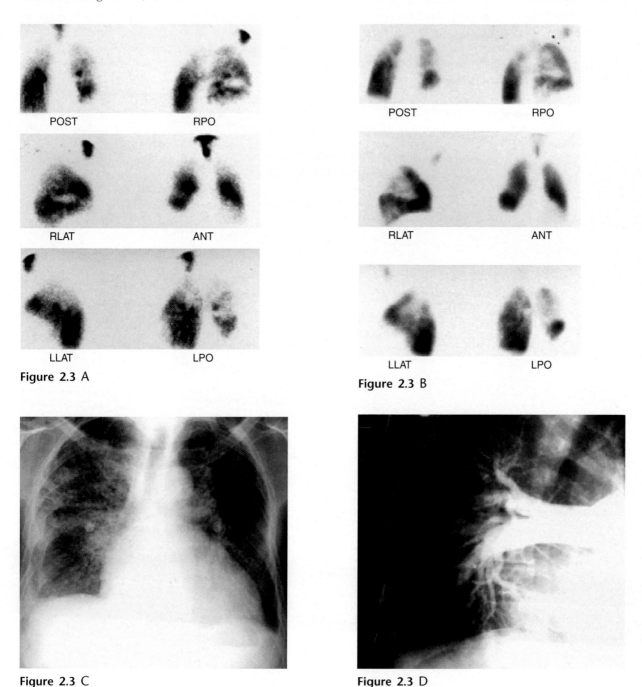

Figure 2.3 A

Figure 2.3 B

Figure 2.3 C

Figure 2.3 D

Findings: There is a large, well-defined, wedge-shaped perfusion defect involving the right upper lobe best seen in the lateral projection (Fig. 2.3 B), in the area in which there is some ventilation (Fig. 2.3 A). The radiographic abnormality (Fig. 2.3 C) is smaller than the perfusion abnormality.

Discussion: A perfusion defect substantially larger than the chest x-ray opacity with preservation of some ventilation is one of the criteria for a high-probability scan.

Given this patient's history of alcohol use and esophageal varices, he is considered to be at high risk for anticoagulation. The PE diagnosis was confirmed by angiography (Fig. 2.3 D) and a Greenfield filter was inserted.

A perfusion defect in an area of pulmonary parenchymal opacity does not mean an intermediate probability for PE in every instance. The scan can be classified as high probability when the criteria are met. In this case, the presence of some ventilation supports the diagnosis of PE. The segmental nature and wedge-shaped defect extending to the pleural surface is also a characteristic pattern for PE and should not be weighed lightly where the diagnosis of PE is concerned.

In patients with a high-probability scan and a relatively high clinical likelihood of PE, there should be no need for further diagnostic tests; however, in patients undergoing more aggressive therapy, such as inferior vena cava filtration, thrombolysis, or embolectomy, pulmonary angiography is indicated and justified.

Diagnosis: High probability of acute PE.

CASE 2.4

History: A 62-year-old man presented to the emergency room with dyspnea, chest pain and hypoxemia. Acute myocardial infarction was excluded and an emergency V/Q scan was performed (Figs. 2.4 A and 2.4 B). An admission chest x-ray was taken (Fig. 2.4 C).

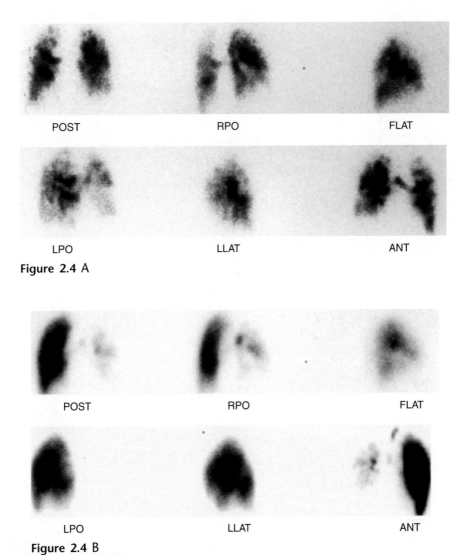

POST | RPO | FLAT

LPO | LLAT | ANT

Figure 2.4 A

POST | RPO | FLAT

LPO | LLAT | ANT

Figure 2.4 B

Findings: The chest x-ray reveals enlargement of the right pulmonary artery but no parenchymal infiltrates. The lung scan shows diffuse heterogeneous distribution of radioaerosol and a large mismatched perfusion defect involving virtually the entire right lung.

Discussion: A scintigraphic finding of near absence of right lung perfusion in an adequately ventilated lung implies a high probability for PE. Other causes of a near absence of unilateral lung perfusion defect include the following: bronchogenic carcinoma causing compression of the pulmonary artery; congenital heart disease and after shunt procedure; fibrosing mediastinitis usually due to histoplasmosis; postradiation fibrosis; unilateral hyperlucent lung (Swyer-James syndrome); pulmonary arterial hypoplasia; giant bullae; mediastinal hematoma resulting from aortic dissection (valve replacement); Marfan's syndrome; and several other uncommon conditions. Most of these entities can be excluded by history and radiographic findings.

In addition to the clinical presentation, the enlargement of the pulmonary artery (Fleischner's sign) seen on this patient's chest x-ray is a supportive finding that the V/Q mismatch represents a pulmonary embolus for which the patient received treatment. Enlargement of the pulmonary artery is due to pulmonary arterial hypertension and/or distention of vessels by bulky thrombosis. It is to be noted that prominence of the pulmonary artery may be seen in 20% of radiographs of patients with or without pulmonary emboli. As such, the sensitivity of Fleischner's sign in predicting PE is low and many patients with PE do not show this sign.

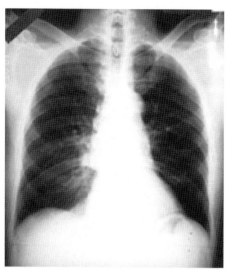

Figure 2.4 C

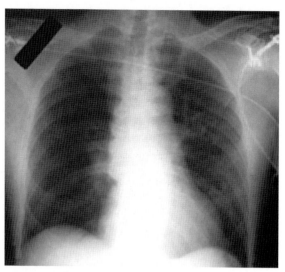

Figure 2.4 D

The patient's chest x-ray (Fig. 2.4 D) taken 2 months after the initial episode of massive right pulmonary artery emboli shows a generalized hyperlucency of the right lung, a manifestation of reduction in the right lung blood volume and pulmonary oligemia (Westermark's sign), and, in this case, a sequela of massive emboli. This will probably persist for a pro-longed period. Westermark's sign is not a common finding and is seen even with lesser frequency than the Fleischner's sign. However, when it is present, it is seen more on the right than on the left side.

Diagnosis: Massive emboli of the right pulmonary artery.

CASE 2.5

History: A 60-year-old man presented with increasing shortness of breath and dyspnea. A V/Q scan was performed to rule out pulmonary embolus (Figs 2.5 A, B) and a chest x-ray was taken (Fig. 2.5 C).

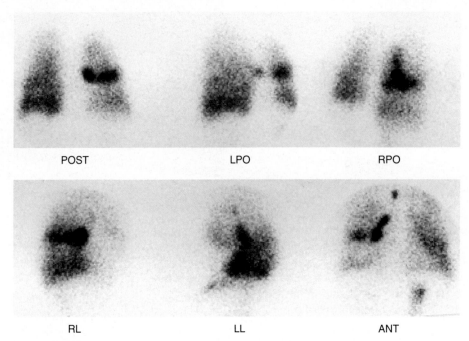

POST   LPO   RPO

RL   LL   ANT

Figure 2.5 A

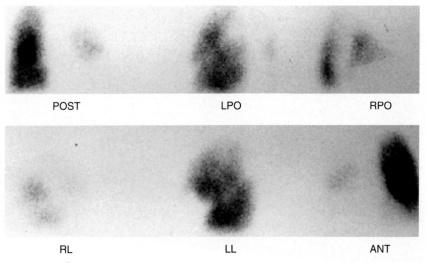

POST   LPO   RPO

RL   LL   ANT

Figure 2.5 B

Findings: The chest x-ray is free from acute infiltrate. There may be an increase in upper-lobe lucency, more on the right than the left. There is tortuosity of the aorta.

The ventilation scan (Fig. 2.5 A) reveals some asymmetry, with minimally reduced ventilation of the right lung compared with the left. Most notable is an intense deposition of radioaerosol in what appears to be the right main-stem bronchus.

The perfusion scan (Fig. 2.5 B) reveals a significant loss of perfusion in the entire right lung.

Discussion: The unilateral loss of perfusion with preservation of ventilation is not common and has a reported incidence of 2%.

Conceptually, a mismatched defect with reduced perfusion and the presence of ventilation is generally considered to be of embolic etiology. However, unilateral absence of perfusion is an infrequent finding in pulmonary emboli. Although a massive embolus involving the right pulmonary artery should be considered, absence of a perfusion defect in the left lung makes this diagnosis unlikely.

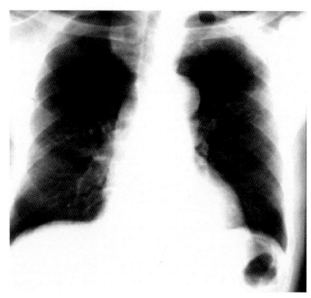

Figure 2.5 C

Among the other causes of unilateral absence or near absence of V/Q abnormalities that have the potential for a false-positive high-probability scan is a previous unresolved pulmonary embolus, a centrally located mass, and endobronchial lesions. Although these are the major causes, other entities such as pneumonectomy, Swyer-James syndrome (unilateral hyperlucent lung), radiation therapy to the lung, fibrosing mediastinitis, congenital pulmonary artery hypoplasia, giant bullae, and pneumothorax should also be considered. Most of these entities can be excluded by history, status of the ventilation scan, and findings on other imaging techniques.

A centrally located intrathoracic mass, by compromising the airway and compressing the blood flow, may cause major asymmetry in the perfusion. A bronchogenic carcinoma is a major cause that might not be easily detectable on the chest radiograph. Bronchogenic carcinoma in 65% of cases causes a matched V/Q defect; in the remaining cases the perfusion defect is usually larger than the ventilatory abnormality, as in this case.

The diagnosis of an endobronchial lesion by chest roentgenogram usually depends on the indirect signs of atelectasis, vascular crowding, or a shift of the anatomic landmarks of the mediastinum and hilar structures. When there is insignificant or only minimal obstruction to airflow, as in this case, the chest x-ray appears normal. The ventilation lung scan is more sensitive than the chest radiograph in detecting bronchial obstruction. The intense, lobulated deposit of radioaerosol in this patient's ventilation scan is most likely related to the turbulent bronchial airflow in the prestenotic segments of the bronchus. The prestenotic bronchial segment becomes dilated, resulting

in turbulent airflow and retention of radioaerosol. Typically this pattern is accompanied by a distal airspace defect. When present, this "prestenotic aerosol deposition sign" may direct attention to an obstructive bronchial lesion.

V/Q scanning is of no value in screening patients for lung cancer. However, demonstration of a perfusion abnormality may lateralize the lesion in patients with an inconclusive CT or radiograph but with positive sputum cytology. Unilateral extensive bullous disease or pneumothorax of one lung in which adjacent lung tissue is compressed also results in unilateral reduction of the perfusion.

It is worth noting that unilateral loss of perfusion when it involves the right lung may, in the proper clinical setting, raise the possibility of an aortic dissection. The right pulmonary artery and aortic root have a common tunica adventitia; therefore the pulmonary artery is susceptible to compression of hematoma resulting from dissected aneurysm. Dissection of the aorta is a rare complication of aortic valve replacement and may be confused with acute pulmonary embolism. The distinction is very important, particularly because anticoagulation is contraindicated in these patients.

Injection of the macroaggregated albumin (MAA) into a central venous line, pulmonary artery catheter, or Swan-Ganz catheter should be considered an artifactual possibility in the differential diagnosis of massive perfusion defect of one lung. Injection of MAA should ideally be made into a peripheral vein.

This patient's diagnosis of a nonocclusive bronchial carcinoma at the junction of the right upper and right middle lobe was confirmed by a bronchoscopic examination.

Diagnosis: Endobronchial mass mimicking PE.

History: A 67-year-old man, bedridden due to multiple sclerosis, presented to the emergency department with shortness of breath. An emergency V/Q lung scan (Figs. 2.6 A, B) was performed to evaluate for possible pulmonary embolism. A duplex Doppler examination of the lower extremities was negative for DVT. An admission chest x-ray (Fig. 2.6 C) was taken.

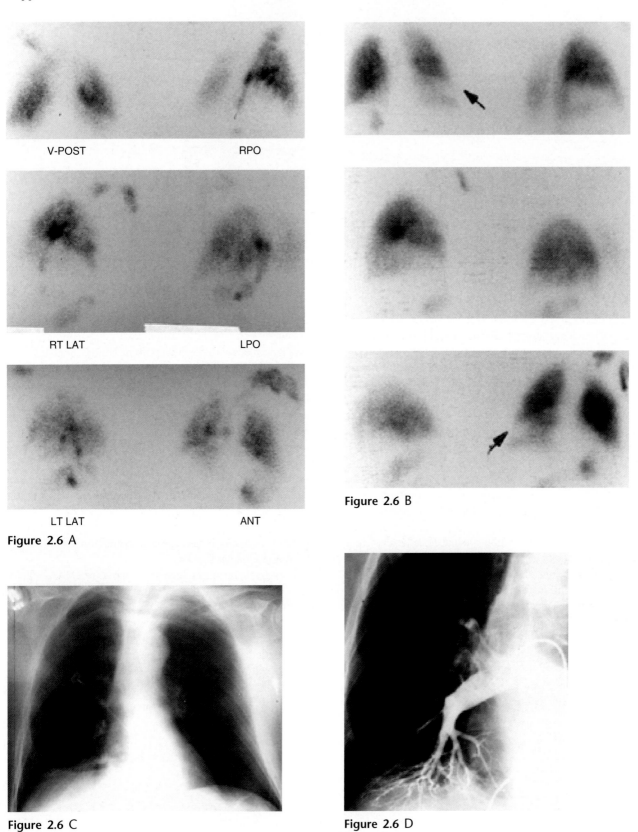

V-POST   RPO

RT LAT   LPO

LT LAT   ANT

Figure 2.6 A

Figure 2.6 B

Figure 2.6 C

Figure 2.6 D

Findings: The chest x-ray is unremarkable except for plate-like atelectasis in the right lower lobe. The V/Q scan reveals a matched defect in the right lower lobe. Although perfusion of the right lobe is reduced, a wedge-shaped defect appears to be present laterally (arrows in Fig. 2.6 B) in the area where ventilation is less disturbed.

Discussion: There is a triple-matched defect occupying the right lower lobe, which corresponds to an intermediate-probability scan and 33% prevalence for PE. The subsequent pulmonary angiogram (Fig. 2.6 D) demonstrates no evidence of PE. There is, however, crowding of the right-lower-lobe vascularity medially owing to the atelectasis and resulting in a splaying out of the lateral vessels, producing a wedge-shaped zone of relative flow deficit peripherally.

A small- to moderate-sized area of atelectasis may be the cause of a nonembolic segmental mismatch and is a potential etiology for a false-positive V/Q scan. The shape and configuration of the defect depends on the extent of reexpansion of the adjacent segments and the size and location of the atelectatic area. Among the long list of causes of nonembolic mismatched defects, the most frequently encountered include previous pulmonary embolism, pneumonia, bronchogenic carcinoma, and previous radiation therapy. However, atelectasis should also be considered.

Diagnosis: Right-lower-lobe segmental atelectasis.

CASE 2.7

History: A 62-year-old man, bedridden, was admitted with acute dyspnea, chest pain, and blood in his sputum. A chest x-ray (Fig. 2.7 A) was taken and a V/Q scan (Figs. 2.7 B, C) was performed.

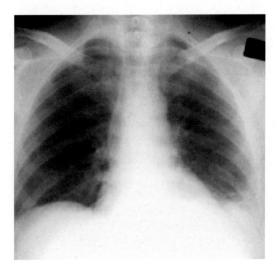

Figure 2.7 A

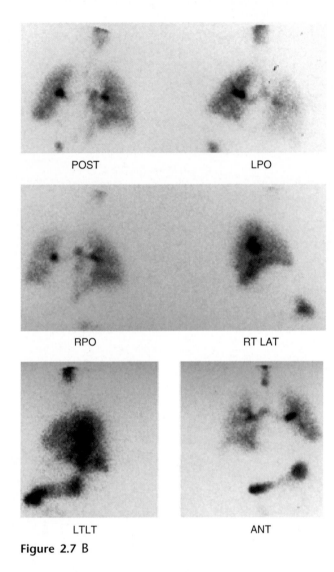

POST   LPO

RPO   RT LAT

LTLT   ANT

Figure 2.7 B

Findings: The chest x-ray demonstrates a left-lower-lobe infiltrate. The V/Q scan shows a matched defect in the posterobasilar segment of the left lower lobe in the area of a pulmonary parenchymal infiltrate (triple-matched). Swallowed radioaerosol is identified in the gastrointestinal tract.

Discussion: A triple-matched defect in the lower lung zone qualifies for an indeterminate-probability scan with an overall 33% prevalence of pulmonary emboli (PIOPED data).

The diagnostic accuracy of the scan can be improved if it is interpreted in light of clinical information and ancillary findings. The finding of an intermediate scan in a patient with or without prior cardiopulmonary disease has a different diagnostic value. For example, in patients with a known history of valvular heart disease, coronary artery disease, heart failure, asthma, chronic obstructive pulmonary disease (COPD), or interstitial lung disease, an intermediate-category scan has a higher probability of 66% for PE when the clinical probability is high (PIOPED data).

In this patient, the presence of PE, represented by a triple-matched defect, is documented by a pulmonary angiography (Fig. 2.7 D).

Parenchymal infiltrate as a result of PE is related to vascular changes and pulmonary infarct. Within 24 to 48 hours after a PE, capillary congestion and hemorrhage into the airspace may occur, resulting in a matching V/Q defect. It is well established that pulmonary scintigraphy is more helpful in diagnosing PE when the radiograph is normal. When the radiograph becomes abnormal secondary to changes of pulmonary embolus, it is

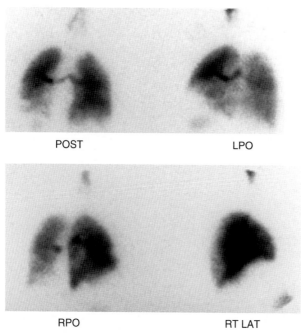

POST   LPO

RPO   RT LAT

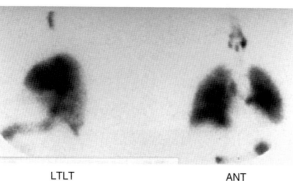

LTLT   ANT

Figure 2.7 C

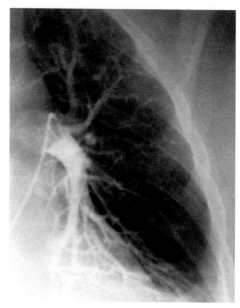

Figure 2.7 D

likely that the disease began several days earlier. Postponement of the V/Q scan until the x-ray becomes abnormal would result in an increase in the number of intermediate-probability interpretations. The V/Q scan should be done as early as possible in the course of the disease. Because the clinical symptoma-tology of PE is not specific, a high level of clinical suspicion must be maintained to proceed with the necessary diagnostic workup.

Diagnosis: Angiographically proven PE in a patient with high clinical suspicion and an intermediate-probability scan.

History: A 46-year-old female with lupus presented with difficulty in breathing, fever, erythema, and swelling of the right calf. The patient was referred for V/Q scintigraphy (Figs. 2.8 A, B). Admission chest x-ray was performed (Fig. 2.8 C).

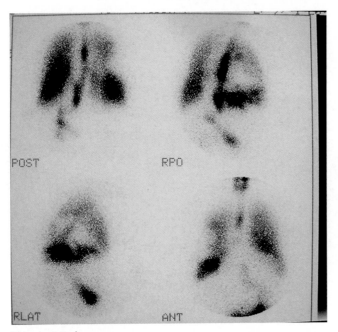

Figure 2.8 A

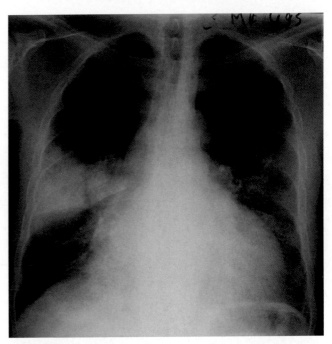

Figure 2.8 C

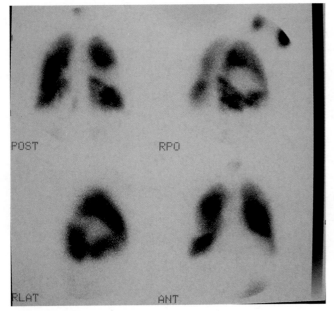

Figure 2.8 B

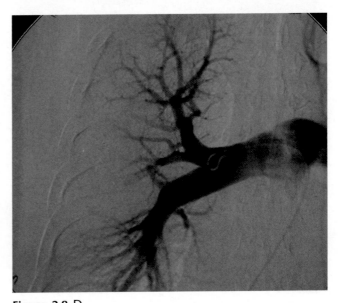

Figure 2.8 D

Findings: There is a large triple-matched defect involving the superior and lateral basal segments of the right lower lobe.

Discussion: A triple match in the lower lobe represents an intermediate-probability scan.

In this patient with a low clinical likelihood of PE in spite of a large triple-matched defect, the prevalence of PE would also be lower (16%) according to the PIOPED data. The absence of PE in this patient is documented by angiography (Fig. 2.8 D).

In the interpretation of a V/Q scan, the importance of a clinical assessment and pretest probability for PE cannot be overemphasized; however, when clinical and chest x-ray findings are such that a clear diagnosis cannot be provided by V/Q scan, CT angiography would be a more effective tool.

Diagnosis: Intermediate-probability scan in a patient with a low pretest probability; negative pulmonary angiogram.

History: An 80-year-old patient who has recently had an acetabular hip fracture developed an acute onset of chest pain, hypoxia, and tachycardia. A chest radiograph (Fig. 2.9 A) and V/Q scan (Figs. 2.9 B, C) were obtained for the evaluation of possible acute pulmonary emboli.

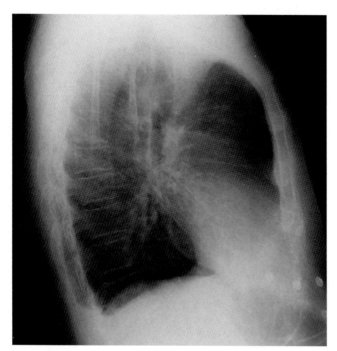

Figure 2.9 A

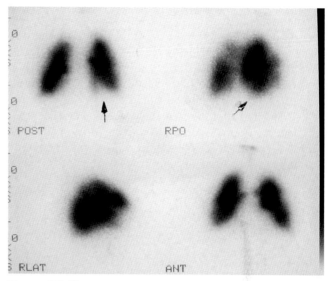

Figure 2.9 C

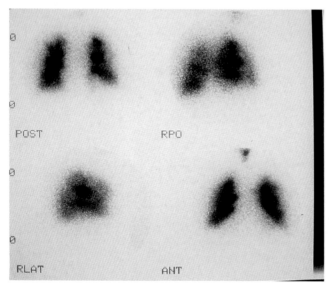

Figure 2.9 B

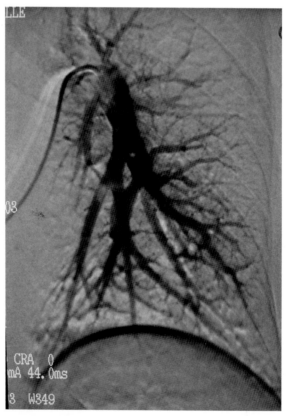

Figure 2.9 D

Findings: The lateral chest x-ray shows a small amount of pleural effusion blunting the right costophrenic angle. The V/Q scan shows a corresponding defect in the posterobasilar segment of the right lower lobe (arrow in Fig. 2.9 C).

Discussion: Performance of a V/Q scan to exclude PE in patients with pleural effusion is not an uncommon clinical request. Pleural effusion and pleural-based density with an elevated hemidiaphragm may be seen in patients with pulmonary emboli. However, the majority of these effusions are small and cause only blunting of the costophrenic angle. On the other hand, pleural effusion not related to PE by compression or displacement of the lung parenchyma can alter the regional pulmonary perfusion and create a perfusion defect. Moreover, shifting of the pleural effusion on chest radiography and V/Q scanning performed with the patient in different positions can create a different size, shape, and position of the defect, leading to difficulty in interpretation. Currently there is no general agreement on interpretive criteria for lung scans of patients with pleural effusions of different sizes.

According to the PIOPED criteria, a small pleural effusion causing blunting of the costophrenic angle is associated with an intermediate probability for pulmonary emboli, while the defect due to a large pleural effusion is commonly classified as a very low probablity scan. Further angiographic investigation (Fig. 2.9 D) in this patient with a high clinical likelihood of PE shows the presence of emboli.

There are reports indicating that PEs are associated with pleural effusion of all sizes. Therefore all should be considered as being of intermediate probability, requiring further investigation.

Diagnosis: Intermediate-probability scan in a patient with a small pleural effusion and high pretest probability; positive pulmonary angiogram.

CASE 2.10

History: A 70-year-old hypertensive, diabetic patient with coronary artery disease and COPD developed shortness of breath and hemoptysis. A perfusion scan (Fig. 2.10 A) and chest radiograph (Fig. 2.10 B) were obtained.

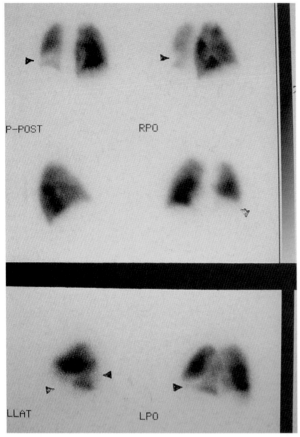

Figure 2.10 A

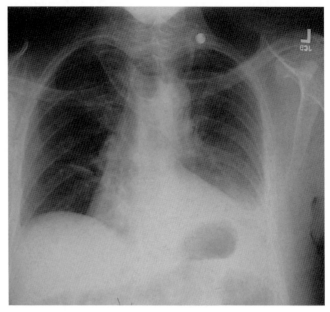

Figure 2.10 B

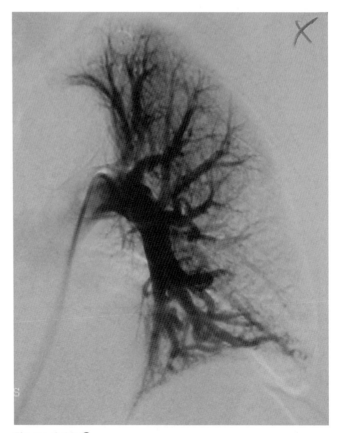

Figure 2.10 C

Findings: Chest x-ray shows a large left-sided pleural effusion. The perfusion scan shows a corresponding defect to the location and size of the pleural effusion.

Discussion: A scan showing a perfusion defect in a patient with pleural effusion is usually classified as being of intermediate probability. Since the frequency of PEs associated with large pleural effusion is less than 30%, they can be placed in the lower portion of the intermediate-probability range. Owing to a low clinical likelihood of PE and the presence of a large pleural effusion, the scan is classified close to the very low probability category; the absence of PE was documented on angiography (Fig. 2.10 C).

It should be emphasized that the interpretation criteria for the lung scan should not be applied blindly and automatically in all patients. The combination of criteria, clinical correlation, and pretest probability is the best approach for diagnosing PE.

Diagnosis: Very low probability scan in a patient with a large pleural effusion and low pretest probability; negative angiogram.

CASE 2.11

History: A 57-year-old HIV-positive male with a sudden onset of dyspnea has a wedge-shaped pulmonary infiltrate on his chest radiograph (Fig. 2.11 A). A V/Q scan was performed to rule out pulmonary emboli (Figs. 2.11 B, C).

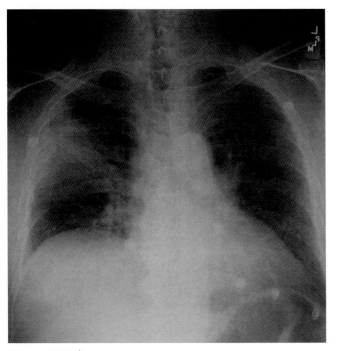

Figure 2.11 A

Figure 2.11 C

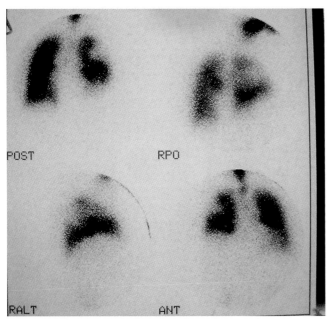

Figure 2.11 B

Figure 2.11 D

Findings: Chest radiography shows elevation of the right hemidiaphragm and a wedge-shaped pulmonary parenchymal infiltrate in the posterior segment of the right upper lobe. The V/Q scan shows a matched V/Q abnormality corresponding to the right-upper-lobe infiltrate.

Discussion: A matched V/Q defect associated with parenchymal opacity on the chest radiograph is defined as a triple-matched defect. Such a defect may result from a pulmonary infarct caused by PE. The pulmonary infarct may be complete, with necrosis of the pulmonary parenchyma, or, more commonly, an incomplete process with transient hemorrhage and edema that resolves over several days. A complete infarct, however, is permanent. When a pulmonary infarct occurs in the lower lobe, a well-defined, pleural-based opacity with a convexed medial border ("Hampton's hump") may appear, which can easily be differentiated from pleural effusion, since the latter has a concave border. Development of Hampton's hump within 2 to 3 days following the onset of symptoms strongly suggests associated PE.

Conceptually, a V/Q defect matched with a parenchymal opacity of the infarct belongs to the category of an intermediate scan, as the pulmonary infarct is not the only entity that can cause a pulmonary parenchymal infiltrate. In fact, the most common opacity appearing in patients with PE is due to atelectasis.

Data from the PIOPED study and its subsequent revision indicate that the prevalence of PE in patients with a triple-matched defect varies based on the location of the abnormality. Data indicate that the positive predictive value for PE when there is a triple match in the upper or middle lung zone is only 4%. Therefore this scan can be assigned to a very low probability category. However, the lower zone triple-match defect should remain in the intermediate category. The result of a pulmonary angiogram in this patient, shown in Figure 2.11 D, excludes the presence of PE. This patient had pneumonia, which resolved with antibiotic therapy.

Diagnosis: Triple-matched defect, upper lobe; very low probability for PE.

CASE 2.12

History: Two days following successful resuscitation from cardiac arrest, suspected to be due to PE, this 55-year-old male who had recently undergone hip arthroplasty received a V/Q lung scan (Figs. 2.12 A, B). His concurrent chest radiograph is shown in Figure 2.12 C.

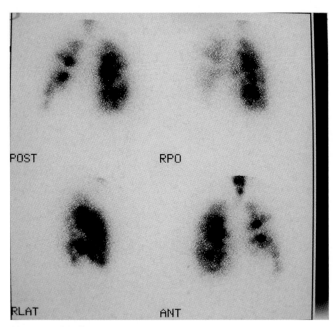

Figure 2.12 A

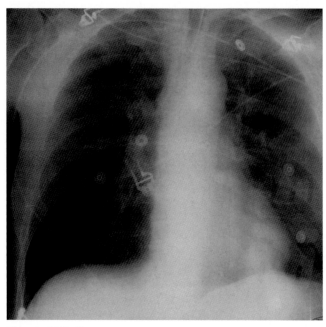

Figure 2.12 C

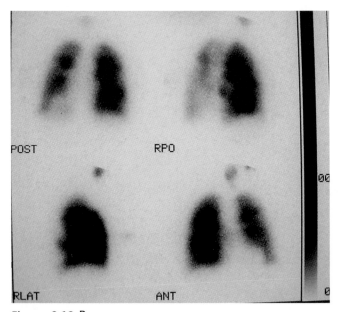

Figure 2.12 B

Findings: The chest radiograph is unremarkable. An ET tube is in place.

The ventilation scan (Fig. 2.12 A) demonstrates generalized inhomogeneity and central airway deposition of radioaerosol consistent with changes of COPD.

The perfusion scan (Fig. 2.12 B) shows inhomogeneity of the perfusion and at least two matched, nonsegmental defects in the right middle and lower lung zones. There are also subsegmental defects, mild in degree, scattered in both lung fields. Overall ventilation appears to be more impaired than perfusion.

Discussion: Small subsegmental mismatched or multiple matched V/Q defect regardless of size in combination with a normal chest radiograph can be classified as being of low probability and in some cases even of very low probability for PE.

The probability of an acute PE in a low-probability scan is as low as 4% when the clinical probability is also low. However, the probability increases to 12% when the pretest probability is indeterminate and to 40% if the pretest probability is high.

This patient, with a history of recent hip arthroplasty and subsequent cardiac arrest suspected to be due to PE, was studied further with bilateral pulmonary angiography (Figs. 2.12 DR, DL) which revealed no evidence of pulmonary emboli.

The low-probability category of V/Q lung scans has been met with some criticism and skepticism as to its value in the management of patients suspected of having PE. It must be remembered that a low-probability interpretation does not exclude the diagnosis of PE but significantly reduces its likelihood. In many clinical settings, the majority of the referrals

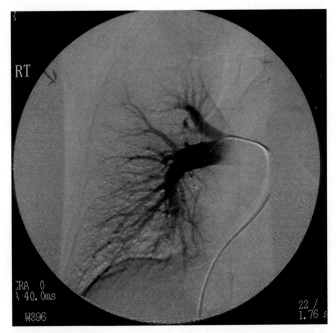

Figure 2.12 DR

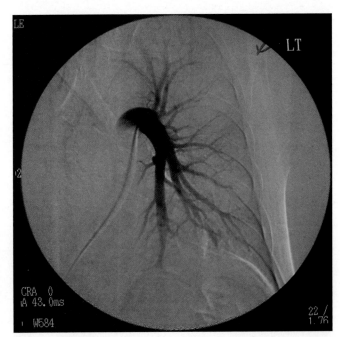

Figure 2.12 DL

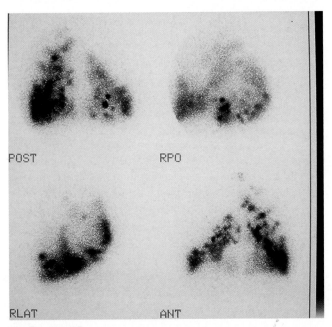

Figure 2.12 E

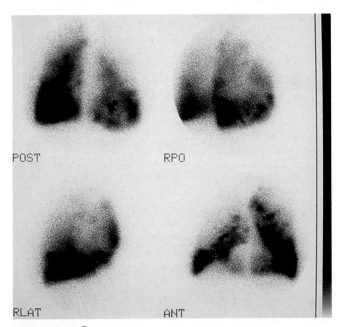

Figure 2.12 F

for lung scan have a relatively low clinical probability for PE. To rule out PE is the clinician's working diagnosis in the hope that a low probability pulmonary perfusion scintigraphy will provide them additional confidence in excluding emboli.

Several studies have shown that in patients with low-probability scans, major morbidity or mortality attributable to PE is quite infrequent. Low-probability and nondiagnostic scans are more frequently caused by the airway and airspace disease.

COPD is a common, frequently debilitating disease with recurrent exacerbation of symptoms mimicking PE. Differentiation of exacerbating COPD from PE can be difficult clinically, since the signs and symptoms of the two conditions overlap.

Patients with COPD invariably show some abnormality in ventilation and perfusion that vary in size and distribution. The defect may be symmetrical, asymmetrical, segmental, or lobar; in some cases the entire lung may be involved.

Figures 2.12 E, F show a V/Q scan of this pattern in a patient who developed an acute onset of shortness of breath, hypoxia, and tachycardia. Note the markedly abnormal pattern of ventilation and perfusion, although perfusion is somewhat less impaired. A chest radiograph (Fig. 2.12 G) shows an overinflated lung and reduction in the number and caliber of peripheral vascular markings, consistent with COPD. However, the lungs are free from infiltrate. Bilateral pulmonary angiograms (Figs. 2.12 HR, HL) are normal.

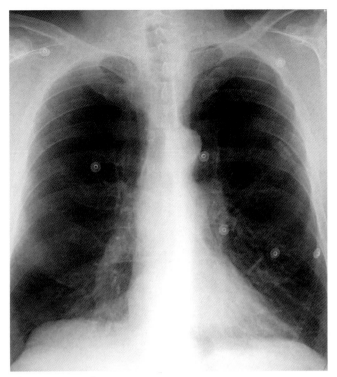

Figure 2.12 G

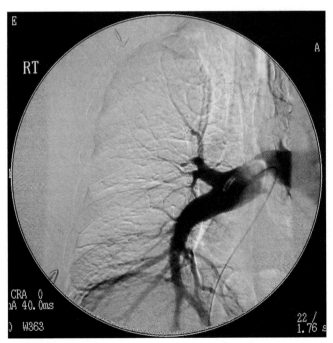

Figure 2.12 HR

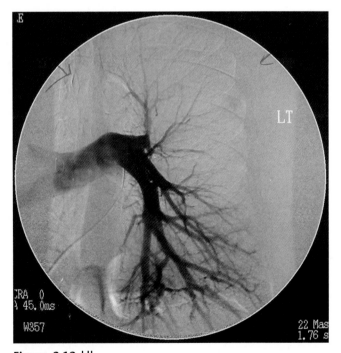

Figure 2.12 HL

A V/Q scan is not often used in the evaluation of COPD. However, the results of the scans in a substantial number of patients with COPD are still conclusive. The scan can provide information contributing to the patient's management.

Demonstration of a regional ventilation abnormality associated with a lesser degree of perfusion defect represents an imbalance in ventilation and perfusion, which may explain worsening of dyspnea in patients with COPD and not necessarily the presence of PE. Therefore a low-probability lung scan in patients with COPD in the proper context not only excludes PE but, with a reasonable degree of certainty, can explain the cause of the patient's worsening dyspnea.

It is to be noted that the prevalence of PE in patients with COPD is comparable to that in those without COPD. However, the frequency of perfusion defects is higher, and these defects are usually larger.

Diagnosis: Low-probability scan; COPD.

CASE 2.13

History: Five days after porcine valve replacement, a 48-year-old man experienced cardiac arrest, requiring mechanical ventilation. An emergency perfusion lung scan (Fig. 2.13 A) was performed and a chest x-ray (Fig. 2.13 B) was taken.

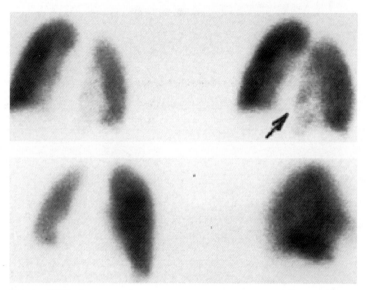

Figure 2.13 A

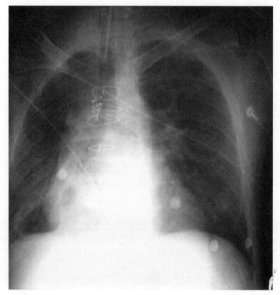

Figure 2.13 B

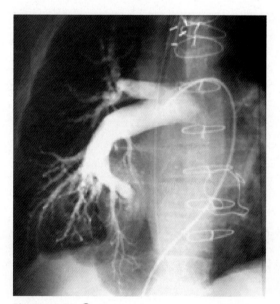

Figure 2.13 C

Findings: The chest x-ray shows proper placement of the endotracheal tube and consolidation of the right lower lobe.

The perfusion lung scan reveals reduced right lung volume with decreased perfusion as compared with the left. In addition, there is a large perfusion defect involving the right lower lobe posteriorly corresponding to the radiographic parenchymal opacity. Closer inspection of the scan, primarily in the right posterior oblique (RPO) view, reveals that there is a rim of activity between the perfusion defect and the adjacent pleural surface known as a stripe sign (arrow in Fig 2.13 A).

Discussion: The stripe sign is a useful adjunct criterion in the interpretation of perfusion lung scans to predict the absence of PE. Proper utilization of this sign not only reduces the number of intermediate-probability categories but commonly allows exclusion of PE, as subsequently confirmed by angiography in this patient (Fig. 2.13 C).

A stripe sign may be seen in many views but is best visualized in the posterior oblique projection. In this particular projection, the pleural surface is seen in tangent without superimposition of surrounding or contralateral lung. A stripe sign related to the involved right middle lobe and lingula is best seen in tangent on anterior oblique projections.

It is important to remember that stripe signs predict the absence of PE only in the specific area of stripe, not in other areas of the lung field. However, exclusion of PE by stripe sign applies to different zones, whether in the upper, middle, or lower lung. The stripe sign is not a frequent finding; it was noted in only 4.7% of the scans in the PIOPED series.

The etiology of the stripe sign is not known. By changing the morphology of the lung, a centrally located emphysema may result in the appearance of a stripe sign, but a ventilation scan would be abnormal in this situation. Also, partial resolution of pleural-based perfusion defects may cause the appearance of a stripe sign. This would be demonstrated on serial lung scans showing changes from perfusion defect to a stripe appearance.

Diagnosis: Partial atelectasis of the right lower lobe.

History: Three days after total hip replacement, a 65-year-old man with multiple preexisting medical problems suddenly developed dyspnea and hypoxia. An emergency V/Q lung scan (Figs. 2.14 A, B) was performed for the evaluation of acute PE.

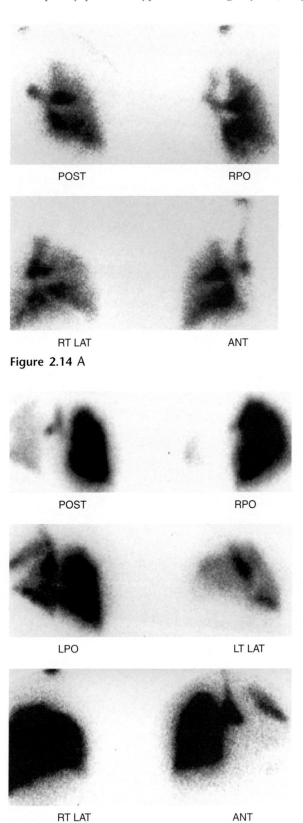

POST   RPO

RT LAT   ANT

Figure 2.14 A

POST   RPO

LPO   LT LAT

RT LAT   ANT

Figure 2.14 B

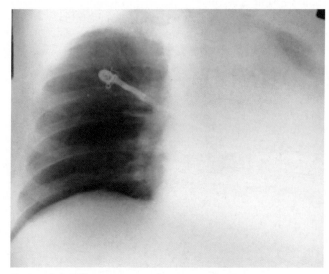

Figure 2.14 C

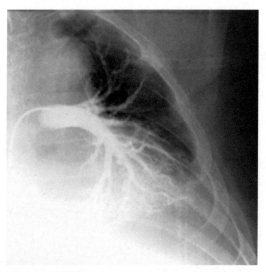

Figure 2.14 D

Findings: There is virtual absence of ventilation to the entire left lung, with matching moderately decreased perfusion.

Discussion: These scintigraphic findings are indicative of early bronchial obstruction and represent only a low probability for PE. A subsequent portable chest radiograph (Fig. 2.14 C) shows complete collapse of the left lower lobe. Despite extraction of mucous plugs by bronchoscopy, his dyspnea and atelectasis persisted. PE was excluded by angiography (Fig. 2.14 D) performed several hours after the V/Q scan.

Mucous plugging of bronchi is one of the more common causes of the reverse mismatched defect in which ventilation is more impaired than perfusion. In an area of obstructed airway, regional hypoxia activates vasoconstrictive reflux, resulting in shunting of blood to the region of better aerated lung, thus leading to diminished perfusion in the obstructed area varying in severity from mild to severe.

Radiographic findings may be subtle and often underestimate the extent of ventilatory compromise. Initially, the chest x-ray findings will lag behind the V/Q scan abnormality. This is due to the time required for air to be absorbed and for obstructed alveoli to collapse.

Further, it must be remembered that the vasoconstrictive reflex–associated regional hypoxia is not an immediate response; therefore reduction of perfusion in a nonventilated region and shunting of blood to a normally oxygenated region is delayed. The effectiveness of this reflex increases with time. In addition, the degree and extent of ventilatory obstruction affect the degree of perfusion defect. Total obstruction produces a more marked perfusion abnormality than partial obstruction. The coexistence of COPD and disease of pulmonary vascular or parenchymal tissue also may play a role in the redistribution of blood toward better oxygenated regions.

From animal studies, it appears unlikely that acute bronchial obstruction would cause any major perfusion abnormality within 2 hours after obstruction. The quantity of redistribution is, at most, 20%.

In the differential diagnosis of reverse mismatched defect, pleural effusion, COPD, pneumonia, and bronchial carcinoma should be considered; however, these can be excluded by history, chest radiograph, and other findings.

Diagnosis: Mucous plug.

CASE 2.15

History: A 62-year-old man admitted with a history of tachypnea, tachycardia, and a PO$_2$ of 40 mm Hg was referred for a V/Q scan to rule out PE (Figs. 2.15 A, B). There were no parenchymal opacities on chest x-ray.

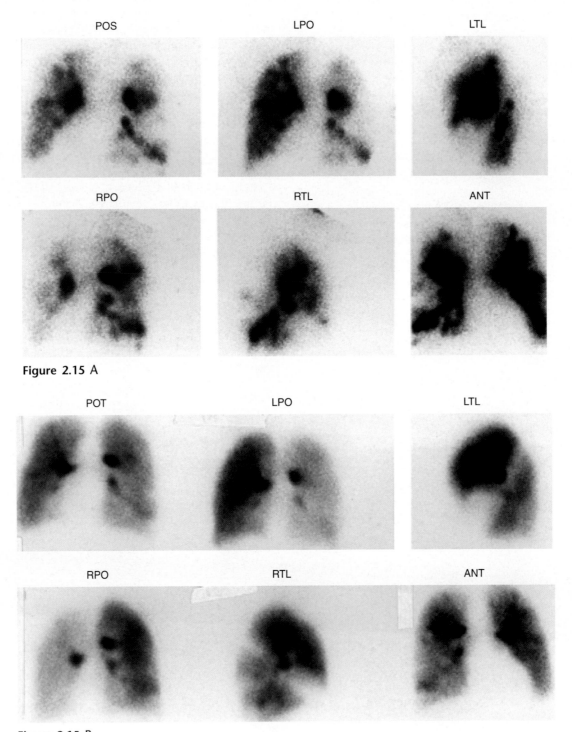

Figure 2.15 A

Figure 2.15 B

Findings: There is heterogeneous ventilation with an area of markedly reduced ventilation in the right lower lobe (Fig. 2.15 A). The distribution of perfusion is more uniform, and perfusion is present in the area of the right lower lobe (Fig. 2.15 B). The pattern of loss of ventilation but preserved perfusion is characterized as a reverse mismatched defect.

Discussion: The pattern of reverse mismatch (perfusion is better than ventilation) is not consistent with PE and can be used to exclude PE. On rare occasions, however, a large PE coexistent with moderately severe COPD may result in a reverse mismatched defect. This occurs when the increased vascular resistance produced by a major PE in the ventilated area shunts blood flow into the nonventilated regions. However, this results in both a reverse mismatched defect and a mismatched defect, leading to the proper diagnosis of PE.

Reverse mismatched defects are related to failure of the vasoconstrictive response to alveolar hypoxia and usually is seen in patients with pulmonary arterial hypertension, pulmonary venous hypertension, respiratory alkalosis, etc. Alveolar hypoxia causes regional vasoconstriction and reduces perfusion to the nonventilated area. Variation in perfusion is related to the degree of airway disease. An incomplete obstruction is more likely to produce near-normal perfusion. Failure of this protective response results in an abnormal V/Q ratio, which is the cause of clinical hypoxemia. In the current case, blood returning from the nonventilated right lower lobe is not saturated with oxygen, thus contributing to the patient's hypoxemia.

Reverse mismatches are usually seen in patients with bronchial obstruction, COPD, pneumonia, collapsed lung, and pleural effusions. Therefore a reverse mismatch is often seen in patients in the intensive care unit, in whom these abnormalities are more common. Most patients in the intensive care unit with reverse mismatched defects have a mucous plug. In intubated patients, the possibility of inserting the oxygen delivery catheter into the lung bronchus (usually the right) exists, which would cause exacerbation of hypoxemia and result in a scan with a reverse mismatched defect. Reverse mismatches may be transitional, but conversion to matched defect could be incomplete.

A reverse mismatched defect is observed in approximately 25% of patients with pulmonary infections. It has been postulated that the local release of inflammatory mediators with vasodilatory properties results in failure of the vasoconstrictive response and causes a reverse mismatched defect. Reverse mismatches may be seen before inflammatory changes become visible on chest x-ray. Reverse mismatch also is seen in unilateral lung transplantation. It is probably due to impairment of the hypoxic vasoconstrictive response in the transplanted lung, so that blood flow in the less ventilated transplanted lung is preserved.

Diagnosis: COPD; no PE.

CASE 2.16

History: A 73-year-old man was admitted with increasing dyspnea and interstitial lung disease of uncertain etiology. After a thorough, essentially negative evaluation, a V/Q scan was performed to evaluate the possibility of recurrent PE (Figs. 2.16 A, B), and a chest x-ray was taken (Fig. 2.16 C).

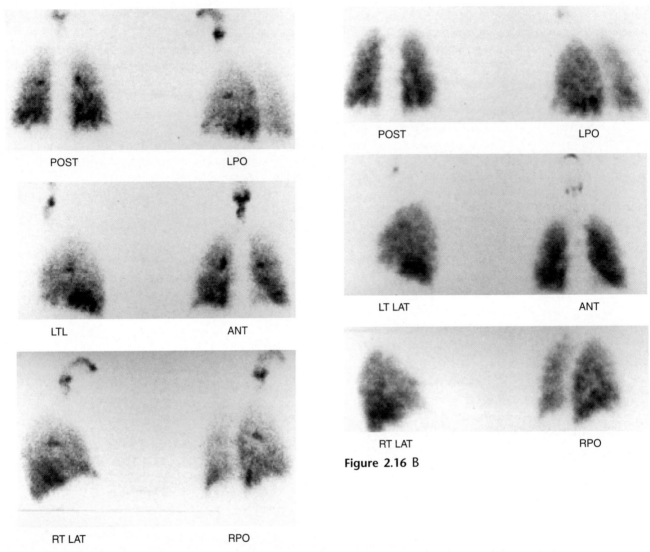

POST LPO

LTL ANT

RT LAT RPO

Figure 2.16 A

POST LPO

LT LAT ANT

RT LAT RPO

Figure 2.16 B

Findings: The chest x-ray shows a prominent interstitial pattern throughout. The ventilation scan is normal; the perfusion scan shows numerous subsegmental defects located peripherally and distributed throughout both lung fields, a pattern termed "contour mapping."

Discussion: The patient died of respiratory failure 7 days after hospitalization. At autopsy, pancreatic adenocarcinoma with extensive small tumor emboli within pulmonary arterioles was noted. There were no gross emboli into major branches of the pulmonary arteries.

PE as the result of occult malignancy should not be confused with tumor emboli. Several malignancies are associated with hypercoagulable states, notably, gastric, pancreatic, colon, breast, ovarian, and prostate carcinoma. Thrombotic disease is

a well-known phenomenon in cancer patients, occurring in approximately 15% of that population.

In patients with a primary malignancy who have clinical signs of major PE associated with a normal or near-normal lung scan, the diagnosis of tumor emboli should be entertained.

Radiologic findings in patients with pulmonary tumor microemboli are minimal. Although the diagnosis may be suspected clinically, it is most often a postmortem diagnosis. The chest radiograph and ventilation scan are usually unremarkable. A contour mapping configuration giving a diffuse mottled appearance to the perfusion scan may be the only positive finding suggestive of pulmonary tumor microembolism. Other causes of the contour mapping pattern include fat, air, or amniotic fluid emboli, collagen vascular disease, congestive

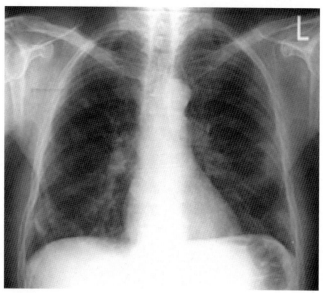

Figure 2.16 C

heart failure, lymphangitic carcinomatosis, and intravenous drug abuse.

A shrunken lung pattern also may represent tumor microemboli. In this pattern, there is an apparent decrease in the size of the lung resulting from lack of visualization of the lung periphery due to embolic obstruction of peripheral vessels.

Pulmonary tumor emboli are not rare. Rates of 2% to 26% have been reported on autopsy in those patients dying of solid tumor. Malignancies of the liver, kidney, and breast are re-sponsible for the majority of larger pulmonary tumor emboli (65%).

A distinction should be made between tumor emboli, metastatic disease to the lung, and lymphangitic spread. Lymphangitic carcinomatosis represents a complication of tumor microemboli and is one of the more common causes of contour mapping configurations.

Diagnosis: Tumor microembolism.

CASE 2.17

History: A 74-year-old man with lung cancer and progressive dyspnea was admitted because of chest pain, hemoptysis, and respiratory distress. A V/Q scan was performed to evaluate the patient for possible PE versus exacerbation of his COPD as the cause of his worsening dyspnea (Figs. 2.17 A, B).

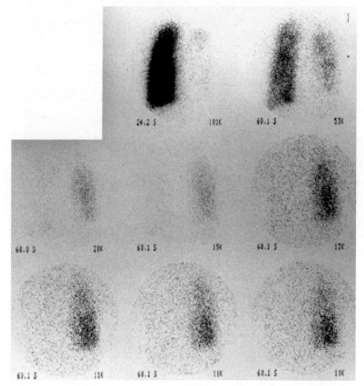

Figure 2.17 A

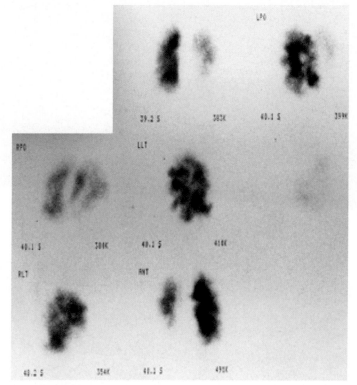

Figure 2.17 B

Findings: The ventilation lung scan using ^{133}Xe shows normal ventilation of the left lung, with reduced ventilation to the right lung. The associated right-lower-lobe retention of ^{133}Xe is consistent with airway trapping.

The perfusion scan shows marked generalized reduced perfusion to the right lung matched with the ventilation abnormality. In addition, multiple subsegmental perfusion mismatched defects are evident on the left.

Discussion: The ventilation abnormality of the right lung is consistent with the patient's right hilar mass causing partial airway obstruction. The mass also is responsible for the perfusion defect of the right lung due to pulmonary artery involvement by invasion, compression, thrombosis, or even regional reflex hypoxia secondary to bronchial compression and poor ventilation.

The multiple subsegmental peripheral perfusion defects on the left without accompanying ventilatory abnormality are suggestive of segmental contour mapping consistent with tumor emboli. Other entities such as primary pulmonary hypertension, intravenous drug abuse, septic emboli from an indwelling venous catheter, fat emboli, or diffuse vasculitis, also may produce this pattern. Clinical assessment and other ancillary findings help to eliminate most of the differential considerations.

Metastatic tumor embolization to the lung is a common manifestation of malignant neoplasm. The most frequent primaries are breast, stomach, prostate, liver, kidney, and choriocarcinoma. Almost all metastatic tumors in the lung develop from tumor emboli to the pulmonary artery. Bronchogenic carcinoma may also be a source of tumor emboli to the lung; adenocarcinoma more frequently embolizes to the lung than does epidermoid.

In as many as 10% of patients with lung cancer, tumor emboli may result in the development of cor pulmonale over a short period of time and will be a significant factor in shortening their life span. The occurrence of severe and unexplained progressive dyspnea in patients with malignancy should raise the question of complicating tumor emboli. The chest x-ray is frequently unremarkable. The characteristic segmental contour mapping pattern seen on perfusion scintigraphy without associated ventilation abnormality is almost diagnostic of this event. Pulmonary angiography usually is negative for evidence of embolism, but it may show tortuosity or pruning of small peripheral vessels.

The pathway for tumor emboli to the lung from bronchogenic carcinoma is via either lymphatic or hematogenous spread. In the lymphatic pathway, the tumor spreads through the lymphatic vessels and thoracic duct to the right heart and hence to the pulmonary arteries. In hematogenous spread, the event starts from an already existing extrapulmonary metastasis, often in the liver or adrenal gland.

The patient died 2 weeks after admission of respiratory failure. Autopsy revealed adenocarcinoma of the right lung with distant metastases, axial node involvement, and tumor emboli to the left lung.

Diagnosis: Pulmonary tumor emboli from bronchogenic carcinoma.

CASE 2.18

History: A 60-year-old man undergoing chemotherapy and radiotherapy for squamous cell carcinoma of the tongue metastatic to the cervical lymph nodes and lung presented to the emergency department with marked shortness of breath. He was intubated and a portable perfusion scan was performed to evaluate for PE as the source of his dyspnea (Fig. 2.18 A). A chest x-ray was also taken (Fig. 2.18 B).

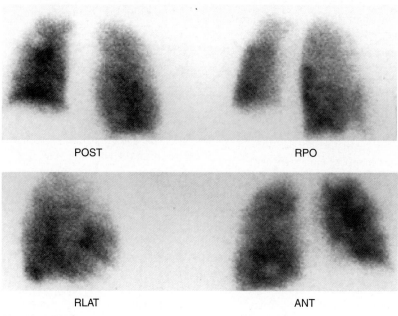

POST   RPO

RLAT   ANT

Figure 2.18 A

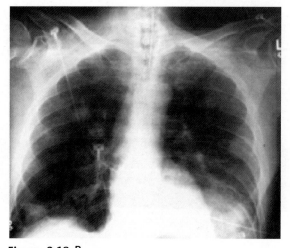

Figure 2.18 B

Findings: The chest radiograph shows multiple nodular densities in both lungs due to pulmonary metastases. The perfusion scan demonstrates multiple spherical perfusion defects in both lungs congruent with the multiple pulmonary metastases seen on chest x-ray. No peripheral wedge-shaped or segmental defects are present

Discussion: The pattern of perfusion defects is not that of PE. They are within the parenchyma, with no segmental pattern or peripheral distribution, and they do not correspond to

the bronchopulmonary boundaries. The perfusion defects are due to metastatic tumors that exist as space-occupying lesions present within the pulmonary parenchyma.

The patient died later the same day; the autopsy revealed a perforated viscus. Eleven separate metastatic masses were identified within the lungs but no PEs were seen.

Pulmonary metastases are perfused via the bronchial artery; therefore they do not accumulate intravenously administered MAA and appear as perfusion defects. Visualization of pulmonary metastases as foci of increased activity on lung scan implies the presence of a pulmonary-to-bronchial artery (or right-to-left) communication.

Metastatic tumor to the lung may result from hematogenous, lymphatic, or intra-alveolar dissemination. At autopsy, at least 20% of patients who die of malignancy have evidence of pulmonary metastasis. There is a high incidence of pulmonary metastasis at the time of diagnosis of certain malignancies, such as renal cell carcinoma, choriocarcinoma, Wilm's tumor, and Ewing's sarcoma. In patients with functioning thyroid carcinoma, multiple pulmonary micrometastases may be detected using ^{131}I scintigraphy. Osteosarcoma metastatic to the lung may be detected on bone scan as an area of increased focal uptake in the lung fields.

Diagnosis: Pulmonary metastases.

CASE 2.19

History: A 37-year-old man presented with a 4-day history of lower extremity swelling and increasing dyspnea on exertion. His chest radiograph (Fig. 2.19 A) is remarkable for borderline cardiomegaly, prominence of the pulmonary artery, and a diffuse reticular nodular pattern. A V/Q scan was performed to evaluate the possibility of chronic PE (Figs. 2.19 B, C).

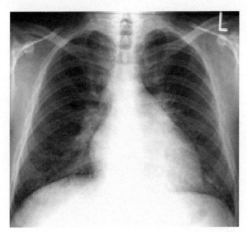

Figure 2.19 A

PERF LUNG

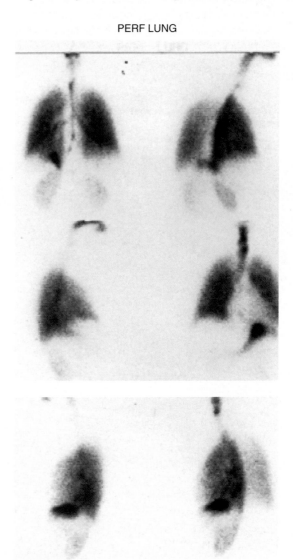

VENT LUNG

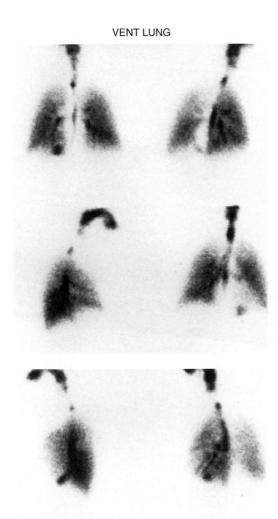

Figure 2.19 C

Figure 2.19 B

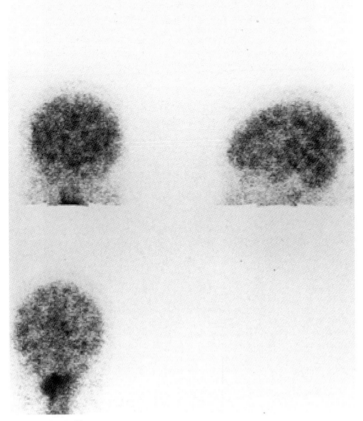

Figure 2.19 D

Findings: The V/Q scan demonstrates a normal pattern of ventilation and perfusion, thus excluding the possibility of PE. Of interest, however, is the presence of radioactivity in the kidneys on the perfusion images. An image of the head (Fig. 2.19 D) reveals intracranial activity.

Discussion: Intravenously administered ^{99m}Tc-MAA normally passes to the right side of the heart and is trapped in the pulmonary bed via the pulmonary artery. Very few particles are small enough to escape pulmonary capillary entrapment. The appearance of radioactivity outside the lung field is a result of right-to-left shunting, commonly intracardiac, but may be extracardiac, as in the case of an intrapulmonary arteriovenous (AV) malformation. In the presence of intracardiac shunting, the MAA particle passes from right-to-left chamber into the systemic arterial circulation and lodges in the capillary bed of the kidneys, brain, and spleen. A right-to-left shunt of more than 10% is readily apparent on the scan by identifying activity in organs with high systemic blood flow, such as the kidneys and brain.

The shunt magnitude can be estimated semiquantitatively by the ratio of systemic (kidney) to pulmonary radioactivity. In this case, the shunt fraction is estimated at 14.78%. However, the shunt may be evaluated more precisely by quantifying the total-body and pulmonary count activity using the following formula:

$$\text{Percent R-L shunt} = \frac{\text{total body count} - \text{total pulmonary count}}{\text{total body count}} \times 100$$

This requires scanning of the patient's whole body 2 minutes after the injection of ^{99m}Tc-MAA and acquiring images in the posterior projection for 15 minutes.

The diagnosis of an extracardiac shunt such as a pulmonary AV malformation may be suggested in patients with no intracardiac shunt but significant radioactivity in the kidney. The AV malformation appears as a lobulated parenchymal mass on x-ray.

The diagnosis of AV malformation requires pulmonary angiography in order to identify a dilated feeding artery and a dilated draining vein. This patient's angiogram did not reveal an AV malformation but did demonstrate small, peripheral, punctuated, opacified vessels suggestive of pulmonary telangiectasia (Fig. 2.19 E). Hereditary hemorrhagic telangiectasia of Osler-Weber-Rendu disease may occur with (30% to 50%) or without associated AV malformation. These patients also exhibit cutaneous and mucosal telangiectasia. They have other congenital anomalies, such as tetralogy of Fallot, Eisenmenger's complex, and tricuspid and pulmonary valve stenosis.

Pulmonary telangiectasia may be acquired, such as that seen in patients with advanced cirrhosis. Telangiectasia in these patients is due to a microscopic arteriovenous malformation and is secondary to hepatopulmonary syndrome. The shunting in these patients is reversible, which suggests that the shunt is functional rather than anatomic. The mechanism of development of pulmonary telangiectasia in cirrhosis and its reversibility is not known. Changes in the circulating vasoactive substances may play a pivotal role.

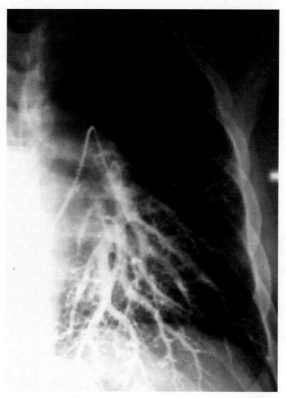

Figure 2.19 E

The patient's clinical status deteriorated gradually and he died 3 months later as a result of respiratory failure and subsequent cardiac arrest. At autopsy, numerous intrapulmonary aggregates of small vessels measuring less than 1 mm to approximately 3 mm in size were noted. Telangiectasias of the small and large bowel were also present, but the brain appeared normal.

In the evaluation of extrapulmonary activity and shunt estimation in patients with right-to-left shunt, attention should be given to the quality of the injected MAA radiopharmaceutical. A 99.6% radiochemical purity of the administered dose is required. A faulty radiopharmaceutical, such as unbound ^{99m}Tc-pertechnetate and small particles, would result in visualization of the kidneys. Unbound technetium impurity can be excluded by the lack of gastric and intense thyroidal uptake; however, some accumulation may be present owing to a normal, relatively high level of systemic blood flow to this organ. Smaller particles, less than an average of 30 μm, pass through the pulmonary arterial capillary bed and localize in the kidney. Both of these impurities would falsely elevate the calculated shunt fractions.

Diagnosis: Pulmonary telangiectasia of Osler-Weber-Rendu disease with right-to-left shunt.

CASE 2.20

History: A 66-year-old male with a right-upper-lobe lung mass and a marginal pulmonary function test was referred to establish operability and predict his postoperative lung function. A perfusion lung scan and fractionated analysis was performed (Fig. 2.20). His forced expiratory volume at 1 second (FEV$_1$) is 1.65 L.

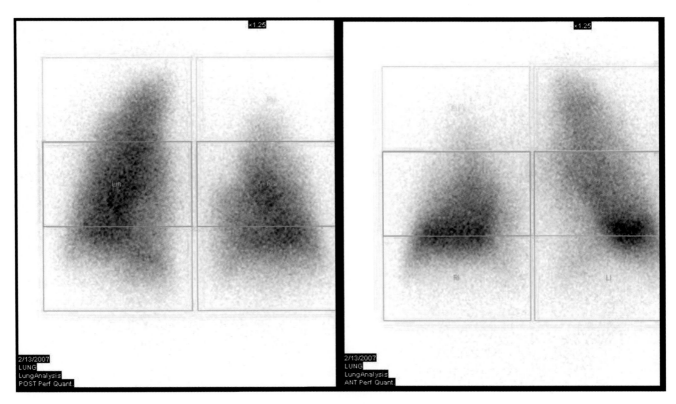

	Posterior Kct				Geometric Mean Kct				Anterior Kct			
	Left		Right		Left Lung		Right Lung		Right		Left	
	%	Kct	%	Kct	%	Kct	%	Kct	%	Kct	%	Kct
Upper Zone:	12.0	58.21	3.2	15.56	12.6	60.88	3.8	18.17	4.4	21.22	13.3	63.66
Middle Zone:	30.3	147.57	21.7	105.72	29.7	142.89	23.9	115.15	26.2	125.42	28.9	138.36
Lower Zone:	16.0	77.68	16.9	82.19	14.1	68.11	15.8	76.25	14.8	70.74	12.5	59.72
Total Lung:	58.2	283.46	41.8	203.47	56.5	271.88	43.5	209.57	45.4	217.38	54.6	261.74

Figure 2.20

Findings: The planar anterior and posterior projections of the perfusion scan show an area of markedly reduced perfusion of the right upper lobe that corresponds to a known lung mass. Fractionated analysis shows 56.5% of the total perfusion to the left lung and 43.5% to the right lung. Segmental perfusion of the right lung is 3.8% to the right upper zone and 39.7% for the remaining right middle and right lower zone.

Discussion: Perfusion lung images by themselves are of limited help in determining the resectability of a tumor; however, fractionated analysis of perfusion is quite reliable in predicting the postoperative loss of pulmonary function.

A pneumonectomy is usually considered feasible if the patient's FEV$_1$ is greater than 2 L, and 1.5 L for lobectomy. However, a minimum value of 0.8 to 1 L FEV$_1$ is required postoperatively to carry out a functional life.

A split perfusion scan with quantitative analysis allows for the calculation of the postoperative FEV$_1$ and predicts the risk of developing chronic ventilatory insufficiency postpneumonectomy.

An anterior and posterior projection of the lung is preferably obtained on a dual-head camera simultaneously following the IV injection of 4 to 5 mCi of ^{99m}Tc-MAA. Three equal-sized regions of interest are marked on each lung. Relative perfusion of the upper, middle, and lower zones of each lung is determined by obtaining geometric mean from the anterior and posterior projections. The patient's postoperative FEV_1 can be estimated as follows:

$$\text{Postop } FEV_1 = \text{preop } FEV_1 \,(1 - \text{percent of the functional contribution of perfusion of the lung to be removed})$$

In this case, removal of the entire right lung would leave the patient with a postoperative FEV_1 of 1.65 (1 – 43.6/100) = 0.93 L.

However, as the result of a right-upper-lobe lobectomy, this patient would lose only 3.8% of his total lung function, and his postoperative FEV_1 would be 1.65 (1 – 3.8/100) = 1.58 L, suggesting that his risk of developing chronic ventilatory insufficiency following lobectomy would be very low.

Although the quantitative split lung function may underestimate the postoperatively measured FEV_1, it is still the simplest and the most reliable method of evaluating a patient scheduled for a pneumonectomy preoperatively and appears to be a good marker of surgical feasibility in patients with lung cancer and ventilatory obstruction.

Fractionated analysis of the perfusion lung scan is also of value in the management of patients with emphysematous bullae. Surgical resection of emphysematous bullae has been shown to improve the patient's overall respiratory status provided that the perfusion images demonstrate a normal pattern in the lung zone adjacent to the bullae. The results of quantitative analysis of the perfusion scan in conjunction with those of spirometry can predict postoperative ventilatory dependency.

Diagnosis: Bronchogenic carcinoma; surgical candidate. Posturgical respiratory insufficiency is unlikely.

History: A 36-year-old woman with easy fatigability, low-grade fever, arthralgia, and night sweats was noted on her chest roentgenogram to have hilar node enlargement (Fig. 2.21 A). A tuberculin skin test was negative. A ^{67}Ga scan was performed to evaluate for possible sarcoidosis (Figs. 2.21 B, C).

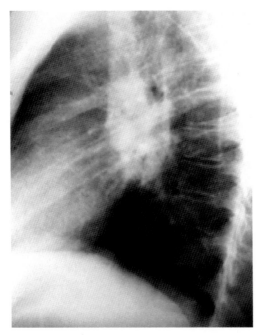

Figure 2.21 A

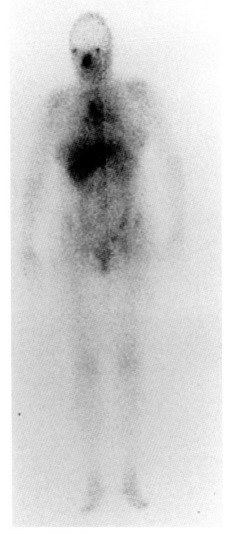

Figure 2.21 B

Findings: There is uptake of gallium in the hilar region corresponding to the x-ray findings. Selected images of the thorax suggest that uptake is present in the right paratracheal as well as right and left hilar regions (Fig. 2.21 C). In addition, there is intense focal uptake in the lacrimal glands bilaterally.

Discussion: Uptake of ^{67}Ga in hilar and mediastinal nodes without pulmonary uptake suggests a lymphoproliferative disorder, most notably Hodgkin's or non-Hodgkin's lymphoma. Of the nonneoplastic disorders that should be considered, chronic granulomatous diseases are more likely than other infectious entities to present similarly.

Owing to its nonspecificity, the value of gallium imaging in the differential diagnosis of an inflammatory process from a neoplastic process is limited; however, the symmetrical pattern of hilar uptake is suggestive of sarcoidosis.

The recognition of a distinct pattern of ^{67}Ga uptake in sarcoidosis has been reported. It is only in this condition that right paratracheal uptake accompanied by symmetrical, bilateral, para- and infrahilar uptake (λ) is seen. This diagnosis is further strengthened by the lacrimal gland uptake. The reported prevalence of salivary and/or lacrimal gland involvement in systemic sarcoidosis varies, but when there is uptake of gallium, sarcoidosis is considered likely. Localization of ^{67}Ga in the salivary and lacrimal glands may also occur in Sjögren's syndrome and tuberculosis as well as after radiation therapy.

Sarcoidosis is a chronic, multisystemic granulomatous disease of uncertain etiology that frequently involves the thorax. Ninety percent of patients show radiographic evidence of thoracic involvement consisting of bilateral symmetrical hilar adenopathy with or without parenchymal disease. There is

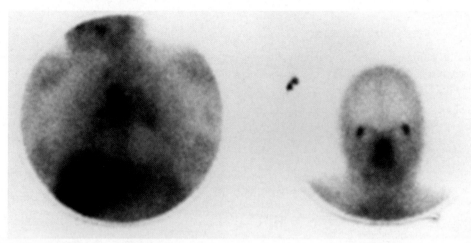

Figure 2.21 C

usually enlargement of the right paratracheal node in a configuration known as a 1–2–3 pattern (Garland's triad). Despite this, the chest radiograph has limitations in detecting sarcoidosis, and radiographic changes do not necessarily represent the sequential progress or activity of the disease. As the x-ray findings change from hilar adenopathy to parenchymal infiltration and fibrosis, the gallium uptake also changes from a hilar to a parenchymal pattern; eventually no uptake is seen in the stage of fibrosis.

Since the clinical and radiologic finding of sarcoidosis is not adequate to differentiate active inflammatory lesion of sarcoid from fibrosis, a gallium scan traditionally has been used to evaluate the activity of the disease. However, the availability of PET and ability of ^{18}F-FDG to accumulate in activated inflammatory cells allows the use of PET for visualization of sarcoid tissue and makes it a promising modality for the management of patients with sarcoidosis. Although clinical studies have shown no significant difference in the detection of the pulmonary sarcoidosis between ^{67}Ga and ^{18}F-FDG, the latter appears to be more sensitive for the evaluation of extrapulmonary involvement (e.g., muscles, spleen, skin, and lymph nodes of the cervical, supraclavicular, axillary, para-aortic, and inguinal regions).

^{111}In pentreotide (Octreoscan) may also be used as an alternative to ^{67}Ga scintigraphy for the evaluation of organ involvement with sarcoid, particularly in patients who have been treated with steroids. Somastatin receptors are known to be present in epitheloid and giant cells of the sarcoid tissue, which accounts for the Octreoscan finding.

Extrapulmonary sarcoid may be seen infrequently in the myocardium. These patients are usually asymptomatic, but they may present with conduction abnormalities such as right-bundle-branch block and AV block. ^{201}Tl scintigraphy of the myocardium may reveal a perfusion defect not related to coronary artery disease, which is secondary to myocardial infiltration by sarcoid. This perfusion defect may concentrate ^{67}Ga, indicative of active disease. The result of the gallium scan would be useful to predict the effect of steroid therapy.

Diagnosis: Pulmonary sarcoidosis.

CASE 2.22

History: A 47-year-old man positive for HIV was admitted with fever and dyspnea. A chest radiograph (Fig. 2.22 A) and ^{67}Ga scan (Fig. 2.22 B) were obtained.

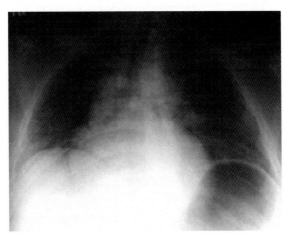

Figure 2.22 A

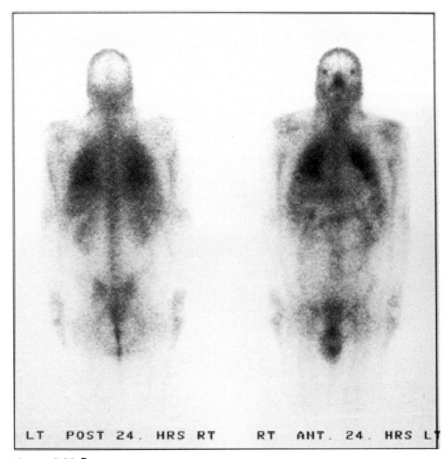

Figure 2.22 B

Findings: The chest x-ray reveals a low lung volume bilaterally, with opacification of the bases most likely secondary to atelectasis. The gallium scan reveals diffuse pulmonary accumulation of gallium.

Discussion: Diffuse gallium uptake with an intensity higher than that of the liver and with clear delineation of the pho-

topenic cardiac silhouette represents an abnormal scan of grade 4 severity. Although there are numerous etiologies of diffuse pulmonary uptake, an acute opportunistic infection must be considered in immunocompromised individuals, including those with AIDS or organ transplants or those receiving chemotherapy.

Pneumonitis due to *Pneumocystis carinii*, typical or atypical mycobacteria, *Cytomegalovirus*, *Actinomyces*, *Cryptococcus*, *Aspergillus*, *Blastomyces*, and filaria, as well as the more typical bacteria, are all known to be associated with diffuse pulmonary uptake of gallium.

In patients with AIDS-related pulmonary disorders, the scan findings precede radiographic changes by days or weeks, which allows earlier diagnosis and implementation of specific treatment for improved prognosis.

There are four distinct patterns in ^{67}Ga scanning of the thorax in patients with AIDS:

1. *Diffuse pulmonary parenchymal uptake.* The pattern of diffuse intense lung uptake in patients with AIDS is most likely related to *P. carinii* pneumonia (PCP), a disease that occurs in more than 80% of patients with AIDS. The sensitivity of this procedure exceeds 90%. The specificity for PCP is particularly high when the chest x-ray is normal. The negative predictive value of the scan for PCP is reported to be 96%. In fact, a negative ^{67}Ga scan, despite clinically progressive respiratory symptoms, carries a grave prognosis. Low-grade diffuse uptake may be due to cytomegalovirus infection or lymphoid interstitial pneumonia, in which case the former may be associated with bilateral eye uptake (retinitis) and the latter with parotid uptake.

2. *Lymphatic node uptake.* Adenopathy may be a manifestation of AIDS and may be infectious, neoplastic, or reactive. Adenopathy may occur anywhere in the body, but it is most often seen in the hilar and mediastinal or para-aortic regions. Nodal uptake of gallium is a common finding in AIDS; however, the differentiation of infectious, neoplastic, or reactive etiologies by gallium is not possible. In reactive adenopathy, however, uptake may be seen in multiple nodal groups, including cervical, inguinal, and axillary as well as mediastinal.

Thoracic nodal uptake of gallium may be due to *Mycobacterium avium-intracellulare* (MAI) or tuberculosis. MAI is a common infection in AIDS, which is associated with mediastinal nodal uptake of gallium and may be accompanied by patchy lung uptake as well. This pattern usually indicates a less treatable process. Whereas MAI is more common than tuberculosis (TB) in homosexual individuals with AIDS, TB is more common than MAI in drug abusers. TB is more frequently accompanied by parenchymal pulmonary uptake. In addition to TB and MAI, coccidioidomycosis, toxoplasmosis, herpes lymphadenitis, and neoplastic entities such as lymphoma (Hodgkin's, non-Hodgkin's, and Burkitt's) and angioimmunoblastic lymphadenopathy should also be considered. Bulky thoracic adenopathy is typical of lymphoma.

3. *Focal pulmonary uptake.* This pattern of gallium uptake is usually due to bacterial pneumonia, usually streptococcal or *Haemophilus* influenza. Fungal infections and actinomycosis also may produce a similar pattern. These entities usually are accompanied by a corresponding radiographic abnormality.

4. *Normal pattern.* Although a negative gallium scan and a negative chest radiograph are strong evidence against an infectious process, a negative gallium scan and an abnormal chest radiograph implies that Kaposi's sarcoma is the most likely cause of the patient's deteriorated respiratory status. Imaging with ^{201}Tl or ^{99m}Tc-sestamibi will usually demonstrate activity at sites of involvement with Kaposi's sarcoma, as reported to occur in patients with AIDS.

Diagnosis: *P. carinii* pneumonia.

CASE 2.23

History: A 36-year-old male who was diagnosed with non-Hodgkin's lymphoma received a ^{67}Ga scan (Fig. 2.23 A) for the initial evaluation and staging.

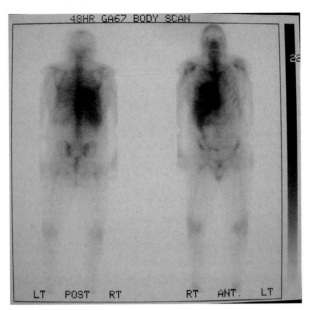

Figure 2.23 A

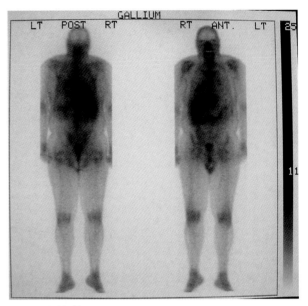

Figure 2.23 B

Findings: This patient's whole-body ^{67}Ga scintigram is remarkable for a large area of intensely increased uptake in the right hilar and midlung region. There is absence of splenic activity (status postsplenectomy). Physiologic activity is seen in the liver, GI tract, and genitalia.

Discussion: Focal accumulation of ^{67}Ga in the thorax can be due to malignancy, infectious or inflammatory process.

Bronchogenic carcinoma and lymphoma are the two malignancies that commonly demonstrate an intense uptake of ^{67}Ga. The other causes of increased ^{67}Ga uptake, which may be focal or diffuse, include inflammatory pneumonitis, drug-induced pneumonitis, radiation pneumonitis, sarcoid, and pneumoconiosis. Pneumonia and pulmonary abscess also take up ^{67}Ga. All of these entities are usually diagnosed by laboratory and other diagnostic imaging procedures.

The use of ^{67}Ga for the diagnosis and staging of lymphoma has decreased significantly, as CT and ^{18}F-FDG PET provide the necessary diagnostic information. The major indication for a ^{67}Ga scan in the initial evaluation of lymphoma is to determine the avidity or nonavidity of the tumor for gallium. Some lymphomas do not take up the gallium. If a scintigram shows a gallium-avid tumor, the scan can be used successfully to monitor the response to therapy and to detect relapse and/or disease progression. The result of ^{67}Ga scanning in monitoring posttreatment lymphoma is quite good and can be successfully used in clinical decision making.

Figure 2.23 B shows a follow-up scan of the patient 8 weeks after a course of chemotherapy. It shows a marked interval reduction in the size and intensity of uptake, indicating a favorable response to therapy. Hence there is no need to change the therapeutic regimen.

The other indication for ^{67}Ga scintigraphy in patients with lymphoma treated with chemotherapy and radiotherapy is to differentiate the viable tumor from fibrotic and necrotic tissue. More than 60% of treated patients will have a mass density on CT that could be an active tumor or a fibrotic mass. There is no relationship between the size of the mass and viability. ^{67}Ga, like ^{18}F-FDG, is taken up by viable cells but not by necrotic masses. Although PET scanning has largely replaced gallium, it may not be available. In such instances, gallium is an effective alternative which can differentiate active tumors from the necrotic and fibrotic radiated masses.

In the interpretation of ^{67}Ga scan, one should note that ^{67}Ga, like ^{18}F-FDG, suffers from a lack of specificity. These agents cannot differentiate one type of tumor from another. In addition, both agents may accumulate in the other nonmalignant entities, as described above.

Interpretation of a ^{67}Ga scan, like one obtained with ^{18}F-FDG, requires a thorough knowledge of its biodistribution. After the IV injection, the gallium binds to the transferrin and distributes similarly to iron bound to transferrin. Physiologic uptake can be seen within 24 to 72 hours in the lacrimal gland, salivary gland, breast tissue, liver, spleen, bone marrow, bowel, kidney, and genitalia. Uptake of ^{67}Ga in hyperplasia of the thymus, which may occur after chemotherapy, should not be considered abnormal.

The usual dose of ^{67}Ga is 5 mCi, but the quality of the scan can be improved by using a higher dose, of 10 mCi, and obtaining additional SPECT images.

Diagnosis: Thoracic lymphoma responding to therapy.

SOURCES AND SUGGESTED READING

1. Kline JA, Jones KL. New diagnostic tests for pulmonary embolism. *Ann Emerg Med* 2000;35:168–180.
2. Mineo TC, Orazio S, Schillaci O, et al. Usefulness of lung perfusion scintigraphy before lung cancer resection in patients with ventilatory obstruction. *Ann Thorac Surg* 2006;82(5):1828–1834.
3. Hunsaker AR, Ingenito EP, Reilly JJ, et al. Lung volume reduction surgery for emphysema: correlation of CT and V/Q imaging with physiologic mechanisms of improvement in lung function. *Radiology* 2002;222: 491–498.
4. Schuster DM, Alazraki N. Gallium and other agents in disease of the lung. *Semin Nucl Med* 2002;32:193–211.
5. Kumar AM, Parker AJ. Ventilation/perfusion scintigraphy. *Emerg Med Clin North Am* 2001;19:957–973.
6. Hatabu H, Uematsu H, Nguyen B, et al. CT and MR in pulmonary embolism: a changing role for nuclear medicine in diagnostic strategy. *Semin Nucl Med* 2002;32:183–192.
7. Stein PD, Gottschalk A. Review of criteria appropriate for a very low probability of pulmonary embolism on ventilation-perfusion lung scans. *Radiographics* 2000;20:99–105.
8. Gottschalk A, Stein PD, Goodman LR, et al. Overview of prospective investigation of pulmonary embolism diagnosis II. *Semin Nucl Med* 2002;32:173–182.
9. Freeman LM, Krynyckyi B, Zuckier LS. Enhanced lung scan diagnosis of pulmonary embolism with the use of ancillary scintigraphic findings and clinical correlation. *Semin Nucl Med* 2001;31:143–157.
10. Stein PD, Woodard PK, et al. Diagnostic pathways in acute pulmonary embolism: recommendations of the PIOPED II Investigators. *Radiology* 2007;242:15–21.
11. Hayashino Y, Goto M, Noguchi Y, et al. Ventilation-perfusion scanning and helical CT in suspected pulmonary embolism: meta-analysis of diagnostic performance. *Radiology* 2005;234:740–748.

CHAPTER THREE

CARDIOVASCULAR IMAGING

João V. Vitola
and Dominique Delbeke

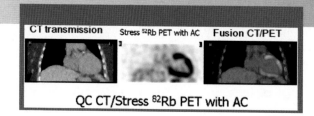

QC CT/Stress ^{82}Rb PET with AC

INTRODUCTION

Evaluation of suspected or known heart disease remains one of the most important applications of nuclear cardiology. This chapter reviews the main basic and clinical concepts involving nuclear cardiology and application of techniques to diagnose heart disease and stratify cardiac risk. In the last decades, technological developments have provided many innovative diagnostic tools for the improved identification and measurement of disease, not only in nuclear medicine but also in cardiac imaging in general. Despite all of these advances, the evaluation of coronary artery disease (CAD) involves a great deal of individual clinical judgment. Before proceeding with any diagnostic test, it is essential to obtain a thorough medical history and to perform a complete physical examination, formulate a diagnostic hypothesis, determine the pretest probability of disease, and define the best strategy of investigation for each patient. Nuclear cardiac studies and other complementary modalities are extremely helpful when well indicated and are invaluable diagnostic tools for evaluating the cardiac patient in current medical practice.

Although the delivery of optimal patient care is the ultimate goal, cost-efficient utilization of limited resources is a growing concern. The goal of avoiding unnecessary use of expensive invasive procedures has focused more attention on the use of noninvasive or less invasive diagnostic and therapeutic modalities, including nuclear imaging. Ultimately, it is the treating physician's responsibility to rationalize the utilization of resources for optimal patient care at reasonable cost.

ATHEROSCLEROSIS AND IMPAIRED CORONARY BLOOD FLOW RESERVE (CBFR)—THE BASIS OF NUCLEAR CARDIOLOGY

Human atherosclerosis is a dynamic process that begins early and progresses throughout life. Risk factors, smoking, hypertension (HTN), hypercholesterolemia, diabetes mellitus (DM), or a positive family history of coronary artery disease (CAD) are well known to accelerate the atherosclerotic process, which naturally affect all human beings (1). Atherosclerotic lesions may or may not affect myocardial blood flow (MBF) to a certain region of the heart, depending basically on the degree of impairment of the dilatory capacity of the coronary arteries and, importantly, the quantity and quality of collateral vessels. In terms of myocardial area at risk, these two factors are more important than the degree of vessel obstruction alone. In this context a moderately obstructive lesion of 50%, involving importantly the vessel wall, to the point of impairing its ability to dilate in response to exercise, may cause more myocardial ischemia than a 90% obstruction with a rich collateral circulation.

With progression, atherosclerotic lesions may impair coronary blood flow reserve (CBFR), initially affecting MBF during stress/exercise and at a later stage at rest. The stress tests most commonly used for evaluation of CBFR include the treadmill test (TMT) alone and rest/stress myocardial perfusion scintigraphy (MPS) using various methods for stress testing, including exercise, dipyridamole, adenosine, or dobutamine. Alternative protocols include low-level physical exercise combined with dipyridamole or adenosine.

TMT FOR EVALUATION OF CAD

A multitude of parameters have been studied and validated over the last four decades. TMT is still useful and several parameters can be measured, including total exercise time, magnitude of increase in blood pressure (BP), indicative of good cardiac function; heart rate (HR), indicative of good perfusion of the conduction system; the magnitude of ST-segment shifts; the presence of chest pain on exertion; and the cardiac rhythm abnormalities during exercise. Prognostic data can be obtained from the TMT using the Duke Treadmill Score (DTS), which can be calculated as follows for the standard Bruce protocol (2):

$$DTS = \text{exercise time} - (5 \times \text{ST deviation}) - (4 \times \text{angina index})$$

Angina index can be classified as: no angina = 0, nonlimiting angina = 1, limiting angina = 2.

The scores typically range from –25 to +15. These values classify patients in the following categories: low risk, $\geq +5$; moderate risk, –10 to +4; and high risk, ≤ -11.

In addition, the prognostic information obtained from a TMT is very important. Failure to achieve 85% of the maximum age-predicted heart rate (MPHR) and a low chronotropic response is predictive of adverse cardiovascular events (3). The average sensitivity and specificity of TMT for the diagnosis of CAD is 67% and 72% respectively, according to two meta-analyses (4,5). In addition to low sensitivity and low specificity, the TMT has additional limitations. The exercise electrocardiogram (ECG) is not interpretable in patients with left-bundle-branch block (LBBB) and pacemakers, which are usually referred to MPS for pharmacologic stress. Furthermore, some baseline ECG abnormalities will make any additional changes during exercise poorly specific (high number of false positives). This includes the changes that may occur in left ventricular hypertrophy (LVH), the effect of digitalis, the presence of preexcitation syndrome (Wolf-Parkinson-White syndrome), or prior myocardial infarction (MI). Furthermore, the sensitivity of TMT is decreased, especially when related to a limited capacity to achieve an adequate increment of myocardial oxygen consumption due either to limited exercise capacity or because of concurrent treatment with some medications such as calcium channel blockers and beta blockers.

TMT is less accurate in women than in men owing to a higher number of false-positive exercise ECG results (6). A meta-analysis determined the weighted average sensitivities and specificities of exercise ECG, exercise ^{201}Tl, and exercise echocardiography in women (7) and demonstrated that the use of cardiac imaging increases overall accuracy. The lower specificities may be due to a digoxin-like effect of circulating estrogens, resulting in varying changes in the ST segment and

TABLE 3.1 Contraindications for various types of stress

Contraindications to all types of stress[d]:
1. High-risk unstable angina[a]
2. Acute myocardial infarction (within 2 days)
3. Uncontrolled symptomatic heart failure
4. Uncontrolled arrhythmias causing symptoms or hemodynamic compromise
5. Unwillingness or inability to give informed consent (legislation-dependent)

Contraindications to exercise[d]:
Absolute
1. Symptomatic severe aortic stenosis
2. Acute pulmonary embolism or pulmonary infarction
3. Acute myocarditis or pericarditis
4. Acute aortic dissection

Relative[b]
1. Left main coronary stenosis
2. Moderate stenotic valvular heart disease
3. Electrolyte abnormalities
4. Severe arterial hypertension[c]
5. Tachyarrhythmias or bradyarrhythmias
6. Hypertrophic cardiomyopathy and other forms of outflow tract obstruction
7. Mental or physical impairment leading to inability to exercise adequately
8. High-degree atrioventricular block

Contraindications to dipyridamole and adenosine:
1. Second- or third-degree AV block or sick sinus syndrome
2. Bronchospastic disease manifested by active wheezing/rhonchi, steroid dependency for asthma/COPD, severely depressed FEV_1 (<40% predicted), a history of respiratory failure requiring hospitalization
3. Hypotension (systolic BP <90 mm Hg)
4. Ongoing transient ischemic attack (TIA) or recent cerebrovascular accident (<6 months)
5. Caffeine intake within the previous 12 hours
6. Theophylline intake within the previous 48 hours

Contraindications to dobutamine:
1. Cardiac arrhythmias, including atrial fibrillation and ventricular tachycardia
2. Severe aortic stenosis or hypertrophic obstructive cardiomyopathy
3. Hypotension (SBP <90 mm Hg) or uncontrolled hypertension (SBP >200 mm Hg)
4. AAA greater than 5 cm is a relative contraindication
5. Presence of LV thrombus is a relative contraindication
6. Presence of an implanted ventricular defibrillator
7. LVEF <25% is a relative contraindication due to increased risk of ventricular arrhythmia

From Vitola and Delbeke (11), by permission from Springer- Verlag.

[a]ACC/AHA Guidelines for the management of patients with unstable angina/non-ST-segment elevation myocardial infarction. From Anderson et al. (10).

[b]Relative contraindications can be superseded if the benefits of exercise outweigh the risks.

[c]In the absence of definitive evidence, the committee suggests systolic blood pressure of >200 mm Hg and/or diastolic blood pressure >100 mm Hg. Modified from Fletcher et al. (12).

[d]Adapted from Gibbons RJ. ACC/AHA 2002 Guideline Update for Exercise Testing. www.acc.org. (9)

leading to a higher false-positive rate of exercise ECG stress testing in women (8).

In summary, the TMT is a good proven modality for diagnosis and determination of prognosis in patients suspected to have CAD, but a wide variety of limitations restricts its utility, requiring the use of alternative or complementary modalities in many patients.

Guidelines for exercise testing are available from the American College of Cardiology (ACC)/American Heart Association (AHA) (9) and contraindications for exercise testing are summarized in Table 3.1 (9,10).

UTILIZATION OF NUCLEAR CARDIOLOGY PROCEDURES

Nuclear cardiology procedures allow evaluation of myocardial perfusion, viability, and function using single photon emission

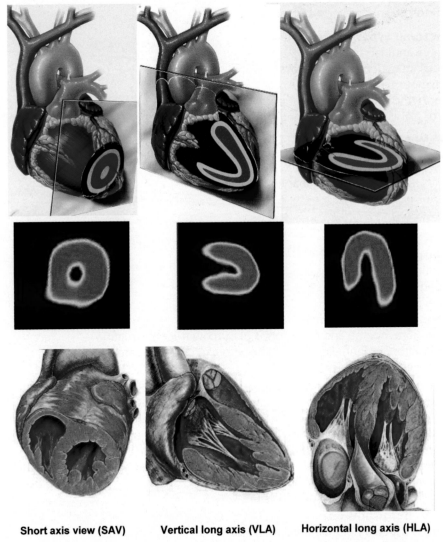

Short axis view (SAV)   **Vertical long axis (VLA)**   **Horizontal long axis (HLA)**

Figure 3.A Schematic representation of tomographic sections through the heart along the short axis, vertical long axis, and horizontal long axis. [From Vitola and Delbeke (11), by permission from Springer-Verlag.]

computed tomography (SPECT) (see Fig. 3.A), gated SPECT, positron emission tomography (PET), and radionuclide ventriculography (RVG). These techniques continue to evolve. The indications for cardiac radionuclide imaging have been extensively reviewed and discussed in the ACC/AHA "Guidelines for the Clinical Use of Radionuclide Imaging" (13) and the American College of Cardiology Foundation/American Society of Nuclear Cardiology (ACCF/ASNC) appropriateness criteria for SPECT MPI (14).

MPS makes it possible to evaluate the CBFR, detect ischemia, and provide risk stratification, including the degree, location, and extent to which CAD is affecting MBF. Since its beginning in 1973 the prognostic and diagnostic value of MPS has been well established in the literature (15).

Many technological developments occurred since then, with progressively improved software and hardware for better performance and interpretation of gated SPECT studies. Excellent reviews discussing the performance of commonly used commercial software packages for SPECT analysis have recently been published (16–18). Normal left ventricular vol-

umes utilizing two commonly used software packages to analyze gated SPECT studies are shown in Table 3.2.

Recent hardware developments include small dedicated cardiac gamma cameras, such as the Digirad Cardiac 3XPO (Digirad, Poway, CA), CardiArc (CardiArc, Lubbock, TX), and D-SPECT (Spectrum Dynamics; Haifa, Israel), that allow fast acquisition protocols (20).

Evaluation of ventricular function is critical in many clinical situations, including patients with CAD and valvular diseases (21). Both global and regional wall motion can be accurately evaluated with gated blood pool studies by radionuclide ventriculography (RVG). In addition, ventricular size, right and left ventricular ejection fractions (RVEF and LVEF), and regurgitation indexes can be calculated. The RVG technology and other nonperfusion applications in nuclear cardiology have been reviewed and summarized in a report by the task force of the ASNC (22). Recent technical developments of SPECT technology applied to gated blood pool studies allow more accurate evaluation of ventricular function, especially right ventricular function and diastolic dysfunction.

TABLE 3.2 Comparison between ECTb and QGS for assessment of left ventricular function from gated myocardial perfusion SPECT

LV functional parameters for subjects at low likelihood for CAD

	All		Men		Women	
	QGS	**ECTb**	**QGS**	**ECTb**	**QGS**	**ECTb**
EF (%)	62 ± 9	67 ± 8	57 ± 7	63 ± 6	69 ± 8	72 ± 8
EDV (mL)	84 ± 26	105 ± 33	101 ± 20	124 ± 29	63 ± 17	84 ± 24
ESV (mL)	33 ± 17	35 ± 17	44 ± 13	46 ± 14	20 ± 10	24 ± 12
EVD (mL/m^2)	31 ± 8	39 ± 10	35 ± 6	43 ± 9	26 ± 6	34 ± 9
ESV (mL/m^2)	12 ± 5	13 ± 6	15 ± 4	16 ± 5	8 ± 4	10 ± 4

EDV$_1$, EDV indexed to body surface area; ESV$_1$, ESV indexed to body surface area.

Source: Reproduced with permission from Nichols et al. (19).

Multimodality imaging with integrated PET/CT and SPECT/CT systems offers the possibility for simultaneous evaluation of anatomy and function and is one of the most exciting new developments in imaging technology. Currently most PET/CT imaging systems are equipped with 16-slice CT scanners, but integrated PET/CT systems with 64-slice CT scanners are available for advanced cardiac applications and SPECT/64-slice multidetector computed tomography (MDCT) systems are under development. Cardiac PET/CT and SPECT/CT technology allows evaluation in one imaging setting of coronary calcium scoring (CCS), coronary artery anatomy with contrast-enhanced coronary CT angiography (CTA), rest/stress MPS, and localization of the hypoperfused regions to specific coronary arteries with the help of fusion images of the coronary tree superimposed on a 3D map of perfusion (23) (see discussion of Case 3.13). The ACC/AHA have recently published guidelines for the use of CCS (24) and cardiovascular CT imaging (25) as well as appropriateness criteria for the use of cardiovascular CT (26). The anatomic and functional information obtained with combined MPS/coronary CTA is complementary. Debate continues regarding the cost-effectiveness of the combined approach and whether the sequential approach of MPS and coronary CTA, with one test guiding the other, would be more cost-effective in specific clinical scenarios.

The choice of one of the tests discussed above to evaluate a specific patient will depend on several factors, including availability of technology, local experience with a given modality, and the pretest probability of disease, as well as patient-specific factors such as body habitus and resting ECG abnormalities. Updated imaging guidelines for nuclear cardiology procedures have been published (27), as well as training guidelines for physicians in training (28), clinical competence for physicians in practice (29), and technologist training in nuclear cardiology (30). Relevant literature on this topic and recent guidelines are discussed further on in this chapter.

COMMONLY USED RADIOPHARMACEUTICALS FOR MPS

^{201}Tl as a Perfusion Agent. ^{201}Tl is an analog of potassium, after the initial experiences using potassium-43 (15), which enters viable myocardial cells by passive diffusion and also by an active mechanism involving the sodium-potassium adenosine triphosphatase pump (31). Only 4% to 5% of the injected dose of 2.0 to 3.5 mCi concentrates in the myocardium, the remainder being distributed to skeletal muscle and other tissues. The physical half-life of thallium 201 (^{201}Tl) is approximately 72 hours, but its half-life in the myocardium is significantly shorter. During its decay, ^{201}Tl emits low-energy x-rays of approximately 70 keV. ^{201}Tl is usually administered at peak stress and distributes in the myocardium proportionally to blood flow at stress.

One of the most clinically important characteristics of ^{201}Tl is its redistribution over time. Redistribution is a phenomenon by which an agent dynamically crosses the cell membrane, recirculates into the coronary vessels, and becomes concentrated in the myocardium proportionally to resting blood flow. This property forms the basis of stress-redistribution imaging protocols used to diagnose CAD with ^{201}Tl. With ^{201}Tl, redistribution is significant, and acquisition of stress images should begin soon after the isotope is injected, preferably within 10 to 20 minutes. The longer the redistribution time, the more likely it is that ^{201}Tl will redistribute within viable cells with an intact cell membrane—cells that were ischemic and had decreased uptake during stress. Therefore ^{201}Tl is often used to differentiate viable tissue from scar tissue. In this regard, ^{201}Tl has advantages over agents labeled with technetium 99m (^{99m}Tc), which do not redistribute significantly (see Case 3.18 for a detailed discussion on the use of ^{201}Tl for viability). The pharmacokinetics of ^{201}Tl have been investigated and discussed by Krahwinkle (32).

^{99m}Tc-Labeled Agents. Cellular uptake of cationic perfusion agents, such as ^{99m}Tc-sestamibi and tetrofosmin, is mediated by a nonspecific charge-dependent transfer of lipophilic cations across the sarcolemma but is independent of Na$^+$/K$^+$ channels. Therefore cellular uptake is not affected by cation channel inhibitors. Intracellularly, ^{99m}Tc-sestamibi appears to bind to the mitochondria in myocardial cells. Damaged nonviable cells do not maintain membrane potential, so ^{99m}Tc-sestamibi does not accumulate within nonviable cells.

^{99m}Tc-sestamibi rapidly clears from the blood pool with a peak activity at 1 minute postinjection. Ninety-five percent of activity is cleared from the plasma at 5 minutes postinjection. Myocardial uptake is 1% of the injected dose following a resting injection and 1.4% following an injection during exercise. ^{99m}Tc-sestamibi has a slow clearance rate from the heart. Its effective half-life is 3 hours. After it binds to the mitochondria, there is very little redistribution, approximately 2% after 1 hour and 5% after 6 hours. Images can be acquired up to 6 hours postinjection. This allows evaluation of patients with acute chest pain syndrome (see Case 3.9) and patients with evolving myocardial infarction (MI) in whom thrombolytic therapy is planned. Although the kinetics of ^{99m}Tc-sestamibi are affected by cell metabolism and viability (33), a disadvantage of ^{99m}Tc-sestamibi is its underestimation of the extent of viable myocardium in comparison with ^{201}Tl studies using a reinjection or 24-hour redistribution protocol. This limitation of ^{99m}Tc-sestamibi to detect viable tissue in some patients has been overcome significantly by treatment with nitrates prior to injecting the tracer (see Case 3.21 for details). Another limitation of ^{99m}Tc-sestamibi is prominent excretion into the bowel via the hepatobiliary system, which occasionally can cause difficulties in the evaluation of the inferior wall. Delayed images, especially after a meal filling the stomach, can be sufficient to improve image quality in these cases.

^{99m}Tc-tetrofosmin is used in a similar way to ^{99m}Tc-sestamibi. The myocardial uptake is approximately 1.2% of the injected dose both at rest and during exercise. Mitochondrial membrane potential plays a major role in the myocardial uptake and retention of tetrofosmin, as it does for ^{99m}Tc-sestamibi (34). Blood clearance and hepatic excretion are rapid compared with ^{99m}Tc-sestamibi. Therefore ^{99m}Tc-tetrofosmin causes less hepatic artifact, but the myocardial uptake plateaus at a slightly lower flow rate than ^{99m}Tc-sestamibi. Overall, in clinical practice these two tracers are felt to be equivalent.

The isotope ^{99m}Tc is widely used in nuclear medicine because the detectors and electronics of conventional gamma cameras are optimized for the 140-KeV photons emitted by ^{99m}Tc. In addition, ^{99m}Tc is inexpensive and readily available. The short 6-hour half-life of ^{99m}Tc permits it to be given in higher dosages than ^{201}Tl, resulting in higher count statistics with resultant better image resolution and quality and less attenuation by intervening soft tissues. The higher count rate also allows high-quality gated images to be acquired in order to assess wall motion and ventricular function simultaneously with perfusion. Owing to the absence of significant redistribution, both supine and prone (or right lateral) imaging can be accomplished in instances where diaphragmatic attenuation artifact may pose a problem.

The energy emitted by the various isotopes may affect the choice of agent. For example, in patients with a large body habitus, it may be wise to use a higher-energy tracer, such as ^{99m}Tc-sestamibi, because there is less soft tissue attenuation than with a lower-energy-emitting tracer such as ^{201}Tl. Owing to the lower dose used (most commonly) for the rest study, more soft tissue attenuation may be noted on the resting images; usually this presents no clinical dilemma.

The disadvantages of ^{99m}Tc-sestamibi and tetrofosmin compared to ^{201}Tl are reduced linearity with flow, increased hepatic and splanchnic uptake, and less common lung uptake as an indicator of LV dysfunction (see Cases 3.2 and 3.5 for more details).

^{18}F-FDG as a PET Agent. ^{18}F-FDG is still considered as the reference standard for evaluation of myocardial viability. This is supported by a large literature, as discussed in Cases 3.19 and 3.20. However ^{18}F-FDG is not as available as the SPECT radiopharmaceuticals (^{201}Tl or ^{99m}Tc isonitriles). In addition, ^{18}F-FDG myocardial imaging requires further preparation, such as glucose loading (see Case 3.20), adding 30 to 60 minutes to the procedure.

^{82}Rb as a PET Agent. Rubidium 82 (^{82}Rb) is a potassium analog and can be eluted from a strontium-82 generator, making it more easily available and more commonly used clinically than nitrogen-13 (^{13}N) ammonia, which requires a cyclotron on site. Although ^{82}Rb-PET cardiac imaging is reimbursed by third-party payers, the generator (CardioGen-82, Bracco Diagnostics, Inc., Geneva) is expensive and must be replaced monthly, limiting the use of ^{82}Rb-PET imaging to large centers that have the volume of referrals to justify the cost. A theoretical limit in resolution of the ^{82}Rb (compared with ^{13}N ammonia) images occurs because the energy of the positrons emitted is higher than that of ^{13}N and the distance traversed by ^{82}Rb positrons is longer than that of ^{13}N before the annihilation process. ^{82}Rb has a short half-life of 78 seconds, allowing acquisition of rest and stress images back to back and completion of the study within 30 to 45 minutes. However, because of the short half-life, the optimal time for acquisition of the images is critical and technically demanding. Occasionally, ^{82}Rb images may be of limited quality because of low count images or blood pool activity. These two factors together explain the lower quality of ^{82}Rb images compared with ^{13}N-ammonia images. Because of the short half-life, stress is limited to pharmacologic agents, which is another limitation of ^{82}Rb.

The resting study should be performed first to reduce the impact of residual stress effects. The dose administered depends of the type of PET system [bismuth germanate oxide (BGO), lutetium oxyorthosilicate oxide (LSO), or gadolinium oxyorthosilicate (GSO) crystals] and imaging mode (the 2D imaging mode requires a higher dose than the 3D). Typically in the 2D imaging mode with a BGO PET system, ~50 mCi of ^{82}Rb is administered intravenously and the images are acquired starting at 70 to 90 seconds after administration for patients with a LVEF >50% and 90 to 120 seconds after administration for patients with a LVEF <50%. The emission images are usually acquired for 5 minutes and are ECG-gated.

^{13}N-Ammonia as a PET Agent. ^{13}N-ammonia requires a cyclotron for its production and has a half-life of 10 minutes, requiring a timely production related to the time of administration. It is rapidly cleared from the blood pool and diffuses intracellularly proportionally to MBF. Its retention depends on its metabolic incorporation into glutamine, thus cellular viability. For ^{13}N-ammonia, the transmission images can be acquired immediately before or after the emission images if the attenuation software can adequately correct for residual emission activity. For the resting study, gated emission images are acquired 1.5 to 3.0 minutes after 10 to 20 mCi of ^{13}N-ammonia is administered intravenously. The images are usually acquired for 5 to 15 minutes. The stress study can be performed using the same protocol during pharmacologic stress after a 1-hour waiting period to allow for decay of the resting ^{13}N-ammonia dose.

^{13}N-ammonia also allows quantitative measurement of CBF and CBFR using compartmental modeling and kinetic analysis. The possibility of evaluating absolute MBF and CBFR using vasodilators also offers a means of investigating endothelial function and vascular smooth muscle relaxation as well as detecting early atherosclerosis. Quantitative measurement of MBF with PET is dependent on accurate attenuation correction (AC) and lack of motion of the patient during the scanning period as well as careful calibration of the imaging system. To measure the absolute myocardial perfusion rate, the arterial input function can be derived from a region of interest placed in the LV cavity. The dose of ^{13}N-ammonia must be infused over 30 seconds and dynamic images must be acquired with varying frame durations for 4 minutes starting at the time of infusion of ^{13}N-ammonia. Various kinetic models have been developed and validated to measure absolute MBF but are not practical in the clinical setting and are beyond the scope of this chapter.

Advantages of PET versus SPECT Radiopharmaceuticals

The advantages of PET over SPECT perfusion radiopharmaceuticals include (a) better resolution and therefore better sensitivity, (b) more accurate attenuation correction (AC); (c) true stress LV EF; (d) shorter imaging protocols; (e) optimal evaluation of perfusion and viability in conjunction with ^{18}F-FDG; and (f) a smaller radiation dose to patients compared to ^{201}TP (23) (see discussion of Cases 3.14, 3.19 and Table 3.3).

STRESS MODALITIES TO TEST CORONARY BLOOD FLOW RESERVE IN NUCLEAR CARDIOLOGY

Exercise Stress

Exercise stress testing is most commonly performed using the TMT and is discussed above, under "TMT for Evaluation of CAD."

Pharmacologic Stress

Dipyridamole as a Stress Agent. Pharmacologic stress represents approximately 40% of the MPS studies performed in the United States (35,36). Dipyridamole inhibits the action of an enzyme called adenosine deaminase, responsible for the degradation of endogenously produced adenosine. Dipyridamole also blocks the reuptake of adenosine by cells, which again will contribute to elevation of adenosine, causing vasodilation. Dipyridamole increases MBF approximately three- to fourfold compared with baseline.

Indications for vasodilator stress are (a) inability to exercise, (b) failure to achieve 85% maximum predicted heart rate (MPHR) in the absence of typical angina or >2 mm ST-segment depression, (c) concurrent beta-blockade (or calcium antagonist) therapy (relative indication), and (d) presence of LBBB or pacemaker. Contraindications are listed in Table 3.1.

Theophylline and other xanthines (i.e., pentoxifylline) should be withheld for at least 72 hours and all caffeine and caffeinated beverages/foods for 24 to 48 hours prior to vasodilator infusion. Special attention should be given to the stopping of coffee, tea, chocolate, and soft drinks. Patients taking oral dipyridamole (as antiplatelet therapy) should stop it for 24 to 48 hours prior to vasodilator infusion. Since caffeine is cleared by the liver, special care should be taken in patients with hepatic failure, especially those evaluated prior to liver transplant. In these cases, exercise or dobutamine stress should be considered.

Dipyridamole is infused over 4 minutes at a dose of 0.56 to 0.84 mg/kg and the radiopharmaceutical is administered 7 minutes after the start of the infusion.

Special care should be taken to watch for the occurrence of severe bronchospasm and higher-degree atrioventricular (AV) block; these may occur with dipyridamole and require prompt discontinuation of the infusion and treatment.

The safety of dipyridamole has been reviewed in a series of 73,806 patients (37). Dipyridamole (at a dose of 0.56 mg/kg) causes side effects in about 50% of individuals, flushing being the most frequent in 43% of patients, chest pain (nonspecific for ischemia) in 20%, and headache in 12% (38). The half-life of dipyridamole is approximately 45 minutes. Patients receiving dipyridamole may experience symptoms after completion of the infusion when they have already left the laboratory. Administration of aminophylline prevents these occurrences in most cases. Aminophylline is administered at 1.0 to 1.5 mg/kg slow IV push until symptoms resolve, with a maximum dose of 250 mg.

The sensitivity and specificity of dipyridamole stress for the detection of CAD (>50%) have been described to be in the same range as those for exercise.

Adenosine as a Stress Agent. Adenosine promotes vasodilation by activation of vascular A_2 receptors, which has an effect on cyclic AMP, reduces the influx of calcium into the intracellular space, and consequently relaxes smooth muscle cells of the coronary arteries. Adenosine increases MBF approximately four- to fivefold above baseline in myocardium supplied by normal arteries, whereas the MBF increases less in myocardium supplied by diseased arteries. The ischemic territories can be identified on MPS as areas of decreased tracer uptake. Ischemic areas can be identified on MPS by heterogenous tracer distribution owing to a differential capacity of vessels to dilate without causing true myocardial ischemia. True myocardial ischemia may occur with administration of adenosine or dipyridamole, when there is a "coronary steal phenomenon." The steal phenomenon occurs in patients who have part of their myocardium supplied by collateral vessels owing to an occluded or critically stenotic coronary artery (39). When there is true ischemia, ST-segment shifts may be observed during the test, as well as clinical evidence of ischemia with typical angina. Wall motion abnormalities may develop as a result of the steal phenomenon during infusion of vasodilators.

Adenosine is infused IV with a pump in a volume of 50 mL of saline at a rate of 140 μg/kg per minute over 4 to 6 minutes; the rate can be decreased to 100 μg/kg per minute without a loss in sensitivity in the event of significant symptoms. BP, HR, and ECG are monitored every minute. If heart block progresses or does not resolve, infusion should be terminated. Studies comparing 4- versus 6-minute infusions of adenosine demonstrated similar sensitivity for detection of CAD, and the 4-minute infusion was better tolerated (40). The radiopharmaceutical is administered IV 3 minutes into the 6-minute adenosine infusion. BP, HR, and ECG are monitored every minute for 10 to 20 minutes or until the patient's hemodynamic status returns to baseline.

Approximately 81% of patients undergoing adenosine infusion have some side effects, flushing being the most frequent and occurring in 37% of patients, which is followed by dyspnea in 35% and AV block in 8%. The safety of adenosine stress has been demonstrated in a large prospective study of 9,256 consecutive patients (41,42).

Adenosine has a very short half-life of less than 10 seconds. This does not necessarily mean that all side effects occurring with adenosine will resolve after cessation of infusion. Once the adenosine receptors have been activated, a cascade of events is triggered, and therefore side effects may be much more prolonged than could be suggested by the drug's short half-life. The antidote to adenosine is aminophylline, 25 mg/min slow IV push, until symptoms resolve, with a maximum dose of 250 mg. In view of the brief half-life of adenosine, termination of the infusion is often (but not always) adequate to manage adverse events. If possible, wait 2 to 3 minutes after radiopharmaceutical injection to terminate adenosine infusion and give aminophylline. In case of very severe ischemic symptoms, administration of sublingual or intranasal nitroglycerin, 0.4 mg, may be necessary following aminophylline administration (43).

For detection of CAD in general, the sensitivity and specificity of adenosine stress have been described in the same range as exercise stress (44–46); however, there is some evidence that a normal SPECT study in patients undergoing vasodilator stress may not have the same negative predictive value as compared with exercise stress (47). This may be related to the higher intrinsic risk of the population usually referred for vasodilator stress. Ischemic ECG changes with normal SPECT images during vasodilator stress is uncommon but may be helpful in identifying patients at an increased risk for future cardiac events (48,49).

Dobutamine as a Stress Agent. When there is a contraindication for using adenosine or dipyridamole, dobutamine is usually utilized. Dobutamine is an inotropic agent frequently used in intensive care units to increase cardiac output, BP, and urinary output. Dobutamine has a mild effect on alpha-1 receptors, strong effect on beta-1 receptors, and moderate effect on beta-2 receptors. In the heart, dobutamine activates beta-1 receptors (50). Dobutamine causes increased HR and myocardial contractility, promoting coronary hyperemia through

mechanisms similar to exercise. It is a fast-acting drug with the effect starting approximately 2 minutes into infusion. Its hemodynamic effects depend highly on the dose infused. At a low-dose of 5 to 10 μg/kg per minute it activates beta-1 and alpha-1 receptors, which increase myocardial contractility without significant effects on HR. Doses above 10 to 20 μg/kg per minute activate alpha-1 receptors, which increases both the HR and myocardial contractility, resulting in an increase of cardiac output. Doses higher than 30 μg/kg per minute increase significantly the development of ventricular arrhythmias. Dobutamine also causes a reduction of systemic vascular resistance mediated by activation of the beta-2 receptors, which may actually cause the BP to decrease in some cases. The hyperemic effect of dobutamine alone increases MBF approximately twofold above baseline, which is an effect considered lower than that obtained with dipyridamole or adenosine. However, it has been demonstrated that the administration of dobutamine combined with atropine has an hyperemic effect similar to that of dipyridamole (51). In the nuclear laboratory, dobutamine infusion has been indicated mainly to evaluate CAD in patients with chronic obstructive pulmonary disease (COPD) who are unable to exercise adequately, as is usually the case in severe COPD. Contraindications for the use of dobutamine are listed in Table 3.1.

The patient should be off beta blockers for 5 to 7 days, preferably slowly discontinuing such medication so as to prevent rebound effects. Other antianginal medications (calcium channel blockers and nitrates) should also be discontinued, as discussed earlier in this chapter. The protocol most commonly used for MPS with dobutamine starts with an infusion rate of 10 μg/kg per minute, increasing by an additional dose of 10 μg/kg per minute every 3 minutes, to a maximum dose of 40 μg/kg per minute. Atropine may be used to increase HR, starting at the second stage (52). Usually, target HR is achieved at the rate of 20 to 30 μg/kg per minute with a small dose of atropine, around 0.5 mg. The higher the dobutamine dose given, the higher the incidence of arrhythmias and side effects; the addition of atropine helps to achieve the target HR at lower dobutamine doses. The radiopharmaceutical is injected once the target HR, preferably maximum HR, is achieved and the infusion of dobutamine is continued for another minute.

Dobutamine leads to side effects in about 75% of patients, 39% having chest pain, which can be treated with sublingual nitroglycerin, and 45% having supraventricular tachycardia or ventricular ectopy (53). Ventricular tachycardia (VT) occurs in 4% to 5% of patients. Other side effects include headache (7%), dyspnea (6%), flushing (<1%), nausea, and anxiety; these are usually well tolerated and do not necessitate interruption of the infusion. Symptomatic hypotension occurs rarely and can be treated with the infusion of saline. Severe side effects of dobutamine can be reversed by beta blockers such as esmolol (0.2 mg/kg over 1 minute) or an IV bolus of metoprolol (2.5 to 5 mg). However, patients undergoing dobutamine infusion often have COPD. Beta blockers, especially at higher doses, are known to worsen COPD and should be avoided if possible. When dobutamine induces VT, amiodarone or electric cardioversion may be necessary, especially if hemodynamic instability is present. Despite the relative high incidence of cardiac arrhythmia with dobutamine, in a study of 3,578 patients reported in the literature, there were no reports of death, MI, or ventricular fibrillation (54). The safety of dobutamine stress has also been reported in the elderly population (55) as well as in heart transplant recipients (56).

Normal myocardial perfusion studies with dobutamine are associated with a good prognosis and low cardiac event rate, less than 0.8% per year. Patients with fixed and reversible perfusion defects have a risk of 6.8% and 8.1% for major cardiac events respectively. If both fixed and reversible cardiac defects are present, the risk is 11.6% (57,58).

A_{2A} Receptor Agonists as Stress Agents. New vasodilator stress agents, called A_{2A} receptor agonists, have been developed. The coronary vasodilatory effect of adenosine and dipyridamole is mediated primarily by A_{2A} receptors present in the vascular wall. Agents that selectively or preferentially stimulate A_{2A} receptors have the advantage of improved patient safety and comfort. A number of highly potent and selective A_{2A}-receptor agonists have now been synthesized and are in various stages of clinical development (59–62). Recently the results of a large first phase III trial evaluating regadenoson became available (63). In this trial 784 patients underwent two sets of gated SPECT MPS. The initial stress MPS study was done with adenosine and patients were subsequently randomized, in a double-blinded fashion, to either regadenoson (two-thirds of patients) or adenosine (one-third of patients). The dose of regadenoson was given as a rapid bolus (<10 seconds) while that of adenosine was 140 μg/kg per minute given as an IV infusion for 6 minutes. A summed symptom score of flushing, chest pain, and dyspnea was lower with regadenoson than with adenosine ($P = 0.018$). There were no serious side effects and no high-degree AV block with regadenoson. Regadenoson as a bolus provides diagnostic information on the presence and severity of reversible defects that is comparable to the information provided by a 6-minute infusion of adenosine. Regadenoson has been recently approved by the FDA in the USA.

Commonly Used Protocols for MPS

Protocols for ^{201}Tl-SPECT MPS (Fig. 3.B)

^{201}Tl migrates intracellularly and begins to be redistributed approximately 20 minutes after its injection. Regions of the myocardium that had decreased uptake of the radiotracer on the poststress images but which are viable will appear normal on resting redistribution images. Areas of nonviable cells resulting from previous MI will have decreased uptake of ^{201}Tl on both the poststress and resting images. These are matched, or fixed, defects. With the stress-redistribution protocol (Fig. 3.B, top), 3 to 4 mCi of ^{201}Tl is injected at peak stress and the images are acquired after 10 to 20 minutes. The redistribution images are then acquired after a 3- to 4-hour interval. Because this protocol overestimates the number of fixed defects by as much as 50%, the reinjection protocol has become the standard. With the reinjection protocol (Fig. 3.B, middle), a second dosage of the tracer (1 to 1.5 mCi) is given 2 to 3 af-

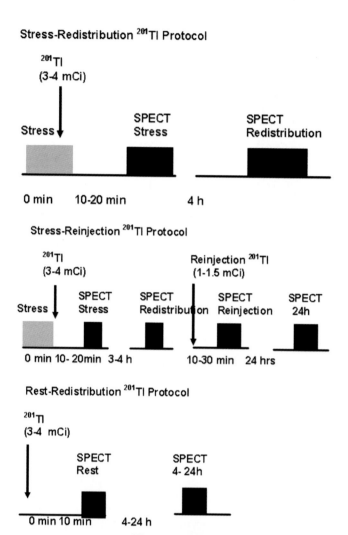

Figure 3.B Protocols for ^{201}Tl-SPECT MPS. [From Vitola and Delbeke (11), by permission from Springer- Verlag.]

ter the stress testing is completed. After 10 to 30 minutes, a second set of images, called reinjection images, is acquired. In extremely ischemic cells, significant uptake of ^{201}Tl into these segments may be seen only when a longer period (24 hours) of redistribution is allowed (64). Often patients evaluated for viability cannot be stressed due to clinical constraints because of symptoms of congestive heart failure (CHF). For these patients, viability can be evaluated using the rest/redistribution ^{201}Tl protocol (Fig. 3.B, bottom). ^{201}Tl (3 to 4 mCi) is injected at rest and images are acquired 4 and sometimes 24 hours later (see Case 3.18 for further details on ^{201}Tl imaging for viability).

Protocols for ^{99m}Tc-Sestamibi and Tetrofosmin SPECT MPS (Figure 3.C)

Two separate administrations of radiopharmaceutical are necessary for the stress-induced and resting images because they are retained in the myocardium without redistribution over time. Ideally, rest and stress studies are performed on two different days (Figure 3.C, top) with a 20- to 30-mCi dose for each study, gating both image acquisitions. However,

Stress-Rest ^{99m}Tc -MIBI or –Tetrofosmin: Separate Day Protocols

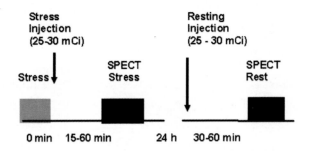

Stress-Rest ^{99m}Tc -MIBI or –Tetrofosmin: Same Day Protocol

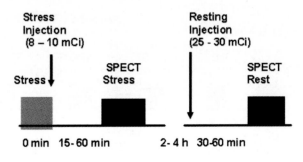

Rest-Stress ^{99m}Tc -MIBI or –Tetrofosmin: Same Day Protocol

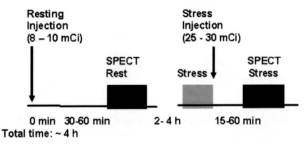

Figure 3.C Protocols for ^{99m}Tc-sestamibi and Tetrofosmin SPECT MPS. [From Vitola and Delbeke (11), by permission from Springer-Verlag.]

in some cases this is not practical, especially for patients needing to travel long distances. A 1-day protocol (Fig. 3.C, middle and bottom) can then be used. A lower dose is administered for the first study (typically 8 to 10 mCi), which can be started by stress or rest as demonstrated. The second study can be performed 1 hour later with a threefold higher dose (25 to 30 mCi). Images are typically acquired 30 to 60 minutes after administration of the radiopharmaceutical at rest and 15 to 30 minutes after physical exercise. After pharmacologic stress using vasodilators, there is also vasodilation of the splanchnic circulation, increasing liver uptake, therefore a longer waiting period of 45 to 90 minutes before acquisition of the images reduces interference of hepatic uptake with the inferior wall of the myocardium. Longer intervals may be necessary in individual cases.

In the rest/stress protocol, there is no contamination on the second study from the previous ^{99m}Tc-sestamibi injection. Despite some limitations of same-day versus separate-day protocols, the rest/stress same-day ^{99m}Tc-sestamibi protocol

provides high diagnostic accuracy for the detection of CAD (65). If stress imaging is performed first and is normal, rest imaging may not be necessary—an advantage of the stress/rest sequence. If a 2-day rest/stress protocol is used with the higher dose (25 to 30 mCi) of ^{99m}Tc-sestamibi, performance of the resting study may be unnecessary if the stress images are normal. However, attenuation artifacts, which are frequent in nuclear medicine and vary from patient to patient, may warrant the acquisition of both rest and stress studies to facilitate accurate interpretation. When stress images are acquired with attenuation correction (AC), rest images may become unnecessary.

Dual-Isotope Rest ^{201}Tl/Stress ^{99m}Tc-Sestamibi or Tetrofosmin SPECT MPS Protocol (Fig. 3.D)

Using the dual-isotope protocol, the resting study is acquired 10 to 20 minutes following administration of 3 mCi ^{201}Tl, after which the patient can be immediately stressed; the ^{99m}Tc-labeled agent (25 to 30 mCi) is administered at peak stress. An additional rest ^{201}Tl image can be obtained at 24 hours if necessary to increase sensitivity to detect viable tissue/hibernating myocardium (see Case 3.18 for further details). The dual-isotope protocol is used less commonly because of the higher radiation dose due to ^{201}Tl compared with rest/stress ^{99m}Tc-radiopharmaceutical protocols (see Table 3.3).

Protocols Using Vasodilator Stress and Low-Level Exercise Combined

Pharmacologic alternatives must be considered in patients with poor exercise tolerance and/or those who are unable to reach at least 85% of their MPHR. Protocols combining vasodilators (dipyridamole and adenosine) with exercise have been established in the past several years (66–68). The vasodilator effect of dipyridamole or adenosine has been described to be greater than that of exercise alone except in cases of nonresponders. There are some data suggesting that exercise can contribute to the identification of these individuals, but this is under investigation (69,70).

Compared with exercise, which is the most physiologic stimulus, dipyridamole or adenosine stimuli alone have several limitations, including low sensitivity of the ECG for ischemia and frequent side effects (38). These vasodilators induce dilatation of the splanchnic vasculature, resulting in a higher concentration of radiopharmaceutical in the liver and intestinal tract (71). Exercise promotes a redistribution of blood flow to the skeletal musculature and away from intra-abdominal organs such as the liver (72). These effects result in a higher ratio of heart-to-liver activity on images obtained after exercise compared with those obtained after vasodilator infusion alone (73). Some studies have shown that the addition of low-workload exercise helps to decrease dipyridamole's side effects (74–77). Other studies, using adenosine, have shown similar effects, reducing side effects (78) and arrhythmias (79) and decreasing ^{99m}Tc-sestamibi concentration in the liver (79), resulting in better image quality. The images can also be acquired earlier, after administration of the radiopharmaceutical, in patients undergoing a combined exercise/vasodilator protocol compared with vasodilator alone (66,80).

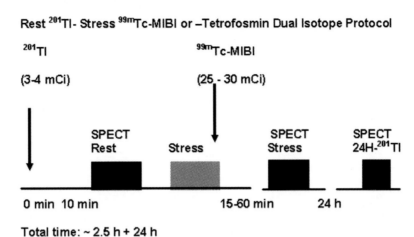

Rest ^{201}Tl- Stress ^{99m}Tc-MIBI or –Tetrofosmin Dual Isotope Protocol

^{201}Tl

(3-4 mCi)

^{99m}Tc-MIBI

(25 - 30 mCi)

SPECT Rest

Stress

SPECT Stress

SPECT 24H-^{201}Tl

0 min 10 min   15-60 min   24 h

Total time: ~ 2.5 h + 24 h

Figure 3.D Dual-isotope rest ^{201}Tl/stress ^{99m}Tc-sestamibi or tetrofosmin SPECT MPS protocol. [From Vitola and Delbeke (11), by permission from Springer-Verlag.]

The indication for this combined protocol include patients unable to exercise to 85% MPHR but able at least to walk and those with concurrent use of medications that may limit HR increase. It is important to note that patients with LBBB or pacemakers should undergo vasodilator stress alone to reduce the false-positive rate associated with exercise (81).

Most patients for the combined protocol are exercised at low workload as per their abilities, such as the first and second stage of a standard or modified Bruce. Some other lower-workload protocols, such as Kattus or Naughton, may be applied. If the patient tolerates it, the workload is increased, but if he or she is unable to exercise at a higher level, then exercise should be maintained at a lower level (limited to stage 1 or 2 of the protocols described). With exercise plus dipyridamole, the maximum action of the drug occurs between 6 and 9 minutes into the infusion; therefore the infusion may start before the exercise (approximately at 3 minutes into the infusion), with the tracer being injected at 6 to 9 minutes from the start of infusion (66). With adenosine, the infusion is started at the same time as the exercise protocol and the radiopharmaceutical is administered at 2 to 3 minutes into the drug infusion while the patient continues to exercise to maximum tolerance (68).

Significant ST-segment changes during low workload (the first 3 minutes of a Bruce protocol) are signs of severe disease and are associated with a higher rate of adverse cardiac events (82). Importantly, the magnitude of ST-segment depression at this low workload can stratify patients into different risk categories, with approximately 80% of patients with 3 mm of ST-segment depression having cardiac events within 6 years.

The impact of adjunctive adenosine infusion during exercise MPS has been studied as part of a multicenter trial where 35 patients were enrolled prospectively and underwent both exercise MPS and exercise MPS with a 4-minute adenosine infusion on a separate day (BEAST trial) (83). The summed stress scores (SSS) and summed difference scores (SDS) were greater in the exercise-plus-adenosine group than the exercise-only group. The study concludes that the combined protocol resulted in a greater amount of myocardial ischemia detected on the SPECT images while allowing for the assessment of functional capacity.

Attenuation Correction

Attenuation correction is recommended when available and improves normalcy rate. In 2001, the ASNC and Society of Nuclear Medicine (SNM) issued a joint position statement after reviewing the literature, using the current transmission maps acquired with radioisotope sources (84). The addition of AC improves specificity from an average of 64% to 81%, and normalcy rates from an average of 80% to 89% without a loss of sensitivity. Attenuation correction can also be performed using CT attenuation maps from integrated imaging systems (see Cases 3.14 and 3.22)

Radiation Dose Considerations

With the technical development of coronary computed tomography angiography (CTA) and hybrid nuclear/CTA procedures, radiation doses from cardiovascular imaging procedures have become a concern to both patients and physicians. In 1998, the ACC has published a consensus document discussing radiation safety in the practice of cardiology (85). The issues regarding radiation dosage from various cardiac nuclear and radiographic procedures have recently been summarized (86). The dual-isotope protocol and other protocols using ^{201}Tl are utilized less commonly nowadays because of the higher radiation dose of ^{201}Tl compared with rest/stress ^{99m}Tc-radiopharmaceutical protocols (Table 3.3).

Choice of Diagnostic Tests Based on Prevalence of Disease

The appropriateness of noninvasive testing must be considered in light of Bayes' theorem, which expresses the posttest likelihood of disease as a function of sensitivity and specificity of the test and the prevalence (or pretest probability) of disease in the population being tested (Fig. 3.E). Algorithms used to evaluate patients for myocardial ischemia depend on the pretest probability of the presence of CAD. Patients can be classified into low, intermediate, or high pretest probability. Placing a patient into one or another category depends greatly on the physician's judgment, taking into account the patient's age, gender, coronary risk factors, and symptoms.

TABLE 3.3 Radiation dosage from cardiovascular procedures

Study	Total-body Effective dose (mSv)
^{99m}Tc-tetrofosmin rest/stress (10 mCi + 30 mCi)	10.6 mSv
^{99m}Tc-sestamibi 1-day rest/stress (10 mCi + 30 mCi)	12.0 mSv
^{201}Tl stress and reinjection (3 mCi + 1 mCi)	25.1 mSv*
Dual-isotope (3 mCi ^{201}Tl + 30 mCi ^{99m}Tc)	27.3 mSv
^{82}Rb PET myocardial perfusion (45 mCi + 45 mCi)	16.0 mSv†
^{18}F-FDG PET viability (10 mCi)	7.0 mSv
^{68}Ge transmission for PET	0.08 mSv
^{137}Cs transmission for PET	0.01 mSv
^{153}Gd transmission for SPECT	0.05 mSv
CT transmission for PET (low-dose CT protocol)	0.8 mSv
MDCT coronary calcium scoring	1.0–3.6 mSv
64-slice MDCT coronary CTA	~10.0 mSv (4.8–21.4)

*^{201}Tl dose based on package insert is 39 mSv/3 mCi.

†^{82}Rb dose based on calculation from package insert is 5.5 mSv for 60 + 60 mCi.

Source: Adapted Thompson et al. (86).

The other important parameter is the absence or presence of symptoms. For asymptomatic patients, risk stratification is commonly evaluated using the Framingham Risk Score (FRS), which is an estimate of 10-year risk for hard coronary events (MI or coronary death). The FRS is calculated based on age, gender, systolic blood pressure, total and HDL cholesterol levels in plasma, and the presence of risk factors including diabetes and smoking (87). Asymptomatic patients with an intermediate FRS (10-year risk of hard coronary events between 10% and 20%) should be considered for coronary calcium scoring (CCS) to further risk-stratify them as recommended by the ACC/AHA (24) and ASNC (88) .

After a review of the literature, including 28,948 patients, Diamond and Forrester (89) have reported the prevalence of CAD based on the patient's age, gender, and symptoms. With respect to symptoms, the patients were classified as asymptomatic, nonanginal, atypical, and typical chest pain according to three characteristics of chest pain (substernal location, induction by exercise, relieved by nitroglycerin). When the three characteristics were present, the patients were classified as having typical chest pain. Their results demonstrated that the prevalence of CAD in the asymptomatic population ranges from 0% to 20%. As another example, the pretest likelihood of disease for men 30 to 60 years of age is much higher than that for women of the same age, of course secondary to the influence of gender on CAD development. If symptoms of typical chest pain are present as opposed to those of atypical chest pain, the pretest probability of CAD is markedly increased. Factors such as smoking, family history of CAD, sedentary lifestyle, or presence of hypercholesterolemia, HTN, or DM are known to contribute to the risk of CAD and increase the pretest probability even further. The aggressiveness of further evaluation depends on the pretest probability.

Once the pretest probability of disease is estimated, an algorithm can be created to evaluate patients with chest pain.

The posttest probability for CAD depends on the sensitivity and specificity of the test being performed (90).

Patients with Low Pretest Probability of CAD

According to Diamond and Forrester, a positive result obtained with MPS study or another method of evaluating myocardial ischemia (e.g., TMT and stress echocardiography) is more likely to be a false positive if the patient has a low pretest probability for CAD. This suggests that a positive MPS study in asymptomatic patients with low risk factors (low pretest probability) does not necessarily establish the presence of CAD, while a negative test effectively excludes the presence of CAD. Several studies do support that theoretical conclusion (91). Therefore the approach to the evaluation of patients with a low-pretest probability is to begin with a resting ECG and a TMT. If there are abnormalities on the resting ECG, making it uninterpretable during a TMT, other options including imaging should be considered. MPS is one of the most sensitive and specific methods for the noninvasive evaluation of myocardial ischemia, considering that MPS evaluates physiology while coronary angiography primarily evaluates anatomy. Pooled data from 19 studies (92) have shown a sensitivity of 83% to 98% (with a mean of 92%) and a specificity of 53% to 100% (with a mean of 77%) for detecting ischemia.

Coronary CTA may become the first test of choice in these low-probability patients because of its high negative predictive value (NPV) excluding CAD. However, when coronary CTA is abnormal, the functional impact on perfusion should be further evaluated with MPS (93).

Patients with Intermediate Probability for CAD

MPS has optimal discriminative value in the patient population with an intermediate pretest probability of CAD in the range of 40% to 70% (Fig. 3.E). This population includes (a) patients with nonanginal chest pain and a positive or nondiagnostic

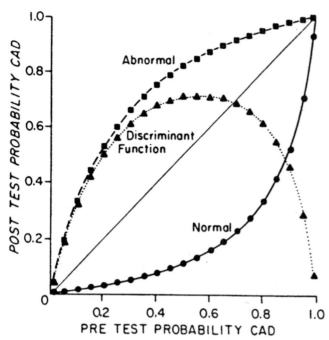

Figure 3.E Probability of CAD and posttest probability of CAD for abnormal and normal results of quantitative ^{201}Tl stress imaging (sensitivity 90%, specificity 95%). The curve describes the difference between posttest probability of a normal and an abnormal test result, indicating the range of disease prevalence for which ^{201}Tl stress imaging discriminates most effectively between the presence or absence of disease. ^{201}Tl stress imaging is most useful when the pretest prevalence of CAD is 40% to 70%. For example, in a patient with a pretest probability of disease of 60%, a positive ^{201}Tl stress test increases the probability of CAD to 90%, while a negative test decreases it to about 15%. ■ = abnormal; ▲ = posttest probability difference; ● = normal. [Reproduced with permission from Hamilton et al. (90).]

exercise ECG; (b) asymptomatic patients with significant risk factors, abnormal resting ECG, or positive exercise ECG; (c) patients with atypical chest pain; and (d) patients with typical chest pain and a negative exercise ECG. For patients in this category, MPS may be more helpful as an initial evaluation than it would be in those with a low or high pretest probability. A positive result is more likely to be a true-positive finding in a patient with intermediate probability than in a patient with low probability. A negative result in a patient with intermediate probability is more likely to be a true-negative finding than in a patient with high pretest probability. This hypothesis was also supported by several studies (94,95).

Coronary CTA may also be considered in this group of patients (25) and may show nonobstructive atherosclerosis when MPS is normal. The presence of atherosclerosis may lead to more aggressive medical therapy and require greater patient compliance with treatment.

Patients with a High Pretest Probability of CAD

Patients with a high pretest probability should almost always be investigated, at least once, more aggressively and invasively. According to Bayes' theorem, a negative MPS in a patient with a high pretest probability for CAD, for example, a symptomatic patient, is more likely to have a false-negative than a true-negative result. Coronary angiography is often used as the initial evaluation in these patients. The advantage of performing nuclear before proceeding to invasive would be to identify the culprit lesion responsible for the patient's symptoms and to document a baseline status useful for therapeutic follow-up.

In some cases, the angiographic findings are already known and the question is whether or not the lesions found compromise MBF and to what extent. Information obtained with MPS allows accurate estimation of the prognosis. It is essential to remember that CAD is not synonymous with myocardial ischemia and that anatomic findings do not always provide information about the physiologic significance of coronary lesions.

This introduction has reviewed some of the basic concepts of how nuclear cardiology, through coronary reserve testing, is able to detect and evaluate CAD, as well as stressing the importance of understanding the patient's pretest probability of CAD before proceeding to any given test and the implications this has for the interpretation of a given result. The remainder of this chapter reviews important topics for the everyday practice of nuclear cardiology using real-life cases as a basis for discussion.

CASE 3.1

History: A 69-year-old male with a 2-year history of progressive typical exertional angina presented for preoperative evaluation prior to excision of a parotid gland tumor. Cardiac risk factors included HTN, DM, tobacco use, age, and gender. The resting ECG was normal. An exercise ^{201}Tl SPECT (Fig. 3.1) was performed. He exercised for 8.5 minutes without chest pain using a standard Bruce protocol. He achieved 78% of his MPHR. His stress ECG was positive for myocardial ischemia.

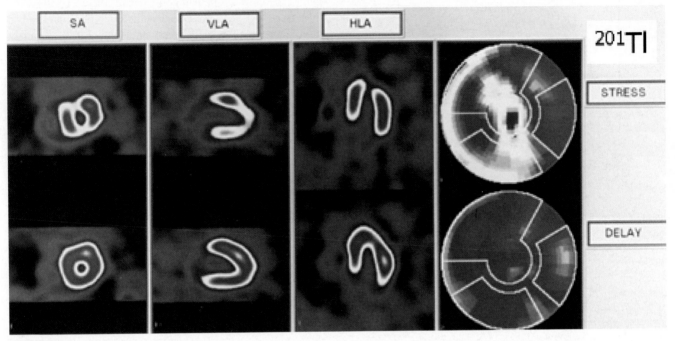

Figure 3.1

Findings: There is a severe reversible defect involving the mid- and distal anteroseptal region, the entire apex, and the inferior wall.

Discussion: A reversible defect indicates myocardial ischemia and is defined as a regional area of relative decreased ^{201}Tl uptake (or other perfusion tracers) with stress that resolves, improves, or is normal at rest. Because of this patient's typical anginal symptoms, age, and numerous cardiac risk factors, he was found to have a high pretest probability of myocardial ischemia and had been referred initially for coronary angiography, which revealed a chronic occlusion of the mid-left anterior descending coronary artery (LAD) with distal filling via collaterals from the right coronary artery (RCA); a 70% lesion was noted at the mid-RCA.

Following the coronary angiography, an exercise ^{201}Tl SPECT study was ordered to determine the extent of myocardial ischemia and viability to the vascular territories found abnormal on angiography. MPS demonstrated significant ischemia, and the patient was referred for treatment with percutaneous coronary angioplasty (PTCA) of the mid-RCA lesion. MPS may often be useful, as in this patient, in determining the physiologic importance of known sites of CAD.

^{201}Tl as a perfusion agent and the different ^{201}Tl protocols are discussed in the introduction to this chapter.

Diagnosis: Myocardial ischemia due to two-vessel CAD detected by ^{201}Tl imaging.

CASE 3.2

History: A 73-year-old woman presented with a 1-month history of recurrent nausea and diaphoresis. She denied chest pain and had no history of CAD. Cardiac risk factors included age, HTN, hypercholesterolemia, and peripheral vascular disease (PVD). The resting ECG was normal. Using a 1-day protocol, an adenosine ^{99m}Tc-tetrofosmin SPECT (Fig. 3.2) was performed. No chest pain occurred, and the stress ECG was negative for myocardial ischemia.

Stress ^{99m}Tc-tetrofosmin

Rest ^{99m}Tc-tetrofosmin

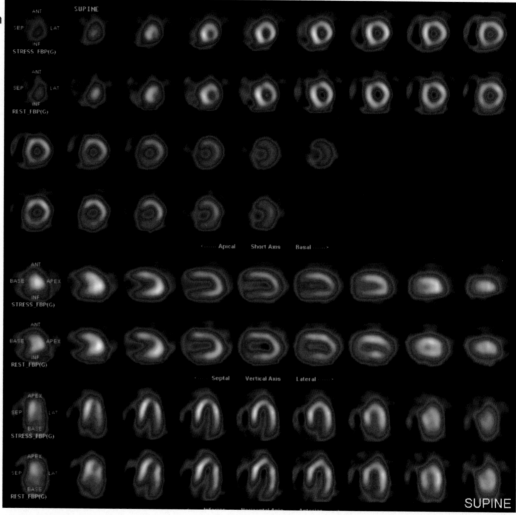

Figure 3.2

Findings: Distribution of the radiopharmaceutical is homogeneous throughout the myocardium on both sets of images, compatible with normal perfusion at both stress and rest. The polar plots reveal similar normal perfusion.

Discussion: The normal MPS is indicative of an excellent prognosis, even in the presence of an abnormal ECG or abnormal coronary angiography (96). A study of 652 patients who had a normal stress SPECT study alone and were followed for 2 years demonstrated that the overall cardiac event rate in these patients was <1% (97).

The overall sensitivity, specificity, and accuracy of ^{99m}Tc-tetrofosmin or ^{99m}Tc-sestamibi SPECT for the detection of myocardial ischemia is similar to that of ^{201}Tl imaging. The normal perfusion scan is indicative of an excellent prognosis, even in the presence of an abnormal coronary angiogram. The shorter half-life of ^{99m}Tc-labeled agents compared with ^{201}Tl allows

a higher dosage to be administered. This, combined with the higher energy of ^{99m}Tc, results in a higher count density than is possible using ^{201}Tl. Image quality is improved, and attenuation artifacts are less frequent and less severe. The higher count rate also allows high-quality gated images to be acquired in order to assess wall motion and ventricular function simultaneously with perfusion. Owing to the absence of significant redistribution, both supine and prone (or right lateral) imaging can be accomplished in instances where diaphragmatic attenuation artifact may pose a problem. A major disadvantage of ^{99m}Tc-labeled agents is that their use underestimates the extent of viable myocardium in comparison with ^{201}Tl imaging using a reinjection or 24-hour redistribution protocol, which can be overcome by nitrate administration (see Case 3.21 regarding the use of nitrate ^{99m}Tc-sestamibi for viability).

Diagnosis: Normal ^{99m}Tc-tetrofosmin rest/stress study.

CASE 3.3

History: A 70-year-old male with no prior history of CAD presented with a 2-week history of atypical chest pain. Cardiac risk factors included age, gender, HTN, and hypercholesterolemia. The resting ECG was normal. An exercise ^{99m}Tc-sestamibi SPECT (Fig. 3.3 A) was performed. The patient exercised for 9.5 minutes on a standard Bruce protocol without chest pain. Target HR was achieved. The stress ECG was suggestive of myocardial ischemia.

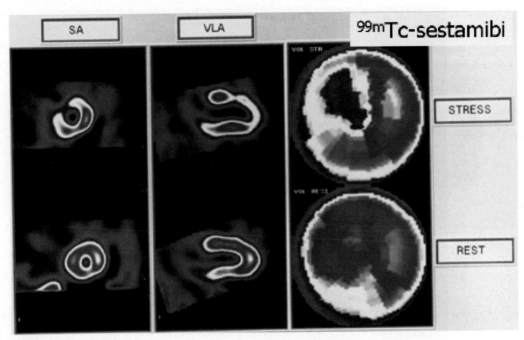

Figure 3.3 A

Findings: There is a reversible large defect involving the mid- and distal anteroseptal region and apex.

Discussion: Although the patient's symptoms were atypical, his advanced age and cardiac risk factors gave him a moderate to high pretest probability of having significant CAD. Upon the discovery of ischemia, the patient was referred for coronary angiography. Looking at the vascular territories and the LV segmentation as represented in Figures 3.3 B and 3.3 C, a large reversible defect, consistent with myocardial ischemia, in the LAD distribution can be clearly identified involving segments 2, 8, 14, and 17 and also partially involving segments 3, 9, 1, 7, 13 and 17. Coronary angiography showed a 90% proximal LAD stenosis. The patient underwent successful PTCA and stenting of the proximal LAD lesion.

^{99m}Tc-labeled perfusion agents and protocols are discussed in the introduction. The images should be interpreted with reference to the coronary anatomy, attempting to identify, from the perfusion image, what is the most likely site of anatomic obstruction. This is easier for the typical anterior, septal, and apical defect corresponding to the LAD distribution or the typical lateral wall defect of the left circumflex (LCX). It may become challenging when anatomic variation may lead to more than one vessel possibly being responsible for a territory. The inferior wall, for example, is usually perfused by the RCA; however, in some cases it is perfused by the LCX.

A popular method allowing quantification of perfusion abnormalities in relation to disease likelihood, prognosis, and viability is segmental analysis using a scoring system to grade the degree of perfusion for each segment of the heart. The current recommendation of the ASNC is division of the heart into 17 segments, adding one apical segment to the 16-segment model typically used for echocardiography (Figs. 3.3 B and 3.3 C) (98).

Coronary Artery Territories

Short Axis

Apical   Mid   Basal

Vertical Long Axis

Mid

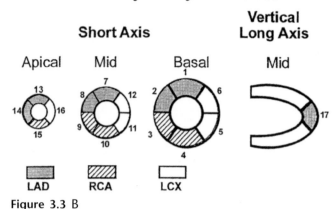

Figure 3.3 B

Left Ventricular Segmentation

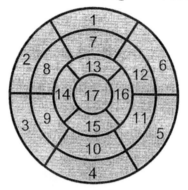

1. basal anterior
2. basal anteroseptal
3. basal inferoseptal
4. basal inferior
5. basal inferolateral
6. basal anterolateral

7. mid anterior
8. mid anteroseptal
9. mid inferoseptal
10. mid inferior
11. mid inferolateral
12. mid anterolateral

13. apical anterior
14. apical septal
15. apical inferior
16. apical lateral
17. apex

Figure 3.3 C Reproduced with permission from Cerqueira et al. (98)

However a large number of studies have been published using the Cedars–Sinai 20-segment model with five-point scoring: it includes six segments per slice, distal, midventricular, and basal, and two apical segments. Each segment is assigned a perfusion score between 0 and 4, 0 being normal and 4 denoting no perfusion. With the 20-segment model, a summed score of 1 to 3 indicates an equivocally abnormal study, a score of 4 to 7 a mildly abnormal study, a score of 8 to 12 a moderately abnormal study, and a score >13 a severely abnormal

study. In currently available software packages, these scores are generated from an analysis of segmental intensity and the standard deviation from that of normal databases. These scores must be corrected when an artifact is suspected, whether it is from motion, attenuation, or other sources. The summed stress score is compared with the summed rest score to generate a summed difference score.

Diagnosis: Anteroseptal and apical reversible defects consistent with myocardial ischemia due to severe LAD stenosis.

CASE 3.4

History: A 32-year-old male with chronic back pain and peptic ulcer disease presented with left-sided chest pain radiating to the arm. A dual-isotope rest ^{201}Tl/exercise ^{99m}Tc-tetrofosmin gated MPS was performed, as demonstrated in Figure 3.4. He exercised for 9 minutes using a standard Bruce protocol and reached 85% of MPHR. He complained of chest pain with deep inspiration but had no ECG changes suggestive of ischemia.

Stress ^{99m}Tc-tetrofosmin

Rest ^{201}Tl

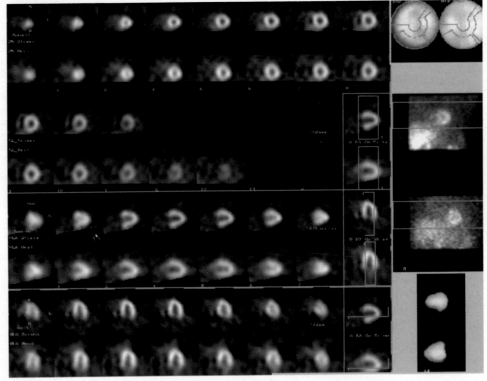

Figure 3.4 (From Vitola JV and Delbeke D, 2004 (11), by permission from Springer- Verlag)

Findings: There is homogenous myocardial perfusion on both stress and rest images. The gated images revealed normal wall motion and wall thickening. The LVEF after stress was 58% and the end-diastolic volume (EDV) and end-systolic volume (ESV) were 49 and 20 mL respectively, both of which are within normal limits.

Discussion: When images obtained with radiopharmaceuticals labeled with isotopes of different energies are compared, such as ^{99m}Tc and ^{201}Tl, the interpreter must take into account the technical differences in image quality. The ^{99m}Tc images have a better resolution than the ^{201}Tl images; therefore the ^{201}Tl images appear fuzzier, the walls of the myocardium are not as well defined and appear thicker, and the LV cavity appears smaller than on the ^{99m}Tc images. For the same reason, a perfusion defect may appear smaller on ^{201}Tl compared with ^{99m}Tc images, and partially reversible defects on dual-isotope studies are sometimes a diagnostic challenge. When semiquantitative analysis of perfusion and motion are performed, normal reference data are different for different isotopes, and the appropriate ones must be selected for accurate interpretation. Different reference values for left-ventricular ejection fraction (LVEF), ESV, EDV, and transient dilatation of the LV must also be taken into account.

Differential attenuation of isotopes of different energies by soft tissues such as diaphragm and breast can also be challenging and cause partially reversible defects that can be confused with ischemia. Imaging in both supine and prone positions is often helpful to assess the persistence of absence of a defect when the source of attenuation projects differently over the myocardium.

The comparison of gated-SPECT data on rest and stress images acquired with radiotracers of different energies is more challenging as well. LVEF is usually accurate, but wall motion analysis is less often interpretable with ^{201}Tl than with the ^{99m}Tc agents.

Advantages of the dual-isotope technique for MPS include faster protocol for rest/stress study, increasing throughput and the possibility of acquiring 24-hour delayed ^{201}Tl images for assessment of viability if fixed defects/hibernating myocardium is present (see Case 3.18).

The disadvantages include (a) the difference in resolution of the images and (b) differential attenuation related to the lower peak energy of ^{201}Tl compared with ^{99m}Tc, making the interpretation of the images more difficult, especially in obese patients. In addition, the dual-isotope protocol requires different filters and separate acquisition of the images. Simultaneous dual-isotope acquisition is complicated by cross-talk of ^{99m}Tc photons in the ^{201}Tl energy window.

The dual-isotope protocol is discussed in the introduction and shown on Figure 3.D.

Diagnosis: Normal dual-isotope rest ^{201}Tl/exercise ^{99m}Tc-tetrofosmin MPS.

History: A 57-year-old man with a prior MI was admitted with chest pain. An adenosine ^{201}Tl myocardial SPECT was performed (Fig. 3.5 A).

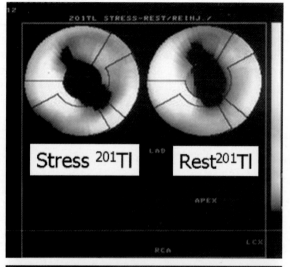

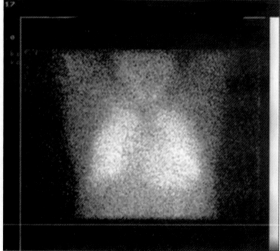

Figure 3.5 A

Findings: The polar plot demonstrates a fixed anteroapical defect. There was no evidence of ischemia on the stress/rest SPECT images (not shown). Increased pulmonary ^{201}Tl activity is present (Fig. 3.5 A), indicating increased pulmonary capillary pressure, extensive poststress dysfunction of the left ventricle (LV), advanced CAD, and high-related coronary risk.

Discussion: In the past, planar acquisitions of ^{201}Tl allowed identification of increased ^{201}Tl lung uptake on stress images and calculation of a lung-to-heart ratio, the upper limit of normal being 0.52. With SPECT acquisitions, planar images are not usually acquired, so increased lung activity must be identified on tomographic views or on the rotating cine display of the normalized data. SPECT data should not be used to calculate a lung-to-heart ratio (L/H), but software is available to calculate an accurate L/H from the cine data. In this case, it was markedly elevated to 0.74.

Increased pulmonary ^{201}Tl uptake is associated with severe LV dysfunction, a reduced LVEF, multivessel disease, and larger, more severe perfusion defects. There is a higher association with LAD disease when only single-vessel disease is present. By inference, poorer survival and increased frequency of cardiac events are associated with increased ^{201}Tl activity within the lung on stress MPS. Two factors identified as important for prognosis are resting LVEF and increased pulmonary uptake of ^{201}Tl with stress MPS. Both ^{201}Tl (99) and ^{99m}Tc-sestamibi can cause increased lung uptake and stress-induced LV dysfunction (100–103). Increased pulmonary uptake of ^{201}Tl reflects the increased pulmonary capillary wedge pressure, which can be caused by CAD but also by mitral valve regurgitation or stenosis, decreased LV compliance, and no-ischemic cardiomyopathy with LV dysfunction. Although both elevated transient ischemic dilatation (TID) and L/H are associated with severe

Stress ^{99m}Tc-sestamibi

Rest ^{99m}Tc-sestamibi

Figure 3.5 B

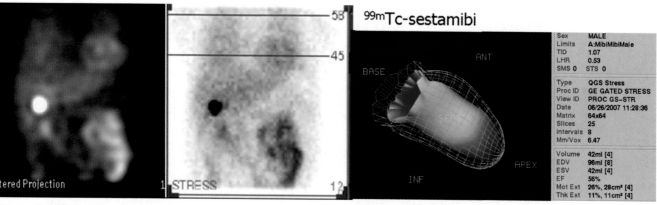

^{99m}Tc-sestamibi

Sex	MALE
Limits	A:MibiMibiMale
TID	1.07
LHR	0.53
SMS 0	STS 0
Type	QGS Stress
Proc ID	GE GATED STRESS
View ID	PROC GS-STR
Date	06/26/2007 11:28:36
Matrix	64x64
Slices	25
Intervals	8
Mm/Vox	6.47
Volume	42ml [4]
EDV	96ml [8]
ESV	42ml [4]
EF	56%
Mot Ext	26%, 28cm² [4]
Thk Ext	11%, 11cm² [4]

Figure 3.5 C

CAD, they have no significant correlation, as demonstrated in a study of 1,129 consecutive patients undergoing pharmacologic stress with dipyridamole and ^{201}Tl (101). Increased L/H on resting ^{201}Tl images is weakly associated with higher LV end-diastolic pressure and pulmonary wedge pressure and lower LVEF (102).

There was a concern that ^{99m}Tc-perfusion radiopharmaceuticals do not accumulate in the lungs to the same extent as ^{201}Tl does in patients with CAD. However, a Phase III multicenter study showed a fair correlation between the two imaging agents when L/H of 0.50 and 0.44 were chosen for ^{201}Tl and ^{99m}Tc-tetrofosmin, respectively (103).

Figures 3.5 B and 3.5 C shows images from another patient, with known CAD, with large areas of moderate to severe ischemia including all three coronary territories, associated with significant transient ischemic dilation (TID) of the LV and increased lung uptake of ^{99m}Tc-sestamibi (L/H ratio of 0.53). On Figure 3.5 C, the level of lung uptake is similar to the uptake seen in the liver.

An automatic algorithm assessing L/H on exercise ^{99m}Tc-sestamibi images correlated well with manually derived values on both ^{99m}Tc-sestamibi images and ^{201}Tl images. An L/H >0.44 yielded a sensitivity and specificity of 63% and 81%, respectively, for identifying severe and extensive CAD (103). A study of 149 patients evaluated with exercise ^{201}Tl scintigraphy demonstrated a higher event rate in patients with an L/H ratio >0.5 (104).

Diagnosis: Diffuse pulmonary uptake of ^{201}Tl and ^{99m}Tc-sestamibi due to severe CAD in two patients.

CASE 3.6

History: A 63-year-old man presents with recent onset of chest pain induced with exercise. However, he reports that his pain resolves as exercise continues. His family history is remarkable for the sudden death of his brother at 50 years of age. He has no other significant risk factors. His baseline ECG (Fig. 3.6 A) demonstrates left anterior hemiblock (LAHB). He was referred for a rest/stress ^{99m}Tc-sestamibi study. He underwent exercise on the TMT, using the Bruce protocol, exercising for 9 minutes. During exercise he had no significant ST-segment changes on his ECG (Fig. 3.6 B). His HR and BP were normal. He was injected at a HR of 139 bpm. During exercise, he developed pain at minute 6 of the Bruce protocol, which progressively subsided until it disappeared at peak exercise (Fig. 3.6 C). SPECT images were acquired (Fig. 3.6 C).

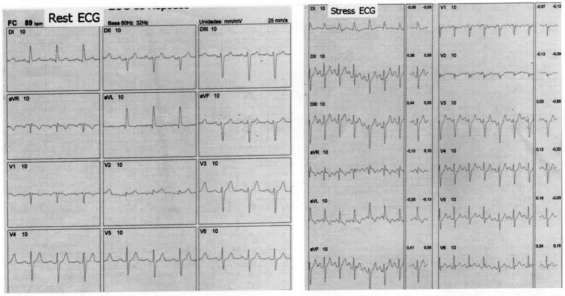

Figure 3.6 A

Figure 3.6 B

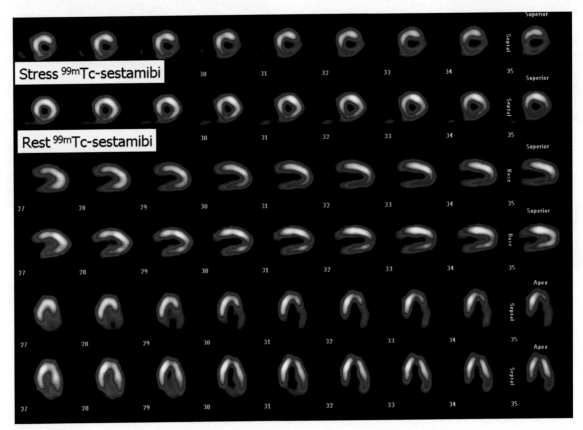

Figure 3.6 C

Findings: There is a reversible defect along the lateral and inferior walls consistent with ischemia.

Discussion: The MPS results prompted coronary angiography, which showed a critical lesion in the LCX. His symptoms, which disappeared as exercise continued, are related to what has been described as "walking through angina" (105). Some controversy exists whether this phenomenon relates to recruitment of collateral circulation, coronary spasm or ischemic preconditioning. In this case, it is clear that this patient was ischemic, and collateral vessels could not explain the relief of his symptoms at peak stress.

The TMT has limitations in both sensitivity and specificity. Additionally, the exercise ECG is uninterpretable in patients with LBBB and pacemakers. Some baseline ECG abnormalities make any additional changes during exercise poorly specific, such as those that may occur in left ventricular hypertrophy (LVH), with the use of some medications such as digitalis, and in the presence of Wolf-Parkinson-White syndrome or prior MI. Furthermore, the sensitivity of TMT is decreased, especially when it is related to a limited capacity to achieve an adequate increment of myocardial oxygen consumption owing either to limited exercise capacity LAHB, (such as in the present case), or because of concurrent treatment with some medications, such as calcium channel blockers and beta blockers.

The sensitivity of the TMT alone is around 60% to 70%, and it can be lower for the diagnosis of single-vessel disease (106). It has been said that TMT sensitivity is even lower for ischemia involving the LCX territory, possibly because of its anatomic location (107,108). The lateral wall of the heart and the inferolateral region are quite posterior anatomically, with the RV positioned more anteriorly, near the sternum. If additional leads were used, extending the evaluation more posteriorly (V7 and V8), ECG sensitivity could be increased slightly. The prevalence of CAD in patients 63 years of age, presenting with atypical symptoms, as in the current case, is about 60% (109) . In cases where there is doubt, MPS should be used for further risk stratification. TMT is also less accurate in women than in men owing to a higher number of false-positive exercise ECG results (110). A meta-analysis determined the weighted average sensitivities and specificities of exercise ECG, exercise ^{201}Tl, and exercise echocardiography in women (111), demonstrating that cardiac imaging increases overall accuracy. The lower specificities may be due to a digoxin-like effect of circulating estrogens, resulting in varying changes in the ST segment and leading to a higher false-positive rate of exercise ECG stress testing in women (112). In summary, the TMT is a good proven modality for diagnosis and the determination of prognosis in patients suspected of having CAD, but a wide variety of limitations restricts its utility, requiring the use of alternative or complementary modalities in many patients.

MPS is one of the most sensitive and specific methods for the noninvasive evaluation of myocardial ischemia. Pooled data from 19 studies (113) have shown a sensitivity of 83% to 98% (with a mean of 92%) and a specificity of 53% to 100% (with a mean of 77%) for detecting ischemia.

In this case, MPS added prognostic information and stratified this patient in the high-risk category. This information changed the patient's management and prompted coronary angiography; this showed the LCX lesion, which had not been diagnosed by the exercise TMT alone. MPS in patients without known CAD adds prognostic information to the TMT, even in patients with a low DTS (114) .

Diagnosis: Severe ischemia in the LCX territory detected by MPS, with no ECG changes during exercise.

CASE 3.7

History: A 58-year-old man with known CAD presented with a 3-week history of occasional exertional chest pain 6 years following coronary artery bypass graft (CABG) surgery. He had stopped smoking cigarettes, and his hyperlipidemia and HTN were well controlled with medications. He remained sedentary owing to chronic low back pain. An adenosine ^{201}Tl SPECT (Fig. 3.7) was performed without the occurrence of diagnostic ECG changes or arrhythmias.

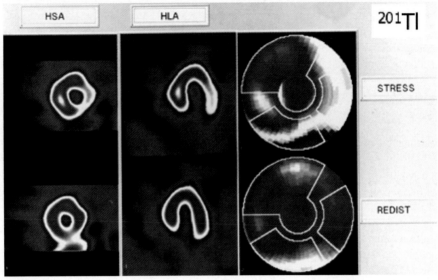

Figure 3.7

Finding: There is a reversible perfusion abnormality along the lateral wall.

Discussion: These findings represent clear evidence of ischemia in the distribution of the LCX, induced with pharmacologic stress and subsequently confirmed at coronary angiography. Pharmacologic stress is an excellent alternative for patients unable to exercise appropriately or those using medications that prevent reaching target HR. Details regarding pharmacologic stress and different protocols are discussed in the introduction to this chapter.

Diagnosis: Lateral wall ischemia, detected on SPECT using pharmacologic stress, due to severe stenosis of the LCX.

CASE 3.8

History: A 66-year-old female, obese and with a history of CAD as well as prior stent placement, presented with sensations of burning in the chest at rest unrelated to exertion. She is referred to nuclear medicine for a rest/stress ^{99m}Tc-sestamibi gated study on separate days (Figs. 3.8 A and 3.8 B). Owing to her limited exercise capacity, a protocol combining standard dipyridamole infusion for 4 minutes and simultaneous exercise on the treadmill (Bruce protocol, limited to stages 1 and 2) was used. The patient was injected at 2 minutes after termination of dipyridamole and while still walking on the treadmill at a HR of 131 bpm (barely reaching 85% of MPHR). During exercise, the patient developed chest pain, tightness, and ST-segment depression on the ECG (not shown).

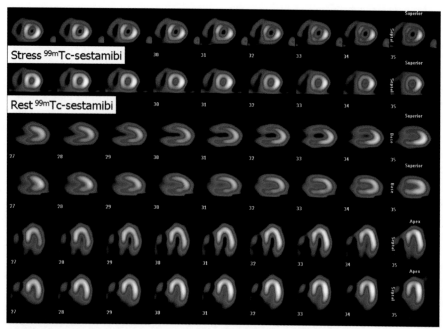

Figure 3.8 A

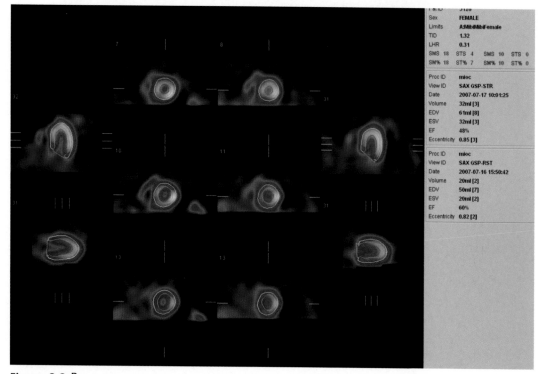

Figure 3.8 B

Findings: SPECT images demonstrated moderate-sized moderately severe reversible defect involving the anterolateral region of the heart. The transient ischemic dilation (TID) index is 1.32.

Discussion: The combination of vasodilator and low-level exercise, also known as DipEx or AdenoEx, is a good alternative for patients requiring pharmacologic stress. Details about this protocol are discussed in the introduction of this chapter. In this case, TID is a marker of severe myocardial ischemia, indicating a poor prognosis (115–119). The dilation represents either subendocardial ischemia or true LV cavity dilation. If there is global subendocardial ischemia on the stress images, the apparent LV dilation is probably due to uptake in a thinner area through the thickness of the myocardium (epicardial region only). It has also been suggested that poststress end-systolic dilation can be due to endocardial postischemic stunning (120). TID can be determined subjectively (see Case 3.5) or from automatically derived stress and rest measurements of ventricular volume. TID must persist poststress during the actual SPECT acquisition to be detected. It has been first described on ^{201}Tl studies (defined as abnormal when the TID ratio > 1.12) and have been shown to have a sensitivity of 60% and a specificity of 95% for identifying patients with multivessel critical stenoses (115). The significance of TID after pharmacologic stress is similar to that of exercise testing (121) with a similar specificity but lower sensitivity. A study of 110 patients with suspected CAD using dipyridamole ^{201}Tl-MPS demonstrated TID more frequently in patients with multivessel disease than those with single vessel disease and that the sensitivity of TID in identifying patients with multivessel disease was 27% and the specificity was 95% (122). In addition, ECG changes were observed more frequently in patients with TID.

Normal thresholds for TID ratio can vary slightly according to the type of stress and type of radiopharmaceutical and protocol used (from <1.14 to <1.40) (123). For dual-isotope rest ^{201}Tl/exercise ^{99m}Tc-sestamibi studies, abnormal TID ratio values correspond to LV endocardial volume ratios greater than 1.20. These criteria identify severe and/or extensive CAD with a sensitivity and specificity of 71% and 95% respectively. An increased TID ratio has also been associated with a poor prognosis and increased cardiac event rate in a study of 512 patients evaluated with dipyridamole and ^{99m}Tc-labeled agents (124). The patient in the present case had a TID of 1.32.

Diagnosis: Myocardial ischemia detected using the combination of vasodilator and low-workload exercise in a patient with limited exercise capacity. Transient ischemic dilation was seen.

CASE 3.9

History: A 37-year-old man with no history of heart disease presented to the emergency department (ED) with moderately severe chest pain. His physical examination was unremarkable. The resting ECG and enzymes were nondiagnostic. While he was in the ED, experiencing severe chest pain, a dose of 24 mCi of ^{99m}Tc-tetrofosmin was injected intravenously and SPECT MPS images were obtained (Fig. 3.9).

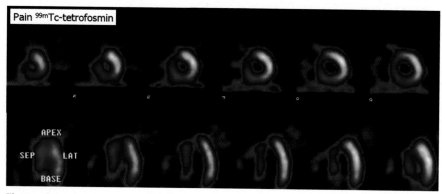

Pain ^{99m}Tc-tetrofosmin

APEX
SEP   LAT
BASE

Figure 3.9

Findings: Images demonstrate a severe perfusion defect along the anteroseptal region, septum, and apex, consistent with a lesion in the LAD territory.

Discussion: There is increasing evidence that ^{99m}Tc-sestamibi or tetrofosmin MPS may be effectively used to triage patients presenting to the ED with chest pain of unclear etiology. If a patient with an acute coronary ischemic syndrome is injected at rest while experiencing chest pain, the distribution of the perfusion agent should demonstrate a zone of diminished perfusion. Of course one cannot differentiate acute ischemia from acute infarction or remote infarction using perfusion imaging data alone. However, when combined with clinical data, this differentiation can usually be accomplished with a reasonable degree of certainty. In equivocal cases, a rest study can be repeated at a later time, after resolution of the chest pain, for further clarification.

In the current case, there was no past history or any ECG evidence of prior infarct, so the perfusion abnormality present at the time of chest pain is most consistent with acute ischemia or acute infarction. The patient was efficiently triaged for admission to the coronary care unit. Coronary angiography was performed early after admission, demonstrating a critical stenosis of the proximal LAD.

Management of patients presenting to the ED with chest pain suggestive of acute MI remains a continuing challenge (125). ED visits for the evaluation of chest pain or other symptoms suggestive of acute coronary symptoms exceed 5 million each year in the United States, and more than 40% of these visits lead to costly hospitalization. Of patients presenting to the ED with acute chest pain, a majority will have an ECG that is normal or nondiagnostic for acute myocardial ischemia or MI; only a minority will eventually be diagnosed with an acute coronary syndrome (ACS) (126). Typically, these patients are admitted to exclude acute myocardial infarction (AMI) despite a very low incidence of ACS. However, missed ACS in patients who are inadvertently sent home from the ED has significant adverse outcomes and associated legal consequences (127,128).

To reduce unnecessary admissions but maintain patient safety and enhance cost-effectiveness, innovative strategies have been applied to the management of patients with chest pain. Many medical centers have developed chest pain centers and are using a wide range of diagnostic strategies to deal with this dilemma. A MPS can play an important role in this setting by providing a safe and efficient means for risk stratification of patients with a low-to-moderate likelihood of unstable angina (129).

The sensitivity of a rest MPS is not the same when patients are injected after cessation of pain as compared with those injected during the pain; therefore, an exercise MPS is warranted for patients who are pain-free and have no perfusion defects at rest. Cardiac markers, particularly the troponin, are very specific for the detection of a larger part of the spectrum of ACS in the ED, including patients with minimal myocardial damage and a higher risk of short-term death and nonfatal AMI (130). However the sensitivity for unstable angina requires additional workup strategies to discharge these patients safely (131).

According to the results of the ERASE trial (132), MPS with ^{99m}Tc-sestamibi in the ED reduces the number of unnecessary admissions without increasing mistaken discharges. ERASE was the first prospective, multicenter, randomized trial to address this issue and its findings are in agreement with those of previous observational studies. In ERASE, 2,475 patients were randomized with chest pain or other ischemia symptoms to either standard ED evaluation strategies or usual care plus acute resting MPS using ^{99m}Tc-sestamibi SPECT. The standard ED assessment was as good as standard care plus ^{99m}Tc-sestamibi study in terms of appropriately determining that these patients should be hospitalized (80% to 90%). Both strategies were equally effective in identifying these true ACS patients (13%).

^{99m}Tc-sestamibi imaging seemed to have some advantages in identifying patients without ischemia who did not need to be hospitalized. In the standard-care group, 52% of nonischemic patients were unnecessarily hospitalized compared with 42% of those who underwent a ^{99m}Tc-sestamibi scan, meaning a 10% absolute reduction.

The ASNC has published a position statement on radionuclide imaging in patients with suspected acute ischemic syndromes in the ED or chest pain center. Six studies including a total of 2,113 patients performed between 1993 and 1999 demonstrated a weighted average negative predictive value of 99.2% for the detection of ACS with MPS during chest pain. The reliability of the resting scan alone is controversial if the ^{99m}Tc perfusion agent is administered after the resolution of chest discomfort. Therefore it is recommended that the radiopharmaceutical be injected during ongoing chest pain and not more than 2 hours after cessation of the symptoms. Stress testing is recommended (when ACS is excluded) to evaluate whether the presence of CAD is a contributor to the symptoms.

Developing strategies that aggressively identify the patient with ACS can shorten the time to therapy and result in improved prognosis. Furthermore, quickly and safely discharging patients in whom the ACS is not present is necessary. MPS can play a pivotal role in achieving these goals.

Diagnosis: Unstable angina with critical LAD lesions diagnosed early in the ED using the rest/perfusion protocol.

CASE 3.10

History: A 57-year-old woman experienced chest pain radiating into her arm and presents for an exercise ^{201}Tl perfusion SPECT study (Fig. 3.10 A). She is a smoker and has hypertension and hypercholesterolemia as well as a positive family history of CAD. She exercised on a treadmill for 8.5 minutes to a HR of 161 bpm, achieving a double product of 32,700. Chest pain occurred at 5 minutes, and a 1.5-mm ST-segment depression developed on her ECG.

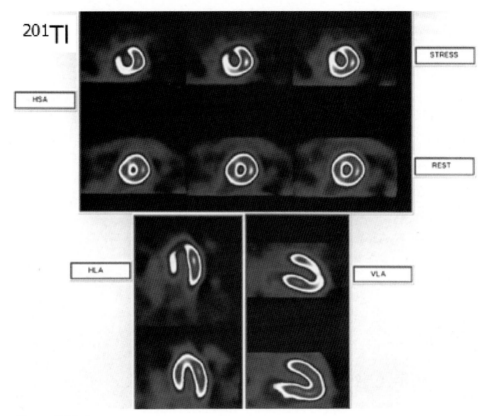

Figure 3.10 A

Findings: There is a severe perfusion defect in the anteroseptal region and a moderate perfusion defect along the septum on the stress images with complete reversibility at rest, consistent with ischemia.

Discussion: The images represent a classic finding of myocardial ischemia in the distribution of the LAD. At coronary angiography, the patient had an 80% stenosis of the LAD that was treated by angioplasty. She returned 4 months later with somewhat atypical exertional chest pain. A repeat exercise ^{201}Tl SPECT (Fig. 3.10 B) was obtained, which revealed normal ho-

mogenous uptake throughout the myocardium. The normal follow-up scan indicated the successful result of PTCA resulting in the patency of the LAD. Therefore repeat angiography was avoided.

At present, there is more percutaneous coronary intervention (PCI) performed in the United States than there are open heart procedures. Myocardial perfusion scintigraphy is an effective tool for evaluating patients after therapy, including revascularization and medical therapy (see Case 3.11 for further discussion).

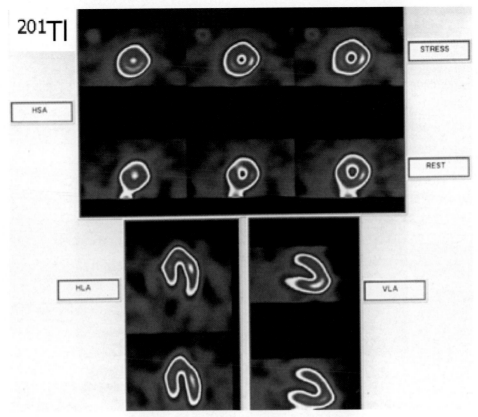

Figure 3.10 B

The issue of CAD in women has been the subject of many investigations. The AHA has made great efforts to bring this issue into awareness for both the general population and physicians. There is generally a misconception that CAD is a disease of the male gender; however, the prevalence of CAD in women, contrary to the general belief, is quite high, although the affected women are usually older than the affected men. There is enough evidence to suggest that CAD in women is more aggressive than in men and that the mortality rate is higher when the disease is established. Annually, approximately 50,000 more women than men die as the result of heart disease. Thirty-eight percent of women die in the first year after an acute MI, as compared with 25% of men. Women suffering from CAD do not necessarily present with typical chest pain; therefore their disease may be overlooked. Their usual presentation consists of nonspecific symptoms such as indigestion, nausea, vomiting, dyspnea, and fatigue. Awareness of the atypical presentation of CAD in women is key to its early diagnosis and timely management. Note should be made that a perfusion abnormality on a woman's SPECT MPI images are associated with a higher rate of cardiac events as compared with the same defect in a man, especially in diabetic women (see discussion of Case 3.20).

Diagnosis: Typical LAD ischemia in a female patient successfully treated with angioplasty.

CASE 3.11

History: A 52-year-old male patient with chest pain and hypercholesterolemia is referred for a rest/stress ^{99m}Tc-sestamibi study. The patient exercised for 10 minutes on the treadmill using the Ellestad protocol. He has a normal HR and BP response. His chest pain was reproduced by exercise during the test. His ECG showed a 1-mm ST-segment depression at peak exercise (V5 and V6). He was injected with ^{99m}Tc-sestamibi at peak exercise and SPECT images were obtained 30 minutes later (Fig. 3.11 A).

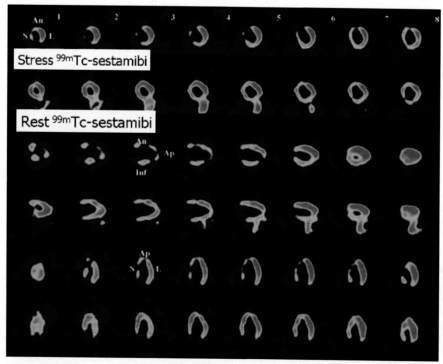

Figure 3.11 A

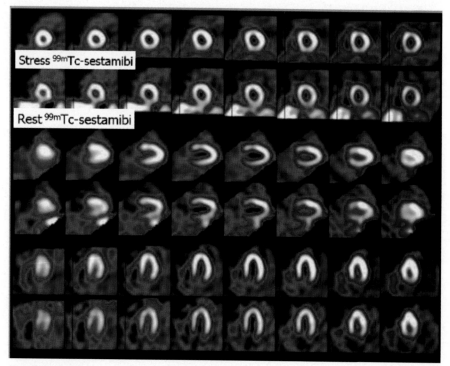

Figure 3.11 B

Findings: Figure 3.11 A reveals a severe, extensive, exercise-induced perfusion defect involving the anteroseptal region, the entire septum and the apex, consistent with LAD disease. The patient underwent coronary angiography, confirming a proximal critical LAD lesion. A drug-eluting stent was placed to treat the lesion. Twelve months after stenting, the patient returned complaining of atypical chest pain. He underwent another rest/stress ^{99m}Tc-sestamibi which was normal (Fig. 3.11 B). The patient's chest pain was not reproducible by exercise and was considered atypical for ischemia.

Discussion: Figure 3.11 A as compared with Figure 3.11 B shows resolution of a previously noted ischemia, illustrating that MPS can be used to evaluate the result of PCI using the new generation of drug-eluting stents. However, the routine use of MPS for the evaluation of patients after revascularization procedures is debatable. According to the guidelines for clinical use of cardiac radionuclide imaging, routine evaluation is not indicated for asymptomatic patients (13). The use of nuclear imaging should be symptom-driven (as in the present case), and early testing for all patients following PCI should be discouraged unless the clinical scenario warrants otherwise, especially when there is a higher risk of silent ischemia.

Compared with balloon angioplasty alone, coronary stenting has been shown to decrease the rate of restenosis significantly (133), supporting the view that the routine evaluation of asymptomatic patients may not be necessary. However, routine evaluation with MPS may be recommended in diabetic patients, as they can have ischemia without symptoms of chest pain, and the rate of restenosis is higher in this population. MPS has been considered a reliable method for the detection of restenosis (134) and has a higher accuracy for the detection of restenosis than for the occurrence of angina or exercise-induced ECG changes (135). Milavetz et al. (136) studied 209 patients within a year of stenting, showing a sensitivity and specificity of 95% and 70% for the detection of significantly angiographically treated stenosis (over 70%). The positive predictive values, negative predictive values, and accuracy of the results are 88%, 89%, and 88% respectively. Ischemia due to endothelial dysfunction can be demonstrated by MPS, whereas coronary angiography may be normal.

Recommendations for MPS post-PCI are as follows (13): (a) For symptomatic patients, MPS may be used if restenosis, occlusion, or subocclusion is suspected, and (b) for asymptomatic patients, the follow-up MPS may be helpful for the

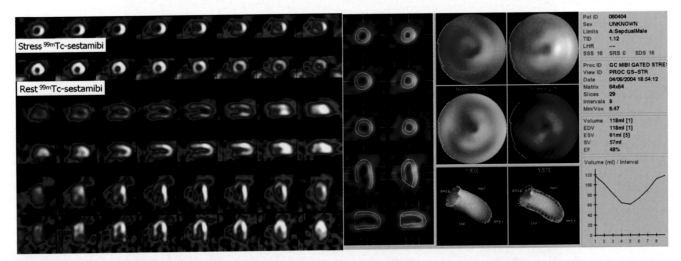

Figure 3.11 C

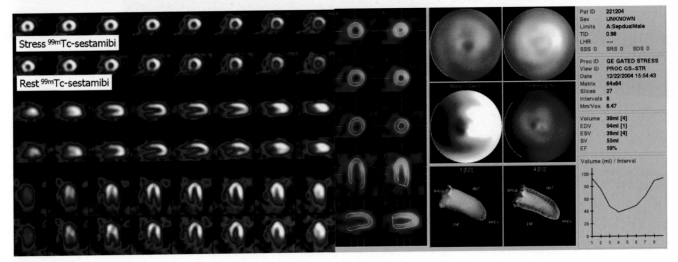

Figure 3.11 D

risk-stratification of patients at risk for silent ischemia (diabetics).

Myocardial perfusion scintigraphy also plays a major role in the follow-up of patients post-CABG procedures. The long-term effectiveness of CABG has been limited owing to graft stenosis and progression of CAD in the native vessels; both of these can be effectively evaluated by MPS (13,137).

Figure 3.11 C represents pre-CABG MPS in a patient with an extensive abnormality in the LAD territory. His gated SPECT demonstrated an ESV of 61 mL, LVEF of 48% (myocardial stunning), and a TID of 1.12. His annual follow-up post-CABG

Recommendations are as follows: (a) For symptomatic post-CABG patients, MPS is indicated, providing diagnostic and prognostic information; (b) for asymptomatic patients, MPS is indicated if the CABG procedure was performed more than 5 years earlier or the patient's exercise capacity is limited (less than 6 METS) regardless of the age of the CABG or if there is a possibility of silent ischemia.

Myocardial perfusion scintigraphy is also helpful for following patients with CAD treated medically. Medical therapy (including anti-ischemic medications and risk-factor modification) is used to treat CAD even in the presence of anatomically significant lesions.

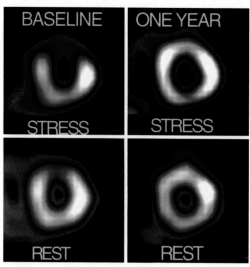

Figure 3.11 E Reproduced with permission from O'Rourke et al. (140).

MPS (Fig. 3.11 D), despite his atypical chest pain, shows a marked improvement in the LAD perfusion abnormality (Fig. 3.11 C and 3.11 D) and improved left ventricular function. The ESV decreased to 39 mL, and the LVEF increased to 59%. The TID noted previously is no longer seen.

A normal MPS in post-CABG patients indicates a good prognosis and a low risk for cardiovascular events. Zellweger et al. (138) suggest that symptomatic patients who are less than 5 years out from CABG would benefit from MPS. The perfusion images would demonstrate the severity and extent of ischemia, if present, and provide guidance to therapy. This same study indicates that all patients, regardless of the symptom, would benefit from MPS if they were more than 5 years post-CABG procedures. Lauer et al. (137) reviewed 873 symptomatic patients who underwent exercise ^{201}Tl SPECT imaging following CABG to evaluate the prognostic value of MPS in predicting the cardiac death and nonfatal MI. They concluded that perfusion defects and impaired exercise capacity (less than 6 metabolic equivalents, or METS) were strong and independent predictors of adverse events and that routine screening exercise MPS post-CABG should be considered in asymptomatic patients.

Figure 3.11 E represents a baseline and 1-year follow-up MPS of a 50-year-old hypertensive patient with hypercholesterolemia who complained of typical exertional angina over the preceding 6 weeks. His baseline MPS shows marked ischemic changes of the anterior wall. Coronary angiography revealed 80% stenosis of the mid-LAD and 50% ostial stenosis of the RCA. One year following aggressive medical therapy to control his hypertension and hypercholesterolemia, the MPS shows complete resolution of the perfusion abnormality.

The COURAGE trial randomized 2,287 patients with objective evidence of myocardial ischemia to medical therapy or PCI plus medical therapy. The 4- to 6-year follow-up revealed no significant difference between the groups regarding the rate of death, MI, stroke, or hospitalization for ACS. However, MPS played a significant role in the COURAGE trial not only as a modality to document the ischemia but also to monitor therapy and identify those high-risk patients requiring coronary angiography and/or PCI (140).

Diagnosis: Severe ischemia in the LAD territory detected and monitored by MPS in 3 patients following PCI with stent, CABG, and aggressive medical treatment.

CASE 3.12

History: A 66-year-old male with no known CAD was referred for preoperative evaluation prior to the surgical correction of a right femoral artery stenosis. The patient reported substernal typical and atypical chest pain partially relieved with nitroglycerin. Cardiac risk factors included HTN, tobacco use, peripheral vascular disease (PVD), cerebrovascular disease, age, and gender. The resting ECG revealed a RBBB. Treadmill exercise was not possible owing to PVD, dipyridamole and adenosine were contraindicated because of recent TIAs. A dobutamine ^{201}Tl SPECT (Fig. 3.12) was performed with an adequate hemodynamic response. The patient did not experience chest pain. His stress ECG was positive for myocardial ischemia.

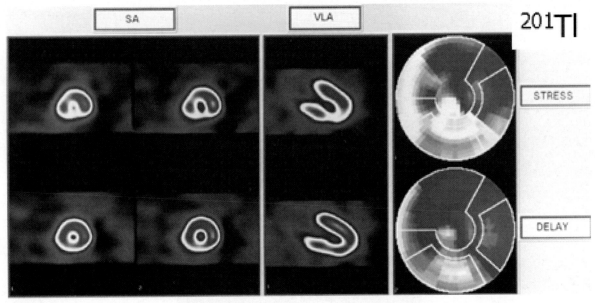

Figure 3.12

Findings: There are moderately severe reversible defects involving the mid-to-basal septum and the distal inferior wall.

Discussion: The scintigraphic findings are positive for severe ischemic changes. The patient was referred for coronary angiography, which revealed a 60% ostial lesion of the left main artery, 40% and 50% tandem lesions of the mid-LAD, 50% to 60% stenosis of the LCX, and 80% of the mid-RCA. The patient's elective surgery was postponed and he underwent CABG.

Myocardial perfusion scintigraphy is used frequently for the preoperative assessment of patients who are scheduled for elective nonvascular and, in particular, vascular surgery. There is a high prevalence of CAD in patients with PVD (141), 60% of whom have associated CAD. This has been documented in a series of 1,000 patients who underwent coronary angiography prior to vascular surgery. The utility of MPS in the preoperative evaluation of patients has been reviewed in a meta-analysis (142). The studies included 1,994 preoperative patients evaluated with dipyridamole ^{201}Tl and revealed ischemia in 26%. Among these, nonfatal MI or cardiovascular death occurred in 9% postoperatively. This is in contrast to the 1.4% event rate noted in 22% of patients who demonstrated a normal MPS preoperatively.

In the preoperative assessment of patients undergoing elective surgery, in particular vascular surgery, MPS can be performed using pharmacologic stress protocols, as these patients commonly are unable to exercise.

Although there are only a few cases of transient or permanent neurologic deficit reported in patients given dipyridamole or adenosine, many investigators advise against their use in patients with recent cerebrovascular accidents (CVAs) or ongoing transient ischemic attacks (TIAs). In the proper clinical setting, dobutamine can be used. Dobutamine increases the cardiac workload (HR and myocardial contractility) and may induce ischemia, as noted in this patient. Should it become necessary, the beta-agonist effect of dobutamine may be reversed quickly by IV administration of a beta blocker such as esmolol.

Diagnosis: Ischemic heart disease detected by MPS during a preoperative evaluation for vascular surgery.

CASE 3.13

History: A 66-year-old male with known three-vessel CAD who underwent CABG 3 years earlier presented with recurrent chest pain. He was referred for rest/stress MPS and coronary CTA. The study was performed using an integrated SPECT/64-slice MDCT system and a common imaging table (Ventri gamma camera and a GE Lightspeed VCT system from GE Healthcare, Waukesha, WI). Resting and gated postadenosine SPECT images were acquired first in the supine position using a low-dose rest/high-dose stress same day ^{99m}Tc-tetrofosmin protocol. After completion of the poststress images and without moving the patient from the imaging table, the HR was controlled with beta blockers and a breath-hold coronary CTA was performed. The rest/stress SPECT images (Fig. 3.13 A), coronary tree from the coronary CTA (Figure 3.13 B), multiplanar reformatted images (MPR) from the coronary CTA images (Figure 3.13 B), and fusion of the coronary tree on the 3D myocardial perfusion maps obtained from MPS (Fig. 3.13 C) are displayed. The fusion image was obtained using a software package (CardIQ Fusion, GE Healthcare, Waukesha, WI).

Stress ^{99m}Tc-tetrofosmin no AC

Rest ^{99m}Tc-tetrofosmin no AC

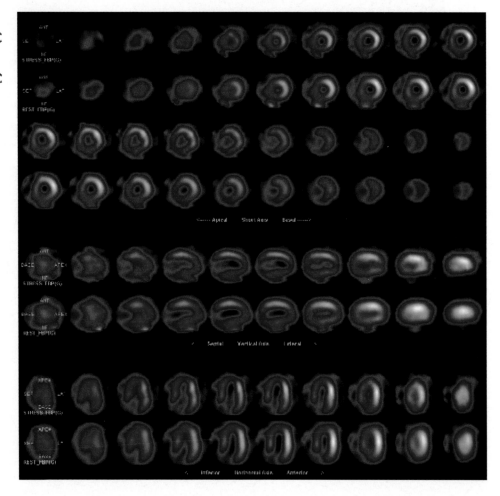

Figure 3.13 A

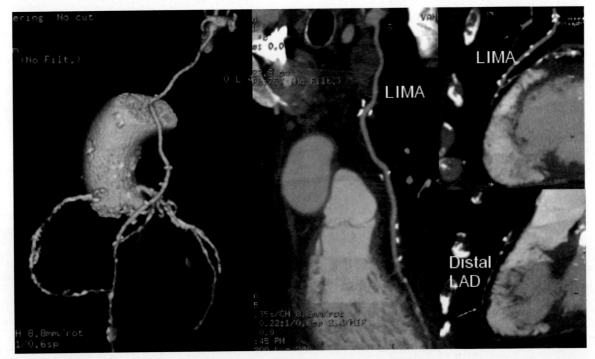

Figure 3.13 B

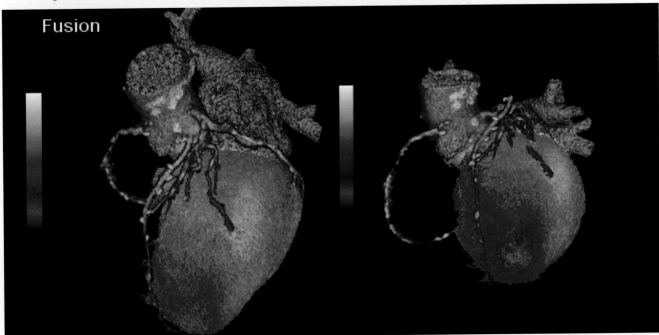

Figure 3.13 C

Findings: The rest/stress MPS demonstrated a fixed inferior wall defect consistent with MI that persisted on prone imaging (not shown) and a questionable reversible apical defect (Fig. 3.13 A). The poststress LVEF was 49%, with hypokinesis of the inferior wall and apex (not shown). The coronary tree clearly demonstrated the left internal mammary artery (LIMA) graft originating from the left subclavian artery and anastomosed into the mid-LAD (Fig. 3.13 B). Multiplanar reformatted images of the coronary CTA demonstrated diffuse narrowing of the RCA, corresponding to the inferior wall defect and moderate diffuse irregularities of the LCX (not shown). There was subtotal occlusion of the LAD, a patent LIMA graft to the middle third of the LAD, and patent anastomosis, but there was also stenosis along the runoff to the apex (Fig. 3.13 C). This stenosis corresponded to the questionable reversible apical defect on the fusion images.

Discussion: For this patient, the combination of MPS and coronary CTA demonstrated diffuse disease in the right coronary system and a patent LIMA graft to the LAD. Diffuse disease in the distal LAD may have been responsible for the recurrent chest pain and the questionable ischemia in the apex.

The fusion image of the coronary tree on the 3D map of perfusion helps identify stenoses with functional impact. The combination of the anatomic and functional studies led to more intense medical therapy and avoided invasive coronary angiography because revascularization was not possible.

The cardiac PET/multidetector CT (MDCT) and SPECT/MDCT technology allows evaluation, in one imaging setting, of (a) calcium scoring, (b) coronary artery anatomy with contrast-enhanced CT coronary angiography, (c) rest/stress MPS and localization of the hypoperfused regions to specific coronary arteries.

MPS and CTA images can be obtained from different systems at different times or from an integrated system, as in this case. Fusion images can be generated using software packages. Good reviews of the potential applications of this new integrated technology are available (143,144).

Detection, description, and characterization of plaque by CT in the early stages of CAD could play an important role in preventing both CAD progression and its complications. Coronary CTA allows noninvasive detection of atherosclerotic plaques, estimation of plaque burden, and characterization of plaques. Various plaques subtype can be characterized using CT density measurements (Hounsfield units).

A study compared data from 64-slice MDCT coronary CTA and invasive coronary angiography in 67 patients and showed that the sensitivity, specificity, and positive and negative predictive values of coronary CTA were 94%, 97%, 87%, and 99%, respectively (145). Two other studies have reported similar sensitivity, specificity, and negative predictive values using 64-slice MDCT (146,147). In these studies, the number of nonevaluable segments ranged from 0% to 12%. However, a multicenter trial using 16-slice CTA reported limited positive predictive value compared to catheter angiography owing to a large number of false-positive studies related to unevaluable segments (148). In addition, quantitative estimates of stenosis severity from 64-slice CTA correlates only modestly with quantitative coronary angiography (146). There is a high degree of agreement in the literature regarding the high negative predictive value of a normal coronary CTA: 97% with 16-slice MDCT (149–151), and 99% with 64-slice MDCT (146). Therefore coronary CTA may be very useful to exclude CAD in a population of patients with equivocal clinical or other findings.

The advantages of coronary CTA compared with catheter coronary angiography include noninvasiveness, true 3D imaging, lower cost, better characterization of plaques (calcium deposits versus soft plaque), and better delineation of ostial stenoses combined evaluation of coronaries, plaque morphology, valves, myocardial mass and function, lungs, and thoracic aorta.

The limitations of coronary CTA are as follows: (a) limited visualization of distal segments, segments of small size, and tortuous segments; (b) overestimation or underestimation of stenosis secondary to coronary arterial calcification; (c) no real-time assessment of flow through vessels; (d) no direct assessment of collateral vessels; (e) no intervention possible during the examination; (f) technological difficulties related to persistent irregular HR, such as atrial fibrillation, resulting in interscan discontinuities prohibiting evaluation of coronary artery stenoses; (g) contraindication in patients with contrast allergy or renal failure.

For the evaluation of patients with CABG, coronary CTA can provide a good roadmap of the coronaries and graft prior to invasive catheter angiography. A good review article is available (152). In planning a coronary CTA of a patient with saphenous venous grafts (SVGs), the field of view should extend from the aortic arch to base of the heart. In planning a coronary CTA of a patient with a LIMA graft, the field of view should extend from thoracic inlet to the base of the heart. Coronary CTA is valuable to assess the patency of bypass grafts. Bypass grafts are relatively motionless and can be imaged fairly easily. The sensitivity and specificity to determine the patency of venous and arterial grafts is in the 90% range and were reported early in the development of spiral CTA.

Coronary CTA has limitations for evaluation of coronary stent patency because of beam-hardening artifact, which limits sensitivity for the detection of in-stent stenosis. However, stent occlusion can be documented by lack of visualization of contrast in the vessel distal to the stent (153–155). Factors that affect the evaluation of stents include not only the type of scanner used but also the size, type, and material of the stent.

Not all stenoses detected on coronary CTA are flow-limiting, and evaluation of the functional impact on MPS is critical. Coronary CTA has a relatively low positive predictive value in evaluating perfusion defects (in the 30% range).

In summary, the anatomic and functional information obtained with combined MPS/coronary CTA is complementary. There is still debate regarding the cost-effectiveness of the combined versus sequential approach and whether MPS and coronary CTA with one test guiding to the other would be more cost-effective in specific clinical scenarios.

Diagnosis: Combined coronary CTA and MPS demonstrating severe three-vessel disease and a patent LIMA graft to the LAD with inferior MI and equivocal apical ischemia not amenable to revascularization.

CASE 3.14

History: A 72-year-old obese female (112 kg) with known CAD and orthostatic hypotension presented with recurrent episodes of syncope. Her medical problems included HTN, type II DM, renal insufficiency, three-vessel CAD, history of non-Q-wave MI, and CABG 3 years earlier. She underwent a rest/stress adenosine ^{99m}Tc-sestamibi SPECT MPS (Fig. 3.14 A). There was a concern for breast attenuation artifact and she was referred for a rest/dipyridamole ^{82}Rb-PET MPS. The rest and stress PET images were acquired 90 seconds following intravenous infusion of approximately 50 mCi of ^{82}Rb. For the stress images, dipyridamole 140 μg/kg per minute was infused over 4 minutes before infusion of ^{82}Rb, and the patient was monitored with ECG. Attenuation correction (AC) was performed using CT transmission images acquired before the rest and after the stress images. The rest/stress ^{82}Rb PET images (Fig. 3.14 B) as well as a selected coronal fusion CT/stress ^{82}Rb image for assessment of the quality of coregistration are displayed (Fig. 3.14 C). The stress ECG was positive for ischemia with 1- to 2-mm ST-segment depression in the lateral leads.

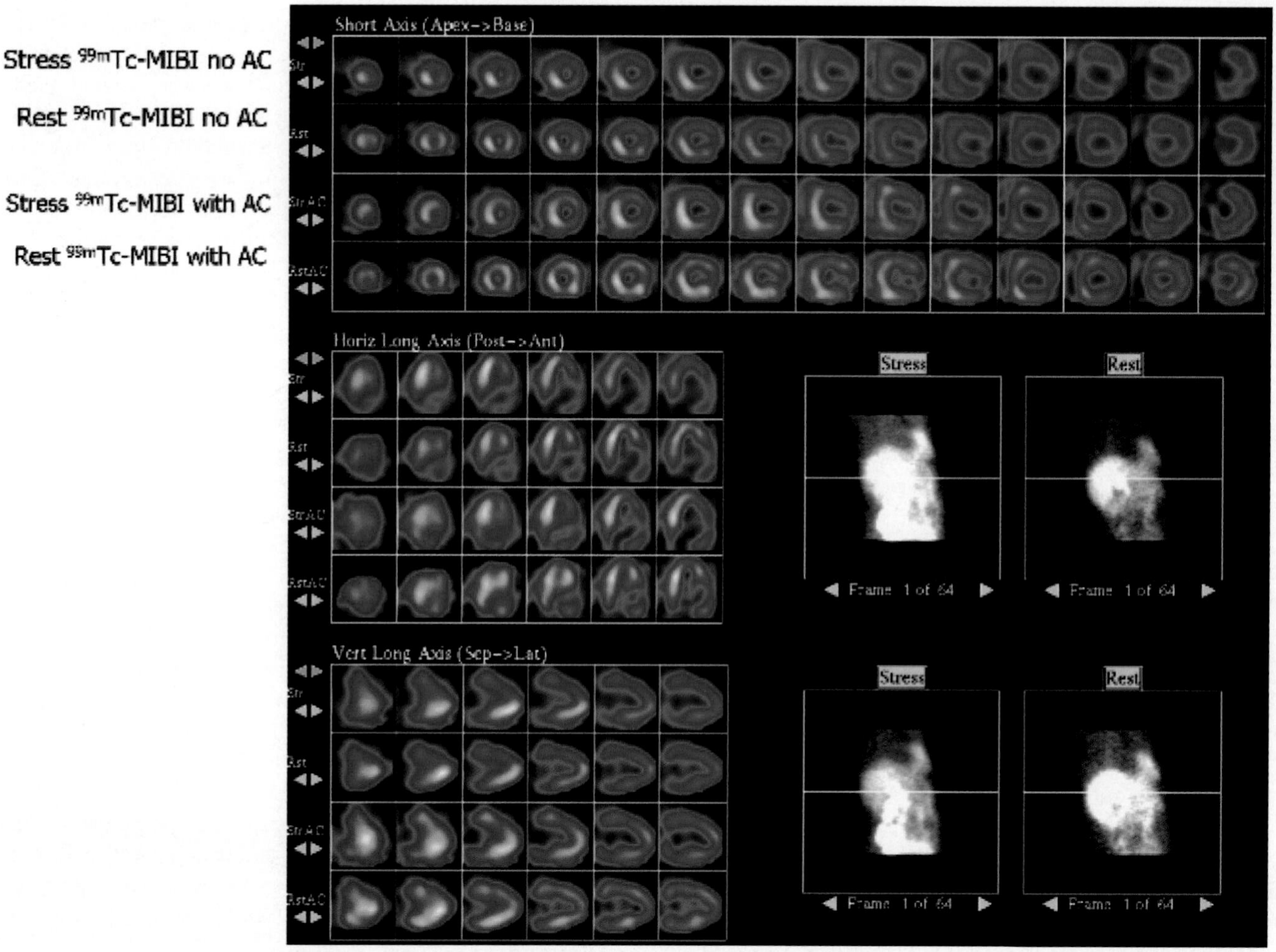

Figure 3.14 A

Stress ⁸²Rb PET with AC

Rest ⁸²Rb PET with AC

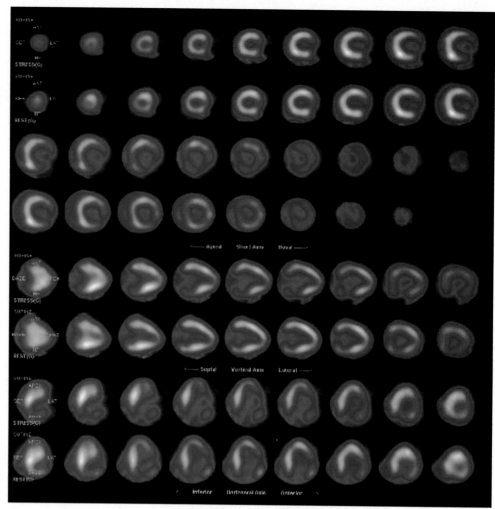

Figure 3.14 B

CT transmission   Stress ⁸²Rb PET with AC   Fusion CT/PET

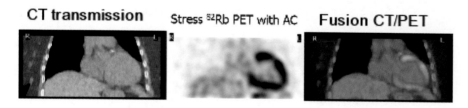

QC CT/Stress ⁸²Rb PET with AC

Figure 3.14 C

Findings: The rest/stress SPECT images (Fig. 3.14 A) demonstrate a large severe fixed defect in the lateral wall on both the images with and without AC, consistent with MI. There is a moderate fixed defect in the anterior wall on the images without AC that partially corrects with AC on the stress images and almost completely corrects with AC on the rest images. The effects of attenuation are more important on PET than SPECT images and PET images are always corrected for AC. Despite the patient's large body habitus, the quality of the ^{82}Rb PET images (Fig. 3.14 B) is good and without attenuation artifacts. The quality-control PET/CT fusion image shows good coregistration between the CT and PET images for both the stress (Figure 3.14 C) study and the rest study (not shown). On the rest/stress PET images (Figure 3.14 B), there is a large, severe perfusion defect in the lateral wall on the stress images with partial reversibility inferolaterally at the base, consistent with MI and peri-infarct ischemia. The perfusion of the anterior wall is normal. The LVEF is globally decreased to 37% on both the rest and stress studies. The patient underwent coronary angiography, which demonstrated total occlusion of the LAD with a patent LIMA to the LAD, subocclusion of the LCX, and occlusion of the SVG to the first and second obtuse marginal branches and occlusion of the RCA with a patent SVG to the RCA.

Discussion: This case illustrates the advantages of PET over SPECT myocardial images. Both ^{82}Rb and ^{13}N-ammonia are positron emitters that accumulate in the myocardium proportional to MBF but require dedicated positron tomographs for imaging. The advantages of PET perfusion radiopharmaceuticals compared with SPECT agents are the following: (1) more efficient rest/stress protocols because of the shorter half-lives; (2) higher resolution (approximately 5 mm for PET versus 10 mm for SPECT) and therefore higher sensitivity of PET than SPECT for the detection of CAD; (3) a more accurate AC algorithm for PET than for SPECT, leading to better image quality and superior accuracy for the detection of CAD in both normal and obese patients; and (4) true stress LVEF, because stress imaging is performed while dipyridamole still has effect. The sensitivity for detecting ischemia using PET perfusion scintigraphy is in the 95% range, with a very high normalcy rate in patients without CAD (156,157). A true stress LVEF increases the sensitivity for detection of ischemia, especially in patients with balanced three-vessel disease. Failure of the LVEF to raise 5 points or a drop of LVEF between rest and stress indicates ischemia (158). In this case, in addition to the perfusion abnormality, the LVEF did not increase with stress. However, a drop in LVEF in the absence of a perfusion abnormality strongly suggests balanced three-vessel disease.

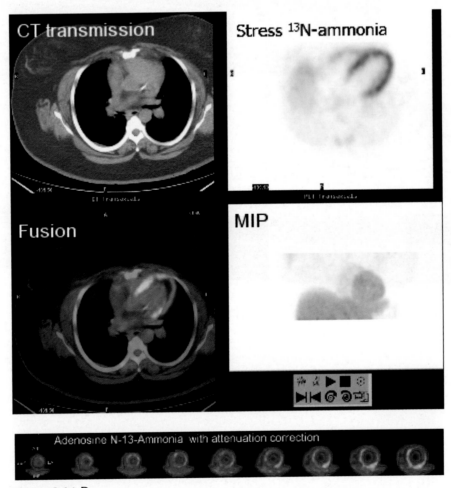

Figure 3.14 D

In the future, nearly all PET tomographs will be obtained with PET/CT systems and CT will be used for AC. During the PET acquisition, the patient is breathing and the diaphragm blurred. Therefore a slow CT acquisition is recommended (>20 seconds) or any CT protocol with the same average position of the diaphragm. It is not unusual that the position of the diaphragm is higher during stress; therefore a CT performed after the stress is usually better coregistered to the PET images. Regardless, the fusion images should be inspected for every acquisition to document proper coregistration. If there is mis-registration, as illustrated in Figure 3.14 D (another patient), an artifactual defect in the anterolateral wall is usually seen on the stress images and can be misinterpreted as anterolateral ischemia. If this happens, the stress acquisition must be repeated. There are software packages allowing reregistration manually, but they are not yet widely available for PET.

Diagnosis: Lateral wall ischemia and infarction demonstrated with rest/stress ^{82}Rb in a patient with a large body habitus and equivocal SPECT.

CASE 3.15

History: A 55-year-old man with non-Hodgkin's lymphoma was referred for a follow-up resting RVG (Fig. 3.15). He had received several courses of combination chemotherapy, including doxorubicin. His prechemotherapy RVG demonstrated a normal-sized LV with normal wall motion and an LVEF of 52%.

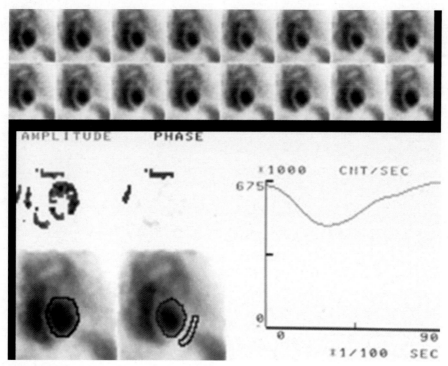

Figure 3.15

Findings: On the follow-up RVG (Fig. 3.15), there is global hypokinesis with a LVEF of 36%. The left and right ventricular chamber sizes are normal.

Discussion: Dropping LVEF from 52% to 36% represents a significant deterioration in systolic myocardial function presumably related to anthracycline (doxorubicin/Adriamycin) cardiotoxicity. The incidence and severity of doxorubicin-induced cardiotoxicity is variable, but approximately 7% of patients receiving a cumulative dose of 550 mg/m^2 experience CHF; this rises to 20% at doses >700 mg/m^2.

A baseline LVEF of less than 50% identifies patients at high risk for developing cardiotoxicity, and patients with a baseline LVEF of less than 30% are generally not treated with cardiotoxic drugs. Although the LV dysfunction is generally irreversible, its incidence and severity may be reduced by monitoring the LVEF and the cumulative received dose. The decline in LVEF may be used to halt the drug therapy before LV function deteriorates significantly. A fourfold decrease in the incidence of overt CHF rate is expected if strict guidelines are observed. These can be accomplished by halting the therapy if LVEF declines by more than 10 percentage points below the level of <50%. The mean difference in LVEF in the same subjects measured on separate days is 4% in patients with normal ventricles and 2% in patients with LV dysfunction. The LVEF criteria noted above may be observed uniformly. Many clinicians will relax these criteria if enough functional reserves can be demonstrated with exercise or dobutamine stress studies. Overall, the equilibrium resting RVG as a noninvasive, accurate, and quantitative study is ideal for serial determination of LV function.

Diagnosis: Doxorubicin-induced LV dysfunction.

CASE 3.16

History: A 49-year-old man with no history of cardiac disease presented with several weeks of progressive dyspnea and cough. He had no cardiac risk factors other than his age and gender. His resting ECG shows a normal sinus rhythm with a nonspecific interventricular conduction delay. An RVG was performed (Fig. 3.16).

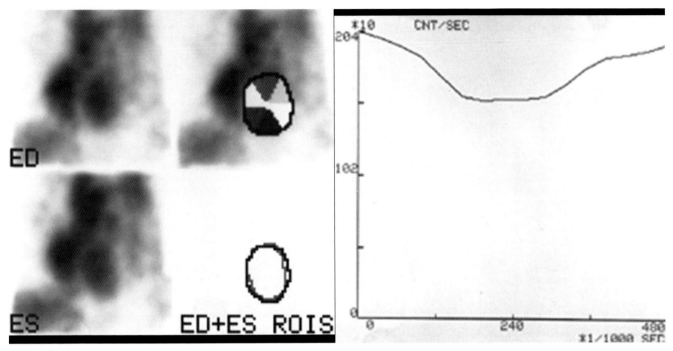

Figure 3.16

Findings: There is a LV enlargement and severe global LV hypokinesis with no segment of akinesis or dyskinesis. The LVEF is 25%.

Discussion: The RVG finding combined with the patient's history would be most consistent with the diagnosis of severe dilated cardiomyopathy. Right ventricular function appears to be preserved and chamber size is not significantly dilated. The absence of segmental wall motion abnormality, akinesis, or dyskinesis is evidence against the diagnosis of ischemic cardiomyopathy. Although the RV is often involved in patients with idiopathic or postviral dilated cardiomyopathy, the absence of RV involvement is inconclusive.

The LVEF determined by equilibrium RVG is a highly accurate and reproducible measure of LV contractility and can be used to follow the response to therapy and aid in the decision regarding the need for transplantation. Although an accurate estimation of RVEF can be calculated similarly, the accuracy is compromised somewhat due to overlying adjacent blood pool. The procedure of choice for determination of RVEF is a first pass RVG, which can be performed on the first several cardiac cycles following the bolus injection of a radiopharmaceutical, either ^{99m}Tc-pertechnetate or ^{99m}Tc-sestamibi.

Diagnosis: Dilated cardiomyopathy with severe LV dysfunction.

History: A 68-year-old male with no history of angina or MI presented with symptoms of CHF. Cardiac risk factors included his age, gender, and long-standing hypertension. Resting ECG was notable for LV hypertrophy. A resting RVG was performed (Fig. 3.17).

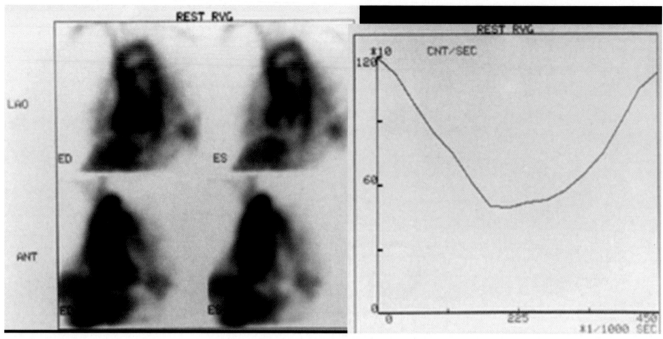

Figure 3.17

Findings: Gated blood pool images with radiolabeled autologous red blood cells in the anterior and LAO projections demonstrate normal LV and RV chamber sizes. No segmental wall motion abnormalities were identified. The end-systolic images show the expected normal decrease in LV activity, and the calculated LVEF is normal at 58%. The time–activity curve demonstrates rapid systolic emptying, consistent with normal LV systolic function. However, the postsystolic slope or peak diastolic filling rate is blunted as compared with normal, with resultant prolongation of the time to peak filling rate.

Discussion: RVG finding combined with the patient's history would be suggestive of LV diastolic dysfunction. Diastole in a cardiac cycle consists of active ventricular relaxation followed by ventricular filling. This latter aspect is characterized by an initial rapid filling phase followed by a period of slow filling and then a brief kick of increased filling due to atrial contraction. As compared with a normal time–activity curve, this patient's curve demonstrates a prolonged time to peak filling rate due to decreased early rapid diastolic filling, resulting in a reduced peak filling rate. These findings are typical for diastolic dysfunction and may be seen in patients with HTN, CAD, aortic stenosis, various cardiomyopathies, and other processes associated with diminished ventricular compliance.

Approximately 30% to 40% of patients presenting with CHF have diastolic dysfunction. These patients usually have a normal systolic function, although systolic dysfunction eventually follows. It is not unusual to see a frank pulmonary edema in a hypertensive patient with an entirely normal systolic function.

The distinction of systolic versus diastolic dysfunction in patients with CHF has therapeutic ramifications. Therapy with calcium antagonists may result in symptomatic improvement and the reversal of the abnormal diastolic parameters, whereas angiotensin converting enzyme (ACE) inhibitor therapy is more useful for systolic dysfunction.

The parameter of the ventricular diastolic dysfunction can be assessed by RVG. If the cardiac cycle is divided into a minimum of 32 frames per cycle (instead of the commonly used 16 to 24 frames per cycle), the quantitative measurement of diastolic parameters such as the peak filling rate and time to peak filling rate may be obtained. However, the qualitative assessment of the shape of the curve and the pattern of diastolic dysfunction is often adequate to suggest a diastolic dysfunction only to be confirmed by echocardiography. Doppler echocardiography is often utilized to measure the systolic and diastolic parameters in patients with symptoms of CHF.

Diagnosis: CHF due to diastolic dysfunction.

CASE 3.18

History: A 55-year-old woman with ischemic cardiomyopathy presented with exacerbation of dyspnea, CHF, and chest discomfort. She was referred for evaluation of myocardial viability. A rest/redistribution ^{201}Tl MPS was performed (Fig. 3.18).

15 min-Rest ^{201}Tl

24 hours-Rest ^{201}Tl

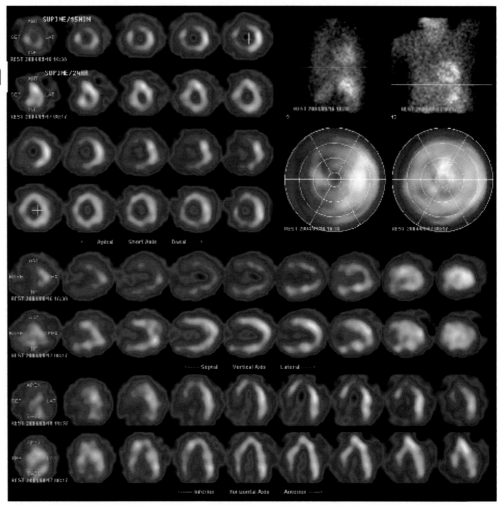

Figure 3.18

Findings: On the 15-minute ^{201}Tl images, there is moderately decreased perfusion in the anterior wall, basal septum, and basal inferior wall of the myocardium that is reversible on the 24-hour images, indicating ischemic but viable myocardium. Coronary angiography revealed ostial stenosis in both the right and left coronary arteries, and the ventriculogram reveals a LVEF of 20%. She underwent CABG with a LIMA graft to the LAD, SVG, RCA, and first obtuse marginal branch. At her 3-month follow-up visit, her symptoms and exercise tolerance showed marked improvement.

Discussion: Chronically ischemic myocardium in which the blood supply is adequate to preserve viability but not enough to maintain a normal functional myocardium can lead to LV dysfunction and regional dyssynergy (hibernated myocardium). Revascularization and restoration of blood supply in these tissues can lead to a significant improvement in wall contractility and LV function, at least in a large number of such patients.

The exact incidence of the viable myocardium in patients with chronic ischemic LV function is not known, but it is in the range of 30% to 50% among patients with ischemic cardiomyopathy.

In chronically dysfunctional myocardium, the resting blood flow is decreased but can be improved by revascularization. However, some data suggest that chronic dysfunctional myocardium is due to impaired CBFR (not resting flow), and accordingly the term "repetitive stunning" has been proposed to describe the disease process. Regardless of the pathogenesis of the process, it is expected that the restoration of the blood supply should improve the functionality of the hibernating segment, which includes contractility and improving the LVEF.

Dysfunctional but viable myocardium invariably demonstrates wall motion abnormality (severe hypokinesis, akinesis, or dyskinesis). There is impaired myocardial perfusion; cell membrane integrity and glucose metabolism characteristic of cellular viability are also impaired. Wall motion can be evaluated noninvasively by echocardiography, radionuclide ventriculography, gated perfusion SPECT, gated CT, gated MRI, or invasively by contrast ventriculography. Perfusion can be evaluated with either SPECT or PET tracers. With PET imaging, perfusion can be evaluated with ^{82}Rb and ^{13}N-ammonia (see Case 3.14). The characteristics of cellular viability include cell membrane integrity evaluated with ^{201}Tl, intact mitochondria evaluated with ^{99m}Tc-isonitriles, preserved glucose metabolism evaluated with ^{18}F-FDG (see Cases 3.19 and 3.20), and contractile reserve evaluated with dobutamine echography or MRI (159). Viability can also be evaluated with fatty acid metabolism using ^{11}C-palmitate and ^{123}I-beta-methyliodophenyl pentadecanoic acid (BMIPP), and oxidative metabolism with ^{11}C-acetate; however, these radiopharmaceuticals are still investigational. The extent of scarring can be evaluated with delayed gadolinium (Gd)-enhanced MRI and is also predictive of improvement of function in patients with chronic ischemic LV dysfunction (160).

^{18}F-FDG is still considered the reference standard for evaluation of myocardial viability because of the large supportive literature, as discussed in Cases 3.19 and 3.20. However ^{18}F-FDG is not as available as the SPECT radiopharmaceuticals (^{201}Tl or ^{99m}Tc-isonitriles). For example, this patient was referred at the end of the day and the ^{18}F-FDG supply has been consumed. In addition, ^{18}F-FDG myocardial imaging requires glucose loading (see Case 3.20), adding 30 to 60 minutes to the procedure. Therefore ^{201}Tl was chosen in this case, using a rest/24-hour redistribution protocol. Typically a 15-minute rest/4-hour redistribution ^{201}Tl SPECT is used; it has a sensitivity of 67% and a specificity of 77% compared with a sensitivity of 89% and a specificity of 81% for ^{18}F-FDG SPECT (161).

The value of routine acquisition of additional images at 24 hours is still debated in the literature. In this case, the 24-hour delay in acquiring the redistribution images was related to patient's availability.

For patients evaluated for stress-induced ischemia with ^{201}Tl, two protocols are commonly used to maximize detection of viability in compromised myocardium: the stress-redistribution–late redistribution and the stress-redistribution–reinjection protocols. Evidence of stress-induced perfusion defects on ^{201}Tl images that redistribute after 4 hours is indicative of ischemic viable myocardium, but fixed defects do not necessarily indicate scarring. The identification of viable myocardium is improved by the addition of a third set of images obtained at 24 hours that allows a longer period of redistribution for ^{201}Tl (162). A prospective study demonstrated that late redistribution occurs in 53% of the patients with fixed defects on stress-redistribution images (163). However, fixed defects at 24 hours do not exclude viability, as 37% of segments that remain fixed on both 4- and 24-hour images also improve after revascularization. Imaging at 24 hours often results in suboptimal count statistics, making the images difficult to interpret even if the acquisition time is increased.

The concept of reinjection of a booster dose of ^{201}Tl (1 to 1.5 mCi) 15 to 30 minutes prior to acquiring the rest redistribution images was introduced in the early 1990s. In a study of 100 patients with 33% of fixed defects after 4-hour redistribution images, Dilsizian et al. (164) demonstrated that there is improvement of ^{201}Tl uptake in 49% of these fixed defects on images obtained after reinjection of 1 mCi of ^{201}Tl. In addition, patients with regions identified as viable improved wall motion after PTCA. ^{201}Tl reinjection protocols have been shown to provide incremental prognostic information compared to clinical, exercise, and stress-redistribution data (165). The degree of severity of the LV dysfunction is important; ^{18}F-FDG imaging can demonstrate viability in fixed defects on stress-reinjection ^{201}Tl SPECT images in patients with an LVEF <20% (166).

Diagnosis: Ischemic viable myocardium identified by rest/redistribution ^{201}Tl SPECT.

CASE 3.19

History: A 65-year-old female with a known ischemic cardiomyopathy presented with worsening CHF. Coronary angiography revealed a 40% stenosis of the LAD, 100% stenosis of the LCX after the take off of the first obtuse marginal branch, occlusion of the RCA with collateral circulation, and global hypokinesis with an LVEF of 20%. A rest ^{13}N-ammonia/^{18}F-FDG PET study was performed for evaluation of myocardial viability. Prior to ^{18}F-FDG administration, the patient was loaded with glucose using an IV infusion of insulin and dextrose (Fig. 3.19).

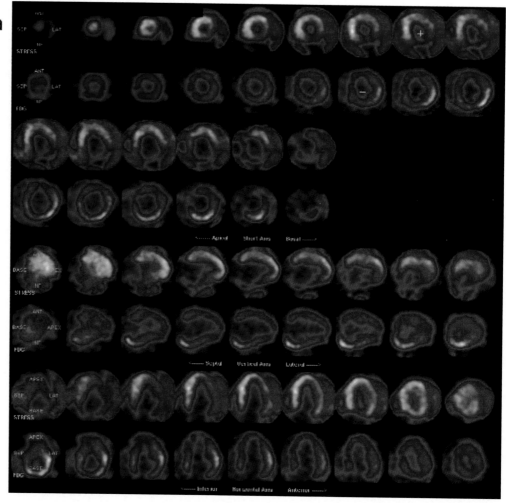

Rest ^{13}N-ammonia

Rest ^{18}F-FDG

Figure 3.19

Findings: The rest ^{13}N-ammonia PET MPS demonstrated a large severe fixed defect in the inferior and inferolateral wall of the myocardium. The gated images demonstrated global hypokinesis, worse in the inferior wall, with an LVEF of 21%. The large area of decreased perfusion in the inferior wall of the myocardium demonstrates intense ^{18}F-FDG uptake and therefore is viable. The area of mismatch represents at least 4 of 17 myocardial segments (>20% of the myocardium). The patient underwent CABG with SVG to the first and second obtuse marginal branches. Six months later, her LVEF was 49%.

Discussion: The mismatched perfusion/metabolism in the inferior wall indicates injured but viable myocardium that will benefit from revascularization. The approach of the combined blood flow/metabolism mismatch has been extensively documented as a good predictor of regional wall motion improvement postrevascularization, as well as improvement of CHF symptoms, exercise capacity, and prognosis (167,168). Long-term prognosis and survival may be the ideal end-point in the clinical setting. A meta-analysis reviewing studies and including 3,088 patients demonstrates a strong association between myocardial viability on noninvasive testing and improved survival in patients with chronic CAD and LV dysfunction who underwent revascularization (169). Absence of viability was associated with no significant difference in outcomes irrespective of treatment strategy.

From a clinical point of view, improvement of global LV function may be more relevant than improvement of regional LV function. The number of studies focusing on improvement of global function postrevascularization is significantly less than those focusing on improvement of regional LV function. The large region of ischemic but viable myocardium in the inferior wall of this patient has an excellent predictive value of good recovery postrevascularization, including improvement of the LVEF of more than 5%. The extent of 25% of the LV being dysfunctional but viable may be the optimal threshold to predict improvement of LVEF postrevascularization (170). The extent of mismatch can be estimated using the extent and severity scoring system in a 17-segmental myocardial model similar to the one used for rest/stress myocardial perfusion and described in the guidelines (171).

There is mounting evidence that myocardial hibernation represents an adaptation to ischemia that cannot be maintained indefinitely. Following this hypothesis, timely revascularization is important, the LVEF is more likely to improve with early (<12 days) than late (>30 days) revascularization (172). LV remodeling (increased LV volumes and cavity size) is also a predictor of poor outcome in patients with ischemic cardiomyopathy undergoing CABG; for example, a preoperative left ventricular end-systolic volume (LVESV) of 70 mL or greater, as assessed by echocardiography, was shown to be a marker of poor outcome postrevascularization (173).

The interpretation of the ^{18}F-FDG images may be somewhat confusing, because the highest level of ^{18}F-FDG uptake is in the inferior wall that is the region with the least perfusion. Because the images are normalized to the pixel with most activity in the myocardium, the remainder of the myocardium appears hypometabolic compared to the region of ischemic myocardium. If the ^{18}F-FDG images were interpreted without perfusion images, the decreased activity along the anteroseptal wall could be misinterpreted as an infarct. This example demonstrates the importance of comparing perfusion and metabolic images for accurate interpretation. The pathophysiologic mechanism underlying this phenomenon is the inhibition of lipolysis and decreased serum levels of fatty acids during ischemia, shifting the metabolism of the myocardium toward glucose. Therefore the ^{18}F-FDG uptake in ischemic regions may be above the level of uptake in normal myocardium. Anaerobic metabolism with severe ischemia results in supraphysiologic ^{18}F-FDG uptake.

Diagnosis: Ischemic but viable myocardium in the inferior and inferolateral wall demonstrated by mismatched resting ^{13}N-ammonia/^{18}F-FDG PET.

History: A 73-year-old male patient with DM, ischemic cardiomyopathy, and an earlier CABG was admitted due to worsening CHF. The patient was referred for viability evaluation using a rest ^{13}N-ammonia/^{18}F-FDG PET protocol (Fig. 3.20). Prior to ^{18}F-FDG administration, the patient was loaded with glucose using an IV infusion of insulin and dextrose.

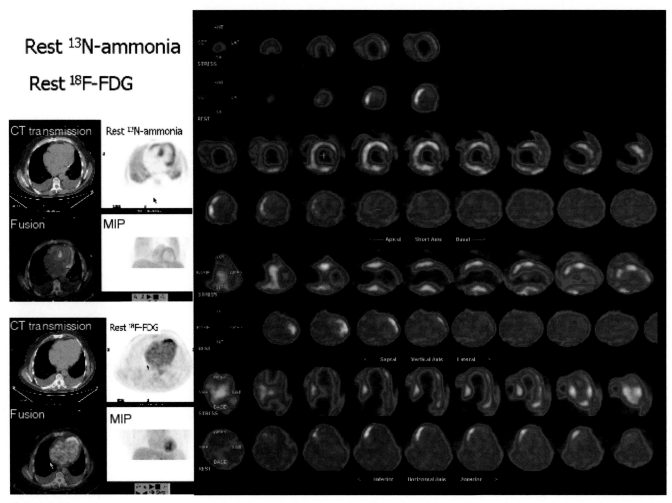

Figure 3.20

Findings: The ^{13}N-ammonia perfusion images demonstrate a large severe perfusion defect in the distal anterior and inferior wall and apex. The ^{18}F-FDG images demonstrate persistent blood pool activity and very poor uptake by the myocardium except for a small region in the distal anteroseptal wall and apex. The mismatch perfusion/metabolism defect is confirmed on the transaxial PET and fusion PET/CT images (Fig. 3.20, left). Poor ^{18}F-FDG uptake is likely related to diabetes and insulin resistance in this patient. The patient was referred for coronary angiography demonstrating severe diffuse three-vessel disease and new occlusion of a stent previously placed in a saphenous graft to the LAD. Revascularization was not possible and the patient was managed medically.

Discussion: This interesting case gives the opportunity to discuss several issues: (a) CAD in DM patients, (b) the importance of evaluating myocardial viability in ischemic cardiomyopathy, and (c) ^{18}F-FDG PET to evaluate viability in patients with DM.

There is a high incidence of premature CAD in patients with diabetes (174). Diabetic patients with normal MPS have a three-fold increase in cardiac events compared to nondiabetic patients (47).

In the evaluation of symptomatic diabetic patients, stress MPS has recently been shown to have diagnostic (175) and prognostic (176,177) accuracy. Stress MPS has a sensitivity of 90% and normalcy rate of 95% for the detection of CAD in patients with diabetes, in the similar range as for nondiabetic patients. The presence and extent of perfusion abnormalities are the strongest predictors of cardiac events among diabetic women with a significantly higher cardiac events rate compared to nondiabetic women (176). The estimate of ischemic burden with stress MPS significantly improved risk stratification in diabetic women compared with clinical assessment alone, and stratification by the number of ischemic vessels demonstrated a significant linear increase in cardiac events.

As data are collected in the asymptomatic diabetic population, it is anticipated that stress MPS will have an increasingly relevant role (178).

In the fasting state, the myocardium uses predominantly fatty acids for its metabolism and the myocardial distribution of ^{18}F-FDG is often heterogenous. Only 50% of PET myocardial images obtained in fasting patients are interpretable (179). Therefore, for evaluation of myocardial viability using ^{18}F-FDG, the levels of circulating substrates/hormones need to favor utilization of glucose by the myocardium. This is accomplished by loading the patient with glucose.

Several protocols are available to promote cardiac ^{18}F-FDG uptake and have been described in the guidelines (180): (a) oral glucose loading, (b) intravenous loading, (c) hyperinsulinemic euglycemic clamping, and (d) the administration of nicotinic acid derivatives. Oral glucose loading is the most frequently used approach, although it results in uninterpretable images in as many as 10% of patients in some studies (181).

The hyperinsulinemic euglycemic clamp allows nearly perfect regulation of metabolic substrates and insulin levels, ensuring excellent image quality in virtually all patients, including diabetics. However, the procedure is laborious and time-consuming. More practical IV glucose/insulin loading procedures have been used with success (180). Oral administration of a nicotinic acid derivative (acipimox) is an alternative but this agent is not available in the United States. Acipimox inhibits peripheral lipolysis, thus reducing plasma free fatty acid levels and indirectly stimulating cardiac ^{18}F-FDG uptake (182).

Diagnosis: Poor ^{18}F-FDG uptake in a diabetic patient but evidence of mismatch perfusion/metabolism indicating viability in the distal anteroseptal wall.

CASE 3.21

History: A 67-year-old man with known CAD, prior MI at 53 years of age, followed by CABG, presented with atypical chest pain. His recent coronary angiography revealed left main (LM) lesion of 70%, RCA lesion of 50%, LAD occluded filled by collateral from the RCA and a patent SVG to the LCX. The graft to the LAD could not be found. Contrasted left ventriculography revealed anteroapical akinesia. A rest/stress ^{99m}Tc-sestamibi study was requested to evaluate ischemic burden and viability (Fig 3.21 A). The patient exercised on the treadmill on the Bruce protocol for 5 minutes; he had ST-segment depression on the ECG but no chest pain.

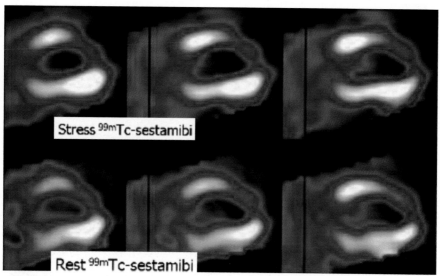

Figure 3.21 A

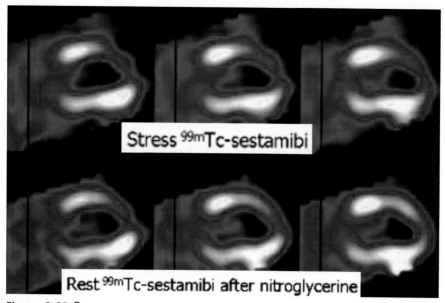

Figure 3.21 B

Findings: Rest/stress ^{99m}Tc-sestamibi (Fig. 3.21 A, vertical long axis) showed a predominantly persistent severe defect, involving the mid- and distal anterior wall and apex, with minimal reversibility suggesting some ischemia in the LAD territory. However, the main feature of the study is that of an anterior scar.

Discussion: Owing to possible underestimation of viability, the study was repeated following the nitrate-enhanced rest ^{99m}Tc-sestamibi protocol (Fig. 3.21 B). There are more reversible areas in the mid-, distal anterior wall and apex in the postnitrate image as compared with Figure 3.21 A, confirming the presence of significant ischemic viable myocardium and a component of associated scar tissue.

The role of ^{99m}Tc-labeled agents for the assessment of viability has been debated over the years (183). Because ^{99m}Tc-sestamibi and tetrofosmin do not redistribute significantly over time as ^{201}Tl does, their use in the evaluation of viability is limited (184,185). However, there are studies indicating that ^{99m}Tc-labeled agents can be used to evaluate both perfusion and viability. The uptake and retention of these tracers is dependent on perfusion, cell membrane integrity, and mitochondrial function, all characteristics of viability.

Several studies have demonstrated that ^{99m}Tc-sestamibi underestimates the presence of viable myocardium as compared to ^{18}F-FDG PET (186–189). Several options have been proposed in the literature to improve the detection of viability using ^{99m}Tc-labeled agents. This includes AC, quantitative evaluation using different threshold of uptake (190), combining the information of perfusion and wall motion (191), and administration of nitrate prior to injection of the perfusion radiopharmaceutical as in the present case.

Nitrate-Enhanced SPECT: Excellent results have been obtained with nitrate-enhanced ^{99m}Tc-sestamibi SPECT imaging for the detection of viable myocardium (192–195). Nitrates enhance blood flow (and tracer uptake) to myocardial regions that are perfused by severely stenosed arteries. For clinical purposes, the best prognostic results may be obtained by comparing poststress images with nitrate-enhanced resting images. Nitrate can be given sublingually or IV. For IV administration, typically 10 mg of isosorbide dinitrate diluted in 100 mL of isotonic saline solution is infused over 20 minutes to the patient lying supine during ECG and blood pressure monitoring. The perfusion radiopharmaceutical is administered as soon as the blood pressure drops >20 mm Hg or 15 minutes after the start of the infusion. ^{99m}Tc-sestamibi or tetrofosmin can be administered 5 to 10 minutes after sublingual administration of 0.4 to 0.8 mg of nitroglycerin, with results similar to those of the IV infusion.

The percent of myocardial segments demonstrating improved uptake on nitrate-enhanced ^{99m}Tc-sestamibi images compared to baseline resting ^{99m}Tc-sestamibi is in the same range as for the ^{201}Tl rest-redistribution protocol and the ^{201}Tl reinjection images compared to 4-hour redistribution ^{201}Tl images (196). Nitrate enhancement has been used with resting ^{201}Tl SPECT as well and compared to the rest/4-hour redistribution ^{201}Tl protocol (197). All the regions identified as viable by the rest/redistribution protocol were identified as viable by the rest/nitrate protocol. Both protocols correctly predicted improvement of regional wall motion after revascularization with a comparable sensitivity (95% and 92%).

Diagnosis: Hibernating myocardium in the LAD territory detected using the rest/nitrate ^{99m}Tc-sestamibi protocol.

CASE 3.22

History: A 67-year-old male with multiple risk factors for CAD presented with atypical chest pain and was referred for rest/stress adenosine ^{99m}Tc-tetrofosmin MPS. His resting ECG was unremarkable and there were no ischemic changes with stress. The stress SPECT supine images were corrected for attenuation correction (AC) using CT transmission maps (Figure 3.22 A). Stress images were also acquired in the prone position in the same patient for comparison (Fig. 3.22 B).

Stress ^{99m}Tc-tetrofosmin with AC

Stress ^{99m}Tc-tetrofosmin no AC

Rest ^{99m}Tc-tetrofosmin no AC

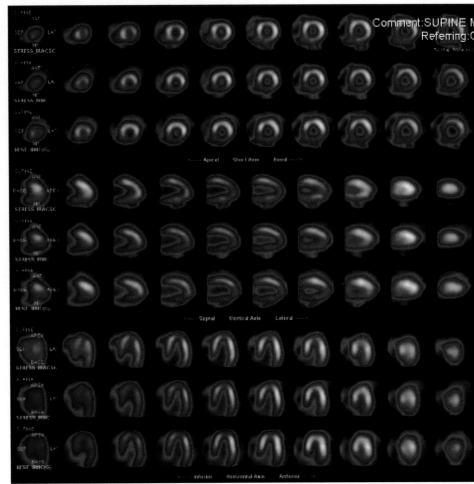

Figure 3.22 A

Stress ⁹⁹ᵐTc-tetrofosmin no AC
Prone

Rest ⁹⁹ᵐTc-tetrofosmin no AC
Supine

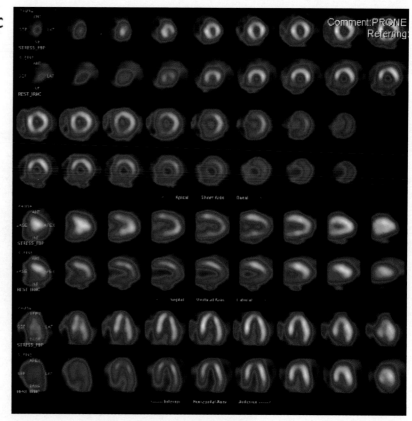

Figure 3.22 B

Findings: The rest/stress images without AC demonstrated a large fixed defect of moderate intensity. The stress images normalize with both AC and prone imaging, indicating diaphragmatic attenuation artifact. The stress LVEF was 50% and the wall motion was normal (not shown).

Discussion: One limitation of MPS is limited specificity due to attenuation artifacts from variable soft tissue attenuation. Attenuation artifacts from breast and diaphragmatic tissue result in anterior and inferior wall defects known to reduce MPS specificity (198,199). Various techniques to improve specificity have been investigated including gating, prone imaging, and AC.

An abnormal wall motion on gated images is indicative of scar and is helpful in the assessment of a fixed defect. However, if the wall motion is normal, the differential diagnosis remains subendocardial scar or attenuation artifacts.

Combined supine and prone imaging improves the diagnostic accuracy of MPS by improving the specificity for detection of CAD and reduces the number of equivocal interpretations (200). The prognostic value of prone imaging in patients with inferior wall defects has been demonstrated in a study of 3,834 patients (201). However, prone imaging has not yet been shown to be helpful for improvement of anterior wall breast attenuation and is not tolerated by all patients.

Improvement of specificity can be accomplished by using AC transmission maps. The topic of AC of MPS has been recently reviewed (202). In 2001, ASNC and SNM issued a joint position statement after reviewing the literature using at that time transmission maps acquired with radioisotopic sources (203): the addition of AC improves specificity from an average of 64% to 81%, and normalcy rates from an average of 80% to 89% without a loss of sensitivity. In 2000, a dual-head gamma camera equipped with an integrated x-ray transmission system was introduced by GE Healthcare, allowing AC using CT-based attenuation maps, anatomic mapping, and image fusion (204). A multicenter clinical trial (205) concluded that CT-based AC of SPECT images improved overall diagnostic performance of interpreters with different interpretative attitudes and level of experience.

A study comparing AC and prone imaging demonstrated that the combination of stress supine SPECT imaging with and without AC decreases the number of equivocal interpretations to a greater extent than the combination of stress supine and stress prone imaging (both without AC), although the combination of all sets of images results in the lowest number of equivocal interpretations (206).

Attenuation correction and prone imaging are more helpful for normalization of inferior wall than anterior wall defect; as such they are less helpful in correcting the breast attenuation artifact.

An anterior defect that does not correct with AC is illustrated in Figure 3.22 C. This is an 18-year-old female presenting with atypical chest pain and referred for suspicion of anomalous coronaries. A coronary CTA demonstrated normal

Stress ^{99m}Tc-tetrofosmin with AC

Stress ^{99m}Tc-tetrofosmin no AC

Rest ^{99m}Tc-tetrofosmin no AC

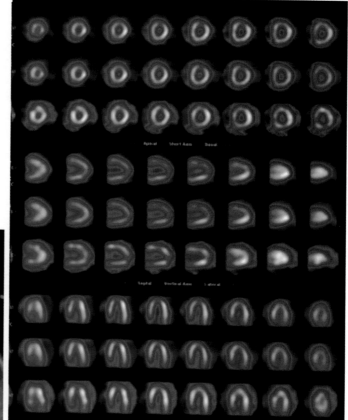

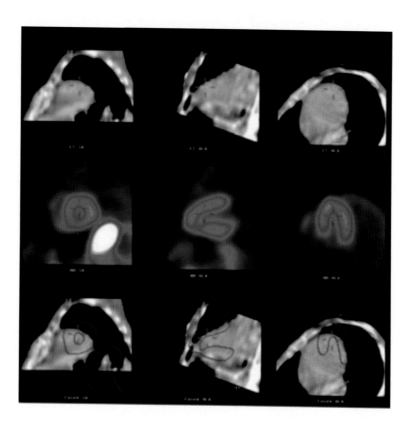

LAD

Figure 3.22 C

Figure 3.22 D

widely patent coronaries (Fig. 3.22 C, left). The defect in the anterior wall and apex on the supine AC images are probably due to overcorrection of the counts in the inferior wall.

Proper interpretation of MPS with AC or acquired in the prone position requires close comparison with conventional non AC images, because new "defect" may occur with prone and/or AC images and also be artifactual.

In the evaluation of CT-based attenuation map, the quality of coregistration CT and SPECT images has to be assessed using the manufacturer's provided software. If there is misregistration identified, for example, as the result of the patient's motion (Fig. 3.22D), the image needs to be reregistered manually. A shift in image greater than 6 mm will result in artifactual defect.

In this case CT-based attenuation maps were acquired using a very low dose CT (Infinia Hawkeye, GE Healthcare).

Diagnosis: Diaphragmatic attenuation artifact, which corrects with AC and prone imaging.

CASE 3.23

History: A 49-year-old man with risk factors for CAD and mental retardation presented with atypical chest pain. He was referred for a rest/adenosine ^{99m}Tc tetrofosmin study (Fig. 3.23 A and 3.23 B).

Stress ^{99m}Tc-tetrofosmin

Rest ^{99m}Tc-tetrofosmin

Projection image

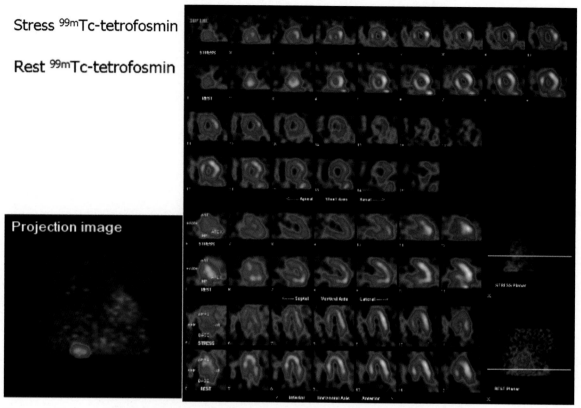

Figure 3.23 A

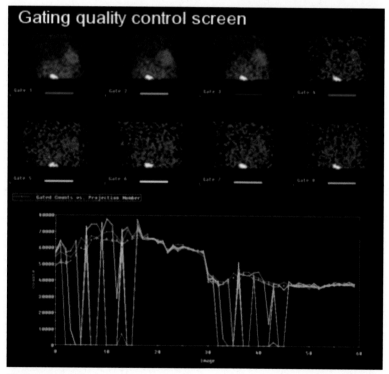

Figure 3.23 B

Stress ^{99m}Tc-tetrofosmin

Rest ^{99m}Tc-tetrofosmin

Projection image

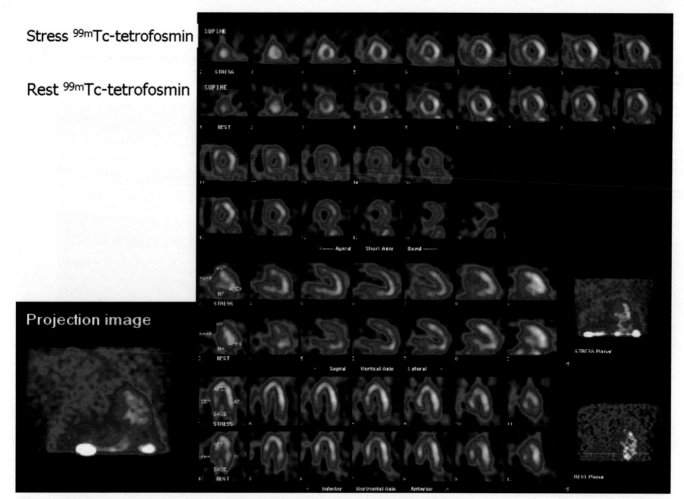

Figure 3.23 C

Findings: The rest/stress SPECT demonstrate a reversible defect in the anterior wall; however, the images appear noisy (Figure 3.23 A). On the cineloop display of the images, there is a flashing artifact (not shown). The selected projection image shown has low counts (Fig. 3.23 A left). On the gating quality control screen (Fig. 3.23 B), the counts/projection vary between projection images and between gates. The technologist reported that some of the ECG leads became loose.

Discussion: When interpreting rest/stress MPS, it is very important to inspect the cineloop display of the projection images to detect gating and motion artifacts. For this patient, the ECG leads were better secured and the images reacquired (Fig. 3.23 C) and interpreted as normal.

The projection images should also be inspected for detection of abnormal extracardiac abnormalities such as neoplasms.

Diagnosis: Normal rest/stress MPS; gating artifact.

CASE 3.24

History: A 53-year-old male with HTN, hypercholesterolemia, and smoking history, presented with a 4-week history of typical chest pain. The resting ECG revealed LBBB. The patient was referred for an exercise/reinjection ^{201}Tl study shown in Figure 3.24 A.

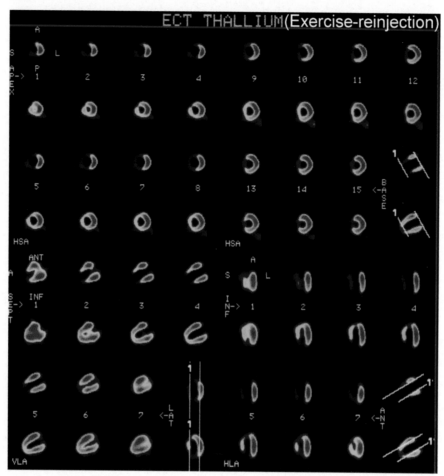

Figure 3.24 A (From Vitola JV and Delbeke D, 2004 (11), by permission from Springer-Verlag)

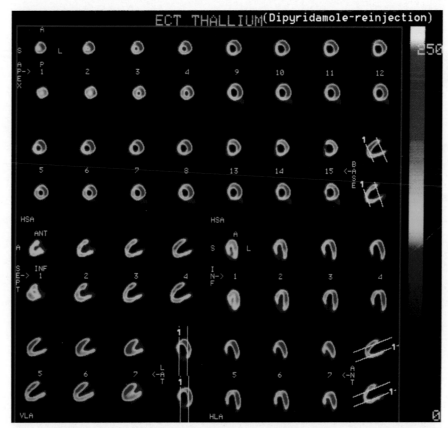

Figure 3.24 B (From Vitola JV and Delbeke D, 2004 (11), by permission from Springer-Verlag)

Findings: The SPECT images demonstrated a large severe anteroseptal, septal, and apical perfusion defect that is reversible on the resting images. Considering the presence of LBBB, this study was repeated using pharmacologic stress with dipyridamole. The images are shown in Figure 3.24 B.

Figure 3.24 B using dipyridamole demonstrated a striking improvement of perfusion in the same areas of severe hypoperfusion previously seen on the exercise study.

Discussion: Conventional exercise stress testing is nondiagnostic in patients with LBBB, because ischemic ST-segment shifts cannot be detected in the presence of LBBB. The Framingham study has shown that the occurrence of LBBB in patients with underlying CAD is a strong predictor of mortality (207), while LBBB in the absence of CAD is associated with a better prognosis (208). Myocardial perfusion scintigraphy offers a sensitive noninvasive diagnostic technique for the detection of ischemia in patients with abnormal resting ECG including LBBB. Reversible defects on exercise MPS can be artifactual in patients with LBBB (209–211). These reversible defects are usually located in the anteroseptal or septal region and are HR-dependent. Therefore vasodilator stress, which does not increase the HR to the same extent as exercise, has been recommended as the method of choice for evaluating these patients (212). Septal wall motion abnormalities occur often in relation to asynchronous contraction of the right and then the left ventricle in patients with LBBB. Exercise may induce perfusion defect involving the anteroseptal and septal region in the absence of significant CAD because the early septal contraction may result in decreased diastolic septal perfusion and result in a reversible septal perfusion defect (213). The most likely explanation for this finding is delayed perfusion of the septum in LBBB and shortening of diastole when HR increases. Myocardial perfusion occurs in diastole and as the HR increases the diastolic period decreases. As the septum would be the last to be filled in patients with LBBB, a decrease in the diastolic period will affect the septum to a greater extent, therefore causing decreased perfusion during exercise. Exercise increases the delay between right and left ventricular activation relative to the duration of systole and would be expected to produce reversible perfusion defects more frequently than dipyridamole or adenosine. In this patient, the exercise stress test was followed by a dipyridamole stress test. By using vasodilation as the mode of stress testing in LBBB, diagnostic accuracy is improved. Therefore patients with LBBB should be evaluated using vasodilators and not with exercise.

Diagnosis: Severe reversible perfusion defect induced by exercise but not vasodilator stress in a patient with LBBB.

CASE 3.25

History: A 66-year-old man presented with a new LBBB, mild CHF, and an acute fracture of his right humeral head. He had experienced a 45-minute episode of moderately severe chest pain a week prior to admission but denied any history of exertional angina. Cardiac risk factors included age, gender, smoking history, and HTN. Cardiac enzymes were normal. Because of the increased preoperative risk in patients with recent MI, a ^{99m}Tc-pyrophosphate "MI" scan (Fig. 3.25) was requested prior to shoulder surgery.

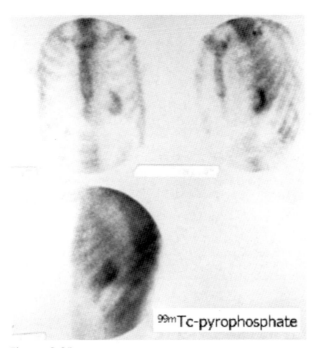

Figure 3.25

Findings: Five-minute planar views of the thorax in various projections acquired 2 hours after injection of 20 mCi of ^{99m}Tc-pyrophosphate reveal diffusely increased activity within the anterior wall and apex of the LV with mildly increased activity throughout the remainder of the myocardium. Physiologic activity is noted within skeletal structures.

Discussion: The increased activity seen in the anterior wall of the LV is consistent with a recent MI. During severe ischemia, there is intracellular deposition of calcium in the mitochondria. ^{99m}Tc-pyrophosphate, initially developed as a bone imaging agent, binds to intracellular calcium in the acutely necrotic myocardium. The maximum uptake occurs at the peri-infarct border, where flow is still present but reduced. This may result in a doughnut pattern with absent uptake in the central zone of necrosis, where flow is essentially absent. It takes 24 to 48 hours before enough calcium is deposited in the infarct to allow adequate complexing of pyrophosphate to produce a positive scan; scans may occasionally be positive as early as 12 hours. Activity gradually diminishes over 5 to 7 days, but in large infarcts it may persist for weeks. Anterior, lateral, and oblique views, with or without SPECT, are obtained 2 to 4 hours postinjection. Normally no myocardial activity other than perhaps faint blood pool activity is observed. Physiologic sternal and rib activity are present; costal cartilage calcification or rib metastases can present a diagnostic dilemma. Activity greater than background is considered positive, although the diagnostic confidence increases as myocardial activity approaches that of the ribs and sternum. Diffusely increased myocardial activity is not infrequently observed in patients with large anterior infarctions.

The sensitivity for the detection of small infarcts is relatively low, but in an autopsy series of patients having undergone ^{99m}Tc-pyrophosphate scintigraphy, the overall sensitivity for infarction was 89%, the specificity 100%, the positive predictive value 100%, and the negative predictive value 72% (214). Within the differential, diagnosis of a positive scan is myocarditis, pericarditis, persistent blood pool activity, doxorubicin cardiotoxicity, radiation therapy, left ventricular aneurysm, and amyloidosis. Owing to the time delay necessary to see a positive scan, this modality is not used routinely in the triage of patients with chest pain. This technique is most useful in the patient with an infarct by ECG findings but with negative enzymes or other confusing factors such as recent trauma, surgery or cardiopulmonary resuscitation.

One limitation of ^{99m}Tc-pyrophosphate is the response time for a disease requiring a quick therapeutic response. Preliminary studies indicate that ^{99m}Tc-glucarate may be a more suitable radiopharmaceutical because it localizes in the necrotic myocardium within hours after the onset of experimental MI but it is still investigational.

Diagnosis: Acute anterior wall MI.

REFERENCES

1. Stary HC, ed. *Atlas of Atherosclerosis: Progression and Regression.* New York: Parthenon, 1999.
2. Shaw LJ, Peterson ED, Shaw LK, et al. Use of a prognostic treadmill score in identifying diagnostic coronary disease subgroups. *Circulation* 1998;98:1622–1630.
3. Lauer MS, Mehta R, Pashkow FJ, et al. Association of chronotropic incompetence with echocardiographic ischemia and prognosis. *J Am Coll Cardiol* 1998;32:1280–1286.
4. Gianrossi R, Detrano R, Mulvihill D, et al. Exercise-induced ST depression in the diagnosis of coronary artery disease: a meta-analysis. *Circulation* 1989;80:87–89.
5. Detrano R, Gianrossi R, Froelicker V. The diagnostic accuracy of the exercise electrocardiogram: a meta-analysis of 22 years of research. *Prog Cardiovasc Dis* 1989;32:173–206.
6. Miller TD, Roger VL, Milavetz JJ, et al. Assessment of the exercise electrocardiogram in women versus men using tomographic myocardial perfusion imaging as the reference standard. *Am J Cardiol* 2001;87:868–873.
7. Kwok Y, Kim C, Grady D, et al. Analysis of exercise testing to detect coronary artery disease in women. *Am J Cardiol* 1999;83:660–666.
8. Morise AP, Dalal JN, Duval RD. Value of a simple measure of estrogen status for improving the diagnosis of coronary artery disease in women. *Am J Med* 1993;94:491–496.
9. Gibbons RJ. Guidelines updated for exercise testing. ACC/AHA 2002. www.acc.org.
10. Anderson JL, Adams CD, Antman EL, et al. ACC AHA guidelines management unstable angina and non ST-segment elevation myocardial infarction. *J Am Coll Cardiol* 2007;50:e.1–e.133.
11. Vitola JV and Delbeke D. Nuclear Cardiology and correlative imaging—a teaching file, Springer-Verlag, 2004.
12. Fletcher GF, Balagy G, Froelicher VF et al. Exercise standards: a statement for healthcare professionals from the American Heart Association writing group-special report. *Circulation* 1995;91:580–622.
13. Klocke FJ, Baird MG, Lorell BH, et al. ACC/AHA/ASNC guidelines for the clinical use of cardiac radionuclide imaging – executive summary: a report of the American College of Cardiology/American Heart Association Task Force on Practice Guidelines (ACC/AHA/ASNC Committee to Revise the 1995 Guidelines for the Clinical Use of Cardiac Radionuclide Imaging). *J Am Coll Cardiol* 2003;42(7):1318–1333.
14. Brindis AG et al. ACCF ASNC Appropriateness criteria for SPECT MPI. *J Am Coll Cardiol* 2005;46:1587–1605.
15. Strauss HW, Zaret BL, Martin ND, et al. Noninvasive evaluation of regional myocardial perfusion with potassium-43: technique in patients with exercise-induced transient myocardial ischemia. *Radiology* 1973;108:85–90.
16. Germano G, Kavanagh PB, Slomka PJ, et al. Quantitation in gated perfusion SPECT imaging: the Cedars-Sinai approach. *J Nucl Cardiol* 2007;14(4):433–454.
17. Garcia EV, Faber TL, Cooke CD, et al. The increasing role of quantification in clinical nuclear cardiology: the Emory approach. *J Nucl Cardiol* 2007;14(4):420–432.
18. Ficaro EP, Lee BC, Kritzman JN, et al. Corridor4DM: the Michigan method for quantitative nuclear cardiology. *J Nucl Cardiol* 2007;14(4):455–465.
19. Nichols K, Santana CA, Folks R, et al. Comparison between ECTb and QGS for assessment of left ventricular function from gated myocardial perfusion SPECT. *J Nucl Cardiol* 2002;9:285–293.
20. Patton JA, Slomka PJ, Germano G, et al. Recent technologic advances in nuclear cardiology. *J Nucl Cardiol* 2007;14(4):501–513.
21. Johnson LL, Tauxe EL. Radionuclide assessment of ventricular function. *Curr Probl Cardiol* 1994;19:590–635.
22. Depuey EG, Port S, Wackers FJT, et al. Nonperfusion applications in nuclear cardiology: report of a task force of the American Society of Nuclear Cardiology. *J Nucl Cardiol* 1998;5:218–231.
23. Di Carli MF, Hachamovitch R. New technology for noninvasive evaluation of coronary artery disease. *Circulation* 2007;115:1464–1480.
24. Greenland P, Bonow RO, Brundage BH, et al. Clinical expert consensus document on coronary artery calcium scoring by computed tomography in global cardiovascular risk assessment and in evaluation of patients with chest pain. *J Am Coll Cardiol* 2007;49(3):378–402/*Circulation* 2007;23:403–426.
25. Budoff MJ, Achenbach S, Blumenthal RS, et al. Assessment of coronary artery disease by cardiac computed tomography: a scientific statement from the AHA Committee on Cardiovascular Radiology and Intervention and Committee on Cardiac Imaging, Council on Clinical Cardiology. *Circulation* 2006;114(16):1761–1791.
26. Hendel RC, Patel MR, Kramer CM, et al. ACCF/ACR/SCCT/SCMR/ASNC/NASCI/SIR: Appropriateness criteria for cardiac computed tomography and cardiac magnetic resonance imaging. *J Am Coll Cardiol* 2006; 48(7):1475–1497.
27. DePuey EG, Berman DS, Garcia EV, et al. Imaging guidelines for nuclear cardiology procedures. *J Nucl Cardiol* 2006;13:e21–e171. www.ASNC.org 2006.
28. Cerqueira MD, Schelbert HR, Wackers FJ, et al. Task force 5: training in nuclear cardiology. *J Am Coll Cardiol* 2006;47(4):898–804.
29. Budoff MJ, Cohen MC, Garcia MJ, et al. ACCF/AHA: Clinical competence on cardiac imaging with computed tomography and magnetic resonance. *J Am Coll Cardiol* 2005;46(2):383–402.
30. Deman P, Eckdahl J, Folks R, et al. Guidelines for technologist training in nuclear cardiology. *J Nucl Cardiol* 1997;4:422–425.
31. Weich HF, Strauss HW, Pitt B. The extraction of Tl-201 by the myocardium. *Circulation* 1977;56:188–192.
32. Krahwinkle W, Herzog H, Feinendegen LE. Pharmacokinetics of thallium-201 in normal individuals after routine myocardial scintigraphy. *J Nucl Med* 1988;29:1582–1586.
33. Beanlands RSB, Dawood F, Wen WH, et al. Are kinetics of technetium-99m methoxyisobutyl isonitril affected by cell metabolism and viability? *Circulation* 1990;82:1802–1814.
34. Younes A, Songadale JA, Maublant J, et al. Mechanism of uptake of technetium-tetrofosmin: uptake into isolated adult ventricular myocytes and subcellular localization. *J Nucl Cardiol* 1995;2:317–326.
35. Travin MI, Wexler JP. Pharmacological stress testing. *Semin Nucl Med* 1999;29:298–318.
36. Cohen MC. A snapshot of nuclear cardiology in the United States. *Am Soc Nucl Cardiol Newsletter* 1998;5:13.
37. Lette J, Tatum JL, Fraser S, et al. Safety of dipyridamole testing in 73,806 patients: the multicenter dipyridamole safety study. *J Nucl Cardiol* 1995;2:3–17.
38. Ranhosky A, Kempthorne-Rawson J. The safety of intravenous dipyridamole thallium myocardial perfusion imaging: intravenous dipyridamole thallium imaging study group. *Circulation* 1990;81:1205–1209.
39. Feldman RL, Nichols WM, Pepine CJ, et al. Acute effects of intravenous dipyridamole on regional coronary hemodynamics and metabolism. *Circulation* 1981;64:333–334.
40. Treuth MG, Reyes GA, He ZX, et al. Tolerance and diagnostic accuracy of an abbreviated adenosine infusion for myocardial scintigraphy: a randomized prospective study. *J Nucl Cardiol* 2001;8:548–554.
41. Abreu A, Mahmarian JJ, Nishimura S, et al. Tolerance and safety of pharmacologic coronary vasodilation with adenosine in association with thallium-201 scintigraphy in patients with coronary artery disease. *J Am Coll Cardiol* 1991;18:730–735.
42. Cerqueira MD, Verani MS, Schwaiger M, et al. Safety profile of adenosine stress perfusion imaging: results from the Adenoscan multicenter trial registry. *J Am Coll Cardiol* 1994;23:384–390.
43. Johnston DL. Hemodynamic responses and adverse effects associated with adenosine and dipyridamole pharmacologic stress testing: a comparison in 2000 patients. *May Clin Proc* 1995;70:331–336.
44. Coyne EP, Belvedere DA, Vande-Streek PR, et al. Thallium-201 scintigraphy after intravenous infusion of adenosine compared with exercise thallium testing in the diagnosis of coronary artery disease. *J Am Coll Cardiol* 1991;17(6):1289–1294.
45. Verani MS, Mahmarian JJ, Hisxon JB, et al. Diagnosis of coronary artery disease by controlled coronary vasodilation with adenosine and thallium-201 scintigraphy in patients unable to exercise. *Circulation* 1990;82(1):80–87.
46. Okeefe JH Jr, Bateman TM, Silvestri R, et al. Safety and diagnostic accuracy of adenosine thallium-201 scintigraphy in patients unable to exercise and those with left bundle branch block. *Am Heart J* 1992;124(3):614–621.
47. Hachamovitch R, Hayes S, Friedman JD, et al. Determinants of risk and its temporal variation in patients with normal stress myocardial

perfusion scans: what is the warranty period of a normal? *J Am Coll Cardiol* 2003;41:1329–1340.

48. Klodas E, Miller TD, Christian TF, et al. Prognostic significance of ischemic electrocardiographic changes during vasodilator stress testing in patients with normal SPECT images. *J Nucl Cardiol* 2003;10:4–8.

49. Abbott BG, Afshar M, Berger AK, Wackers FJ Th. Prognostic significance of ischemic electrocardiographic changes during adenosine infusion in patients with normal myocardial perfusion imaging. *J Nucl Cardiol* 2003;10:9–16.

50. Geleijnse ML, Elhendy A, Fioretii PM, Roelandt JR. Dobutamine stress myocardial perfusion imaging. *J Am Coll Cardiol* 2000;36(7):2017–2020.

51. Tadamura E, Iida H, Matsumoto K, et al. Comparison of myocardial blood flow during dobutamine-atropine infusion with that after dipyridamole administration in normal men. *J Am Coll Cardiol* 2001;37:130–136.

52. Cancer B, Karanfil A, Uysal U. Effect of an additional atropine injection during dobutamine infusion for myocardial SPECT. *Nucl Med Comm* 1997;18:567–573.

53. Picano E, Mathias W, Bigi R, Previtali M. Safety and tolerability of dobutamine-atropine stress echocardiography: a prospective, multicenter study. *Lancet* 1994;344:1190–1192.

54. Elhendy A, Bax JJ, Poldermans D. Dobutamine stress myocardial perfusion imaging in coronary artery disease. *J Nucl Med* 2002;43:1634–1646.

55. Elhendy A, van Domburg RT, Bax JJ, et al. Safety, hemodynamic profile, and feasibility of dobutamine stress technetium myocardial perfusion single-photon emission CT imaging for evaluation of coronary artery disease in the elderly. *Chest* 2000;117:649–656.

56. Elhendy A, van Domburg RT, Vantrimpont P, et al. Impact of heart transplantation on the safety and feasibility of the dobutamine stress test. *J Heart Transplant* 2001;20:399–406.

57. Geleijnse ML, Elhendy A, Domburg RT, et al. Prognostic value of dobutamine-atropine stress technetium-99m sestamibi perfusion scintigraphy in patients with chest pain. *J Am Coll Cardiol* 1996;28(2):447–454.

58. Schinkel AFL, Elhendy A, van Domburg RT, et al. Prognostic value of dobutamine-atropine stress 99mTc-tetrafosmin myocardial perfusion SPECT in patients with known or suspected coronary artery disease. *J Nucl Med* 2002;43:767–772.

59. He ZX, Cwajg E, Hwang W, et al. Myocardial blood flow and myocardial uptake of (201)Tl and (99m)Tc-sestamibi during coronary vasodilation induced by CGS-21680, a selective adenosine A(2A) receptor agonist. *Circulation* 2000;102:438–444.

60. Glover DK, Ruiz M, Yang JY, et al. Pharmacological stress thallium scintigraphy with 2-cyclohexylmethylidenehydrazinoadenosine (WRC-0470). A novel, short-acting adenosine A2A receptor agonist. *Circulation* 1996;94:1726–1732.

61. Trochu JN, Zhao G, Post H, et al. Selective A2A adenosine receptor agonist as a coronary vasodilator in conscious dogs: potential for use in myocardial perfusion imaging. *J Cardiovasc Pharmacol* 2003;41:132–1329.

62. Glover DK, Ruiz M, Takehana K, et al. Pharmacological stress myocardial perfusion imaging with the potent and selective A(2A) adenosine receptor agonists ATL193 and ATL146e administered by either intravenous infusion or bolus injection. *Circulation* 2001;104:1181–1187.

63. Iskandrian AE, Bateman TM, Belardinelli L, et al. Adenosine versus regadenoson comparative evaluation in myocardial perfusion imaging: results of the advance phase III multi-center international trial. *J Nucl Cardiol* 2007;14:645–658.

64. Dilsizian V, Smeltzer WR, Freedman NMT, et al. Thallium reinjection after stress-redistribution imaging: does 24H delayed imaging following reinjection enhance detection of viable myocardium? *Circulation* 1991;83:1247–1255.

65. Heo J, Powers J, Iskadrian AE. Exercise–rest same-day SPECT sestamibi imaging to detect coronary artery disease. *J Nucl Med* 1997;38: 200–203.

66. Vitola JV, Brambatti JC, Caligaris F, et al. Exercise supplementation to dipyridamole prevents hypotension, improves electrocardiogram sensitivity, and increases heart-to-liver activity ratio on Tc-99m sestamibi imaging. *J Nucl Cardiol* 2001;8:652–659.

67. Elliot MD, Holly TA, Leonard SM, Hendel RC. Impact of an abbreviated adenosine protocol incorporating adjunctive treadmill exercise on adverse effects and image quality in patients undergoing stress myocardial perfusion imaging. *J Nucl Cardiol* 2000;7:584–589.

68. Samady H, Wackers FJTh, Joska TM, et al. Pharmacologic stress perfusion imaging with adenosine: role of simultaneous low-level treadmill exercise. *J Nucl Cardiol* 2002;9:188–196.

69. Stein L, Burt R, Oppenheim B, et al. Symptom-limited arm exercise increases detection of ischemia during dipyridamole tomographic thallium stress testing in patients with coronary artery disease. *Am J Cardiol* 1995;75:568–572.

70. Verzijlbergen JF, Vermeersch PHMJ, Laarman Gert-Jan, et al. Inadequate exercise leads to suboptimal imaging after dipyridamole combined with low-level exercise unmasks ischemia in symptomatic patients with non-diagnostic thallium-201 scans who exercise submaximally. *J Nucl Med* 1991;32:2071–2078.

71. Taillefer R. Technetium-99m sestamibi myocardial imaging: same day rest-stress studies and dipyridamole. *Am J Cardiol* 1990;66:80E–84E.

72. Bergman H, Bjorntorp P, Conradson TB, et al. Enzymatic and circulatory adjustments to physical training in middle aged men. *Eur J Clin Invest* 1973;3:414–418.

73. Primeau M, Taillefer R, Essiambre R, et al. Technetium 99m sestamibi myocardial perfusion imaging: comparison between treadmill, dipyridamole and transoesophageal atrial pacing "stress" tests in normal subjects. *Eur J Nucl Med* 1991;18:247–251.

74. Casale PN, Guiney TE, Strauss W, et al. Simultaneous low level treadmill exercise and intravenous dipyridamole stress thallium imaging. *Am J Cardiol* 1988; 62:799–802.

75. Ignaszewski AP, McCormick LX, Heslip PG, et al. Safety and clinical utility of combined intravenous dipyridamole/symptom-limited exercise stress test with thallium-201 imaging in patients with known or suspected coronary artery disease. *J Nucl Med* 1993;34:2053–2061.

76. Laarman G, Niemeyer MG, Van Der Wall EE, et al. Dipyridamole thallium testing: noncardiac side effects, cardiac effects, electrocardiographic changes and hemodynamic changes after dipyridamole infusion with or without exercise. *Int J Cardiol* 1988;20:231–238.

77. Hashimoto A, Palmer EL, Scott JA, et al. Complications of exercise and pharmacologic stress tests: differences in younger and elderly patients. *J Nucl Cardiol* 1999;6:612–619.

78. Thomas GS, Prill NV, Majmundar H, et al. Treadmill exercise during adenosine infusion is safe, results in fewer adverse reactions, and improves myocardial perfusion image quality. *J Nucl Cardiol* 2000;7(5):439–446.

79. Pennell DJ, Mavrogeni SI, Forbat SM, et al. Adenosine combined with dynamic exercise for myocardial perfusion imaging. *J Am Coll Cardiol* 1995;25(6):1300–1309.

80. Vitola JV, Ludwig V, Cunha Pereira Neto C, et al. Exercise and dipyridamole combined myocardial scintigraphy allows early evaluation of perfusion and function. *J Nucl Cardiol* 2003;10(1): S-87.

81. Ebersole, MDG, Heironimus LCJ, Toney LCMO, et al. Comparison of exercise and adenosine technetium–99m sestamibi myocardial scintigraphy for diagnosis of coronary artery disease in patients with left bundle branch block. *Am J Cardiol* 1993;71:450–453.

82. Ellestad MH. *Stress Testing: Principles and Practice.* Philadelphia: Davis, 1996.

83. Holly TA, Satran A, Bromet DS, et al. The impact of adjunctive adenosine infusion during exercise myocardial perfusion imaging: Results of both exercise and adenosine stress test. *J Nucl Cardiol* 2003;10:291–296.

84. Hendel RC, Corbett JR, Cullom SJ, et al. The value and practice of attenuation correction for myocardial perfusion SPECT imaging: a joint position statement from the American Society of Nuclear Cardiology and the Society of Nuclear Medicine. *J Nucl Med* 2002;43(2):273–280.

85. Limacher MC, Douglas PS, Germano G, et al. ACC expert consensus document: radiation safety in the practice of cardiology. *J Am Coll Cardiol* 1998;31(4):892–913.

86. Thompson RC, Cullom SJ. Issues regarding dosage of cardiac nuclear and radiography procedures. *J Nucl Cardiol* 2006;13(910):19–23.

87. NCEP (National Cholesterol Education Program) Expert Panel on ATP III. Executive Summary. http://www.nhlbi.nih.gov/index.htm.

88. Shaw LJ, Berman DS, Bax JJ, et al. The complementary roles of nuclear cardiology and cardiac CT in the current healthcare environment. *J Nuc Cardiol* 2005;12:131–142.

89. Diamond GA, Forrester JS. Analysis of probability as an aid in the clinical diagnosis of coronary artery disease. *N Engl J Med* 1979;300:1350–1358.

90. Hamilton GW, Trobaugh G, Richie JC, et al. Myocardial imaging with ^{201}Tl: an analysis of clinical usefulness based on Bayes' theorem. *Semin Nucl Med* 1978;8:358.

91. Uhl GS, Kay TN, Hickman JR Jr. Computer-enhanced thallium scintigram in asymptomatic men with abnormal exercise tests. *Am J Cardiol* 1981;101:657–666.

92. Verani MS. Myocardial perfusion imaging versus two-dimensional echocardiography: comparative value in the diagnosis of coronary artery disease. *J Nucl Cardiol* 1994;1:399–414.

93. Goldstein JA, Gallagher MJ, O'Neill WW, et al. A randomized controlled trial of multi-slice coronary computed tomography for evaluation of acute chest pain. *J Am Coll Cardiol* 2007;49(8):863–871.

94. Melin JA, Piret LJ, Vanbutsele RJ, et al. Diagnostic value of exercise electrocardiography and thallium myocardial scintigraphy in patients without previous myocardial infarction: a Bayesian approach. *Circulation* 1981;63:1019–1024.

95. Melin JA, Wijns W, Vanbutsele RJ, et al. Alternative diagnostic strategies for coronary artery disease in women: demonstration of the usefulness and efficiency of probability analysis. *Circulation* 1985;71:535–542.

96. Brown KA, Atland E, Rowen M. Prognostic value of normal technetium 99m sestamibi cardiac imaging. *J Nucl Med* 1994; 35:554–557.

97. Gibson PB, Demus D, Hudson W, Johnson LL. Low event rate for stress-only perfusion imaging in patients evaluated for chest pain. *J Am Coll Cardiol* 2002;39:999–1004.

98. Cerqueira MD, Weissman NJ, Dilsizian V, et al. Standardized myocardial segmentation and nomenclature for tomographic imaging of the heart: a statement for healthcare professionals from the cardiac imaging committee of the council on clinical cardiology of the American Heart Association. *J Nucl Cardiol* 2002;105:539–542.

99. Homma S, Kaul S, Boucher CA. Correlates of lung/heart ratio of thallium-201 in coronary artery disease. *J Nucl Med* 1987;28:1531–1535.

100. Bacher-Stier C, Sharir T, Kavanagh PB, et al. Postexercise lung uptake of 99mTc-sestamibi determined by a new automatic technique: validation and application in detection of severe and extensive coronary artery disease and reduced left ventricular function. *J Nucl Med* 2000;41:1190–1197.

101. Hansen CL, Cen P, Sanchez B, et al. Comparison of pulmonary uptake with transient cavity dilation after dipyridamole Tl-201 perfusion imaging. *J Nucl Cardiol* 2002;9:47–51.

102. Sanders GP, Pinto DS, Parker JA, et al. Increased resting Tl-201 lung-to-heart ratio is associated with invasively determined measures of left ventricular dysfunction, extent of coronary artery disease, and rest myocardial perfusion abnormalities. *J Nucl Cardiol* 2003;10:140–147.

103. Barr SA, Jain D, Wackers FJ, et al. Tetrofosmin Phase III multicenter study group: Are there correlates of increased thallium uptake on planar tetrofosmin perfusion imaging? *Circulation* 1993;88(Suppl I):582.

104. Kaminek M, Mysliveck M, Skvarilova M, et al. Increased prognostic value of combined myocardial perfusion SPECT imaging and the quantification of lung Tl-201 uptake. *Clin Nucl Med* 2002;27:255–260.

105. Gavazzi A, De Servi S, Cornalba C, et al. Significance of the walk-through angina phenomenon during exercise testing. *Cardiology* 1986;73(1):47–53.

106. Ellestad MH. *Stress Testing: Principles and Practice*, 5th ed. Oxford and New York: Oxford University Press 2003:307.

107. Chauhan A, Thuraisingham SI, Stone DL. Exercise electrocardiogram and single vessel coronary artery disease. *Postgrad Med J* 73(864):655.

108. Schmitt C, Lehmann G, Wailersbacher M, et al. Problems of electrocardiographic diagnosis of occlusion of the left circumflex coronary artery. *Dtsch Med Wochenschr* 2001;126(45):1257–1260.

109. Diamond GA, Forrester JS. Analysis of probability as an aid in the clinical diagnosis of coronary artery disease. *N Engl J Med* 1979;300:1350–1358.

110. Miller TD, Roger VL, Milavetz JJ, et al. Assessment of the exercise electrocardiogram in women versus men using tomographic myocardial perfusion imaging as the reference standard. *Am J Cardiol* 2001;87:868–873.

111. Kwok Y, Kim C, Grady D, et al. Analysis of exercise testing to detect coronary artery disease in women. *Am J Cardiol* 1999;83:660–666.

112. Morise AP, Dalal JN, Duval RD. Value of a simple measure of estrogen status for improving the diagnosis of coronary artery disease in women. *Am J Med* 1993;94:491–496.

113. Verani MS. Myocardial perfusion imaging versus two-dimensional echocardiography: comparative value in the diagnosis of coronary artery disease. *J Nucl Cardiol* 1994;1:399–414.

114. Hachamovitch R, Berman DS, Kiat H, et al. Exercise myocardial perfusion SPECT in patients without known coronary artery disease. *Circulation* 1996;93(5):905–914.

115. Weiss AT, Berman DS, Lew AS, et al. Transient ischemic dilatation of the left ventricle on stress thallium-201 scintigraphy: a marker of severe and extensive coronary artery disease. *J Am Coll Cardiol* 1987;9:752–759.

116. McLaughlin MG. Transient ischemic dilation: a powerful diagnostic and prognostic finding of stress myocardial perfusion imaging. *J Nucl Cardiol* 2002;9(6):663–667.

117. Noriyuki assessment of transient left ventricular dilatation on rest and exercise on Tc-99m tetrofosmin myocardial SPECT. *Clin Nucl Med* 2002; 27:34–39.

118. Mazzanti M, Germano G, Kiat H, et al. Identification of severe and extensive coronary artery disease by automatic measurement of transient ischemic dilatation of the left ventricle in dual-isotope myocardial perfusion SPECT. *J Am Coll Cardiol* 1996;27(7):1612–1620.

119. Daou D. Identification of extensive cornary artery disease: incremental value of exercise Tl-201 SPECT to clinical and stress test variables. *J Nucl Cardiol* ;9(2):161–168.

120. Besletti A, Di Leo C, Alessi A, et al. Post-stress end-systolic left ventricular dilation: a marker of endocardial post-ischemic stunning. *Nucl Med Commun* 2001;22:685–698.

121. Chouraqui P, Rodriguez EA, Berman DS, et al. Significance of dipyridamole-induced transient dilatation of the left ventricle during thallium-201 scintigraphy in suspected coronary artery disease. *Am J Cardiol* 1990;66:689–694.

122. Toyama T, Caner BE, Tamaki N, et al. Transient ischemic dilatation of the left ventricle observed on dipyridamole-stressed thallium-201 scintigraphy. *Kaku Igaku* 1993;30:605–611.

123. Kristman JN, Ficaro EP, Corbett JR. Post-stress LV dilation: the effect of imaging protocol, gender and attenuation correction. *J Nucl Med* 2001;42(Suppl):50P.

124. McClellan JR, Travin MI, Herman SD, et al. Prognostic importance of scintigraphic left ventricular cavity dilation during intravenous dipyridamole technetium-99m sestamibi myocardial tomographic imaging in predicting coronary events. *Am J Cardiol* 1997;79:600–605.

125. Kirk JD, Diercks DB, Turnipseed SD, et al. Evaluation of chest pain suspicious for coronary syndrome: use of an accelerated diagnostic protocol in a chest pain evaluation unit. *Am J Cardiol* 2000;85(5A):40B–48B; discussion 49B.

126. Abbott BG, Jain D. Nuclear cardiology in the evaluation of acute chest pain in the emergency department. *Echocardiography* 2000;17: 597–560.

127. Lee TH, Rouan GW, Weisberg MC, et al. Clinical characteristics and natural history of patients with acute myocardial infarction sent home from the emergency room. *Am J Cardiol* 1987;60:219–224.

128. Pope JH, Aufderheide TP, Ruthazer R, et al. Missed diagnoses of acute cardiac ischemia in the emergency department. *N Engl J Med* 2000;342:1163–1170.

129. Abbott BG, Wackers FJ. The role of radionuclide imaging in the triage of patients with chest pain in the emergency department. *Rev Port Cardiol* 2000;19(Suppl 1):153–161.

130. Zalenski RJ, Shamsa FH. Diagnostic testing of the emergency department patient with chest pain. *Curr Opin Cardiol* 1998;13(4):248–253.

131. Kontos MC, Jesse RL, Anderson FP, et al. Comparison of myocardial perfusion imaging and cardiac troponin I in patients admitted to the emergency department with chest pain. *Circulation* 1999;99(16):2073–2078.

132. Udelson JE, Beshansky JR, Ballin DS, et al. Myocardial perfusion imaging for evaluation and triage of patients with suspected acute cardiac ischemia. A randomized controlled trial. *JAMA* 2002; 288: 2693–2700.

133. Fischman DL, Leon M, Baim DS, et al. A randomized comparison of coronary stent placement and balloon angioplasty in the treatment of coronary artery disease. *N Engl J Med* 1994;331:496–501.

134. Georgoulias P, Demakopoulos N, Kontos A, et al. Tc-99m –Tetrofosmin myocardial perfusion imaging before and six months after percutaneous transluminal coronary angioplasty. *Clin Nucl Med* 1998;23:678–682.

135. Galassi AR, Rosario F, Azzarelli S, et al. Usefulness of exercise tomographic myocardial perfusion imaging for detection of restenosis after coronary stent implantation. *Am J Cardiol* 2000;85:1362–1364.

136. Milavetz JJ, Miller TD, Hodge DO, et al. Accuracy of single-photon emission computed tomography myocardial perfusion imaging in patients with stents in native coronary arteries. *Am J Cardiol* 1998;82:857–861.

137. Lauer MS, Lytle B, Pashkow F, et al. Prediction of death and myocardial infarction by screening with exercise-thallium testing after coronary-artery-bypass grafting. *Lancet* 1998; 351:615–622.

138. Zellweger MJ, Lewin HC, Lai S, et al. When to stress patients after coronary artery bypass surgery? Risk stratification in patients early and late post-CABG using stress myocardial perfusion SPECT: implications of appropriate clinical strategies. *J Am Coll Cardiol* 2001;37:144–152.

139. Berman DS, Boden WE, O'Rourke RA, et al. Optimal medical therapy with or without pci for stable coronary disease. *N Engl J Med* 2007;356:1–14.

140. O'Rourke RA, Chaudhuri T, Shaw L, et al. Resolution of stress-induced myocardial ischemia during aggressive medical therapy as demonstrated by single photon emission computed tomography imaging. *Circulation* 2001;103:2315.

141. Gersh BJ, Rihal CS, Rooke TW, et al. Evaluation and management of patients with both peripheral vascular and coronary artery disease. *J Am Coll Cardiol* 1991;18:203–214.

142. Hertzer NR, Beven EG, Young JR, et al. Coronary artery disease in peripheral vascular patients: a classification of 1,000 coronary angiograms and results of surgical management. *Ann Surg* 1984;199:223–233.

143. Di Carli MF, Dorbala S, Meserve J, et al. Clinical myocardial perfusion PET/CT. *J Nucl Med* 2007;48:783–793.

144. Di Carli MF, Hachamovitch R. New technology for noninvasive evaluation of coronary artery disease. *Circulation* 2007;115:1464–1480.

145. Leschka S, Alkadhi H, Plass A, et al. Accuracy of MSCT coronary angiography with 64-slice technology: first experience. *Eur Heart J* 2005; 26(15):1482–1487.

146. Leber AW, Knez A, von Ziegler F, et al. Quantification of obstructive and non-obstructive coronary lesions by 64-slice computed tomography. A comparative study with quantitative coronary angiography and intravascular ultrasound. *J Am Coll Cardiol* 2005;46:147–154.

147. Raff GJ, Gallagher MJ, O'Neill WW, et al. Diagnostic accuracy of noninvasive angiography using 64-slice spiral computed tomography. *J Am Coll Cardiol* 2005;46:552–557.

148. Garcia MJ, Lessick J, Hoffmann MH. Accuracy of 16-row multidetector computed tomography for the assessment of coronary artery stenosis; CATSCAN Study Investigators. *JAMA* 2006;296(4):403–411.

149. Kopp AF, Schroeder S, Kuetteer A, et al. Non-invasive coronary angiography with high resolution multi-detector–row computed tomography: results in 102 patients. *Eur Heart J* 2002;23:1714–1725.

150. Ropers D, Baum U, Pohle K, et al. Detection of coronary artery stenoses with thin-slice multi-detector row spiral computed tomography and multiplanar reconstruction. *Circulation* 2003;107:664–666.

151. Knetz A, Becker C, Leber A, et al. Usefulness of multislice spiral computed tomography angiography for determination of coronary stenoses. *Am J Cardiol* 2001;88:1191–1194.

152. Frazier AA, Qureshi F, Read KM, et al. Coronary artery bypass grafts: assessment with multidetector CT in the early and late post-operative settings. *Radiographics* 2005;25:881–896.

153. Nieman K, Cademartiri F, Raajimakers R, et al. Non-invasive angiographic evaluation of coronary stents with multi-slice spiral computed tomography. *Herz* 2003;28:136–142.

154. Schuijf JD, Bax JJ, Jukema JW, et al. Feasibility of assessment of coronary stent patency using 16-slice computed tomography. *Am J Cardiol* 2004;94:427–430.

155. Gilard M, Cornly JC, Rioufol G, et al. Noninvasive assessment of left main coronary stent patency with 16-slice computed tomography. *Am J Cardiol* 2005;95:110–112.

156. Bateman TM, Heller GV, McGhie AI, et al. Diagnostic accuracy of rest/stress ECG-gated Rb-82 myocardial perfusion PET: comparison with ECG-gated Tc-99m sestamibi SPECT. *J Nucl Cardiol* 2006;13(1):24–33.

157. Sampson UK, Dorbala S, Limaye A, et al. Diagnostic accuracy of rubidium-82 myocardial perfusion imaging with hybrid positron emission tomography/computed tomography in the detection of coronary artery disease. *J Am Coll Cardiol* 2007;49:1052–1058.

158. Dorbala S, Vangala D, Sampson U, et al. Value of vasodilator left ventricular ejection fraction reserve in evaluating the magnitude of myocardium at risk and the extent of angiographic coronary artery disease: a 82Rb PET/CT study. *J Nucl Med* 2007;48(3):349–358.

159. Bax JJ, Van Eck-Smit BLF, Van der Wall EE. Assessment of tissue viability: clinical demand and problems. *Eur Heart J* 1998;19:847–858.

160. Kim RJ, Wu E, Rafael A, et al. The use of contrast-enhanced magnetic resonance imaging to identify reversible myocardial dysfunction. *N Engl J Med* 2000;343:1445–1453.

161. Bax JJ, Cornel JH, Visser FC, et al. Comparison of fluorine-18-FDG with rest-redistribution thallium-201 SPECT to delineate viable myocardium and predict functional recovery after revascularization. *J Nucl Med* 1998;39:1481–1486.

162. Marwick TH. The viable myocardium. Epidemiology, detection, and clinical implications. *Lancet* 1998;351:815–819.

163. Yang LD, Berman DS, Kiat H, et al. The frequency of late redistribution in SPECT thallium-201 stress-redistribution studies. *J Am Coll Cardiol* 1990;15:334–340.

164. Dilsizian V, Rocco TP, Freedman NMT, et al. Enhanced detection of ischemic but viable myocardium by the reinjection of thallium after stress-redistribution imaging. *N Engl J Med* 1990;323:141–146.

165. Cuocolo A, Petretta M, Nicolai E, et al. Successful coronary revascularization improves prognosis in patients with previous myocardial infarction and evidence of viable myocardium at thallium-201 imaging. *Eur J Nucl Med* 1998;25:60–68.

166. Dilsizian V, Bonow RO. Current diagnostic techniques of assessing viability in patients with hibernating and stunned myocardium. *Circulation* 1993;87:1–20.

167. Bax JJ, Wijns W, Cornel JH, et al. Accuracy of currently available techniques for prediction of functional recovery after revascularization in patients with left ventricular dysfunction due to chronic coronary artery disease: comparison of pooled data. *J Am Coll Cardiol* 1997;30:1451–1460.

168. Allman KC, Shaw LJ, Hachamovitch R, Udelson JE. Myocardial viability testing and impact of revascularization on prognosis in patients with coronary artery disease and left ventricular dysfunction: a meta-analysis. *J Am Coll Cardiol* 2002;39:1151–1158.

169. Bax JJ, Visser FC, Poldermans D, et al. Relationship between preoperative viability and postoperative improvement in LVEF and heart failure symptoms. *J Nucl Med* 2001;42:79–86. Imaging guidelines for nuclear cardiology procedures . *J Nucl Cardiol* 2006;13:e21–e171.

170. Bax JJ, Visser FC, Poldermans D, et al. Relationship between preoperative viability and postoperative improvement in LVEF and heart failure symptoms. *J Nucl Med* 2001;42:79–86.

171. Imaging Guidelines for Nuclear Cardiology Procedures. *J Nucl Cardiol* 2006;13:e21–171.

172. Beanlands RSB, Hendry PJ, Masters RG, et al. Delay in revascularization is associated with increased mortality rate in patients with severe left ventricular dysfunction and viable myocardium on fluorine 18-fluorordeoxyglucose positron emission tomography. *Circulation* 1998;98:II-51–II-56.

173. Louie HW, Laks H, Milgalter E, et al. Ischemic cardiomyopathy. Criteria for coronary revascularization and cardiac transplantation. *Circulation* 1991;84:III290–III295.

174. Grundy SM, Benjamin IJ, Burke GL, et al. Diabetes mellitus: a major risk factor for cardiovascular disease: a joint editorial statement by the American Diabetes Association; the National Heart, Lung, and Blood Institute; the Juvenile Diabetes Foundation International; the National Institute of Diabetes and Digestive and Kidney Disease, and the American Heart Association. *Circulation* 1999;100:1134–1146.

175. Kang X, Berman DS, Lewin H, et al. Comparative ability of myocardial perfusion single-photon emission computed tomography to detect coronary artery disease in patients with and without diabetes mellitus. *Am Heart J* 1999;137:949–957.

176. Giri S, Shaw LJ, Murthy DR, et al. Impact of diabetes on the risk stratification using stress single-photon emission computed tomography myocardial perfusion imaging in patients with symptoms suggestive of coronary artery disease. *Circulation* 2002;105:32–40.

177. Kang X, Berman DS, Lewin HC, et al. Incremental prognostic value of myocardial perfusion single photon emission computed tomography in patients with diabetes mellitus. *Am Heart J* 1999;138:1025–1032.

178. Wackers FT, Zaret BL. Editorial: detection of myocardial ischemia in patients with diabetes mellitus. *Circulation* 2002;105:5–7.

179. Ding HJ, Shiau YC, Wang JJ, et al. The influences of blood glucose and duration of fasting on myocardial glucose uptake of [18F]fluoro-2-deoxy-D-glucose. *Nucl Med Commun* 2002;23:961–965.

180. Imaging Guidelines for Nuclear Cardiology Procedures. *J Nucl Cardiol* 2006;13:e119–e127.

181. Martin WH, Jones RC, Delbeke D, et al. A simplified intravenous glucose loading protocol for fluorine-18 fluorodeoxyglucose cardiac single-photon emission tomography. *Eur J Nucl Med* 1997;24:1291–1297.

182. Knuuti MJ, Yki-Järvinen H, Voipio-Pulkki LM, et al. Enhancement of myocardial [fluorine-18] fluorodeoxyglucose uptake by a nicotinic acid derivative. *J Nucl Med* 1994;35:989–998.

183. Bonow RO, Dilsizian V. Thallium-201 and technetium-99m-MIBI for assessing viable myocardium. *J Nucl Med* 1992;33:815–818.

184. Matsunari I, Fujino, Taki J, et al. Quantitative rest technetium-99m tetrofosmin imaging in predicting functional recovery after revascularization: Comparison with rest–redistribution thallium-201. *J Am Coll Cardiol* 1997;29:1226–1233.

185. Matsunari I, Böning G, Ziegler SI, et al. Attenuation-corrected ^{99m}Tc-tetrofosmin single-photon emission computed tomography in the detection of viable myocardium: comparison with positron emission tomography using 18F-fluorodeoxyglucose. *J Am Coll Cardiol* 1998;32:927–935.

186. Cuocolo A, Pace L, Ricciardelli B, et al. Identification of viable myocardium in patients with chronic coronary artery disease: comparison of thallium-201 scintigraphy with reinjection and technetium-99m-methoxyisobutyl isonitrile. *J Nucl Med* 1992;33:505–511.

187. Soufer R, Dey HM, Ng CK, et al. Comparison of MIBI single-photon emission computed tomography with positron emission tomography for estimating left ventricular myocardial viability. *Am J Cardiol* 1995;75:1214–1219.

188. Sawada S, Allman KC, Muzik O, et al. Positron emission tomography detects evidence of viability in rest technetium-99m MIBI defects. *J Am Coll Cardiol* 1994;23:92–98.

189. Altehoefer C, Vom Dahl J, Biedermann M, et al. Significance of defect severity in technetium-99m-MIBI SPECT at rest to assess myocardial

viability: comparison with fluorine-18-FDG PET. *J Nucl Med* 1994;35: 569–574.

190. Schneider CA, Voth E, Gawlich S, et al. Significance of rest technetium-99m sestamibi imaging for the prediction of improvement of left ventricular dysfunction after Q wave myocardial infarction: importance of infarct location adjusted thresholds. *J Am Coll Cardiol* 1998;32:648–654.

191. Smanio PEP, Watson DD, Segalla DL, et al. Value of gating of technetium-99m sestamibi single-photon emission computed tomographic imaging. *J Am Coll Cardiol* 1997;30:1687–1692.

192. Bisi G, Sciagra R, Santoro GM, et al. Rest technetium-99m sestamibi tomography in combination with short-term administration of nitrates: feasibility and reliability for prediction of postrevascularization outcome of asynergic territories. *J Am Coll Cardiol* 1994;24:1282–1289.

193. Senior R, Kaul S, Raval U, et al. Impact of revascularization and myocardial viability determined by nitrate-enhanced Tc-99m sestamibi and Tl-201 imaging on mortality and functional outcome in ischemic cardiomyopathy. *J Nucl Cardiol* 2002;9:454–462.

194. Sciagra R, Bisi G, Santoro GM, et al. Comparison of baseline-nitrate technetium-99m sestamibi with rest-redistribution thallium-201 tomography in detecting viable hibernating myocardium and predicting postrevascularization recovery. *J Am Coll Cardiol* 1997;30:384–391.

195. Sciagra R, Leoncini M, Marcucci G, et al. Technetium-99m sestamibi imaging to predict left ventricular ejection fraction outcome after revascularization in patients with chronic coronary artery disease and left ventricular dysfunction: comparison between baseline and nitrate-enhanced imaging. *Eur J Nucl Med* 2001;28:680–687.

196. Batista JF, Pereztol O, Valdes JA, et al. Improved detection of myocardial perfusion reversibility by rest-nitroglycerin Tc-99m-MIBI: comparison with Tl-201 reinjection. *J Nucl Cardiol* 1999;6:480–486.

197. Oudiz RJ, Smith DE, Pollack AJ, et al. Nitrate-enhanced thallium-201 single photon emission tomography imaging in hibernating myocardium. *Am Heart J* 1999;138:206–209.

198. Pitman AG, Kalff V, Van Every B, et al. Contributions of subdiaphragmatic activity, attenuation, and diaphragmatic motion to inferior wall artifact in attenuation-corrected Tc-99m myocardial perfusion SPECT. *J Nucl Cardiol* 2005;12(4):401–419.

199. Corbett JR, Kritzman JN, Ficaro EP. Attenuation correction for single photon emission computed tomography myocardial perfusion imaging. *Curr Cardiol Rep* 2004;6(1):32–40.

200. Nishina H, Slomka P, Abidov A, et al. Combined supine and prone quantitative myocardial perfusion SPECT: method development and clinical validation in patients with no known coronary artery disease. *J Nucl Med* 2006;47:51–58.

201. Hayes SW, Lorenzo AD, Hachamovitch R, et al. Prognostic implication of combined prone and supine acquisitions in patients with equivocal or abnormal supine myocardial perfusion SPECT. *J Nucl Med* 2003;44:1633–1640.

202. Bateman TM, Cullom SJ. Attenuation correction single photon emission computed tomography myocardial perfusion imaging. *Semin Nucl Med* 2005;35:37–51.

203. Hendel RC, Corbett JR, Cullom SJ, et al. The value and practice of attenuation correction for myocardial perfusion SPECT imaging: A joint position statement from the American Society of Nuclear Cardiology and the Society of Nuclear Medicine. *J Nucl Med* 2002;43(2):273–280.

204. Patton JA, Delbeke D, Sandler MP. Image fusion using an integrated dual-head coincidence camera with x-ray tube based attenuation maps. *J Nucl Med* 2000;41:1364–1368.

205. Masood Y, Liu HY, Depuey G, et al. Clinical validation of SPECT attenuation correction using x-ray computed tomography-derived attenuation maps: multicenter clinical trial with angiographic correlation. *J Nucl Cardiol* 2005;12(6):676–686.

206. Malkerneker D, Brenner R, Martin WH, et al. CT-based attenuation correction versus prone imaging to decrease equivocal interpretations of rest/stress 99mTc-tetrafosmin SPECT MPI. *J Nucl Cardiol* 2007;14:314–323.

207. Schneider JF, Thomas Jr HE, Sorlie P, et al. Comparative features of newly acquired left and right bundle branch block in the general population: the Framingham study. *Am J Cardiol* 1981;47:931–9340.

208. Fahy GJ, Pinski SL, Miller DP, et al. Natural history of isolated bundle branch block. *Am J Cardiol* 1996;77:1185–1190.

209. Patel R, Bushnell DL, Wagner R, et al. Frequency of false-positive septal defects on adenosine/201Tl images in patients with LBBB. *Nucl Med Commun* 1995;6:137–139.

210. Hirzel HO, Senn M, Nuesch K, et al. Thallium 201 scintigraphy in complete LBBB. *Am J Cardiol* 1984;53:764–769.

211. DePuey EG, Guertler-Krawczynska E, Robbins WL. Thallium 201 SPECT in coronary artery disease patients with LBBB. *J Nucl Med* 1988;29:1479–1485.

212. Larcos G, Brown ML, Gibbons RJ. Role of dipyridamole thallium-201 imaging in patients with LBBB. *Am J Cardiol* 1991;68:1097–1098.

213. Hirzel HO, Senn M, Nuesch K, et al. Thallium-201 scintigraphy in complete left bundle branch block. *Am J Cardiol* 1984;53:764–769.

214. Poliner LR, Buja LM, Parkey RW, et al. Clinicopathologic findings in 52 patients studied by technetium-99m stannous pyrophosphate myocardial scintigraphy. *Circulation* 1979;59:257–267.

CHAPTER FOUR

NEUROLOGIC IMAGING

Dominique Delbeke
and Carlos Cunha

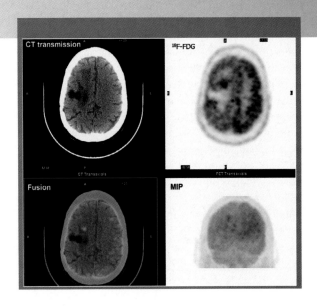

RADIOPHARMACEUTICALS

Any radiopharmaceutical injected as a bolus in a dose ~20 mCi of technetium-99m (^{99m}Tc) for an adult—that provides a high enough count rate to perform dynamic imaging—will allow evaluation of blood flow to the brain. A dynamic flow study is performed by acquiring sequential images rapidly over time, typically every 2 seconds. A flow study can be performed in only one projection—the anterior projection when the brain is evaluated. Technically, the bolus injection can be suboptimal if the patient is hypotensive or bradycardic. If the camera is started too late into the injection, the critical arterial phase of the flow study may be missed.

Two categories of radiopharmaceuticals are used to image the brain: the conventional radiopharmaceuticals, which do not cross the blood–brain barrier and the lipophilic chelate tracers, which do cross it and fix in the brain proportionally to perfusion.

The functional basis of conventional brain imaging is that most intracranial lesions will alter the blood–brain barrier and the radiopharmaceutical will leak from the capillaries into or around the lesion. The lesion appears as a "hot spot" in the normal low background of the brain. A conventional brain study with glucoheptonate includes a dynamic flow followed by immediate static images and, up to 4 hours, delayed images in anterior, posterior, and both lateral projections.

^{99m}Tc-hexamethylpropylene amine oxime exametazime (^{99m}Tc-HMPAO, Ceretec, GE Healthcare), and ^{99m}Tc-ethyl cysteinate dimmer (^{99m}Tc-ECD, Neurolite, Merck Dupont Inc.) are lipophilic chelate radiopharmaceuticals of cerebral perfusion that are now available and approved by the Food and Drug Administration (FDA). They have a high extraction fraction and are taken up by the brain proportionally to perfusion. There is a very stable pattern of uptake within a few minutes and slow or no washout from the brain over time. Cerebral uptake of ^{99m}Tc-HMPAO correlates well with cerebral perfusion measured with labeled microspheres up to 200 mL/100 g per minute. A limitation of ^{99m}Tc-ECD is that the uptake does not increase linearly with perfusion at high flow rates—a limitation for indications such as ictal imaging of epileptic patients. ^{99m}Tc-ECD is stable for 6 hours after preparation, an advantage over ^{99m}Tc-HMPAO, which must be injected within 30 minutes after preparation. The stability of ^{99m}Tc-HMPAO can be increased to 4 hours by the addition of methylene blue, which is required for ictal imaging. The procedure to prepare the ^{99m}Tc-HMPAO stabilized with methylene blue is explained in the kit's package insert (Ceretec, GE Healthcare).

When a brain perfusion study is indicated, 20 mCi of ^{99m}Tc-HMPAO or ^{99m}Tc-ECD is injected intravenously, and SPECT images are acquired between 10 minutes and 2 hours after injection.

Iodine-123 (^{123}I)-iodo-amphetamine (IMP) and xenon-133 (^{133}Xe) are also tracers of cerebral perfusion. ^{123}I-IMP is not widely available and therefore is rarely used for clinical purposes. ^{133}Xe is a gas and less practical to use than ^{99m}Tc-radiopharmaceuticals; in addition ^{133}Xe images are of relatively low resolution with conventional gamma cameras.

^{133}Xe has the advantage of short acquisition time, true quantitation of cerebral perfusion, and rapid washout time—a useful feature in performing challenge tests.

The glucose metabolism of the brain can be evaluated using fluorine-18 (^{18}F)-fluorodeoxyglucose (^{18}F-FDG) as radiopharmaceutical. ^{18}F is a positron emitter that requires coincidence imaging by positron emission tomography (PET) to obtain optimal images. ^{18}F-FDG is transported into the cells by the same mechanism as glucose; it is then phosphorylated by a hexokinase into FDG-6-phosphate. As the brain tissue does not have a glucose-6-dephosphatase, FDG-6-phosphate does not progress into further glycolytic pathways; it accumulates in proportion to the glycolytic rate of the cells. The cortex of the brain normally uses only glucose as its substrate; therefore ^{18}F-FDG accumulation is high. Because PET systems provide for soft tissue attenuation and are calibrated with an external source of known activity of germanium-68 (^{68}Ge), true count rates can be measured over a region of interest. Quantification of the actual metabolic rate using kinetic modeling is possible but requires dynamic scanning after injection of ^{18}F-FDG and dynamic arterial blood sampling to obtain both tissue and plasma tracer concentration.

True quantitative measurements are extremely useful in the investigation of the physiopathologic mechanisms of neuropsychiatric diseases and can be performed with ^{18}F-FDG but also a variety of radiopharmaceuticals labeled with positron emitters. This approach, however, is time-consuming, cumbersome, and more invasive than obtaining a static image after ^{18}F-FDG reaches a plateau, usually 45 minutes following IV injection. Measurement of the absolute metabolic rate is rarely performed clinically. Semiquantitative evaluation using asymmetry indices or ratios to reference structures of the brain are usually satisfactory for diagnostic purposes. When an ^{18}F-FDG study is indicated, 10 mCi of ^{18}F-FDG is injected intravenously and PET images of the brain are acquired after 45 minutes of distribution time. The images are corrected for attenuation with a transmission scan using an external source of ^{68}Ge (measured attenuation) or x-ray source (CT transmission) or with a calculated attenuation using the ellipse model.

To interpret tomographic images (both SPECT and PET), it is critical to have the software to reorient the images along the anterior commissure–posterior commissure (AC–PC) line and to examine the three projections (axial, coronal, and sagittal). If two scans have to be compared (ictal and interictal, baseline and acetazolamide, pre- and posttherapy or intervention, etc.), similar orientation slice thickness and windowing is critical. Comparison with the current MRI or CT films is also critical if there is a structural abnormality.

Cerebrospinal fluid (CSF) dynamics can be studied by intrathecal injection of radiopharmaceuticals. Indium-111 (^{111}In)-DTPA is used to evaluate hydrocephalus and CSF leaks, both requiring 24 and possibly 48 hours of imaging. To evaluate the CSF dynamics, 0.5 mCi of ^{111}In-DTPA is injected intrathecally and images are obtained immediately over the spinal canal to document the quality of the injection and then at 4, 24, and 48 hours over the head in the anterior, posterior, and both lateral projections until the radiopharmaceutical reaches the convexity. ^{99m}Tc-DTPA can be used to evaluate the patency of shunts because of the shorter imaging time.

NORMAL DISTRIBUTION AND VARIANTS

Perfusion and glucose metabolic images of the brain have a similar appearance except in pathologic circumstances when there is decoupling of perfusion and metabolism. The adult pattern of uptake is established by the age of 20. The normal perfusion of the gray matter is approximately 70 mL/min per 100 g and that of the white matter 20 mL/min per 100 g. In the newborn, the perfusion and metabolism of basal ganglia, visual cortex, and sensorimotor cortex is close to that of an adult; there is, however, decreased perfusion to the frontal and parietotemporal cortex, giving an immature pattern of perfusion and metabolism (1).

The weight of the brain decreases approximately 10% between the ages of 30 and 75, and cerebral blood flow decreases by 20%, probably because of neuronal loss and replacement by gliosis. On CT and MRI, this is demonstrated by progressive cortical atrophy with age.

In normal individuals, both the blood flow pattern and metabolism are influenced by certain drugs. Methylxanthines, such as caffeine, and sedatives decrease the blood flow and brain metabolism. If a patient needs sedation for the scanning period, sedatives should be administered no earlier than 20 minutes after the administration of the radiopharmaceutical.

The CSF is secreted by the choroid plexus and flows from the lateral ventricles into the third and fourth ventricles and out into the posterior compartment of the spinal subarachnoid spaces through the foramen of Lushka and Magendie. The CSF then flows in the cephalad direction into the anterior compartment of the spinal canal to reach the basal cisternae. When it reaches the convexities, it is reabsorbed by the arachnoid granulations. When a radiopharmaceutical is injected by lumbar puncture, it normally reaches the basal cisternae by 1 hour, the frontal poles and sylvian fissure by 2 to 6 hours, the cerebral convexities by 12 hours, and the arachnoid granulation in the sagittal sinus region by 24 hours. There is normally no reflux into the ventricular system.

INDICATIONS

Brain Death (2)

Brain death is a clinical diagnosis taking into account both cerebral and brainstem function. Confirmatory tests such as electroencephalography (EEG) and imaging studies assessing blood flow to the brain give evidence for or against the clinical impression. With the widespread use of brain metabolic suppressive therapy, cerebral blood flow imaging is more accurate than EEG. The guidelines published in *JAMA* in 1981 recommend a test of cerebral blood flow to confirm brain death. Radionuclide blood flow imaging is noninvasive and can be done portably, giving it two major advantages over angiography (2–5).

If ^{99m}Tc-glucoheptonate is used as a radiopharmaceutical, the interpretation relies entirely on the dynamic flow scan and the quality of the bolus injection. As the flow scan is obtained in the anterior projection, only flow to the anterior and middle cerebral arteries can be assessed. The posterior circulation must be evaluated clinically. In most cases, however, brain death is due to increased intracranial pressure, and the circulation of the entire brain is affected to the same extent.

^{99m}Tc-HMPAO and -ECD offer the advantage of accumulating within the brain tissue itself. If the dynamic flow images are of poor quality, delayed images can be obtained in multiple projections; even single photon emission tomography (SPECT) can be performed if necessary, offering the advantage of assessing perfusion to the entire brain, including the posterior fossa (6).

Herpes Encephalitis

It is important to make the diagnosis early in the disease because there is a treatment available with acyclovir. Nowadays, this may be the only indication remaining for brain imaging with ^{99m}Tc-glucoheptonate, because the images are abnormal days before the CT scan. The most specific sign of herpes encephalitis is focal temporal uptake, but uptake in this location is found in only 50% of the patients. The remainder have more diffuse frontal or parietal uptake.

Cerebrovascular Disease (7,8)
Infarction

The etiologies of a cerebral infarction are multiple: thrombotic, embolic, and hemorrhagic, among others. CT and MRI have replaced radionuclide imaging with the conventional radiopharmaceuticals for several decades. Functional images are usually abnormal before anatomic images, because the physiologic dysfunction of an organ precedes the resulting anatomic changes. Positron emitters include oxygen-15 (^{15}O, half-life = 2 minutes), nitrogen-13 (^{13}N, half-life = 10 minutes), carbon-11 (^{11}C, half-life = 20 minutes), and fluorine-18 (^{18}F, half-life = 2 hours) and require coincidence detection with a PET scanner for imaging. These radioisotopes have the advantage of being naturally part of the molecular structure of endogenous substrates. PET studies using ^{15}O-H$_2$O to evaluate perfusion, ^{15}O-O$_2$ to evaluate oxygen metabolism, and ^{18}F-FDG to evaluate glucose metabolism have contributed to the understanding of the physiopathology of cerebral infarction. Because of the short half-lives of the positron emitters, these PET radiopharmaceuticals are not practical for clinical use except for ^{18}F-FDG. ^{99m}Tc-HMPAO and -ECD, however, allow evaluation of cerebral perfusion using the SPECT technique. SPECT images with perfusion radiopharmaceuticals can demonstrate a defect of perfusion as early as 2 hours after the onset of symptoms and before the appearance of positive findings on CT or MRI, which can take a day or more. The CT scan becomes abnormal immediately only in case of hemorrhagic stroke. The size of the defect on early SPECT perfusion images (6 hours after the onset of symptoms) seems to have the best prognostic value for the outcome of these patients.

Within the first hours to days after a stroke, there is decreased relative perfusion compared to the glucose and oxygen metabolism, a phenomenon called "misery perfusion." Twenty-four hours to a week after infarction, the perfusion usually improves but the symptoms and crossed cerebellar diaschisis persist. There is decoupling of metabolism and perfusion, a phenomenon called "luxury perfusion," which may last 1 to 10 days and is thought to be due to local accumulation of radicals. The luxury perfusion has usually resolved a month after the onset of infarction. In addition, there is a "penumbral zone" surrounding the infarcted area, which is ischemic and demonstrates decreased perfusion but increased oxygen extraction fraction. If perfusion to the penumbral zone can be restored, irreversible damage will not occur.

There are regions that show decreased perfusion and metabolism that are distant to the region of infarction. For example, cortical infarcts are usually associated with decreased uptake in the contralateral cerebellar hemisphere (crossed cerebellar diaschisis) owing to deafferentation, a phenomenon that occurs when the impulses through the corticopontocerebellar fibers fail to be transmitted and stimulate the contralateral cerebellar hemisphere. Other areas that can demonstrate decreased perfusion and metabolism are the ipsilateral thalamus and caudate nucleus. Infarction of specific nucleus from the thalamus results in cortical hypometabolism, while infarction of other nuclei does not, owing to specific thalamocortical tracts.

Transient Ischemic Attack

Transient ischemic attacks (TIAs) can produce the symptoms of a stroke but resolve within 24 hours. However, 60% of patients with TIAs will develop a stroke later. CT images are usually normal after a TIA, but SPECT perfusion images can be abnormal in as many as 60% of the patients in the first 24 hours and 40% a week later. In patients with TIA and a normal baseline SPECT (^{99m}Tc-HMPAO, ^{99m}Tc-ECD) perfusion scan, evaluation of the cerebral vascular reserve using the acetazolamide challenge test may show the ischemic area.

Estimation of Cerebrovascular Reserve (8)

Evaluation of cerebral perfusion reserve can be performed using acetazolamide (Diamox), an inhibitor of carbonic anhydrase, to vasodilate the capillaries of the brain. Acetazolamide is administered at a dose of 1 g intravenously 30 minutes before administration of the radiopharmaceutical. CO_2 can be used as well but is less practical. In normal individuals, perfusion to the brain increases by 30%. The perfusion increases to a lesser extent in regions of the brain supplied by abnormal vessels that cannot vasodilate. An absolute decrease in perfusion does not occur unless there is a steal phenomenon (e.g., arteriovenous malformation).

Arteriovenous Malformation

Arteriovenous malformations are not seen on SPECT perfusion images but can shunt blood from the normal vasculature and create a steal phenomenon that can induce ischemia. The ischemic zone can be demonstrated on SPECT (^{99m}Tc-HMPAO, ^{99m}Tc-ECD) perfusion images. After treatment, restoration of normal perfusion pressure in vessels previously submitted to

low pressure, because of the steal phenomenon, may lead to their rupture. A challenge test with acetazolamide helps identify territories with enhanced vasoreactivity that are at risk for hyperemic disturbances. SPECT perfusion images can also help monitor the treatment with embolization (8).

Evaluation of Adequacy of Collateral Flow during Balloon Occlusion Test before the Projected Sacrifice of a Large Vessel

Occasionally, it is necessary to sacrifice a large vessel such as a carotid artery. This may occur due to trauma, large tumor encasing the vessel, or treatment of arteriovenous malformation. To assess the adequacy of collateral flow, an intra-arterial balloon catheter is inflated in the vessel at the level of projected ligation. The patient is observed for neurologic deficits with the balloon inflated for 45 minutes, and if signs and symptoms of ischemia develop, the balloon is deflated. Some patients who do not develop symptoms during the balloon occlusion test do develop neurologic deficits after permanent sacrifice of the vessel. Therefore assessment of brain perfusion with ^{99m}Tc-HMPAO or ^{99m}Tc-ECD during balloon occlusion has been added to the evaluation of these patients (8,10).

Subarachnoid Hemorrhage

Subarachnoid hemorrhage is often due to rupture of an aneurysm. A delayed complication is vasospasm of major vessels, which can lead to ischemia and stroke. SPECT (^{99m}Tc-HMPAO, ^{99m}Tc-ECD) perfusion images can demonstrate regions of decreased perfusion secondary to vasospasm when the CT images are still normal. SPECT perfusion images can also help to monitor therapy following treatment with balloon angioplasty (9).

Evaluation of Cerebral Distribution of Amobarbital Sodium in the Intracarotid Wada Test

The intracarotid amobarbital, or Wada, test is performed to lateralize both language and memory in patients considered for temporal lobectomy. Amobarbital sodium (Amytal) is injected into a carotid artery to sedate one hemisphere, and neurologic testing is performed. One mCi of ^{99m}Tc-HMPAO or ^{99m}Tc-ECD can be injected together with the amobarbital sodium to monitor the distribution of amobarbital (11,12).

Head Trauma

In closed head injury, perfusion SPECT images demonstrate perfusion deficits in a larger percentage of patients than CT images, even at remote time from the trauma (13,14).

Seizures

Seizures may be due to epilepsy or to the presence of an irritating focus such as a neoplasm or infectious process. There are two types of epilepsy: (a) generalized seizures (grand mal and petit mal), thought to be due to abnormal impulses between the neocortex and the thalamic reticular system, and (b) partial seizures, due to sudden depolarization of a focal group of neurons. The partial seizures are called complex if the patient loses awareness or simple if not. Most partial seizures arise from the temporal lobe. More than half of the patients with partial seizures become refractory to medical therapy. If the seizure focus can be localized and resected surgically, the symptoms improve or are cured. MRI scanning is helpful to localize a structural lesion that may be responsible for the seizure or to demonstrate hippocampal sclerosis. However, often both the MRI and EEG fail to localize the seizure focus. Functional imaging using both SPECT (99mTc-HMPAO, 99mTc-ECD) and PET (18F-FDG) has been demonstrated helpful in predicting the postsurgical outcome of these patients. Both flow and metabolism are increased during the ictal and decreased during the interictal period. 18F-FDG PET imaging appears more sensitive in demonstrating the seizure focus in the interictal state, but 99mTc-HMPAO SPECT imaging is more suitable for ictal administration because it is rapidly taken up by the cells (7,14,15,16,17,18,19,20,21,22,23).

Brain Tumors

After being treated for high-grade brain tumors with a combination of surgery, radiation therapy, and chemotherapy, patients often develop neurologic symptoms that may be related to edema and radiation necrosis or recurrent tumor. The changes on CT and MRI are very similar for both etiologies. In the early 1980s, Di Chiro and collaborators were the first investigators to demonstrate the potential for metabolic imaging with 18F-FDG PET in differentiating recurrent high-grade from radiation necrosis (14,24,25). 18F-FDG PET can also differentiate high-grade (uptake well above the level of the white matter) from low-grade glioma (uptake close to that of white matter), and the degree of uptake in high-grade gliomas has a prognostic value (26–32). In patients with AIDS and brain lesions, 18F-FDG PET can differentiate lymphoma (high 18F-FDG uptake) from toxoplasmosis (low 18F-FDG uptake) (33–35).

The SPECT radiopharmaceuticals that can be used to differentiate radiation necrosis from recurrent high-grade tumor and high-grade from low-grade gliomas are thallium-201 (201Tl)-chloride and 99mTc-sestamibi.

Dementias and Neuropsychiatric Diseases (36–38)

In degenerative dementia, structural imaging will either be normal or demonstrate nonspecific cortical atrophy. Functional imaging with PET usually demonstrates a pattern of hypoperfusion or hypometabolism that correlates with different syndromes. A first step in evaluating dementing syndromes is to separate patients on the basis of whether they have signs and symptoms of motor dysfunction (cortical dementias) or not (subcortical dementias). In cortical dementia, the cortex is usually affected and the subcortical structures are spared; the patients do not have motor dysfunction but present with apraxia, aphasia, memory loss, abnormal affect (Alzheimer's or Pick's disease). In subcortical dementias, the basal ganglia, thalami, and brainstem are affected; the patients do have motor dysfunction (disorder of posture and tone, tremor, gait disturbance) as well as memory loss, slowing of cognition, and depression. This includes extrapyramidal syndromes (e.g., Parkinson's disease and syndromes, Huntington's disease, and Wilson's disease), white matter disease (e.g., multiple sclerosis), HIV encephalopathy, and normal-pressure hydrocephalus. A mixed category includes conditions that involve both cortical and subcortical structures, such as vascular dementias (e.g., multi-infarct dementia and Biswanger's disease), infectious dementias (e.g., Creutzfeldt–Jakob), and hypoxic encephalopathy.

Alzheimer's disease (AD) accounts for 75% of the dementias in the elderly. These patients present with short-term memory loss and visuospatial problems. However, clinically the diagnosis is unclear in a large proportion of these patients. In advanced disease, CT and MRI demonstrate more pronounced atrophy in the temporoparietal and anterior frontal cortex, and sometimes the atrophy is severe in the hippocampus. On both 18F-FDG PET and perfusion SPECT images, there is a characteristic pattern of decreased uptake in the posterior parietotemporal cortex, probably related to neuronic depletion in these areas. These functional changes precede the atrophy seen on structural imaging. Thirty percent of the patients present with a unilateral defect first (often the left); some present with a bilateral defect. Later in the disease, there is also decreased uptake in the frontal cortex (39,40). AD can occur in conjunction with Parkinson's and Lewy body disease. In these cases, the imaging findings are indistinguishable from AD; histopathologically, the findings are those of AD in addition to Parkinson's or Lewy body disease. The sensitivity and specificity of posterior perfusion defect for AD are in the range of 90% (41). Posterior perfusion defects mimicking AD can be seen in other pathologies such as normal-pressure hydrocephalus, Creutzfeldt–Jakob disease, and AIDS, among others.

Frontal metabolic and perfusion deficits are a landmark for Pick's disease but can also be found in multiple-system atrophy, progressive supranuclear palsy, nonspecific frontal gliosis, and chronic alcoholism. Pick's disease presents clinically with personality changes, emotional disturbances, and deterioration in behavior and judgment.

In Huntington's disease, there is decreased flow and metabolism in the caudate nucleus. These findings are present in some patients with a positive family history; therefore functional imaging may be helpful in identifying the disease before it is expressed clinically.

PET and SPECT images of multi-infarct dementia usually show multiple cortical defects. The large defects follow a vascular distribution. Sometimes vascular dementia and AD can coexist in one patient.

Numerous studies have been published to investigate various neuropsychiatric diseases—such as affective disorders, schizophrenia, obsessive-compulsive disorder, chronic fatigue syndrome, and chronic pain syndrome—mainly with PET, using 18F-FDG and labeled brain receptors. To date, there are few clinical applications, but they may develop in the future.

Normal-Pressure Hydrocephalus

Normal-pressure hydrocephalus (NPH) is associated with the triad of dementia, incontinence, and ataxia. The ventricles are enlarged and the CSF pressure is normal. On radionuclide cysternography, the classic findings are early entry of the radiopharmaceutical in the lateral ventricles, which persists on 24- and 48-hour images, and impairment of flow over the convexities. Because only 40% to 87% of these patients improve after ventriculoperitoneal shunting and owing to the high complication rate of this therapy (up to 31%), the diagnosis of NPH using radionuclide cysternography has become debatable (42).

Cerebrospinal Fluid Leak

About 80% of cases involving CSF rhinorrhea are the result of direct head trauma, 16% are iatrogenic due to surgery, and 4% are spontaneous. The major complication of CSF leakage is meningitis, occurring in 25% to 50% of untreated cases. Meningitis can occur immediately or several years after the fistula. Therefore treatment of a CSF leak is indicated as soon as it is diagnosed. Radionuclide cysternography with pledget placement is the most sensitive and specific imaging test to detect CSF leakage, especially in symptomatic patients with small or intermittent leaks (42).

Ventriculoperitoneal Shunt Patency

To evaluate shunt patency, ^{99m}Tc-DTPA is a satisfactory radiopharmaceutical because images are usually not obtained later than 1 hour after administration into the reservoir of the shunt. If the shunt is patent, the radiopharmaceutical should be seen free in the peritoneal cavity within 30 minutes (42).

CASE 4.1

History: This 12-year-old female was admitted for multiple trauma and a history of smoke inhalation. Brain death was suspected, but the patient was in a barbiturate coma. A nuclear medicine brain flow study was performed using ^{99m}Tc-glucoheptonate (^{99m}Tc-GH) (Fig. 4.1).

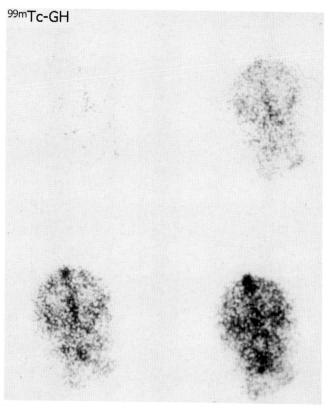

Figure 4.1

Findings: On the dynamic flow images, both anterior and middle cerebral arteries are visualized. There is high background activity present in the brain itself.

Discussion: The findings are indicative of perfusion to the brain. "Brain death" is the irreversible cessation of brain function, including the brainstem. Over the years, there have been alterations in the guidelines based on the Harvard criteria for the diagnosis of brain death. The clinical diagnosis requires the persistence of the following for 6 hours: (a) unreceptivity and unresponsiveness, (b) no spontaneous movements or breathing, (c) no reflexes (including fixed, dilated pupils as well as absence of brainstem reflexes and deep tendon reflexes), and (d) an isoelectric EEG. Current guidelines require exclusion of hypothermia, drug-induced coma/drug intoxication, or reversible metabolic-induced coma, as these conditions can potentially mimic all signs of brain death clinically and are associated with an isoelectric EEG.

A confirmatory test is necessary if the patient suffers from one of the conditions that can mimic brain death; it is also desirable to abbreviate the observation period required to determine the irreversibility of the patient's condition, which is highly desirable in potential organ donors. The "gold standard" in evaluating cerebral blood flow is a four-vessel contrast angiogram, but this is an invasive and nonportable technique. Radionuclide angiography is a widely accepted and well-established method of determining the presence or absence of intracerebral blood flow. It has the advantage of being an accurate, noninvasive, and rapid test. The study involves only a peripheral venous injection and lasts less than 10 minutes; moreover, the radiopharmaceutical is easily stored and readily available. A clear advantage is the ability to image at the bedside using a portable gamma camera, because the patient is usually in critical condition, requiring intense nursing care, mechanical ventilation support, and a multitude of catheter lines and monitor wires.

Diagnosis: Brain flow present.

CASE 4.2

History: A 13-year-old female presented with refractory complex partial seizures and a normal MRI of the brain. The ictal scalp EEG showed ictal discharges predominantly in the right temporal region. An ictal and interictal ^{99m}Tc-HMPAO SPECT study of the brain was performed to localize the seizure focus (Fig. 4.2 A).

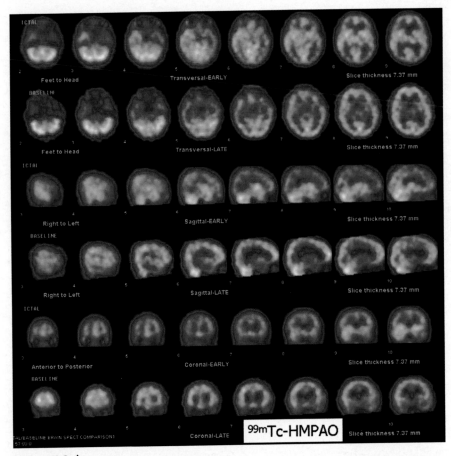

Figure 4.2 A

Findings: On the ictal SPECT images, a focus of increased uptake is seen in the right temporal lobe anteriorly. The interictal SPECT images were obtained 2 days later and demonstrate symmetrical uptake in the temporal lobes.

Discussion: The combination of interictal symmetrical flow and ictal high flow point to the right temporal lobe as the probable site of the seizure focus, especially with concordant scalp EEG findings.

Epilepsy affects 1% of the population in the United States. The seizures can be partial or generalized. If the patient does not lose awareness, the seizures are called "simple partial"; if awareness is lost, they are "complex partial." When the seizures become refractory to medical therapy, surgical removal of the seizure focus can be curative. In patients considered for surgery, precise localization of the seizure focus is critical. CT and MRI can identify focal lesions responsible for the seizure in 40% to 60% of these patients, most commonly low-grade astrocytoma, hamartomas, and ganglioglioma/neuroma. In the remaining patients, correlation of functional imaging using radionuclides with the clinical presentation of the seizure and the EEG findings plays a pivotal role in identifying patients

who will improve following surgery. The temporal lobe is the most common focus of partial seizures, and mesial temporal sclerosis is the most common pathologic lesion.

Both ^{18}F-FDG PET and ^{99m}Tc-HMPAO SPECT imaging are helpful in evaluating patients with refractory complex partial seizures. ^{18}F-FDG evaluates the glucose metabolic rate and ^{99m}Tc-HMPAO evaluates the perfusion. During a seizure, both metabolism and perfusion are increased in the seizure focus; between seizures, both are decreased. Functional imaging in combination with other noninvasive techniques has made monitoring with invasive intracranial electrodes unnecessary in 50% or more patients with temporal lobe epilepsy. Identification of a single focus of interictal temporal lobe hypometabolism on ^{18}F-FDG PET images (asymmetry index greater than 15%) is an excellent predictor of seizure control after surgery (Fig. 4.2 B). The sensitivity of interictal ^{18}F-FDG PET in detecting temporal lobe epileptic foci is in the range of 80%, greater than that of interictal ^{99m}Tc-HMPAO SPECT, which is in the range of 60%. Therefore interictal ^{18}F-FDG PET is the functional study of choice.

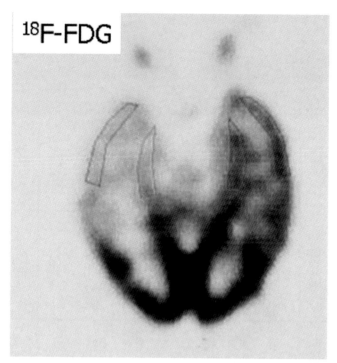

Figure 4.2 B

When interictal ^{18}F-FDG PET imaging is nondiagnostic, an ictal study is indicated. ^{99m}Tc-HMPAO is better suited for ictal imaging because the uptake of ^{99m}Tc-HMPAO reaches a maximum within a minute after injection. Thereafter, up to 15% is eliminated by 2 minutes postinjection, after which little activity is lost except by physical decay. On the other hand, the uptake of ^{18}F-FDG in the brain occurs slowly, reaching a maximum between 30 and 50 minutes after intravenous injection. To perform ictal imaging, ^{99m}Tc-HMPAO must be injected intravenously as a bolus; uptake into the brain occurs within seconds of the start of ictal electrical activity on EEG. Of course the patient must be monitored by EEG, and the syringe with the radiopharmaceutical must be hooked up to the intravenous line and shielded to limit radiation exposure to both the patient and medical staff. Ictal SPECT study will detect an additional 20% to 30% of temporal seizure foci compared with interictal SPECT. The combination of increased flow during an ictal injection and decreased flow during an interictal injection is highly predictive of a seizure focus, with a sensitivity in the range of 90% (18).

Other important technical considerations are the half-life of the radioisotope and the stability of the radiopharmaceutical because seizures cannot be scheduled. The stability of ^{99m}Tc-HMPAO is 30 minutes after reconstitution, which is obviously not practical. This stability, however, can be extended to 4 hours with methylene blue. The physical 6-hour half-life of ^{99m}Tc requires calibration of the dose in the high range (20 + mCi) so as to ensure enough radioactivity when the patient has a seizure.

The temporal lobe is the most common location for seizure foci, and the frontal lobes are the next most common. Frontal seizure foci are often located in the medial or inferior aspect of the frontal lobes; therefore scalp EEG recordings are often nonlocalizing. Interictal PET was found to be a useful modality to localize frontal lobe foci but appears less sensitive than for the detection of interictal temporal lobe foci. The combination of increased uptake on ictal images and decreased uptake on interictal images is particularly helpful in detecting extratemporal seizure foci. Occasionally functional images demonstrate multiple seizure foci, which is a contraindication to surgery.

Several pediatric syndromes are associated with intractable seizure of extratemporal neocortical origin, often refractory to medical therapy. In infants and children, the progressive nature of epileptic syndrome can lead to cortical maldevelopment and focal sclerosis. The psychological effects of intractable epilepsy are disastrous as well. The recent development of surgical techniques with smaller standard resection (amygdalohippocampectomy, modified anterior temporal lobectomy sparing the lateral cortex, computerized lesionectomy, subpial cortical transection, and corpus callosum partial or total transection) has increased the number of patients contemplated for surgery early in the course of their disease. These syndromes include but are not limited to infantile spasms, Lenox-Gastaut syndrome, and Sturge-Weber syndrome. Infantile spasms can be due to an identifiable cause or cryptogenic. Lenox-Gastaut syndrome is defined by the triad of a 1- to 2.5-Hz spike-wave pattern on the EEG, intellectual impairment, and a multiple seizure pattern. Sturge-Weber syndrome is characterized by facial capillary nevus and ipsilateral leptomeningeal angiomatosis. In all these syndromes, PET, in combination with CT and MRI, has proven useful in localizing the seizure foci and guiding placement of semi-invasive (foramen ovale and epidural) and invasive (subdural grids) electrodes as well as in ultimately deciding the best type of surgery for these patients.

Diagnosis: Seizure focus in the right temporal lobe.

CASE 4.3

History: A 60-year-old male with worsening dementia was referred for ^{18}F-FDG PET imaging (Fig. 4.3). The MRI showed mild cortical atrophy (not shown).

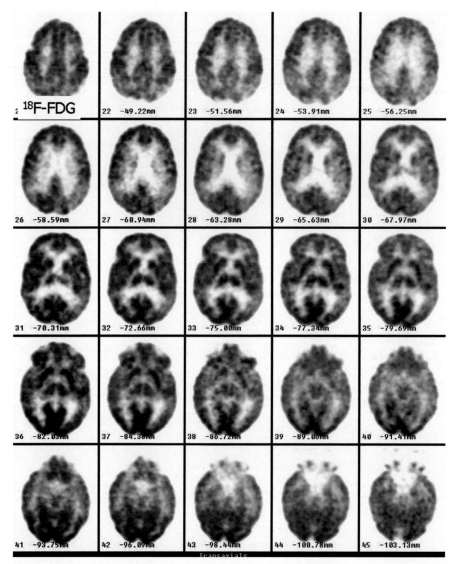

Figure 4.3

Findings: Decreased uptake is seen in the posterior parietotemporal cortex bilaterally. The uptake is preserved in the sensorimotor cortex, subcortical gray matter (basal ganglia and thalami), and cerebellum.

Discussion: Decreased uptake in the posterior parietotemporal cortex is consistent with a degenerative disorder, most likely Alzheimer's disease (AD). Ten percent of the population over 65 years of age is demented and 50% of those are evaluated in hospitals. The cost of long-term care is tremendous. Over half of these demented patients have AD. These patients present with impairment of memory as well as visual and spatial skills. From the physiopathologic point of view, there is accelerated neuronal death, affecting mainly the hippocampus and the posterior parietal and temporal cortex. It has been demonstrated that variants of the apolipoprotein E allele appear to account for most cases of late-onset AD.

^{18}F-FDG is a glucose analog labeled with a positron emitter that allows direct evaluation of glucose metabolism with a PET scanner. This functional imaging technique makes it possible to diagnose degenerative neurologic diseases that do not produce typical findings on CT or MRI. Although there is a large overlap between the pattern of uptake of different degenerative dementias, this patient has a pattern typical of AD. The degree of decreased ^{18}F-FDG uptake seems to correlate with the severity of the symptoms. Histopathologic observation of postmortem brains from patients with AD has revealed the presence of abundant senile plaques and neurofibrillary tangles in the regions with decreased ^{18}F-FDG uptake.

Other patterns of uptake can also be related to AD.

The probability of AD is the following, with different patterns of metabolism and perfusion: bilateral parietotemporal (82%), unilateral temporoparietal more often on the left (57%), frontal (43%), other (18%), normal (19%) (43).

Decreased uptake in the posterior parietotemporal cortex bilaterally is the typical pattern of AD; however, it is not pathognomonic. It may also be seen in patients with Parkinson's disease, bilateral parietal hematomas, bilateral parietal stroke, bilateral parietal radiation therapy, and NPH. The symptoms characterizing Parkinson's disease are bradykinesia, rigidity, and tremor; this condition affects 1% of the population over 60 years of age. It is caused by the degeneration of dopaminergic neurons in the substantia nigra and the locus ceruleus, leading to decreased dopamine production, decreased dopamine storage, and nigrostriatal dysfunction. About 10% to 30% of patients with Parkinson's disease develop dementia; their pattern of ^{18}F-FDG uptake is indistinguishable from the Alzheimer's pattern.

For further readings on this topic, please see references 44, 45, and 46.

Diagnosis: Alzheimer's disease.

CASE 4.4

History: A 7-year-old male patient presented with closed head injury due to a motor vehicle accident. A CT of the head showed a subarachnoid hemorrhage and brain edema (not shown). The patient was hyperventilated, mannitol was given, and he was placed in a pentobarbital coma with epinephrine and dopamine drip. Despite these measures, on the fourth day of hospitalization the intracranial pressure started to rise rapidly, with cerebral perfusion pressures of zero. A portable nuclear medicine brain flow study was performed using ^{99m}Tc-glucoheptonate as radiopharmaceutical (Fig. 4.4 A).

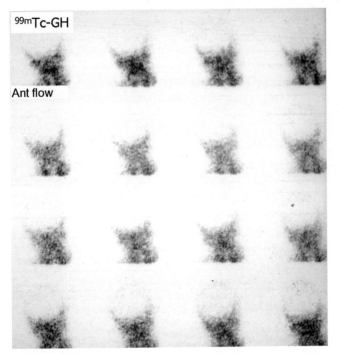

99mTc-GH

Ant flow

Figure 4.4 A

99mTc-GH

Figure 4.4 B

Findings: The anterior and middle cerebral arteries are not visualized in dynamic sequence of images (Fig. 4.4 A). There is no activity in the brain.

Discussion: Based on this study, can we conclude that there is no flow to the brain? The answer is no.

A flow study can be performed with any radiopharmaceutical if the activity is injected as a bolus and is sufficiently high to allow dynamic imaging every 2 seconds. It usually requires 20 to 25 mCi of ^{99m}Tc in an adult; ^{99m}Tc-glucoheptonate was used in this case. Glucoheptonate, however, does not cross the blood–brain barrier and does not fix in the brain. Therefore it is critical to evaluate the arterial phase of the flow study. The images in Figure 4.4 A could represent the end of the venous phase. The only way to be sure is to look at the arterial phase of the study, looking for a background image of the brain first and then an image with the bolus in the carotid arteries; if the cerebral arteries are not then seen, there is no flow to the brain. In this case, faulty camera timing (imaging was started too late after injection of the bolus) led to obtaining images of the venous phase only; the arterial phase was missed. The brain flow study was therefore repeated, starting the camera just before injecting the radiopharmaceutical (Fig. 4.4 B). Now you can report that there is no flow in the anterior and middle cerebral arteries.

To diagnose brain death, the brain flow study must be interpreted in conjunction with the clinical assessment of brainstem

function, because dynamic images can be acquired in only one projection—in practical terms, the anterior projection. Therefore the posterior circulation is not evaluated on a brain flow study. When brain death occurs because of high intracranial pressure, it is very likely that perfusion of the entire brain is affected the same way.

It is also prudent to ascertain whether there is an open skull defect or ventricular drain, as there have been case reports of false-negative studies—for example, visible flow in the presence of clinical brain death (47–49).

If ^{99m}Tc-HMPAO is used as radiopharmaceutical, it does cross the blood brain barrier and fix into the brain. This allows evaluation of the brain itself with static imaging, in addition to the flow portion of the scan. If there is flow through the posterior cerebral arteries, uptake will be present in the posterior fossa and can be seen on immediate static lateral or posterior views. If a doubt remains about the presence of uptake in the brain versus scalp activity, SPECT images may be helpful.

Disadvantages of ^{99m}Tc-HMPAO are its cost and more limited availability than ^{99m}Tc-glucoheptonate on an emergency basis.

Diagnosis: No flow to the anterior and middle cerebral arteries.

CASE 4.5

History: A 30-year-old male, HIV-positive, presented with mental status changes. A CT of the brain was performed and showed a 2-cm ring-enhancing lesion in the right parieto-occipital region (Fig. 4.5 A). In a patient with AIDS, the main differential diagnosis is toxoplasmosis versus lymphoma. ^{18}F-FDG PET imaging of the brain was performed (Fig. 4.5 B).

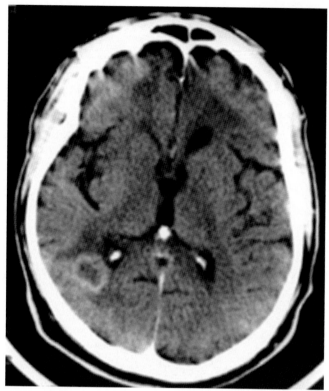

Figure 4.5 A

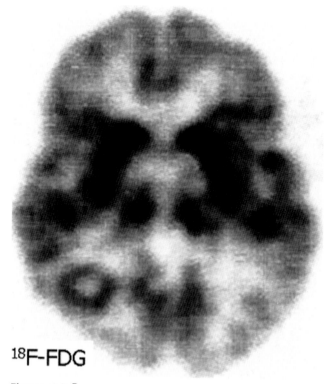

Figure 4.5 B

Findings: On the PET images (Fig. 4.5 B), there is ^{18}F-FDG uptake in the ring-enhancing lesion. The uptake is approximately twice that of white matter, indicating a high-grade tumor rather than toxoplasmosis. In addition, there is a global decrease of the cortical uptake compared to the basal ganglia and thalami.

Discussion: High ^{18}F-FDG uptake in the lesion indicates that it is most likely a lymphoma, and the general pattern of uptake is typical of AIDS-related dementia complex.

HIV-positive patients are immunosuppressed and have a tendency to develop opportunistic infections and malignant tumors such as lymphoma. The opportunistic infection that most commonly involves the central nervous system (CNS) is due to *Toxoplasma gondii*. This infection may produce a diffuse meningoencephalitis or focal lesions. CT and MRI are used to detect and localize the lesions, which often appear as multifocal ring-enhancing lesions. It is, however, not possible to differentiate toxoplasmosis from lymphoma on the basis of CT or MRI findings. Primary CNS lymphoma has increased accumu-

lation of ^{18}F-FDG to the same degree as high-grade gliomas, while toxoplasmosis does not. ^{18}F-FDG PET imaging is an accurate imaging modality to differentiate CNS toxoplasmosis from CNS lymphoma in HIV-positive patients.

AIDS-related dementia is a frequent complication of HIV infection and is sometimes difficult to distinguish from the simple depression or psychiatric problems that these patients experience. It is the result of direct HIV infection into the cerebral matter; therefore multinucleated giant cells can be found in the white matter and to a lesser extent the gray matter. The viral infection also results in demyelination. The pattern of ^{18}F-FDG uptake is helpful in the differential diagnosis, with the limitation that these patients are often polydrug abusers, and there is some overlap between the pattern of uptake due to HIV infection, cocaine abuse, and alcohol abuse, among others.

Diagnosis: (a) CNS lymphoma. (b) AIDS-related dementia complex.

CASE 4.6

History: A 33-year-old male presented with a history of episodic dizziness and loss of consciousness. An MRI showed a relatively large lesion in the left temporal lobe. The lesion has a low signal on T1-weighted images (Fig. 4.6 A), a high signal on T2-weighted images (not shown), and does not enhance with gadolinium. The MRI appearance favors a low-grade neoplasm. ^{18}F-FDG PET imaging of the brain was performed for further evaluation (Fig. 4.6 B).

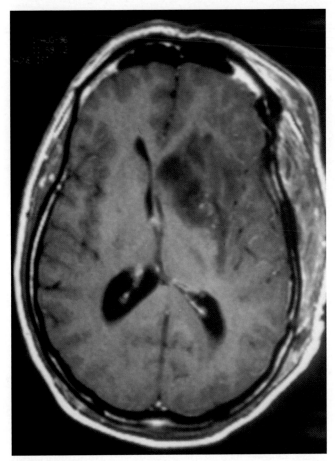

Figure 4.6 A

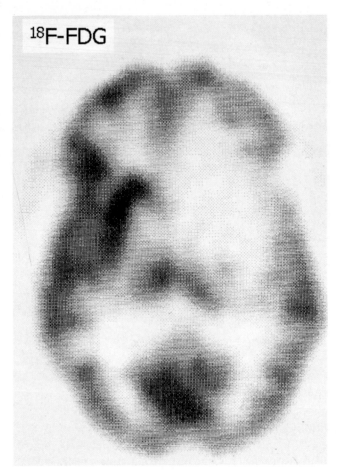

Figure 4.6 B

Findings: On the ^{18}F-FDG PET, the uptake in the lesion is at the same level as white matter.

Discussion: Low ^{18}F-FDG uptake is most consistent with a low-grade tumor.

The incidence of intracranial neoplasms is approximately 10% of all neoplasms. Cerebral metastases represent 25% to 30% of intracranial neoplasms and primary brain tumor 70% to 75%. Fifty percent of primary brain tumors are gliomas (60% of which are low-grade and 40% are high-grade), 12% to 15% are meningiomas, and 1% to 2% are lymphomas. When a patient presents with personality changes, seizures, or a neurologic deficit suggesting a brain lesion, a CT or MRI is usually performed first. The finding of a nonenhancing lesion favors a low-grade glioma. Because most high-grade gliomas develop in the setting of a low-grade glioma, there is debate in the literature about the therapeutic approach to presumably low-grade astrocytoma. Some oncologists favor early biopsy and treatment with resection when possible and radiation therapy. Others favor a more conservative approach until the lesion enlarges or enhances on CT and MRI. Enhancement indicates increased permeability of the blood-brain barrier and is more commonly seen in high-grade tumors, which are treated with resection when possible followed by radiation and chemotherapy.

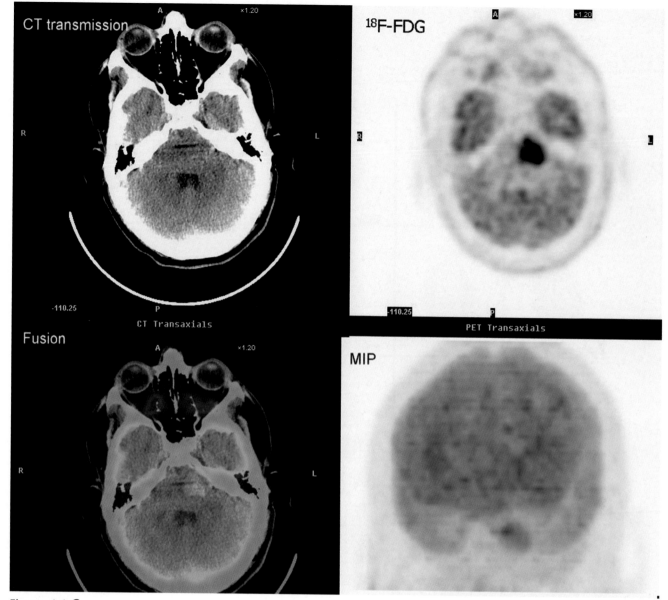

Figure 4.6 C

One of the first clinical applications that emerged for ^{18}F-FDG PET in the early eighties was its ability to differentiate low- from high-grade gliomas. For semiquantitative analysis, different regions of the brain have been used for reference uptake. Because gliomas are tumors that arise from the white matter, it is logical to use the white matter as reference in evaluating the degree of uptake. Most low-grade gliomas should have uptake at the same level as the white matter.

Most high-grade gliomas have uptake greater than twice the level of white matter, which can still be below the level of cortical uptake. An example of a high-grade glioma is shown in Fig 4.6 C. This degree of ^{18}F-FDG uptake supports the diagnosis of high-grade tumor. PET may also help provide guidance at the more metabolically active site, as some tumors, such as cerebral gliomas, may be well differentiated in some regions and contain highly atypical cells in others. Several investigators have demonstrated that the degree of ^{18}F-FDG uptake in high-grade tumors constitutes a prognostic factor. Patients with tumors that have a lesion/cortex ^{18}F-FDG uptake ratio greater than 1.4 have an extremely poor prognosis.

Diagnosis: The lesion was resected and pathologic examination of the surgical specimen demonstrated an oligodendroglioma.

History: This 75-year-old man presented with cognitive loss and memory impairment. An MRI showed cortical atrophy normal for age (not shown). ^{18}F-FDG PET imaging was performed to evaluate the presence of a degenerative dementia (Fig. 4.7).

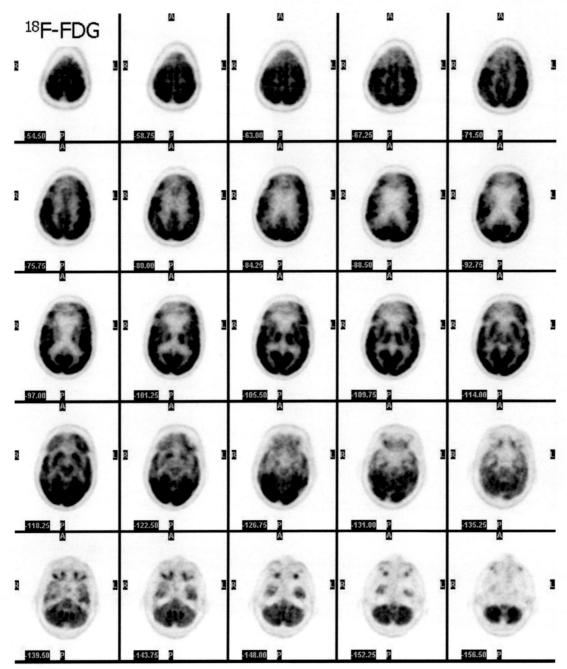

Figure 4.7

Findings: On the PET images, there is severely decreased uptake in the frontal cortex bilaterally as well as to a lesser degree in the basal ganglia.

Discussion: The finding of markedly decreased uptake in the frontal cortex suggests Pick's disease or frontal lobe dementia. Alzheimer's and Pick's disease are very difficult to differentiate clinically. As Alzheimer's disease (AD) is more frequent, a clinical diagnosis of AD is usually made rather than Pick's. Pathologically the two diseases are very different. Alzheimer's disease is characterized by the presence of tangles and plaques primarily in the cortex. Pick's is characterized by swollen neurons and neurons containing Pick's bodies in the cortex, basal ganglia, thalami, and sometimes other regions of the brain. AD tends to present with general cortical atrophy, and Pick's disease demonstrates more circumscribed atrophy located in the frontal and sometimes temporal cortex. On functional imaging with ^{18}F-FDG or HMPAO, AD typically shows decreased uptake in the posterior parietotemporal cortex, and Pick's more frequently affects the frontal cortex and anterior temporal cortex. Studies have shown that the degree of decreased metabolism correlates better with the degree of gliosis than the concentration of Pick's bodies (50).

Studies suggest that Pick's disease may be one member of a larger clinicopathologic syndrome called frontal lobe dementia. In frontal lobe dementia the pattern of uptake is the same as in Pick's disease. These patients typically present with early symptoms of social withdrawal and behavioral inhibition; several years later, they develop progressive dementia. Pathologic examination of the brain demonstrates frontal lobe atrophy with varying degrees of frontal gliosis and neuronal loss. One type of frontal lobe dementia presents in association with clinical features of motor neuron disease. This type progresses more rapidly and pathologically demonstrates mild frontal gliosis and spongiform changes.

Other dementing conditions, such as amyotrophic lateral sclerosis, also involve the frontal lobes but can usually be differentiated from frontal lobe dementia on clinical grounds. For further readings on this topic, please see references 51 and 52.

Diagnosis: Probable Pick's disease or frontal lobe dementia.

CASE 4.8

History: This 69-year-old male has a history of glioma, reported grade II on the initial biopsy, and is now 7 months status post radiation therapy. He has presented with new corticospinal tracts deficits on the right side. An MRI showed an area of enhancement in the right frontoparietal lobe that has slightly increased in size compared with the MRI taken 3 months previously (not shown). ^{18}F-FDG PET/CT imaging was performed to differentiate postradiation necrosis from recurrent tumor (Fig. 4.8 A).

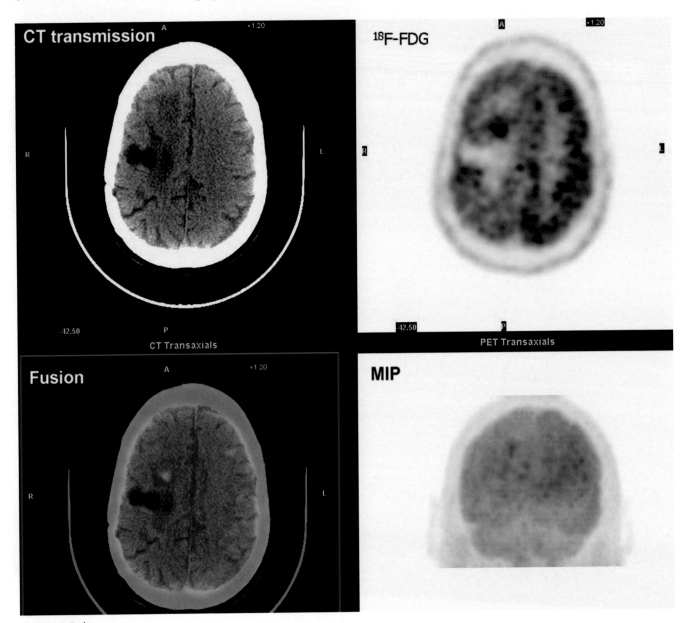

Figure 4.8 A

Findings: On the PET images, there is increased ^{18}F-FDG uptake above the level of cortical uptake corresponding to the area of enhancement on MRI.

Discussion: This indicates high-grade tumor recurrence.

High-grade gliomas (anaplastic astrocytoma and glioblastoma multiforme) are usually treated by resection when possible and a combination of radiation and chemotherapy. Evaluation of the response to therapy and tumor recurrence is a clinical challenge. Necrosis of the tumor and surrounding brain tissue is associated with conventional radiation therapy and is seen in a large proportion of patients following stereotactic radiosurgery. These areas of necrosis have the appearance of edematous masses on CT and MRI that enhance because there is increased permeability of the blood-brain barrier typically occurring 6 to 18 months after therapy. Similar changes follow intra-arterial infusion of chemotherapy and high doses of methotrexate given intravenously after radiation. These changes on CT and MRI are indistinguishable from residual or recurrent high grade tumor.

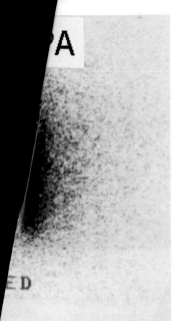

A

ale had a transphenoidal hypophysectomy 3 years earlier and now presents with rhinorrhea. A
performed following placement of nasal pledgets to evaluate the presence of cerebrospinal fluid

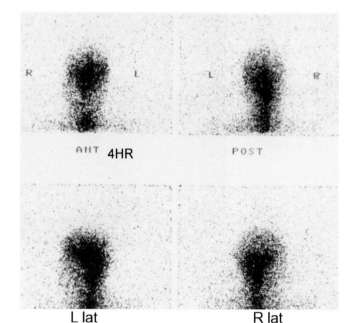

R | L   L | R

ANT 4HR   POST

L lat   R lat

Figure 4.11 B

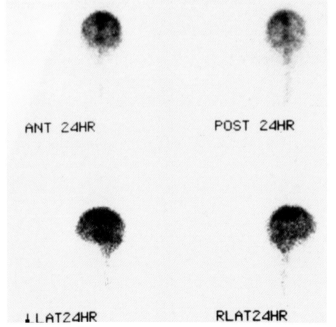

ANT 24HR   POST 24HR

LLAT24HR   RLAT24HR

Figure 4.11 C

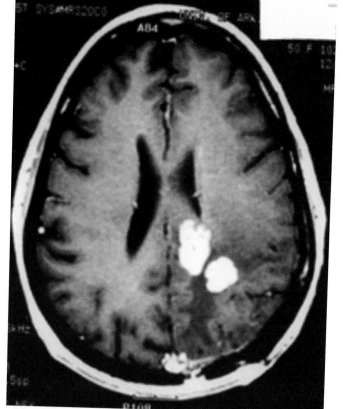

Figure 4.8 B

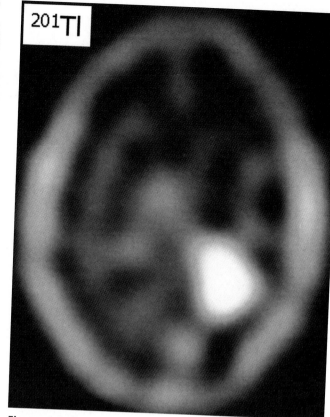

201Tl

Figure 4.8 C

Metabolic imaging with ^{18}F-FDG can differentiate recurrent brain tumor from radiation necrosis. Because most tumors recur as high-grade, they demonstrate marked ^{18}F-FDG uptake. On the other hand, radiation injury leads to tissue necrosis that does not accumulate FDG.

SPECT tumor radiopharmaceuticals have been investigated for the same purpose. ^{201}Tl has been found to localize in various malignant tumors, including malignant gliomas and cerebral metastases; there is little ^{201}Tl uptake in the normal brain. The actual uptake of ^{201}Tl is probably related to a combination of factors including regional blood flow, permeability of the blood-brain barrier (BBB), and cellular uptake. Since nonneoplastic cerebral lesions with breakdown of the BBB (such as most cases of radiation necrosis or resolving hematomas) have little thallium uptake, the increased BBB permeability is probably not an important factor. Experimental data support that ^{201}Tl (like potassium) is transported actively intracellularly through an ATP cell membrane pump and that ^{201}Tl uptake is related to cellular growth. Several semiquantitative indexes of uptake have been investigated to differentiate low-grade from high-grade gliomas. The most popular index is the ratio of uptake in the lesion (maximum counts/pixel) compared with a homologous region in the contralateral cerebral hemisphere (average counts/pixel) on attenuated images. For high-grade gliomas, this ratio averages 3.5/1; for low-grade gliomas, it is approximately 1.99/1. ^{201}Tl may give false-positive findings in radiation necrosis, presumably owing to increased permeability of the BBB. An example of high-grade tumor recurrence is shown in Figures 4.8 B and 4.8 C.

Diagnosis: Recurrent high-grade tumor.

CASE 4.9

History: A 69-year-old black male with non-insulin-dependent diabetes mellitus was referred for an ^{18}F-FDG PET scan as part of an evaluation for dementia (Fig. 4.9 A). He has a known intrasellar mass discovered 2 years prior to this evaluation. An MRI performed at that time showed a mass isointense on both T1- and T2-weighted images but enhancing with gadolinium. The CT scan showed calcifications (Fig. 4.9 B). Both the CT and MRI appearance support that this lesion was probably a craniopharyngioma.

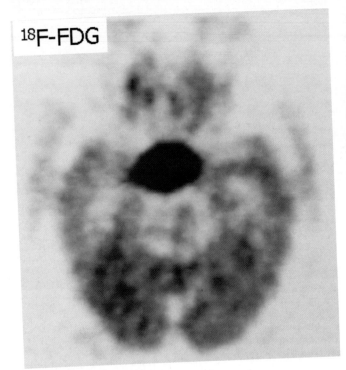

Figure 4.9 A

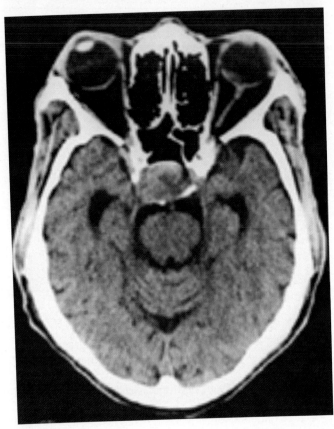

Figure 4.9 B

Findings: There is marked uptake by the intrasellar lesion. There is also very poor uptake globally in the brain. This is probably due to hyperglycemia in a diabetic patient. The poor uptake makes the images suboptimal for the evaluation of dementia.

Discussion: The normal pituitary gland does not accumulate ^{18}F-FDG, but the most common intrasellar tumors—pituitary adenoma and craniopharyngioma—accumulate ^{18}F-FDG to a high degree, even though they are benign (53,54). Because pituitary adenomas accumulate ^{18}F-FDG to a high degree, ^{18}F-FDG PET may be more accurate than CT and MRI in detecting microadenomas in the pituitary (54).

Other low-grade tumors can have marked ^{18}F-FDG uptake. Pilocytic astrocytomas, usually found in children, have a distinct histology and biological behavior compared with the forms of astrocytoma found in adults. They represent approx-

imately 10% of pediatric brain tumors and are usually located in the posterior fossa. Although they behave like low-grade tumors, they usually demonstrate marked ^{18}F-FDG accumulation. Ependymomas represent 2% to 8% of pediatric brain neoplasms and have variable ^{18}F-FDG uptake.

Since ^{18}F-FDG competes with glucose for cellular transport, high levels of plasma glucose will competitively inhibit ^{18}F-FDG transport into all cells, including the neurons. This is one reason why patients must fast for 4 hours prior to ^{18}F-FDG injection. It is a good idea to check the glucose plasma level prior to ^{18}F-FDG injection in every patient so as to assess both the fasting state and identify patients with glucose intolerance. For further readings on this topic, please see reference 55.

Diagnosis: (a) Pituitary adenoma or craniopharyngioma. (b) Poor FDG uptake due to hyperglycemia.

CASE 4.10

History: This 45-year-old male was referred for eva... acetazolamide challenge was requested to evaluate cer...

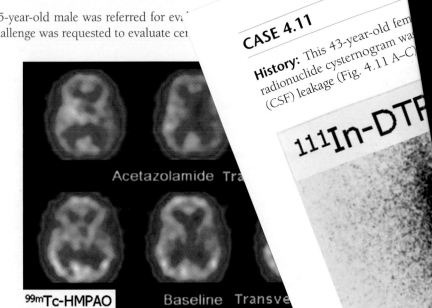

Figure 4.10

Findings: For the acetazolamide challenge, a slow IV injection of 1 g of acetazolamide is given 30 minutes prior to administration of 20 mCi of ^{99m}Tc-HMPAO. The baseline study was performed 2 days later. On the acetazolimide SPECT images, there is decreased uptake in the left cerebral cortex in the distribution of the anterior and middle cerebral artery as compared with the right. The perfusion is symmetrical on the baseline SPECT images.

Discussion
territory of th...
of the carbon...
vasodilates the ...

Diagnosis: Isch...
dle cerebral artery...

CASE 4.11

History: This 43-year-old fem...
radionuclide cysternogram wa...
(CSF) leakage (Fig. 4.11 A–C...

Figure 4.11 A

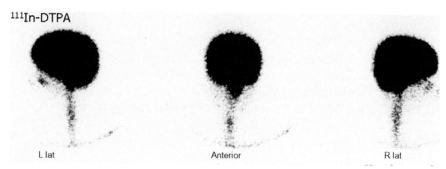

^{111}In-DTPA

L lat   Anterior   R lat

Figure 4.11 D

Findings: An immediate image was obtained over the spinal canal to assess the quality of the intrathecal injection (Fig. 4.11 A). Then images were obtained over the brain with the pledgets in place at 4 (Fig. 4.11 B) and 24 hours (Fig. 4.11 C) after intrathecal administration of 0.5 mCi ^{111}In-DTPA. There is normal dynamics of the CSF moving along the spinal canal to the basal cisternae at 4 hours and to the convexity at 24 hours after injection. The images do not show abnormal uptake at the level of the pledgets.

On the images, a CSF leak is usually better seen on the lateral images, as demonstrated in another case, shown in Figure 4.11 D. The pledgets were then removed and counted *in vitro*. The radioactivity in the pledgets was 20 times above background.

Discussion: The high counts in the pledgets indicate CSF leakage. The patient underwent surgical closure of the leakage and had no evidence of recurrent rhinorrhea 6 months later.

About 80% of cases of CSF rhinorrhea are the result of direct head trauma, 16% are iatrogenic due to surgery, and 4% are spontaneous. Iatrogenic postoperative leaks usually occur following nasal and transphenoidal surgery. The major complication of CSF leakage is meningitis, occurring in 25% to 50% of untreated cases. Meningitis can occur immediately or several years after the fistula. Therefore treatment of a CSF leak is indicated as soon as it is diagnosed.

The diagnosis is a clinical challenge. Helpful laboratory tests include the measurement of glucose (>60% of a concomitant serum level) and protein levels (<200 mg/dL). However, it is difficult to obtain a good sample, and false positives are frequent owing to contamination by lacrimal and nasal secretions. The absence of glucose excludes CSF rhinorrhea. Immunoelectrophoresis to identify CSF B-2 transferrin bands is the most specific laboratory test, independently of contamination with blood, saliva, or nasal secretions. High-resolution CT with intrathecal iopamidol or iohexol contrast is currently the first line of radiographic evaluation because it has a relatively high sensitivity (81% to 87%) for CSF leak

localization and is necessary preoperatively to delineate the anatomy.

Radionuclide cysternography with pledgets placement is more sensitive and specific in detecting CSF leakage, especially in symptomatic patients with small or intermittent leaks. It has the advantage of evaluating the patient for a longer period of time (up to 72 hours) as well as being able to detect spinal leaks, which would require extensive time and cost using CT. Indium-111 (^{111}In)-DTPA is the radiopharmaceutical of choice to evaluate CSF leakages. DTPA is a hydrophilic compound; it does not accumulate in the brain tissue and is quickly eliminated from the plasma (its $T_{1/2}$ is less than 2 hours), keeping the background low. ^{111}In has a half-life of 2.8 days, allowing imaging up to 72 hours. The images are less sensitive in detecting the leak than the *in vitro* counting of the pledgets, as demonstrated in this case. Various protocols have been described for the timing of placement (before or after) and removal (4 to 6 hours) of the pledgets compared with the time of administration of the radiopharmaceutical. The protocols vary as well for the number and location of the pledgets. The radioactivity in the pledgets can be reported as counts per minute (cpm) per gram to account for differences in size and amounts of absorbed fluid. Because the CSF is absorbed by the arachnoid villi into the plasma, some activity may be present in normal nasal secretions. Therefore some investigators have recommended obtaining a plasma sample (0.5 mL) at the time of placement and removal of the pledgets and evaluating the radioactivity. The normal ratio of intranasal pledget to plasma value is 1.3 (56). A value greater than 1.5 is considered abnormal, and most leaks have a ratio between 2 and 10. Leaving the pledgets in place for a longer period of time increases the sensitivity in detecting intermittent leaks, but as the plasma values fluctuate over time, the ratio is not helpful. CSF leakage can also be documented by delayed images over the abdomen, demonstrating activity in the colon due to swallowed nasal fluid.

Diagnosis: Normal cisternography but a CSF leak, as demonstrated by counting the radioactivity in the pledgets.

CASE 4.12

History: This 65-year-old male patient presented with a 1-year history of left facial pain. He was found to have a squamous cell carcinoma of the left maxillary sinus extending into the left orbit and involving the cavernous sinus portion of the carotid artery. Because sacrifice of the left carotid artery was considered for a curative resection of the tumor, a balloon occlusion test was performed with injection of ^{99m}Tc-HMPAO to assess the adequacy of the collateral circulation in perfusing the left cerebral hemisphere (Fig. 4.12).

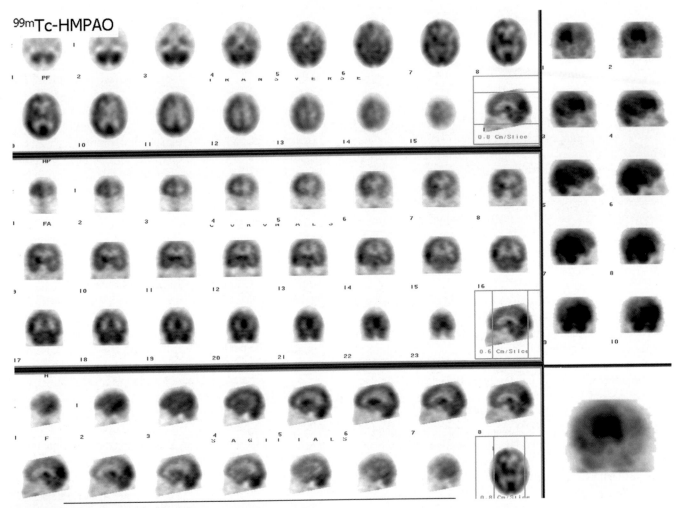

Figure 4.12

Findings: During the balloon occlusion test, the patient progressively became lethargic and had difficulty following commands. After 10 minutes, it was decided to inject the radiopharmaceutical and deflate the balloon. The patient's symptoms immediately resolved. On the SPECT images, there is definite decreased perfusion in the distribution of the left anterior and middle cerebral arteries (Fig. 4.12).

Discussion: The patient developed neurologic symptoms during the inflation of the balloon, and the SPECT images documented inadequate cerebral perfusion. Therefore the left carotid artery cannot be sacrificed without leaving the patient with major neurologic deficits and the decision was made to resect as much tumor as possible but to leave the left carotid artery in place with some residual tumor.

Occasionally it is necessary to sacrifice a large vessel such as a carotid artery. This may occur due to trauma, large tumor encasing the vessel, or treatment of arteriovenous malformation. To assess the adequacy of collateral flow, an intra-arterial balloon catheter is inflated in the vessel at the level of projected ligation. The patient is observed for neurologic deficits with the balloon inflated for 45 minutes; if signs and symptoms of ischemia develop, the balloon is deflated immediately. Some patients who do not develop symptoms during the balloon occlusion test do develop neurologic deficits after permanent sacrifice of the vessel. Therefore assessment of the brain perfusion with ^{99m}Tc-HMPAO or ^{99m}Tc-ECD during balloon occlusion has been added to the evaluation of these patients. The radiopharmaceutical is injected intravenously approximately

20 minutes after the balloon has been inflated. The timing of injection is critical to avoid a false positive. If the tracer is injected too early, the collateral may not have opened completely. As there is no redistribution of ^{99m}Tc-HMPAO over time, the SPECT images can be acquired at some time after the end of the test. If a cortical perfusion deficit occurs, it is usually accompanied by a crossed cerebellar diaschisis, and the patient is at risk for developing a neurologic deficit if permanent occlusion of the vessel is performed.

Patients who do not have perfusion deficits during balloon occlusion can have the vessel sacrificed without major consequences.

Diagnosis: Inadequate cerebral perfusion during balloon occlusion test of the left carotid artery.

History: This 23-year-old male presented with headaches that had been worsening for a month. These were low-pressure headaches, relieved in the supine position and reaching a maximum intensity after 30 minutes in the sitting position. The patient reported doing heavy weight training and recalls that 2 weeks prior to the start of his headaches, he had an episode of nausea and vomiting during a workout. Brain MRI and CT myelogram were normal (not shown). A cysternogram was performed to assess for the presence of a CSF leak (Figs. 4.13 A and 4.13 B).

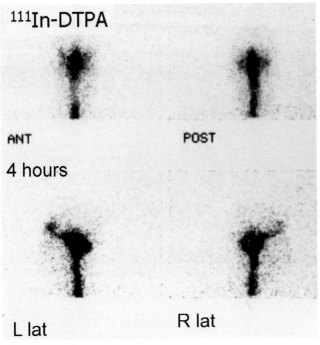

Figure 4.13 A

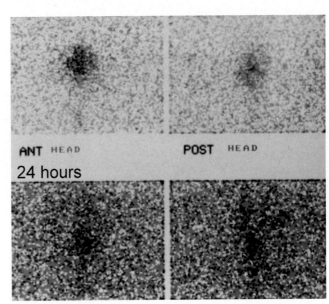

Figure 4.13 B

Findings: ^{111}In-DTPA was injected intrathecally by lumbar puncture and images were obtained over the entire neuroaxis up to 24 hours after injection. The immediate image confirms a successful intrathecal injection (not shown). On the 4-hour images, there is normal flow of the CSF from the site of injection to the basal cisternae (Fig. 4.13 A). Over the next 20 hours, there was a progressive decrease of radioactivity in the CSF and an increase in the background, as illustrated on the 24-hour images (Fig. 4.13 B). The kidneys were visualized as well.

Discussion: The findings are compatible with a leakage of ^{111}In-DTPA from the CSF, reabsorption into the plasma, and excretion by the kidneys. In this case, the site of the leak could not be identified on the images. The patient was treated with an epidural blood patch and bed rest for 10 days, which led to improvement of the headaches.

The syndrome of postural headaches associated with low CSF pressure is well known and usually occurs following a diagnostic lumbar puncture. Similar symptoms can occur when a tear develops in the spinal theca, usually in the midthoracic spine, resulting from coughing, lifting weight, or sometimes spontaneously. The headaches can be accompanied by auditory and vestibular symptoms such as nausea, vomiting, and dizziness, and are worse during a Valsalva maneuver. A complication of low CSF pressure is bilateral subdural hematomas, most probably due to rupture of bridging veins, when the brain pulls away from the dura as the CSF volume decreases. If a lumbar puncture is performed, the opening pressure is usually below 50 mm Hg; often there is an increase in erythrocytes count and increased protein content. A radionuclide cysternogram can document a CSF leak directly by demonstrated accumulation of the radiopharmaceutical outside the subarachnoid space or indirectly by its rapid disappearance from the subarachnoid space and early appearance in the urinary system (57). Bed rest for 2 to 4 weeks usually allows the tear to heal. An epidural blood patch can speed the relief of symptoms. It consists of injecting 5 to 10 mL of the patient's own blood in the epidural space close to the site of the tear. This prevents further leakage by increasing the pressure in the epidural space and coagulation of the blood.

Diagnosis: Low-pressure headaches probably due to CSF leakage through a tear in the spinal theca following weight lifting.

History: This 38-year-old male presented with progressive cognitive disorder. A brain MRI was normal (Fig. 4.14 A, T2-weighted image shown). ¹⁸F-FDG PET imaging was performed (Fig. 4.14 B).

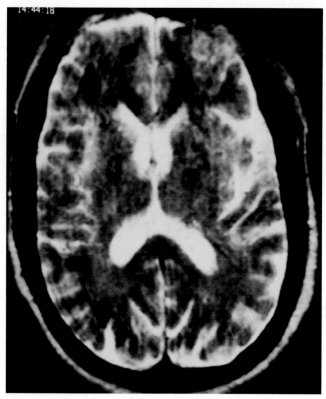

Figure 4.14 A

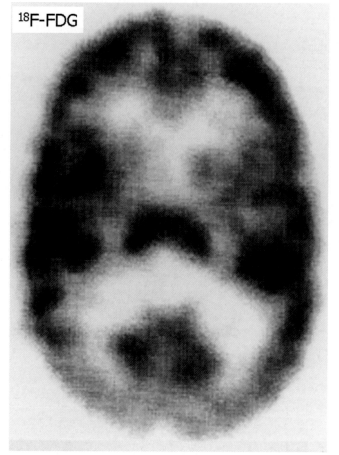

Figure 4.14 B

Findings: The ¹⁸F-FDG PET images show markedly decreased ¹⁸F-FDG uptake in the head of the caudate nuclei bilaterally and normal cortical uptake.

Discussion: In this age group, Huntington's disease is number one in the differential diagnosis. Genetic testing confirmed the diagnosis in this patient.

Huntington's disease (HD) is an autosomal dominant disorder that in most cases presents in the third or fourth decade by progressive cognitive decline and extrapyramidal or choreiform movements. The genetic anomaly is located in the short arm of chromosome 4. The more profound pathologic changes are in the putamen and the caudate nuclei. In advanced disease, atrophy of the caudate nuclei can be demonstrated on CT and MRI. PET imaging of ¹⁸F-FDG identify decreased metabolism in the caudate nuclei in subjects with Huntington's disease or at risk for the disease before atrophy can be seen in symptomatic patients. Therefore PET may be valuable in presymptomatic screening for the detection of gene carriers in the at-risk population (58,59).

The differential diagnosis of decreased perfusion and metabolism in the basal ganglia includes Wilson's disease, progressive supranuclear palsy, and multiple system atrophy. Wilson's disease is an autosomal recessive disorder of copper metabolism that can lead to movement and psychiatric disorders due to the accumulation of copper in the brain. Patients with Wilson's disease have decreased glucose metabolism in the striatum and cerebellum. Patients with progressive supranuclear palsy present with paralyzed gaze, dystonia, axial rigidity, and sometimes dementia. On functional images, the most striking finding is decreased uptake in the frontal cortex, but uptake in the basal ganglia and thalami is also decreased. Multisystem atrophy (Shy-Drager syndrome) includes the syndromes of striatonigral degeneration, pallidopyramidal degeneration, olivopontocerebellar atrophy, and pure autonomic dysfunction. ¹⁸F-FDG PET images usually show decreased metabolism in the striatum. The striatonigral degeneration variant resembles Parkinson's disease clinically but without tremor; on PET images there is striatal and prefrontal hypometabolism. The olivopontocerebellar atrophy variant begins clinically with gait disturbances and progresses to dysarthria and limb ataxia. There is degeneration of the neurons from the cerebellar cortex, pons, and inferior olives, which demonstrates hypometabolism on ^{18}F-FDG images.

The differential diagnosis of decreased uptake in the basal ganglia also includes atypical Parkinson's disease, atypical Creutzfeldt–Jacob disease, prior viral encephalopathy (particularly herpes zoster), toxic encephalopathies (such as ethylene glycol), and a variety of other degenerative neurologic diseases.

Diagnosis: Huntington's disease.

CASE 4.15

History: This 78-year-old man presented with a 4- to 6-month history of "spells" and increasing left-sided weakness. The spells consist of flushing of the head, sweating, rapid heart rate, and increased blood pressure. They were preceded by a smell of oil and a taste in his mouth. They could occur several times a day and lasted several minutes. The clinical differential diagnosis was possible tumor versus transient ischemic attack versus pheochromocytoma. A CT of the brain was performed and demonstrated a heterogeneous mass involving the right frontal lobe, right basal ganglia, right midbrain, and pons. The frontal portion of the mass appeared hemorrhagic (Fig. 4.15 A, black arrow). The rest of the mass appeared to have central necrosis and an enhancing rim suggestive of a primary central nervous system tumor (Fig 4.15 A, white arrow). The lesion was biopsied by fine-needle aspiration, which showed fragments of necrotic brain with hemorrhage consistent with a hemorrhagic infarct but no evidence of malignancy. FDG PET imaging was then performed (Fig. 4.15 B).

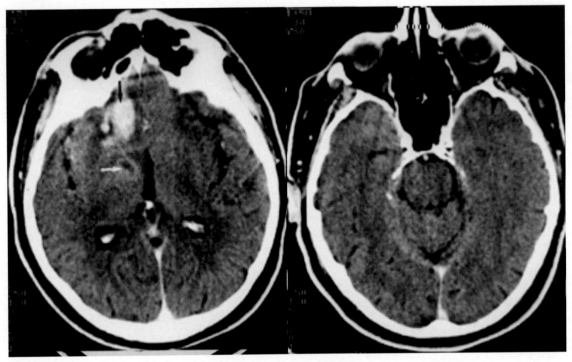

Figure 4.15 A

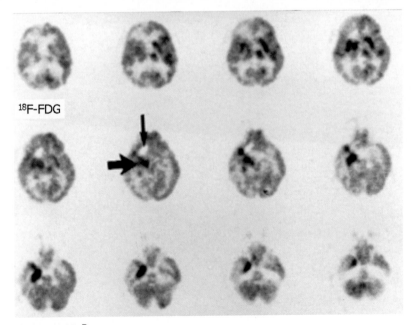

Figure 4.15 B

Findings: The images demonstrate no ^{18}F-FDG uptake in the frontal portion of the mass consistent with hemorrhage (Fig. 4.15 B, thin arrow). In the region of the right basal ganglia, midbrain, and pons, there is ^{18}F-FDG uptake matching the region of enhancement on the CT scan (Fig. 4.15 B, thick arrow). The level of uptake is close to the cortical uptake. In addition there is ^{18}F-FDG uptake at twice the level of cortical uptake in the right hippocampus adjacent to the lesion.

Discussion: These findings are consistent with a high-grade tumor with necrosis and hemorrhage and an adjacent ictal seizure focus in the right hippocampus. Based on the PET scan, the patient underwent a stereotactically guided biopsy, which showed an anaplastic astrocytoma.

This case illustrates that brain tumors are often heterogeneous, and sampling error is not a rare occurrence. PET is an accurate imaging modality to differentiate a low-grade process from high-grade tumors based on the glucose metabolism. PET is particularly helpful when access to the lesion for biopsy is difficult or, as in this case, it provides guidance for the biopsy at the site of maximum activity.

Lesions (both benign and malignant) located in the region of the temporal lobe can present with seizures as the first symptom. If seizures are frequent during the ^{18}F-FDG uptake phase (the first 20 minutes after injection of ^{18}F-FDG), the ictal seizure focus has increased ^{18}F-FDG uptake, usually above the level of cortical uptake. This high uptake, if not recognized as due to seizure, may lead to a wrong interpretation of high-grade tumor. Therefore it is important to recognize that the interpretation of ^{18}F-FDG images cannot be accurate without the appropriate clinical information as well as correlation with anatomic images. The interpreter must evaluate in precisely what anatomic structure the abnormal ^{18}F-FDG uptake is present.

Diagnosis: High-grade tumor with adjacent ictal seizure focus.

CASE 4.16

History: This 57-year-old man was found unconscious and brought to the emergency room. A CT scan of the head showed subarachnoid hemorrhage in the left sylvian fissure, basal cisternae, and third ventricle (not shown). A ventricular drain was placed, and the next day a cerebral arteriogram was performed, showing an anterior communicating artery aneurysm. He was taken to the operating room for aneurysm clipping via craniotomy. During surgery, the aneurysm ruptured, leading to a significant hemorrhage. Postoperatively, he had right hemiparesis. A postoperative CT scan showed the postoperative changes, a left ventricular drain in place, an intracranial pressure monitor over the right frontal region, and some persistent intraventricular and subarachnoid blood but no definite infarction (Fig 4.16 A). A ^{99m}Tc-HMPAO cerebral perfusion study was performed (Fig 4.16 B).

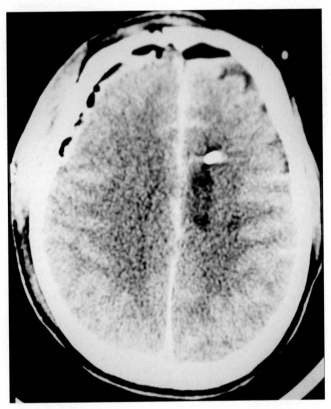

Figure 4.16 A

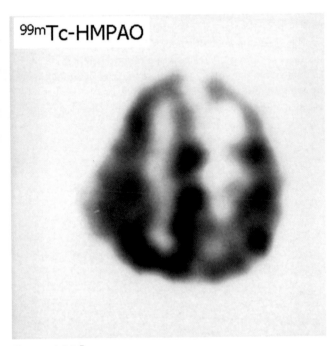

Figure 4.16 B

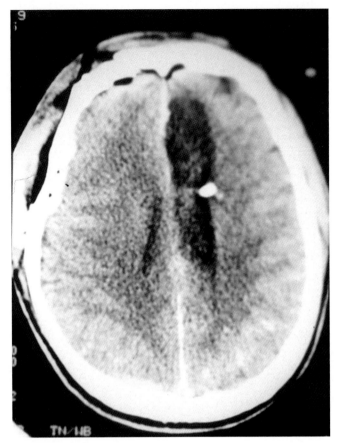

Figure 4.16 C

Findings: The SPECT images demonstrate markedly decreased perfusion in a focal region of the left frontal cortex. In addition, there is milder decreased uptake in the remainder of the left frontal cortex compared with the right.

Discussion: These findings suggest an infarct in the left frontal cortex and possibly a larger region of ischemia. A follow-up CT scan performed 3 days later showed development of an infarct in the territory of the left anterior cerebral artery (Fig. 4.16 C).

This case illustrates that functional changes occur before anatomic changes. When the cerebral blood flow to a region of the brain is jeopardized, decreased perfusion can be visualized on ^{99m}Tc-HMPAO images within 2 hours of the event. Resulting anatomic changes can be seen on CT or MRI, sometimes only several days later.

Diagnosis: Infarct of the left anterior cerebral artery.

CASE 4.17

History: This 69-year-old male presented with dementia, gait disturbance, and incontinence. A CT scan of the brain showed enlargement of the ventricles; there was also cortical atrophy (not shown). A radionuclide cisternography was performed following intrathecal administration of 0.5 mCi ^{111}In-DTPA to evaluate the presence of normal-pressure hydrocephalus (Figs. 4.17 A, 4.17 B, and 4.17 C).

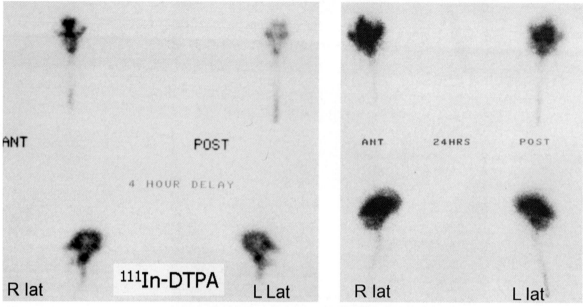

Figure 4.17 A

Figure 4.17 B

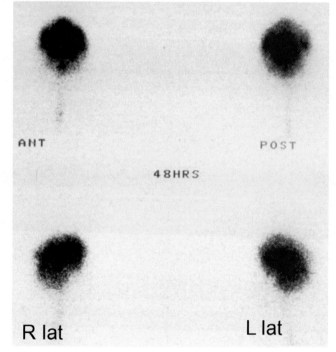

Figure 4.17 C

Findings: On the 4-hour images (Fig. 4.17 A), there is early entry of the radiopharmaceutical into the ventricular system, which persists at 24 hours (Fig. 4.17 B) and 48 hours (Fig. 4.17 C). In addition, there is delayed migration of the CSF over the convexities.

Discussion: These findings are seen in normal-pressure hydrocephalus. Both hydrocephalus and atrophy are characterized by ventricular enlargement on CT and MRI. In hydrocephalus, the ventricular enlargement is out of proportion compared with the atrophy. The etiologies for hydrocephalus are the following: (a) overproduction of CSF (choroid plexus tumors), (b) decreased reabsorption of CSF, (c) obstructive hydrocephalus (both communicating extraventricular obstruction, such as subarachnoid hemorrhage or inflammation, and noncommunicating intraventricular obstruction due to tumors or congenital malformation), and (d) normal-pressure hydrocephalus.

Normal-pressure hydrocephalus is characterized by the triad of dementia, ataxia, and incontinence. The physiopathology of the syndrome is still not well understood, but there is impairment of the CSF dynamics, which can be demonstrated by radionuclide cisternography, as in this patient. Various semiquantitative measurements have been investigated to try to predict the outcome of ventriculoperitoneal shunting, but with limited success.

On ^{99m}Tc-HMPAO or ^{18}F-FDG images, patients with normal-pressure hydrocephalus can have a pattern of uptake similar to that seen in Alzheimer's disease.

Diagnosis: Normal-pressure hydrocephalus.

History: This 13-year-old boy presented with seizures and confusion. A cerebral CT was normal (not shown). A cerebral ^{99m}Tc-glucoheptonate study was performed (Fig. 4.18 A).

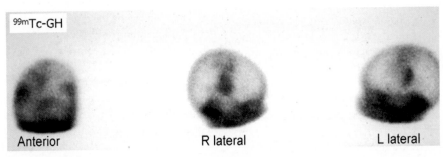

Figure 4.18 A

Findings: The anterior and both lateral projections of a 4-hour delayed scan are shown (Fig. 4.18 A). They demonstrate increased uptake in both temporal lobes.

Discussion: These findings are highly suggestive of herpes encephalitis.

Patients with viral infections of the brain usually present with global deficits such as seizures, confusion, coma, or delirium. Focal deficits, such as involuntary movements or ocular palsies, can also be present. Various viral agents can cause encephalitis; they can be classified in six broad categories: (a) arbovirus (eastern and western equine encephalitis, often lethal), (b) enterovirus (poliomyelitis), (c) respiratory virus, (d) virus from childhood infections (measles, mumps, rubella, chickenpox), (e) other viruses (cytomegalovirus, herpes simplex and zoster, Epstein-Barr virus), and (f) slow viruses. The true slow viruses include subacute sclerosing panencephalitis, often preceded by measles; progressive rubella panencephalitis; and progressive multifocal encephalopathy occurring in patients who are chronically debilitated (tuberculosis, sarcoidosis, and rheumatoid arthritis), or immunosuppressed (including AIDS). The unconventional slow viruses include kuru and Creutzfeldt–Jakob, which cause spongiform changes in the gray matter.

Herpes simplex can produce a number of diseases depending on the organ involved. Both herpes simplex I (labialis) and II (genitalis) can cause encephalitis in neonates, which usually involves the entire brain. Herpes simplex I is also responsible for most cases of encephalitis (acute necrotizing encephalitis) in older children and adults, typically involving the temporal lobes and orbitofrontal cortex. If left untreated, many cases are fatal, and some patients survive with severe dementia and memory deficits. The recently discovered effective therapy with acyclovir has generated a need for early diagnosis.

The blood-brain barrier is often abnormal in viral infections of the brain, and blood-brain barrier imaging is usually abnormal several days before the changes are seen on CT or MRI. There is increased uptake on the dynamic images and extensive areas of diffuse uptake on the delayed images.

Functional cerebral images of perfusion and glucose metabolism demonstrate increased uptake in the temporal lobes in acute herpes encephalitis. These changes also precede by several days the changes on CT and MRI. In the chronic phase, when damage to the brain has occurred, the uptake may be decreased, as seen on the MRI and ^{18}F-FDG images shown in Figures 4.18 B and 4.18 C.

Diagnosis: Herpes encephalitis.

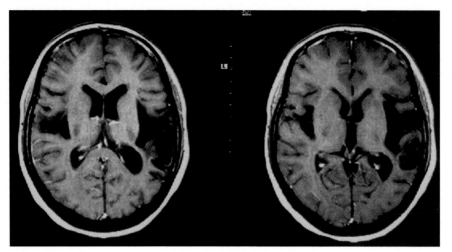

Figure 4.18 B

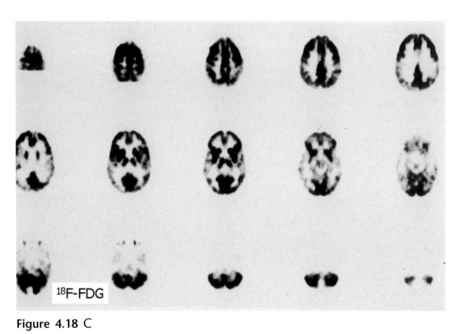

Figure 4.18 C

CASE 4.19

History: This patient presented with a malfunctioning ventriculoperitoneal shunt by physical examination. A shuntogram was performed after administration of 0.5 mCi ^{99m}Tc-DTPA into the shunt reservoir to assess shunt patency (Fig. 4.19 A).

Anterior 20 min   25 min

Figure 4.19 A

Findings: Sequential images obtained up to 25 minutes after administration of the radiopharmaceutical are shown (Fig. 4.19 A). The focus of marked uptake corresponds to the location of the reservoir. The radiopharmaceutical is present in the ventricular system and in a portion of the shunt tubing. The radiopharmaceutical is not seen free in the peritoneal cavity, even on the 25-minute image.

Discussion: These findings indicate obstruction of the distal limb of the shunt.

There are several shunt types, including ventriculoperitoneal, ventriculojugular, ventriculoatrial, and lumboperitoneal. Familiarity with the type of shunt is critical before performing a shuntogram. Several complications can result from CSF shunting: infection, thromboembolism, and overdrainage of CSF. Ventriculoatrial shunts are associated with a higher complication rate than ventriculoperitoneal shunts, including also superior vena cava syndrome and immune glomerulonephritis.

The patency of these shunts can be assessed by administering a radiopharmaceutical percutaneously into the shunt reservoir under aseptic conditions. ^{99m}Tc-DTPA is the radiopharmaceutical of choice to evaluate ventriculoperitoneal shunts. The background is low owing to excretion by the kidneys, and the physical characteristics of ^{99m}Tc provide high-quality images during the time frame of imaging. ^{99m}Tc-MAA is preferred to evaluate ventriculoatrial shunts because the shunt patency is demonstrated by pulmonary uptake. A normal shuntogram is shown in Figure 4.19 B. The distal catheter is usually occluded during administration of the radiopharmaceutical, so that it refluxes into the ventricles. There should be free flow into the peritoneal cavity if the shunt is functioning properly.

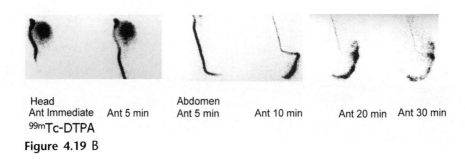

Head
Ant Immediate   Ant 5 min
^{99m}Tc-DTPA

Abdomen
Ant 5 min

Ant 10 min

Ant 20 min   Ant 30 min

Figure 4.19 B

Resistance at the time of injection always indicates malfunction of the shunt. If there is proximal limb malfunction, either no activity will reflux into the ventricle and there will be rapid transit of the radiopharmaceutical through the distal shunt into the peritoneal cavity, as seen in another patient (shown in Fig. 4.19 C), or—if the radiopharmaceutical refluxes into the ventricles—there will be slow clearing, taking several hours. If the one-way valve is located proximal to the port, the pattern will mimic a proximal shunt obstruction.

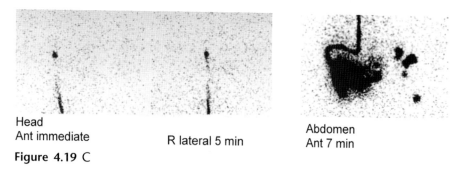

Head
Ant immediate   R lateral 5 min

Figure 4.19 C

Abdomen
Ant 7 min

Obstruction of the distal limb of ventriculoperitoneal shunts is indicated by lack of free radiopharmaceutical into the peritoneal cavity or a loculated collection at the distal tip (Fig. 4.19 A). Obstruction of the distal limb may be due to tip occlusion from fibrous adhesions, distal tubing kinking (more frequent in children), perforation of a viscera, shunt tip migration, peritonitis preventing reabsorption of the CSF, and increased intra-abdominal pressure.

Diagnosis: Occluded ventriculoperitoneal shunt.

CASE 4.20

History: This 42-year-old male was admitted for new-onset tonic-clonic seizures. He has a history of alcohol and intravenous drug abuse and of tuberculosis. He is HIV-negative. A cerebral MRI was performed and showed an enhancing mass in the right frontal lobe centered in the deep white matter, surrounded by edema, but with no significant mass effect (Fig. 4.20 A). ^{18}F-FDG PET imaging was performed to assess the glucose metabolism of the lesion (Fig. 4.20 B).

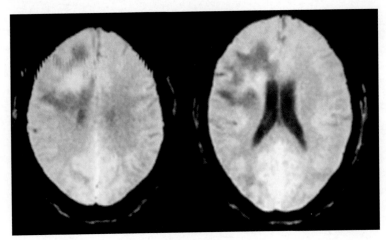

Figure 4.20 A

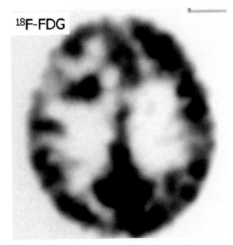

Figure 4.20 B

Findings: The ^{18}F-FDG uptake in the lesion is close to that of cortical level.

Discussion: The level of cortical uptake is consistent with a high-grade tumor, such as a high-grade glioma or lymphoma. The lesion was resected surgically and pathologic examination demonstrated an aspergilloma. Fungal infections are usually associated with granulomatous inflammation, and inflammatory cells (particularly macrophages) are known to have significant accumulations of ^{18}F-FDG (60). Therefore active granulomatous processes such as fungal and yeast infections (especially with *Aspergillus, Nocardia,* and *Candida*), tuberculosis, and sarcoidosis have been reported to accumulate high levels of ^{18}F-FDG and to cause false-positive studies in the evaluation of malignancy.

Aspergillosis involving the central nervous system is rarely encountered and usually affects patients debilitated by neoplasms or collagen vascular diseases, drug addiction, alcoholism, or immunosuppression. Infection of the brain usually presents as abscesses. The gross appearance is often that of a necrotic and hemorrhagic lesion with central cavitation. Infection by *Aspergillus* may be found in HIV-positive patients but is extremely rare. Sixty percent of HIV-positive patients with cerebral lesions have toxoplasmosis, 30% have cerebral lymphoma, and only 10% will have another pathologic process. Therefore a cerebral lesion with high ^{18}F-FDG uptake is likely a lymphoma. In debilitated or immunosuppressed patients that are HIV-negative, granulomatous abscesses should be considered in the differential diagnosis. For further readings on this topic, please see reference 41.

Diagnosis: Aspergilloma.

CASE 4.21

History: This 40-year-old male presented with a history of complex partial seizures, which he had had since the age of 18 years. A cerebral MRI showed cortical dysplasia involving nearly the entire left hemisphere, with a possible closed-lip schizencephalic cleft in the rolandic region (Fig. 4.21 A). The patient was admitted twice at a 1-year interval for EEG-CCTV monitoring. The EEG suggested bitemporal discharges. Interictal 18F-FDG PET imaging was performed (Fig. 4.21 B). The following week, ictal and interictal 99mTc-HMPAO cerebral SPECT images were obtained (Figs. 4.21 C and 4.21 D).

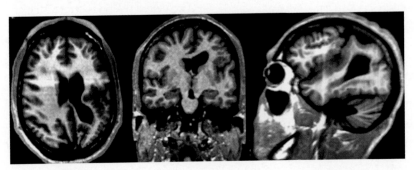

Figure 4.21 A

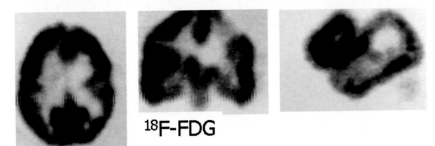

18F-FDG

Figure 4.21 B

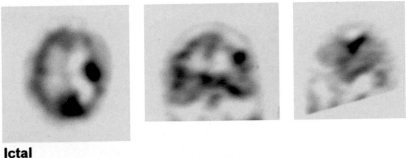

Ictal

Figure 4.21 C

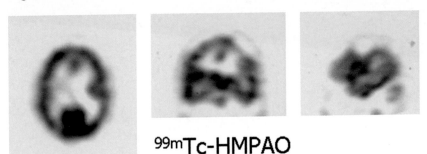

99mTc-HMPAO

Interictal

Figure 4.21 D

Findings: Corresponding transaxial, coronal, and sagittal slices through the left parietal lobe are shown for the four sets of images. Both SPECT and PET images demonstrate marked asymmetry between the right and left hemispheres, the left being atrophic and dysmorphic. On both ^{99m}Tc-HMPAO and ^{18}F-FDG, the pattern of cortical uptake matches the pattern of cortical dysplasia seen on the MRI. HMPAO and ^{18}F-FDG uptake is present along the lining of the cleft. On the ictal SPECT scan, there is increased uptake along that lining, which extends inferiorly in the temporal lobe. On both the interictal SPECT and PET images, there is decreased uptake in that region.

Discussion: The functional images are helpful in two respects. The presence of uptake along the lining of the cleft identifies cortex lining the cleft, which is critical in differentiating schizencephaly from porencephaly. This differentiation is important because of the poor prognosis of schizencephaly compared with porencephaly. Porencephalic cysts develop in fetal life or infancy and are believed to be secondary to an ischemic insult. Schizencephaly is a rare embryologic developmental malformation characterized by gross and microscopic structural defects of neural migration. A primitive four-layer cortical lamination lines a well-defined pial-ependymal cleft extending from the pia arachnoid to the ventricle primarily in the rolandic and parasylvian areas. They are called "closed-lip" when the edges of the cleft are close together, as in this case. Schizencephaly is associated with microgyria and other developmental abnormalities. The clinical manifestations include mental retardation, hemiparesis, hemiplegia, and cerebral seizures. The incidence in subsequent siblings is increased and rare cases of familial incidence have been reported.

The findings of increased uptake on ictal and decreased uptake on interictal functional images are consistent with a seizure focus arising from the cortical dysplasia. The localization of the seizure focus in a region of cortical dysplasia or heterotopia is extremely useful in planning surgery in these patients.

Diagnosis: (a) Cortical dysplasia and closed-lip schizencephaly. (b) Seizure focus arising from the closed-lip schizencephaly.

CASE 4.22

History: This 65-year-old male presented with progressive dementia. The MRI showed diffuse atrophy and old infarcts in the occipital cortex bilaterally (Fig. 4.22 A). ^{18}F-FDG PET imaging was performed to exclude a degenerative dementia (Fig. 4.22 B).

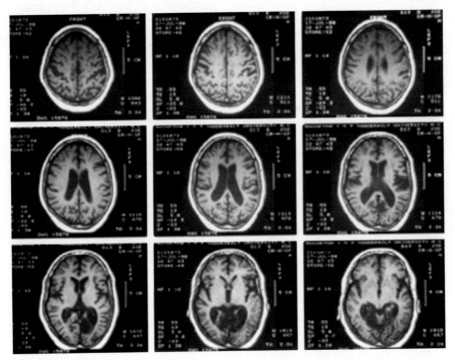

Figure 4.22 A

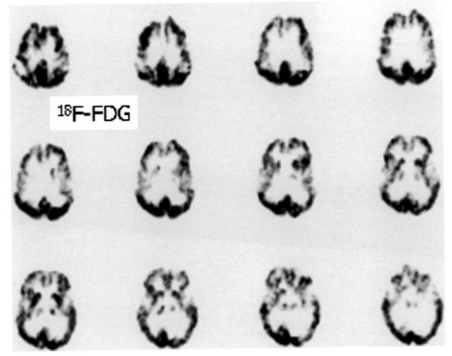

Figure 4.22 B

Findings: The ^{18}F-FDG images demonstrate multiple focal areas of decreased uptake that are scattered throughout the brain. There is also decreased uptake in the occipital cortex bilaterally, corresponding to the infarcts seen on the MRI.

Discussion: These findings are typical of multi-infarct dementia.

Multi-infarct dementia represents only about 10% to 15% of the dementias. It is characterized clinically by a stepwise progression of the symptoms due to separate episodes of infarction. Sometimes this stepwise progression is subtle and the clinical presentation is similar to that of AD. AD and vascular dementia can also coexist. Usually patients with multi-infarct dementia have evidence of infarcts on CT or MRI, and the presence of infarcts of different age is highly suggestive of that diagnosis. On functional scans, their global cerebral perfusion and glucose metabolism are reduced to a greater extent than in patients with AD. In multi-infarct dementia, the sensorimotor cortex can be involved, while it is almost invariably spared in AD.

Diagnosis: Multi-infarct dementia.

REFERENCES AND SUGGESTED READING

1. Chugani HT, Phelps ME, Mazziotta JC. Positron emission tomography study of human brain development. *Ann Neurol* 1987;22:487–497.
2. Guidelines for the determination of death: report of the medical consultants on the diagnosis of death to the president's committee for the study of ethical problems in medicine and biomedical and behavioral research. *JAMA* 1981;246:2184–2188.
3. Nordlander S, Wiklund PE, Asard PE. Cerebral angioscintigraphy in brain death and in coma due to drug intoxication. *J Nucl Med* 1973;14:856–857.
4. Goodman JM, Heck LL, More BD. Confirmation of brain death with portable isotope angiography: a review of 204 consecutive cases. *Neurosurgery* 1985;16:492–496.
5. Korein J, Braunstein P, George A, et al. Brain death: angiographic correlation with the radioisotope bolus technique for evaluation of critical deficit of cerebral blood flow. *Ann Neurol* 1977;2:195–201.
6. Okuyaz C, Gucuyener K, Karabacak NI, et al. Tc-99m-HMPAO SPECT in the diagnosis of brain death in children. *Pediatr Int* 2004;46(6):711–714.
7. Bonte FJ, Devous MD. SPECT brain imaging. In: Sandler MP et al, eds. *Diagnostic Nuclear Medicine*, 4th ed. Baltimore: Lippincott Williams & Wilkins, 2003:757–781.
8. Mountz JM, Liu H, Deutsch G. Neuroimaging in cerebrovascular disorder: measurement of cerebral physiology after stroke and assessment of stroke recovery. *Semin Nucl Med* 2003;33;56–76.
9. Soucy JP, McNamara D, Mohr G, et al. Evaluation of vasospasm secondary to subarachnoid hemorrhage with technetium-99m-hexamethyl-propyleneamine oxime (HMPAO) tomoscintigraphy. *J Nucl Med* 1990;31:972–977.
10. Van Heerden BB, Monsein LH, Jeffrey PJ, et al. Brain SPECT imaging to assess collateral circulation during trial balloon occlusion of internal carotid artery. *J Nucl Med* 1990;31:878.
11. Hietala SO, Silfvenious H, Asaly J, et al. Brain perfusion with intracarotid injection of 99mTc-HMPAO in partial epilepsy during amobarbital testing. *Eur J Nucl Med* 1990;16:683–687.
12. Jeffery PJ, Monsein LH, Szabo Z, et al. Mapping of the distribution of amobarbital sodium in the intracarotid Wada test by use of Tc-99m HMPAO with SPECT. *Radiology* 1991;178:847–850.
13. Reid RH, Gulenchyn KY, Ballinger JR, et al. Cerebral perfusion imaging with technetium-99m HMPAO following cerebral trauma: initial experience. *Clin Nucl Med* 1990;15:383–388.
14. Newberg AB, Alavi A. Role of positron emission tomography in the investigation of neuropsychiatric disorders. In: Sandler MP et al, eds. *Diagnostic Nuclear Medicine,* 4th ed. Baltimore: Lippincott Williams & Wilkins, 2003:783–819.
15. Devous MD Sr, Leroy RF, Homan RW. Single photon emission computed tomography in epilepsy. *Semin Nucl Med* 1990;20:325–341.
16. Engel J Jr, Wiebe S, French J, et al. Practice parameter: temporal lobe and localized neocortical resections for epilepsy: report of the Quality Standards Subcommittee of the American Academy of Neurology in association with the American Epilepsy Society and the American Association of Neurological Surgeons.[erratum appears in *Neurology*. 2003;60(8):1396]. *Neurology* 2003;60:538–547.
17. Newton MR, Berkovic SF, Austin MC, et al. Ictal postictal and interictal single-photon emission tomography in the lateralization of temporal lobe epilepsy. *Eur J Nucl Med* 1994;21:1067–1071.
18. Knowlton RC. The role of FDG-PET, ictal SPECT, and MEG in the epilepsy surgery evaluation. *Epilepsy Behav* 2006;8:91–101.
19. Duncan R, Patterson J, Roberts R, et al. Ictal/postictal SPECT in the presurgical localization of complex partial seizures. *J Neurol Neurosurg Psychiatry* 1993;56:141–148.
20. Marks DA, Katz A, Hoffer P, Spencer SS. Localization of extratemporal epileptic foci during ictal single photon emission computed tomography. *Ann Neurol* 1992;31:250–255.
21. Zubal IG, Spencer SS, Imam K, et al. Difference images calculated from ictal and interictal technetium-99m-HMPAO SPECT scans of epilepsy. *J Nucl Med* 1995;36:684–689.
22. Delbeke D, Lawrence SK, Abou-Khalil BW, et al. Postsurgical outcome of patients with uncontrolled complex partial seizures and temporal lobe hypometabolism on 18FDG positron emission tomography. *Invest Radiol* 1996;31:261–265.
23. Van Paesschen W. Ictal SPECT. *Epilepsia* 2004;45(Suppl 4);35–40.
24. Patronas NJ, Di Chiro G, Brooks RA, et al. Work in progress: [18F] fluorodeoxyglucose and positron emission tomography in the evaluation of radiation necrosis of the brain. *Radiology* 1982;144:885–889.
25. Di Chiro G, Oldfield E, Wright DC, et al. Cerebral necrosis after radiotherapy and/or intraarterial chemotherapy for brain tumors: PET and neuropathologic studies. *AJR* 1988;150:189–197.
26. Di Chiro G, DeLapaz RL, Brooks PA, et al. Glucose utilization of cerebral gliomas measured by [18F] fluorodeoxyglucose and positron emission tomography. *Neurology* 1982;32:1323–1329.
27. Patronas NJ, Brooks RA, DeLaPaz RI, et al. Glycolytic rate (PET) and contrast enhancement (CT) in human cerebral gliomas. *AJNR* 1983;4:533–535.
28. Kim CK, Alvi JB, Alavi A, et al. New grading system of cerebral gliomas using positron emission tomography with F-18-fluorodeoxyglucose. *J Neurooncol* 1991;10:85–91.
29. Delbeke D, Meyerowitz C, Lapidus RL, et al. Optimal cut-off level of F-18-fluorodeoxyglucose uptake in the differentiation of low grade from high grade brain tumors with PET. *Radiology* 1995;195:47–52.
30. Patronas NJ, Di Chiro G, Kufta C, et al. Prediction of survival in glioma patients by means of positron emission tomography. *J Neurosurg* 1985;62:816–822.
31. Alavi JB, Alavi A, Chawluk J, et al. Positron emission tomography in patients with gliomas: a predictor of prognosis. *Cancer* 1988;62:1074–1078.
32. Barker FJ, Chang SM, Valk PE, et al. 18-Fluorodeoxyglucose uptake and survival of patients with suspected recurrent malignant glioma. *Cancer* 1997;79:115–126.
33. Rosenfeld SS, Hoffman JM, Coleman RE, et al. Studies of primary central nervous system lymphoma with fluorine-18-fluorodeoxyglucose positron emission tomography. *J Nucl Med* 1992;33:532–536.
34. Hoffman JM, Waskin HA, Schifter T, et al. FDG-PET in differentiating lymphoma from nonmalignant central nervous system lesions in patients with AIDS. *J Nucl Med* 1993;34:567–575.
35. Kessler RM, Pierce M, Maciunas R, et al. Accuracy of FDG PET studies in distinguishing cerebral infections from lymphoma in patients with AIDS. *J Nucl Med* 1993;34:37P.
36. Tien RD, Felsberg GJ, Ferris NJ, et al. The dementias: correlation of clinical features, pathophysiology, and neuroradiology. *Am J Roentgenol* 1993;161:245–255.
37. Van Heertum RL, Tikofsky RS: PET and SPECT brain imaging in dementia. *Semin Nucl Med* 2003;33:77-86.
38. Van Heertum RL, Greenstein EA, Tikofsky RS. 2-Deoxy-fluorglucose-positron emission tomography imaging of the brain: current clinical applications with emphasis on the dementias. *Semin Nucl Med* 2004;34;300–312.
39. Friedland RP, Budinger TF, Ganz E, et al. Regional cerebral metabolic alterations in dementia of the Alzheimer type: positron emission tomography with F-18-fluorodeoxyglucose. *J Comput Assist Tomogr* 1983;7(4):590-598.
40. Reiman EM, Caselli RJ, Yun LS, et al. Preclinical evidence of Alzheimer's disease in persons homozygous for the E4 allele for apolipoprotein E. *N Engl J Med* 1996;334:752–758.
41. Zakzanis KK, Graham SJ, Campbell Z. A meta-analysis of structural and functional brain imaging in dementia of the Alzheimer's type: a neuroimaging profile. *Neuropsychol Rev* 2003;13:1–18.
42. Lawrence SK, Delbeke D, Partain CL et al. Cerebrospinal fluid imaging. In: Sandler MP et al, eds. *Diagnostic Nuclear Medicine*, 4th ed. Baltimore: Lippincott Williams & Wilkins, 2003:835–1176.
43. Holman BL, Johnson KA, Gerada B, et al. The scintigraphic appearance of Alzheimer's disease. *J Nucl Med* 1992;33:181–185.
44. Kuhl DE, Small GW, Riege WH, et al. Abnormal PET-FDG scans in early Alzheimer's disease. *J Nucl Med* 1987;28:645.
45. Johnson KA, Mueller ST, Walshe TM, et al. Cerebral perfusion imaging in Alzheimer's disease. *Arch Neurol* 1987;44:165–168.
46. Tyrell PJ, Warrington EK, Frackowiak RS, et al. Heterogeneity in progressive aphasia due to cortical atrophy. *Brain* 1990;113:1321–1336.
47. Alvarez LA, Lipton RB, et al. Brain death determination by angiography in the setting of a skull defect. *Arch Neurol* 1988;45:225–230.
48. Petty GW, Mohr JP, Pedley TA, et al. The role of transcranial Doppler in confirming brain death. *Neurology* 1990;40:300–307.
49. Hansen AVE, Lavin PJM, Moody EB, et al. False-negative cerebral radionuclide flow study in brain death caused by a ventricular drain. *Clin Nucl Med* 1993;18:502–505.

50. Kamo H, McGeer PL, Harrop R, et al. Positron emission tomography and histopathology in Pick's disease. *Neurology* 1987,37:439–445.

51. Kumar A, Shapiro MB, Haxby JV, et al. Cerebral metabolic and cognitive studies in dementia with frontal lobe behavioral features. *J Psychiatr Res* 1990, 24:97–109.

52. Miller BL, Cummings JL, Villanueva-Meyer J, et al. Frontal lobe degeneration: clinical, neuropsychological, and SPECT characteristics. *Neurology* 1991;41;1374–1382.

53. Komori T, Martin WH, Graber AL, et al. Serendipitous of Cushing's disease by FDG positron emission tomography and a review of the literature. *Clin Nucl Med* 2002;27:176–178.

54. De Souza B, Brunetti A, Fulham MJ, et al. Pituitary microadenomas: a PET study. *Radiology* 1990;177:39–44.

55. Bergstrom M, Muhr C, Lundberg PO, et al. PET as a tool in the clinical evaluation of pituitary adenomas. *J Nucl Med* 1991;32:610–615.

56. McKusick KA. The diagnosis of traumatic cerebrospinal fluid rhinorrhea. *J Nucl Med* 1977;18:1234–1235.

57. Benamor M, Tainturier C, Graveleau P, Pierot L. Radionuclide cisternography in spontaneous intracranial hypotension. *Clin Nucl Med* 1998;23:150–151.

58. Mazziotta JC, Phelps ME, Pahl J, et al. Reduced cerebral glucose metabolism in asymptomatic subjects at risk for Huntington's disease. *N Engl J Med* 1987; 316:357–362.

59. Feigin A, Leenders KL, Moeller JR, et al. Metabolic network abnormalities in early Huntington's disease: an [(18)F]FDG PET study. *J Nucl Med* 2001;42(11):1591–1595.

60. Kubota R, Yamada S, Kubota K, et al. Intratumoral distribution of fluorine-18-fluorodeoxyglucose *in vivo*: high accumulation in macrophages and granulocytes studied by microautoradiography. *J Nucl Med* 1992;33:1972–1980.

61. Lawrence SK, Kessler RM. Hypermetabolic cerebral fungal infections with PET FDG studies. *J Nucl Med* 1993;34:38P.

CHAPTER FIVE

GASTROINTESTINAL AND CORRELATIVE ABDOMINAL NUCLEAR MEDICINE IMAGING

M. Reza Habibian
and Chirayu Shah

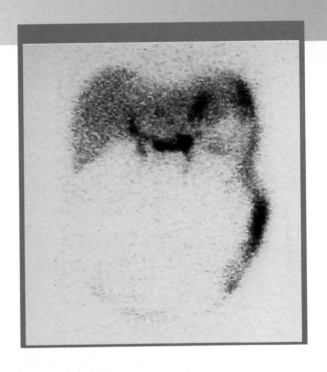

Diverse radionuclide imaging procedures are available for studying the morphology and function of the gastrointestinal (GI) tract.

Although the details of anatomic alterations are demonstrable more reliably by conventional radiographic techniques, such as computed tomography (CT), ultrasound (US), and magnetic resonance imaging (MRI), radionuclide scintigraphy remains a unique noninvasive modality with quantitative capability for the evaluation of equally important functional disorders of the GI tract.

The recent development, acceptance, and integration of functional and structural images has resulted in redefining the role of scintigraphy in diagnosis of the various disorders of liver, GI tract, and abdominal organs.

Scintigraphic approaches using various radiopharmaceuticals can provide important complementary and supplementary information to CT, US, and MRI for further categorization of liver and other abdominal mass lesions, particularly in difficult clinical situations.

The technical aspects of nuclear medicine GI procedures are well described in standard textbooks; however, several of the currently available and clinically used procedures are reviewed briefly, as follows:

Gastric emptying scintigraphy
Gastrointestinal bleeding scintigraphy
Abdominal scintigraphy for bleeding of Meckel's diverticulum
Hepatobiliary scintigraphy
Liver–spleen scintigraphy
Hepatic artery perfusion scintigraphy
Peritoneal venous shunt scintigraphy
Correlative abdominal nuclear medicine imaging
    Hepatic hemangioma
    Focal nodular hyperplasia
    Hepatic adenoma
    Focal fatty metamorphoses
    Hepatoma
    OncoScint immunoscintigraphy
    Octreotide scintigraphy
    MIBG imaging
    Abdominal PET imaging
Scintigraphic detection of abdominal abscesses and inflammatory process
Salivary gland scintigraphy

GASTRIC EMPTYING SCINTIGRAPHY

Gastric emptying scintigraphy is a well-established procedure for the assessment of gastric motility disorder, sometimes called functional obstruction of the stomach.

"Functional obstruction" refers to an abnormality of gastric motility associated with the stomach's inability to grind solid food into the small particle size necessary for emptying or the stomach's inadequate contractility to generate enough GI pressure gradient to propel the gastric contents across the pylorus into the duodenum.

The grinding process occurs in the stomach's antrum, which acts as a grinder to triturate the ingested food through rhythmic contraction at the rate of 30 cycles per minute.

The emptying pattern for solid food is biphasic, initiated by lag phase and followed by continuous emptying, usually in a linear fashion. The lag phase is the time required for the antrum to grind food.

The conventional protocol for gastric emptying scintigraphy involves measuring the rate of transit of radiolabeled liquid or solid food (commonly 300 to 500 μCi of ^{99m}Tc sulfur colloid in scrambled eggs in a volume of approximately 125 mL) through the stomach.

Using a modern dual-head camera system, a series of 1-minute dynamic images is obtained in the anterior and posterior projections for at least 90 minutes (the use of infrequent static images rather than continuous dynamic images is discouraged).

The entire 90-minute gastric emptying data can be displayed as a time–activity curve using geometric mean counts from the anterior and posterior projections. The geometric mean is the square root of the product of anterior and posterior projection counts. The curve is corrected for decay; otherwise gastric emptying would be overestimated.

Several quantitative data can be approximated from the time–activity curve:

1. The time it takes for half of the meal to leave the stomach, or the half-time ($T_{1/2}$). Using the published data, the $T_{1/2}$ of 60 ± 30 minutes for solid food and 30 ± 15 for the liquid phase is considered to be within normal limits. It should be noted that the normal value for the $T_{1/2}$ varies depending on the content of the meal, the patient's position, the protocol used, and the method by which the $T_{1/2}$ is calculated. Also, it should be noted that although the $T_{1/2}$ for emptying is often used clinically, the emptying process is not exponential; instead, it is continuous and linear. Therefore, in a physiologic sense, the use of "$T_{1/2}$" may not be correct.
2. The percent of gastric emptying at 90 minutes [(maximum count − minimum counts)/(maximum counts × 100)], which takes into consideration the physiologic parameters of both the lag phase and the rate of linear emptying. A value of <35% is considered abnormal.
3. The length of the lag phase is approximated by visual inspection of the image as the time before the appearance of radiolabeled meals in the proximal small bowel or time when linear emptying is established on the time–activity curve. The duration of the lag phase may vary; however, a delay of more than 45 minutes is considered abnormal and indicates a grinding-phase abnormality.
4. The percent of the radiolabeled meal remaining in the stomach at 90 minutes. Retention of greater than 50% represents a delay in gastric emptying.

GASTROINTESTINAL BLEEDING

Scintigraphy of the abdominal blood pool following IV administration of a patient's red blood cells (RBCs) tagged with technetium-99m (^{99m}Tc)-pertechnetate is a well-established diagnostic procedure that is complementary to endoscopy and angiography for the detection of GI bleeding.

The procedure is well tolerated and easy to perform. The images provide a high sensitivity for the detection of a low bleeding rate and allow continuous monitoring of the GI tract for several hours. The detection and localization of bleeding sites has been improved significantly by the adoption of the cine scintigraphic technique and use of the improved *in vitro* labeling procedure, which results in greater than 98% labeling efficiency.

Bleeding at the rate of 0.40 mL/min is easily detected as a focus of intense activity outside the vascular blood pool. Although contrast angiography provides exquisite anatomic detail, bleeding at a rate greater than 1 mL/min must be present at the time of contrast injection; therefore scintigraphy may be useful in many circumstances, particularly in view of the inherently intermittent nature of GI bleeding.

ABDOMINAL SCINTIGRAPHY FOR BLEEDING OF MECKEL'S DIVERTICULUM

Abdominal scintigraphy with ^{99m}Tc-pertechnetate is the technique of choice for detecting ectopic gastric mucosa as the cause of GI bleeding. The most common site of ectopic mucosa is in a Meckel's diverticulum.

^{99m}Tc-pertechnetate is taken up predominantly by the mucin-producing cells of the gastric mucosa, which allows for visualization not only of gastric but also heterotopic gastric mucosa.

Visualization of Meckel's diverticulum usually occurs as a focus of intense activity in the right lower quadrant, approximately 20 minutes after the injection of ^{99m}Tc-pertechnetate, in concert with gastric visualization with same intensity of uptake.

Although the detection of a Meckel's diverticulum by ^{99m}Tc-pertechnetate depends on the presence of gastric mucosa, occurring in approximately 30% of cases, GI bleeding from a Meckel's diverticulum also requires the presence of gastric mucosa.

HEPATOBILIARY SCINTIGRAPHY

Hepatobiliary scintigraphy or cholescintigraphy, with or without pharmacologic intervention using cholecystokinin (CCK) and morphine, is used primarily for the assessment of diseases affecting the gallbladder, cystic duct, common bile duct, and sphincter of Oddi.

Diagnosis of acute cholecystitis by far is the most common clinical indication for cholescintigraphy.

A dose of 2 to 6 mCi of ^{99m}Tc-iminodiacetic acid (IDA) derivative is injected IV and serial images of the abdomen are obtained for 1 hour at 10-minute intervals.

Normal examination exhibits homogeneous liver uptake with uniform washout, resulting in visualization of the gallbladder and bowel within 30 to 60 minutes.

A gallbladder not seen by 60 minutes and not visualized by 20 to 30 minutes after IV injection of 0.05 mg/kg morphine strongly suggests acute cholecystitis.

Postcholecystectomy complications such as bile leak, cystic duct remnant, biliary ductal strictures, and stenosis are among other clinical indications for cholescintigraphy. Hepatobiliary images can be used to differentiate biliary atresia from neonatal hepatitis. Hepatobiliary images are also of value in the evaluation of complications associated with liver transplantation.

As a noninvasive procedure, cholescintigraphy is used for the evaluation of functional hepatobiliary disorder. Chronic acalculous gallbladder and biliary disease as a functional abnormality is diagnosed by the lack of response to CCK as measured by gallbladder ejection fraction in an otherwise normally visualized gallbladder and no abnormality on ultrasound.

The gallbladder ejection fraction is determined by IV infusion of 0.02 μg/kg CCK over a period of 30 minutes. Although a gallbladder normally ejects more than 80% of its contents in response to CCK, an ejection fraction that does not exceed 35% at 20 to 30 minutes postintervention is considered abnormal and represents biliary tract dyskinesis.

It is worth remembering that opioids reduce the gallbladder ejection fraction. Exclusion of opium intake is therefore important in order to avoid a false-positive study.

LIVER–SPLEEN SCINTIGRAPHY

Liver–spleen scan using ^{99m}Tc sulfur colloid is a simple procedure that is useful in detecting space-occupying lesions and evaluating diffuse liver disease.

Following the intravenous injection of ^{99m}Tc–sulfur colloid, the colloid particles are phagocytized by reticuloendothelial cells normally distributed in the liver (Kupffer cells, 85%), spleen (10%), and bone marrow (5%). The usual dose is 2 to 6 mCi.

A normal scan shows homogeneous distribution of radioactivity within a normal-sized liver and spleen with normal contour. The liver has relatively more uptake than the spleen.

Performance of a dynamic study as part of the liver–spleen scan procedure may provide additional information of great value for further definition of liver lesions and may reveal other intra-abdominal abnormalities, such as aortic aneurysm, cystic lesions, collateral circulation, and superior vena cava obstruction. Although the liver blood flow study cannot separate a benign from a malignant liver lesion detected on static images, it can help in identifying the vascular nature of the focal defect.

Space-occupying lesions in the liver or spleen are indicated as areas of reduced or absent radioactivity on the ^{99m}Tc–sulfur colloid scan. Space-occupying lesions in the liver may be single, multiple, or even diffuse in distribution. The etiologic origins vary from congenital (cyst), infectious (abscess), trauma (laceration, radiation), degenerative (cirrhosis), benign neoplasm (adenoma, cavernous hemangioma), and malignant neoplasms (primary hepatoma or secondary metastasis).

Contrast-enhanced CT is superior to scintigraphy for the detection of metastatic liver disease with perhaps the exception of endocrine, colon, and ovarian metastasis.

HEPATIC ARTERY PERFUSION SCINTIGRAPHY

Intra-arterial infusion of chemotherapeutic agents through a catheter placed in the hepatic artery for treatment of hepatic tumor may be more effective than systemic IV chemotherapy because a higher dose of agent can be delivered directly to the tumor with a low incidence of systemic toxicity. A misplaced arterial catheter or a catheter tip displaced from the hepatic artery is not an uncommon occurrence and may be seen in 15% to 40% of cases. Infusion of the chemotherapeutic agent through such a catheter results in visceral misperfusion, with the potential for serious clinical toxicity due to inadvertent perfusion of other organs with a high dose of chemotherapy.

Hepatic arterial perfusion scintigraphy with ^{99m}Tc–macroaggregated albumin (MAA) is used to predict the distribution of a subsequently administered chemotherapeutic agent within the liver.

A dose of 1 to 2 mCi of ^{99m}Tc-MAA in a volume of 0.2 to 0.5 mL is injected at a slow rate into the catheter. The distribution of MAA particles reflects hepatic artery blood flow to the tumor and liver. Also, any area of undesired extrahepatic perfusion—such as stomach, pancreas, or bowel—may be detected, necessitating readjustment of catheter placement.

Hepatic artery perfusion scintigraphy may also be used to detect liver metastases in areas of the liver that appear normal by CT. Liver metastases, even avascular ones, are perfused from the hepatic artery; therefore a metastasis may appear as focally increased uptake. A focal defect seen by ^{99m}Tc–sulfur colloid imaging that shows hyperperfusion by hepatic artery perfusion scan is considered to be indicative of a metastatic lesion.

PERITONEAL VENOUS (LAVEEN) SHUNT SCINTIGRAPHY

Insertion of a LaVeen shunt has been shown to be useful in controlling the accumulation of ascites in patients with cirrhosis. The shunt operates by a one-way pressure-activated valve, which helps to reduce ascites by recirculating the ascitic fluid. However, it has a high incidence of spontaneous blockage.

The patency of a peritoneal venous shunt can be studied by injecting 3 to 5 mCi of ^{99m}Tc–MAA directly into the fluid accumulated in the abdominal cavity. The appearance of radioactivity in the lung field represents trapping of MAA particles in the precapillary bed of the lung, indicating shunt patency. Lack of lung activity would be conclusive for a nonfunctional (obstructed) shunt.

CORRELATIVE ABDOMINAL NUCLEAR MEDICINE IMAGING SCINTIGRAPHY

Hepatic Hemangioma

Cavernous hemangioma is the most common benign tumor of the liver and is found about 20% of the time in autopsy series.

Histologically, the mass consists of vascular channels enclosed within the fibroelastic stroma.

^{99m}Tc–tagged RBC hepatic blood pool imaging is extremely useful in the identification of hepatic hemangioma.

The classic finding of hepatic hemangioma is represented by decreased perfusion and increased blood pool (perfusion–blood pool mismatch) activity in suspected areas of the liver.

A flow study is performed following IV injection of the patient's RBCs labeled *in vitro* with ^{99m}Tc-pertechnetate. This is followed by serial planar images looking for a hypoperfused area that progressively accumulates RBCs. The specificity of ^{99m}Tc–tagged RBC scintigraphy for the diagnosis of cavernous hemangioma is extremely high (approximately 100%), but its sensitivity is high only when the lesion is larger than 2.5 to 3.0 cm. Using single photon emission computed tomography (SPECT), the sensitivity remains high for lesions smaller than 2 cm in diameter. SPECT is superior for detecting hemangiomas that are small, multiple, or adjacent to large vessels, heart, spleen, or the renal blood pool.

Focal Nodular Hyperplasia (FNH)

FNH is a benign hepatic mass and is usually an incidental finding. It is the second most common benign mass after hemangioma and occurs in approximately 3% of the population. Histologically the mass is a hypertrophic nodule consisting of Kupffer cells, hepatocytes, and disorganized bile ducts.

Although practically any space-occupying lesion within the liver appears as a cold area on ^{99m}Tc–sulfur colloid scan, a focal nodular hyperplasia, due to the hyperplastic nature of the mass containing all the liver elements, may appear hotter than the surrounding liver tissue. However, in many cases (~70%), the FNH shows uptake equal to that of the liver. On hepatobiliary imaging, the FNH containing hepatocytes and biliary canaliculi takes up the agent and appears as a normal scan or as an area of focal increased uptake.

FNH can have a higher uptake of fluorine-18 (^{18}F)-FDG than the surrounding liver tissue; as such, it may be mistaken for a hypermetabolic focus of metastasis, particularly in patients with a known primary cancer. However, this is a very rare occurrence; as a rule, FNH is not an FDG-avid lesion.

Hepatic Adenoma

Hepatic adenoma typically occurs in women using oral contraceptives or hormone therapy; it is usually asymptomatic. However, it may rupture or bleed, causing right-upper-quadrant pain. Rarely, rupture may lead to hemorrhagic shock. On histologic examination, hepatic adenoma appears to be composed of monoclonal hepatocytes devoid of bile duct and Kupffer cells.

Hepatic adenoma usually appears photopenic on ^{99m}Tc–sulfur colloid scan. However, it may be isodense, but never hotter than the liver. Hepatic adenoma, having no biliary radicals, also appears photopenic on IDA hepatobiliary images.

Focal Fatty Metamorphosis

Focal fatty metamorphosis (FFM) of the liver is a reversible disorder that may be seen in obese patients, diabetics, users of steroids, or alcoholics. FFM may be detected as a vague focal mass on ultrasound or CT. Differentiation from hepatoma or metastatic lesions may be difficult by anatomic studies. Focal fatty metamorphosis in the liver contains Kupffer cells in the perisinoidal space; therefore any area that appears as a focal mass on CT or ultrasound but appears normal or as an area of slightly nonuniform uptake of ^{99m}Tc–sulfur colloid most likely represents a minimally infiltrated fatty liver and not malignancy. However, biopsy may be needed if the diagnosis is still in doubt.

Hepatoma

Hepatocellular carcinoma is usually diagnosed by anatomic study, and there is no need for the functional images. However, gallium-67 (^{67}Ga)-SPECT imaging may be used in the evaluation of an indeterminate liver mass suspected for hepatoma, particularly in a patient with an elevated alpha-fetoprotein level. Typically, a hepatoma concentrates ^{67}Ga and can be detected with a sensitivity of 70% to 90%. However, uptake is not specific, as other lesions—such as lymphoma, metastatic melanoma, infection, and even macroregenerating nodule of cirrhosis—may take up ^{67}Ga.

OncoScint Immunoscintigraphy

OncoScint, a radiolabeled monoclonal antibody, may outperform contrast-enhanced CT in the detection of colon and ovarian cancer metastasized outside the liver (node). The positive predictive value for detection of colon and ovarian cancer is high (83% and 90%, respectively); however, a negative scan does not exclude malignancy.

Available OncoScint is an indium-111 (^{111}In) radiolabeled monoclonal antibody directed against the antigen found in ovarian and colon cancer. A patient with elevated carcinoembryonic antigen (CEA) and a previous history of ovarian or colorectal cancer is a candidate for OncoScint scintigraphy.

The usual dose is 1 mg of antibody labeled with 5 mCi ^{111}In for intravenous administration. A whole-body scintigram is usually acquired at 48 to 72 hours. Interpretation of an OncoScint scan requires close correlation with CT or MRI images.

Normal distribution of OncoScint includes liver, spleen, bone marrow, blood pool, and genitalia. Nonspecific uptake may be seen in the kidneys, bladder, breasts, nipples, and bowel. Further discussion of immunoscintigraphy may be found in Chapter 8.

Octreotide Scintigraphy

Octreotide, a small peptide of eight amino acids, is an analog of the endogenously secreted neuropeptide hormone somatostatin.

Somatostatin is found in various tumors and nontumoral tissue, with the highest concentration in the central nervous system, endocrine pancreas, and GI tract.

^{111}In-labeled octreotide (Octreoscan) can be used to visualize any tumor bearing the somatostatin receptors. The list includes pituitary tumor, endocrine pancreatic tumor (gastrinoma, insulinoma, and glucagonoma), carcinoid, paraganglioma, medullary thyroid carcinoma, and Merkel cell carcinoma of the skin. Other disorders—such as pheochromocytoma, neuroblastoma, small cell lung cancer, breast cancer,

malignant lymphoma, even granulomatous disease and Graves' disease—may be visualized by Octreoscan. Nevertheless, Octreoscan is most effective in the detection and evaluation of carcinoid, islet cell tumor of the pancreas, and abdominal metastatic disease from small cell carcinoma of the lung.

The administered dose of ^{111}In-octreotide is 6 mCi. Whole-body scan is acquired at 4 and 24 hours with optional 24-hour SPECT images. Whole-body scanning is especially useful for the detection of metastases or multiple tumors that may be seen in patients with paraganglioma or multiple endocrine neoplasms.

The normal distribution of Octreoscan includes liver, spleen, kidneys, and bladder. Images provide specific functional information; however, scintigram images complement rather than compete with anatomic studies such as CT or MRI.

The result of an Octreoscan can be used to select patients with neuroendocrine tumors who may benefit from Octreotide treatment.

MIBG (Meta-Iodo-Benzyl-Guanidine) Imaging

Radiolabeled MIBG has been used successfully for visualizing benign and malignant pheochromocytoma, adrenal medullary hyperplasia, and other tumors such as carcinoid, neuroblastoma, and paravertebral paraganglioma.

MIBG performs better than octreotide for differentiating pheochromocytoma and abdominal metastases from medullary thyroid carcinoma.

MIBG is a small molecule that is an analog of guanethidine. It resembles norepinephrine structurally and is taken up by adrenergic tissue. Many medications interfere with MIBG uptake, including tricyclic antidepressants, over-the-counter cold medications (containing phenylephrine, pseudoephedrine, and ephedrine), certain antipsychotics, and cocaine among others. The tumor uptake is not inhibited by adrenergic blocking agents other than labetalol.

Normal distribution of MIBG following IV injection includes the salivary gland, liver, spleen, and urinary bladder. Organs that are visualized less frequently and less intensely include myocardium, kidneys, and normal adrenal glands. Thyroid is not typically visualized as it is blocked by necessary pretreatment with saturated solution of potassium iodine (SSKI).

MIBG image is generally obtained at 48 to 72 hours following IV injection of 1 mCi of iodine-131 (^{131}I)-MIBG or at 24 hours after injection of 10 mCi ^{123}I-MIBG. ^{131}I-MIBG has also been employed as a therapeutic agent for some endocrine tumors. MIBG imaging is reviewed in more detail, along with case presentations, in Chapters 1 and 8.

Abdominal PET Imaging

Oncologic positron emission tomography (PET) imaging and combined PET-CT imaging are the most recent advancements in nuclear medicine. PET imaging typically is a survey covering the neck through the pelvis. When it is combined with CT, the preselected regional anatomy becomes the focus of evaluation.

In oncologic PET imaging, ^{18}F-labeled flurodeoxyglucose (^{18}F-FDG) is the most commonly used radiopharmaceutical at present. The rationale behind the use of ^{18}F-FDG for the imaging of malignant tissue is based on the observation that malignant cells have an elevated rate of glycolytic activity; therefore they exhibit an increased uptake of glucose relative to the normal surrounding cells.

^{18}F-FDG has a half-life of 110 minutes. The usual dose is approximately 10 mCi, which is injected intravenously 1 hour prior to scanning.

Evaluation of the abdomen on PET CT requires a thorough familiarity with the normal distribution of ^{18}F-FDG. Physiologic uptake is seen in the kidneys, urinary collecting system, bowel, and stomach wall. Colonic activity, particularly in the cecum and rectosigmoid, may be intense. Liver uptake is moderate, and the spleen has less uptake than the liver. Skeletal muscles may also demonstrate intense uptake if they were being used during the uptake. Physiologic brown fat uptake may also be seen in paraspinal and perirenal regions. Physiologic ovarian uptake in premenopausal women should not be confused with malignancy.

^{18}F-FDG PET has been used successfully in the assessment of colorectal cancer, metastatic disease of the liver, and evaluation of ovarian cancer (see Chapter 8).

SCINTIGRAPHIC DETECTION OF ABDOMINAL ABSCESSES

Abdominal abscesses may be detected by abdominal scintigraphy using WBCs labeled with indium-111 (^{111}In-WBC), ^{99m}Tc-hexamethylpropyleneamine oxime (HMPAO), or a monoclonal antigranulocyte antibody labeled with ^{99m}Tc-pertechnetate. Utilization of ^{67}Ga-citrate is limited in the evaluation of abdominal abscesses owing to its normal excretory bowel pathway, which may obscure an infected area within the abdominal cavity.

The scintigraphic technique can be supplementary or complementary to CT or ultrasound. Differentiating infected from noninfected abdominal fluid collections is not possible using anatomically oriented modalities, but WBC scintigraphy would be expected to be positive only in the infected sites.

The ^{111}In-WBC scan images are usually obtained 24 hours after reinjection of the patient's WBCs labeled with approximately 500 to 700 μCi of ^{111}In-oxime. For evaluation of inflammatory bowel disease, an early image at 1 and 4 hours is necessary. Whole-body images are important, particularly when localizing signs of abdominal abscess are not present. The scan may show the source of infection to be outside the abdomen. Even when abdominal abscess is present, whole-body scintigraphy may reveal extra-abdominal foci.

A normal scan demonstrates distribution of radioactivity in the liver, spleen, and bone marrow (reticuloendothelial system). Activity outside of these compartments is abnormal or requires a physiologic or technical explanation. A sensitivity of 85% to 95% for the detection of infection and inflam-

matory processes has been reported for ^{111}In-labeled–WBC scintigraphy. Controversy exists as to the effects of antibiotic therapy and chronicity of infection on the sensitivity of this technique.

HMPAO is a lipophilic complex that can penetrate the membranes of WBCs and permit labeling with ^{99m}Tc. The distribution of HMPAO-labeled WBCs is similar to that of ^{111}In-labeled WBCs except that there is significant excretion of activity into the GI and genitourinary tracts.

In imaging with ^{99m}Tc-HMPAO labeling, bowel activity does not appear until 2 hours after the reinjection of labeled WBCs; therefore whole-body scanning should be performed at 1 hour and followed by another set of images at 4 hours.

^{99m}Tc-HMPAO-labeled–WBC images are useful, particularly in the diagnosis of inflammatory bowel disease. Activity rapidly localizes in the involved bowel within 1 hour and provides good-quality images. Segmental involvement of the bowel, skipped areas, and small bowel versus large bowel involvement may easily be demonstrated, often allowing differentiation of Crohn's disease from ulcerative colitis, and can accurately determine the extent of the disease.

Monoclonal antigranulocyte antibody–labeled ^{99m}Tc-pertechnetate (NeutroSpec) has been used for the early diagnosis of appendicitis. In this procedure, 15 mCi of radiopharmaceutical is injected intravenously, which binds to the surface antigen of granulocytes. Activity is distributed in the blood pool, reticuloendothelial system, and urinary excretory organs. The scan done at 2 hours shows liver, spleen, kidney, and bone marrow activity. A positive scan is usually seen within 30 to 60 minutes. It should be noted that Netruspect is currently not available, as its use was suspended by the FDA because of safety concerns.

SALIVARY GLAND SCINTIGRAPHY

Radionuclide scanning with ^{99m}Tc-pertechnetate is a simple, noninvasive method for the evaluation of salivary gland function.

The parotid gland is imaged following IV injection of 10 to 15 mCi of ^{99m}Tc-pertechnetate. Serial images are obtained in the anterior and both lateral projections within the first 20 minutes. The scan is followed by a washout image after oral stimulation with lemon juice.

The scan is evaluated for symmetrical gland accumulation, drainage, and areas of increased or decreased uptake that may suggest neoplasm, inflammation, or avascular lesions.

A washout image is very important in the detection of Warthin's tumor, which does not communicate with the ductal system and therefore cannot excrete its accumulated activity even after lemon juice, resulting in a focus of persistently increased activity.

CASE 5.1

History: A 71-year-old man with anorexia, early satiety, and a history of poorly controlled diabetes is referred for a gastric emptying study in order to evaluate the possibility of gastric outlet obstruction or diabetic gastroparesis.

A solid food gastric emptying study was performed following the ingestion of a sample food of scrambled eggs containing 400 μCi of ^{99m}Tc–sulfur colloid (Fig. 5.1).

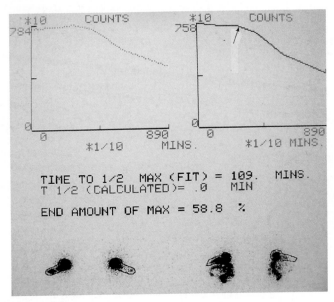

Figure 5.1

Findings: Figure 5.1 displays the gastric emptying curve over a period of 90 minutes generated from geometric mean counts obtained from the anterior and posterior images outlining the stomach as an area of interest.

There is delayed gastric emptying with prolongation of the gastric emptying $T_{1/2}$ exceeding 90 minutes, with 58.8% of radiolabeled meal remaining in the stomach at 90 minutes. There is an apparent 45-minute lag phase before the curve assumes a linear emptying pattern (arrow).

Discussion: Gastric emptying of solid foods, as depicted in Figure 5.1, is a biphasic pattern that initiates with a lag phase and is followed by a continuous linear pattern of emptying.

Delay in gastric emptying may be due to gastric outlet obstruction—commonly seen in patients with chronic duodenal ulcer, carcinoma of the stomach, gastric polyps, and hypertrophic pyloric stenosis—which may be associated with narrowing of the gastric lumen. These disorders should be studied and excluded by contrast radiographic examination or upper GI endoscopy.

Delay in gastric emptying may be functional, and etiologies vary from diabetes, vagotomy, collagen vascular disease, hypothyroidism, celiac disease, progressive systemic sclerosis, brain tumor, electrolyte abnormalities, and effect of medications. Delayed gastric emptying of functional origin, as measured by radionuclide gastric emptying and depicted on the time–activity curve, usually reflects the combination of prolongation of both the lag phase and continuous linear emptying process. However, delayed gastric emptying may be solely due to a prolonged lag phase, as seen in certain diseases such as diabetic gastroenteropathy and morbid obesity.

Prolongation of the lag phase reflects the functional abnormality of the gastric antrum and represents the stomach's inability to grind food in a normal timely fashion. Drugs such as erythromycin improve the gastric emptying rate by shortening the lag phase.

Quantification of the gastric emptying rate and the lag phase are of particular clinical importance in follow-up and evaluation of the effectiveness of treatment. Response to treatment can be judged based on the quantitative results of the gastric emptying study.

In evaluating the gastric emptying curve, it is not unusual to observe an initial transient increase in the count rate. This is due to a reduction in the self-absorption of radiation in food. As the grinding process continues, food triturates into small particles of reduced thickness; therefore there will be fewer barriers to self-absorption and attenuation of gamma rays, resulting in more photons reaching the detector and causing the observed transient increase in count rate.

Accelerated gastric emptying may also be encountered. Duodenal ulcer, Zollinger-Ellison syndrome, hyperthyroidism, postvagotomy dumping syndrome, and medications such as erythromycin have been noted to be associated with accelerated gastric emptying.

Diagnosis: Delayed gastric emptying consistent with diabetic gastroparesis.

CASE 5.2

History: This patient is an 84-year-old man who underwent cystectomy and ileal conduit for bladder cancer 2 weeks earlier. His history is pertinent for partial colectomy 2 years previously for colon cancer. He is now referred for a ^{99m}Tc–tagged RBC abdominal scintigram for the detection of a bleeding site in the setting of painless passage of bloody stool over the preceding 5 days.

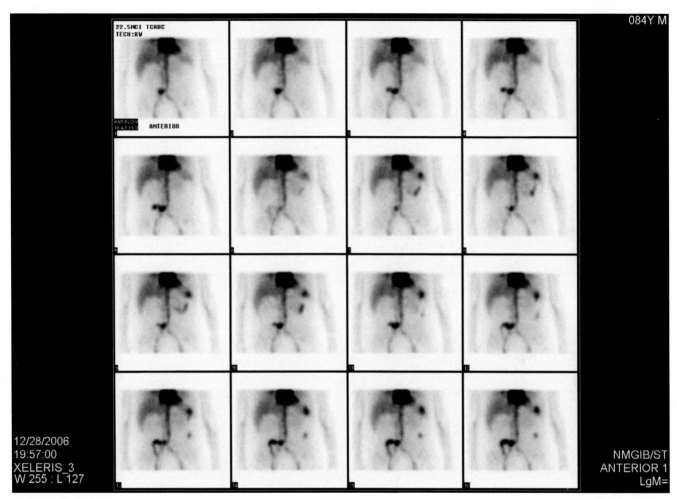

Figure 5.2 A

Findings: Images from the ^{99m}Tc–tagged RBC abdominal scintigram (Fig. 5.2 A) show a focus of radioactivity in the right lower quadrant with rapid changes in configuration and migration to the left upper quadrant. This finding is most consistent with GI bleed originating in the terminal ileum.

Discussion: The patient's bleeding site was confirmed angiographically (Fig. 5.2 B) as a focus of active extravasation from the distal branches of the SMA. He was subsequently taken to the operating room and found to have bled from the anastomotic site that had been repaired.

The detection of a focus of radiolabeled RBCs outside the normal area of expected vascular blood pool which moves within the bowel in either the antegrade or retrograde direction are the two important criteria for the diagnosis of GI bleeding.

Although RBC scintigraphy is a sensitive technique for the detection of a GI bleed, localization of the bleeding site is as important as detection. There are inconsistent reports in the literature as to the accuracy of scintigraphy for detecting and localizing a bleeding site. Variables to be considered for these inconsistencies are the rate of bleeding (massive versus minimal), pattern of bleeding (active versus intermittent), location (large bowel versus small bowel), length of study (60 minutes versus imaging over a longer time period), labeling procedures (*in vitro* versus *in vivo*), and the imaging technique (static images versus rapid dynamic imaging with movie display mode).

The current state-of-the-art in RBC scintigraphy is to use the high labeling efficiency (98%) of the *in vitro* technique and acquisition of the images in a rapid cine scintigraphic mode. The combination of these two techniques provides an overall

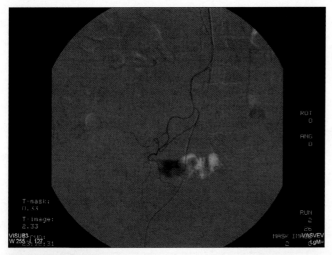

Figure 5.2 B

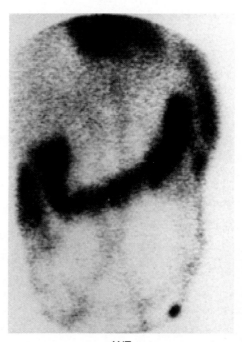

ANT
21-HR DELAY

Figure 5.2 C

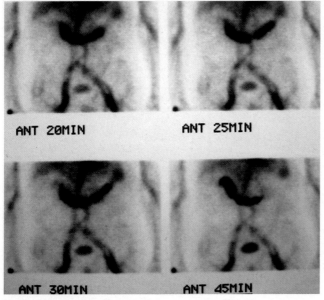

Figure 5.2 D

improvement in the quality of the blood pool image and the test's accuracy.

An abdominal scintigram obtained with ^{99m}Tc-tagged RBCs enables the detection of a bleeding of a rate as low as 0.1 to 0.4 mL/min; with angiography, the bleeding rate must be at least 0.5 mL/min to be detectable. However, clinical studies indicate that, in the majority of patients, the bleeding can be detected angiographically when the rate is greater than 1 mL/min.

More than 80% of the patients with active bleeding have a positive scan within the first 90 minutes of the study. If the initial image is negative, the patient can be reimaged at an interval up to 24 hours. Some patients who are not actively bleeding during the time of early imaging may bleed several hours later, resulting in a positive delayed scan. Up to 60% of patients with a negative RBC scan of 90 minutes will have a positive scan on delayed images at 4 to 24 hours. A delayed positive scan is commonly due to migration of blood through the small bowel

and accumulation in the colon. Intense colonic activity on the delayed image where the early image is normal should be considered evidence of proximal GI hemorrhage and should not be mistaken for large bowel bleeding. This error in localization occurs because extravasated blood originating from the stomach, duodenum, ileum, or jejunum migrates rapidly to the colon and may pool there. Blood in the bowel is an irritant and has a cathartic effect that causes rapid movement of blood both antegrade and retrograde.

Figure 5.2 C represents a delayed 21-hour image of an abdominal blood pool scintigram in a patient with intermittent bleeding. Intense colonic activity is due to pooling of the blood originating from the patient's jejunal arteriovenous malformation detected angiographically. Lack of radioactivity in the stomach and renal collecting system helps to exclude unbound ^{99m}Tc (free technetium) as the cause of colonic activity.

Overall, detection and localization of bleeding in the large bowel is easier than in the small bowel. The well-known anatomic location of the cecum, flexures, and transverse colon facilitates the localization of bleeding, making it more identifiable than bleeding within the highly peristaltic and moving small bowel. On Figure 5.2 D, the GI bleed within the transverse colon is easily recognizable, with the blood moving in both directions.

Selection of patients for noninvasive RBC scintigraphy versus other invasive diagnostic procedures for providing the most favorable outcome is based on the clinical presentation. Upper GI endoscopy is usually used with an accuracy of about 90% for the diagnosis of upper GI bleeding commonly caused by gastric ulcer, duodenal ulcer, gastric erosion, and varices.

Colonoscopy and sigmoidoscopy may disclose the source of lower GI bleeding commonly caused by neoplasm, polyps, diverticula, and angiodysplasia in 60% to 77% of cases. However, owing to the intermediate nature of GI bleeding, endoscopy and angiography may fail to identify the sources of bleeding. Colonic examination may be very difficult when active, perfuse bleeding is present.

^{99m}Tc–tagged RBC scintigraphy can play a major role in triaging and screening the patient for GI bleed. Patients who are actively bleeding and are bleeding intermittently are good candidates for scintigraphic evaluation.

A positive scan can not only make the diagnosis but also identify patients who would benefit from angiography. When the scan is not positive, it is unlikely that angiography will demonstrate a bleeding site. In addition, a positive scan can be helpful in directing the angiographic approach to a specified vascular territory.

A scan can also be used to predict the need for surgery versus medical therapy. Patients who show extensive extravasation of labeled RBCs in the first hours of the study, with the intensity of the extravasated blood pooling being greater than pooling in the liver, usually find their way to the operating room.

Diagnosis: Active small bowel bleeding from the postsurgical anastomotic site in the terminal ileum.

CASE 5.3

History: This 80-year-old male with multiple medical problems—including coronary artery disease, COPD, obstructive uropathy, and bilateral above-knee amputation—presents with GI bleeding requiring eight units of packed RBCs over the previous 24 hours. He was referred for a ^{99m}Tc-tagged RBC abdominal scintigram for detection of the bleeding site.

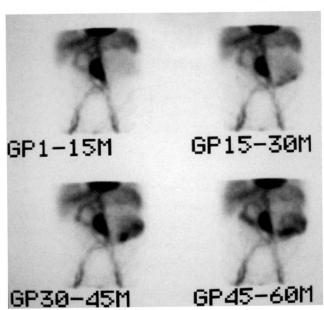

Figure 5.3 A

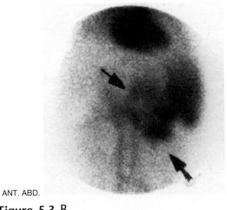

ANT. ABD.

Figure 5.3 B

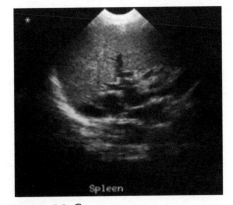

Figure 5.3 C

Findings: Sequential dynamic images of the abdomen over a period of 60 minutes (Fig. 5.3 A) show abnormal distribution of the labeled RBCs in the epigastrium outlining the duodenal loop (GP 1 -15 M), seen repeatedly throughout the hours of examination with some changes in configuration and intensity. On the second group of images (GP 15-30 M), another collection of labeled RBCs appears in the left lower quadrant, which persists throughout the sequence with some changes in intensity and configuration. A large area of stable and nonmobile activity is also present in the midabdomen.

Discussion: Diagnosis of GI bleed in duodenum and sigmoid colon was made based on the observation of activity outside the normally expected vascular blood pool with changes in shape, location, and intensity, even though minimal. The patient was subsequently taken to the operating room, and bleeding from a duodenal ulcer as well as sigmoid colon diverticula was noted.

Application of the rapid sequence cine scintigraphic technique in this case facilitated not only the early detection of bleeding in the duodenum but also bleeding from another site in the sigmoid colon. Otherwise, the sigmoid bleeding might

have been mistaken for the phenomenon of rapid movement of blood originating from the duodenum and pooling in the sigmoid.

In RBC abdominal scintigraphy, a variety of abnormalities may be detected incidentally. The large fusiform area of intense but stable activity in the midabdomen seen in Figure 5.3. A represents a large abdominal aortic aneurysm. The activity there is stable and does not change in location, configuration, or intensity and does not represent bleeding.

Figure 5.3 B represents a selected image of an abdominal blood pool in a 47-year-old patient with hepatic cirrhosis who presents with hemoptysis and guaiac-positive stool. The image is notable for markedly reduced hepatic blood pool activity consistent with this patient's known hepatic cirrhosis and associated reduced portal blood flow. There is a region of increased activity (arrow) within the midabdomen medial to an enlarged spleen. This activity, which did not migrate or change in configuration or intensity on subsequent serial images, does not fulfill the criteria for acute GI bleeding. Further evaluation of this area by ultrasound (Fig. 5.3 C) reveals multiple dilated mesenteric veins secondary to portal hypertension; pooling

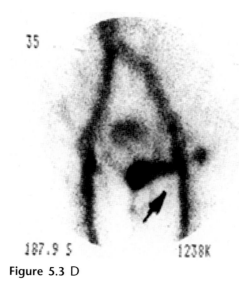 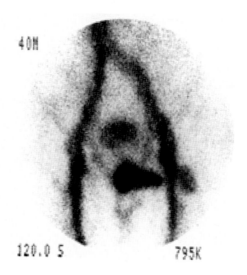

Figure 5.3 D

of tagged RBCs within these varicose veins accounts for the scintigraphic abnormality.

On an abdominal blood pool scintigram, in addition to the well-known lesion of the hepatic cavernous hemangioma, increased activity may be identified in an accessory spleen, ectopic kidney, vascular graft, and pseudo-aneurysm. Increased activity in these structures should not be mistaken for GI bleed, as these areas are stationary and do not demonstrate changes in their appearance.

As in most imaging procedures, recognition of physiologic and anatomic variants is important for the accurate interpretation of blood pool scintigraphy. There are several normal structures visualized on the ^{99m}Tc-RBC scintigram that might easily be confused with bleeding. In addition to the aorta, inferior vena cava, and iliac vessels, the smaller vascular structures—such as the portal and splenic veins—are often visualized and may be mistaken for bleeding in the transverse colon, duodenum, or stomach. Occasionally, the superior mesenteric vein and inferior epigastric vein are visualized. Vessel visualization usually is more pronounced on the early images and later fades slightly. Also, the lack of migration of radioactivity should help

in their differentiation from bleeding. If no movement occurs, no active GI bleeding is present.

A vascular blush not uncommonly appears in the left lower quadrant and represents the mesenteric vascular bed; it should not be erroneously diagnosed as GI bleeding. Uterine blush also may be seen as a result of uterine hyperemia. A penile blood pool overlying the lower abdomen may be mistaken for bleeding. Figure 5.3 D shows intense focal and linear uptake over the left lower pelvis (arrow) in a 65-year-old man with history of duodenal ulcer and melena, mimicking sigmoid bleeding. Error in the diagnosis was avoided by repeating the images following a change in penile position.

In abdominal blood pool imaging, trace amount of activity may be seen in the stomach, kidney, collecting system, and bladder. Visualization of the urinary collecting system is more pronounced on the later images. This artifactual activity is due to the presence of a small amount of unbound ^{99m}Tc (free technetium) and should not occur to any significant degree with the currently used improved in vitro RBC labeling.

Diagnosis: Active GI bleed in the duodenum and sigmoid.

History: A 5-year-old otherwise healthy child presents with an unexplained GI bleed. He undergoes an abdominal radionuclide scintigram following the IV injection of 3 mCi of ^{99m}Tc-pertechnetate (Fig. 5.4).

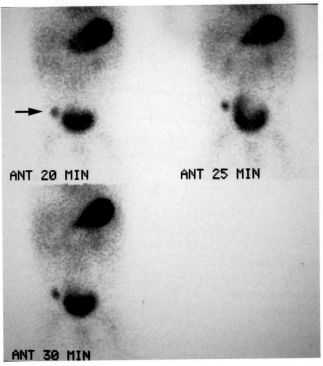

Figure 5.4

Finding: The anterior projection of the abdomen (Fig. 5.4) shows a focal area of increased uptake (arrow) in the right lower quadrant superior and lateral to the visualized urinary bladder on the images obtained at 20, 25, and 30 minutes.

Discussion: The anatomic location, persistent activity, and synchrony with gastric visualization are consistent with the diagnosis of Meckel's diverticulum containing gastric mucosa.

Meckel's diverticulum is a congenital anomaly of the GI tract occurring in 2% to 3% of the population and is the result of incomplete atrophy of the omphalomesenteric duct. It is a true diverticulum composed of all layers of intestinal ileum occurring on the antimesenteric border of the ileum within 100 cm of the ileocecal valve. Heterotopic gastric and pancreatic tissue is seen in approximately 50% of resected Meckel's diverticula, with gastric mucosa being the most common finding.

In the majority of patients, Meckel's diverticulum is asymptomatic. Clinical symptoms arise from complications of the diverticulum such as peptic ulceration and hemorrhage, which commonly occur before the patient reaches 10 years of age. Ectopic gastric mucosa produces gastric acid and pepsin, which can cause mucosal ulceration and hemorrhage. Bleeding is brisk and painless.

Bleeding from a Meckel's diverticulum can be diagnosed by labeled RBC scintigraphy; however, the procedure is less sensitive and less specific than the Meckel's scan.

A Meckel's scan is performed following IV injection of ^{99m}Tc-pertechnetate. Serial images of the abdomen are obtained over a period of 30 minutes. The mucous cells of the gastric epithelium, when present in the diverticulum, accumulate and excrete the pertechnetate; therefore the diverticulum appears as an area of focal accumulation of radioactivity, usually in the right lower quadrant.

In the diagnosis of Meckel's diverticulum, attention should be paid to the timing of the appearance of focal uptake. It should be in synchrony with visualization of the stomach.

Ectopic gastric mucosa may also be found in enteric duplication (located on the mesenteric side) and duplicated cysts. Therefore these anomalies should be entertained in the differential diagnosis, although differentiation is not possible by scan. But the distinction is not as important, as all will be treated surgically.

In the pediatric population, the Meckel's scan has a sensitivity, specificity, and accuracy of 85%, 95%, and 90% respectively. The result would be significantly lower in the adult population, as the prevalence of hypertrophic gastric mucosa declines with age.

A false-positive scan may occur as a result of inflammation and local hyperemia, ulcerative colitis, Crohn's disease, intussusception, retention of radioactivity in the distal right ureter, and arteriovenous malformation of the bowel. A false-negative scan occurs in the diverticulum that does not contain gastric mucosa, or there may be inadequate tissue to concentrate ^{99m}Tc-pertechnetate.

Diagnosis: Meckel's diverticulum.

CASE 5.5

History: A 52-year-old man presents to triage with the complaint of right-upper-quadrant pain and tenderness over the past 3 days. He denies nausea or vomiting. There are no chills or fever. He is referred for a hepatobiliary scan (Fig. 5.5 A).

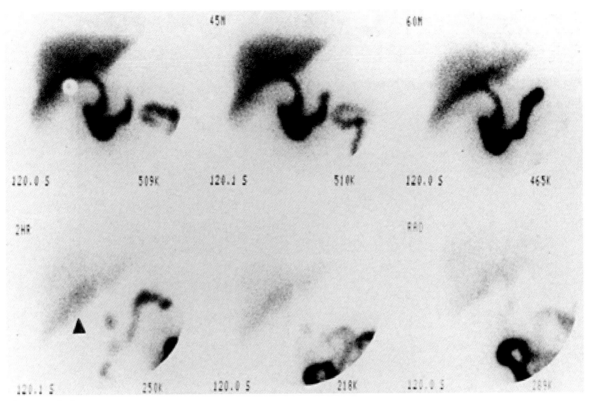

Figure 5.5 A

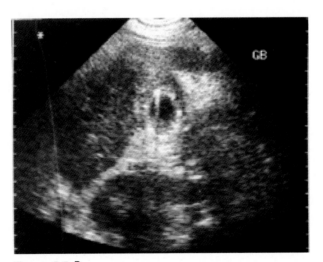

Figure 5.5 B

Findings: There is persistent nonvisualization of the gallbladder up to 3 hours. There is enhanced activity (arrowhead) along the inferior hepatic border, known as the rim sign, which is best seen on the delayed 2-hour image.

Discussion: Persistent nonvisualization of the gallbladder under proper clinical conditions is most consistent with acute cholecystitis. The rim sign, in association with nonvisualiza-tion of the gallbladder, is highly specific for acute cholecysti-tis and was originally described with acute gangrenous chole-cystitis.

Figure 5.5 B shows an ultrasound image of the right up-per quadrant demonstrating multiple echogenic foci within a thickened gallbladder wall that cast (dirty) acoustic shadows consistent with gas and emphysematous cholecystitis.

Acute gangrenous cholecystitis may also appear as a large area of photopenia in the gallbladder fossa with or without the rim sign. This appearance usually represents a relatively late and more severe stage of the disease process.

The rim sign has a high positive predictive value (95%) for acute cholecystitis; when it is present, there should be no need for delayed 3- to 4-hour images. Demonstration of the rim sign, even in the presence of a visualized gallbladder, should be considered as indicating a high probability for acute cholecystitis.

The rim sign should not be confused with normal anatomic variants. In patients with a prominent porta hepatis, the portal area appears as a photopenic region surrounded by normal liver tissue mimicking a rim sign. To avoid misinterpretation, ultrasound correlation should be considered for this atypical appearance.

The rim sign may also be seen along the inferior hepatic border in a patient with recent cholecystectomy. This should not be mistaken for inflammation. It is related to surgical manipulation and retraction of the liver during the surgery.

The rim sign is probably related to the prolonged transition and slow clearance of radioactivity from the edematous and hyperemic liver tissue adjacent to the inflamed gallbladder. Theoretically, the sign occurs throughout the hepatobiliary sequences, including scintiangiography, but it is more easily detected on delayed images as the activity of normal liver tissue disappears and the rim sign activity stands out. It is to be noted that high-count, high-intensity images should be obtained so as not to overlook the rim sign.

Diagnosis: Acute gangrenous cholecystitis.

CASE 5.6

History: A 62-year-old chronically ill patient on total parenteral nutrition (TPN) complains of right-upper-quadrant pain and tenderness. Gallbladder ultrasound (Fig. 5.6 A) shows a moderately distended gallbladder with sludge. Figure 5.6 B is a hepatobiliary scan done to exclude acute cholecystitis.

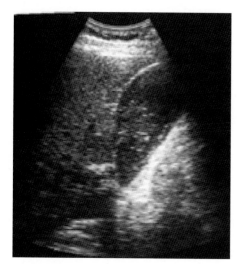

Figure 5.6 A

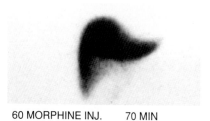

60 MORPHINE INJ.   70 MIN

Figure 5.6 B

Findings: The hepatobiliary images show uniform hepatic uptake of hydroxy iminodiacetic acid (HIDA) radiotracer with excretion into the bile duct and small intestine. There is no visualization of the gallbladder by 60 minutes. Ten minutes after IV injection of 2.5 mg of morphine sulfate, the gallbladder is visualized (arrow).

Discussion: Nonvisualization of the gallbladder prior to administration of morphine could be the result of acute cholecystitis, chronic cholecystitis, hyperalimentation, prolonged fasting, physiologic distention of the gallbladder, pancreatitis, or chronic alcoholism.

Visualization of the gallbladder following IV injection of morphine confirms the patency of the cystic duct, excludes cholecystitis, and suggests the diagnosis of a sludge-filled gallbladder with chronic cholecystitis.

Morphine enhances the tone of the sphincter of Oddi and causes increased intraluminal bile duct pressure severe enough to overcome resistance to bile flow into the sludge-filled gallbladder. Therefore there will be a diversion of bile flow into the gallbladder if the cystic duct is patent.

Morphine augmentation cholescintigraphy helps to avoid 3- to 4-hour delayed imaging without compromising the accuracy of the test. There are studies indicating that the results of morphine-augmented procedures are superior to conventional 3- to 4-hour delayed imaging for including or excluding acute cholecystitis.

Morphine should not be injected before 60 minutes into the study. If the gallbladder is not visualized by 60 minutes, morphine is injected and imaging is continued for an additional 30 minutes. Nonvisualization of the gallbladder at that time, in an appropriate clinical setting, is diagnostic for acute cholecystitis. If the gallbladder is not visualized by 60 minutes but is seen by 30 minutes following morphine injection, the diagnosis of abnormal gallbladder function can be made.

A technical note is that a sufficient amount of radiotracer must be present within the hepatobiliary system at the time of morphine injection to allow visualization of the gallbladder. If it is not, then a booster dose may be used.

It is to be noted that there may be a higher frequency of false-positive (nonvisualized gallbladder) diagnoses in a morphine-augmented study in severely ill patients as well as those receiving TPN. Therefore complementary ultrasound should be used liberally. In this group of patients, the greatest value of the ultrasound lies in the very high negative predictive value of the procedure.

Rarely, false-negative cases (visualized gallbladder) may occur. Forced entry of bile into a gallbladder that is filled with sludge may cause perforation, thus relieving the obstruction. Dislodgement of the stone in the cystic duct by increased pressure allows entry of bile into the gallbladder, which may also cause a false-negative study. The use of cholecystokinin and preemptying of gallbladder sludge is controversial. Its routine use is probably undesirable and has not been recommended.

A dilated cystic duct, the so-called cystic duct sign, may be mistaken for gallbladder visualization, leading to a false-negative study. A segment of cystic duct proximal to the obstruction may be distended. This dilatation becomes accentuated by increased volume and pressure of bile in the cystic duct secondary to morphine and mimics the appearance of the gallbladder. The location of activity medial to the gallbladder fossa and the temporary appearance–disappearance of the focus should help to avoid misinterpretation.

Diagnosis: Chronic cholecystitis.

CASE 5.7

History: A 37-year-old man, status post renal transplant, had been on TPN for several weeks and now complains of upper abdominal pain. A hepatobiliary scan (Fig. 5.7 A) was obtained to evaluate the possibility of acute cholecystitis.

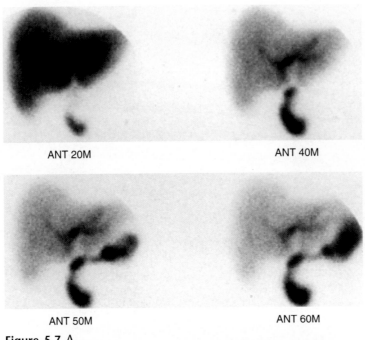

ANT 20M   ANT 40M

ANT 50M   ANT 60M

Figure 5.7 A

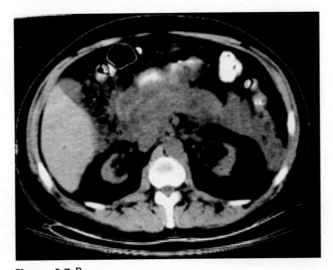

Figure 5.7 B

Findings: There is nonvisualization of the gallbladder by 60 minutes. There is enterogastric reflux of radiotracer outlining the stomach. Radiotracer activity terminates abruptly at the second portion of the duodenum, the so-called duodenal cutoff sign.

Discussion: The most significant cause of nonvisualization of the gallbladder by 60 minutes in patients with no history of cholecystectomy is acute cholecystitis. Although this finding is very sensitive (greater than 90%), it is not specific. There are a variety of other causes that should be considered; among

the most notable are chronic cholecystitis, acute pancreatitis, hyperalimentation, nonfasting state, alcoholism, severe intercurrent disease, and obstruction of the common bile duct. Of these, there is a higher incidence of gastric reflux in association with pancreatitis. In addition, the presence of the duodenal cutoff sign bears the same significance as a radiographic colon cutoff sign seen in patients with acute pancreatitis. Figure 5.7 B is the patient's abdominal CT, which reveals an enlarged, edematous pancreas with loss of normal tissue planes consistent with acute pancreatitis, which was confirmed on autopsy a few days later and believed to be postoperative pancreatitis.

Enterogastric reflux allows the entrance of bile and intestinal enzymes into the stomach. This occurs as a result of pyloric sphincter incompetency. Enterogastric reflux has been implicated in the pathogenesis of gastric ulcer; however, chronic gastritis is more closely associated with reflux. A minimal amount of reflux may be seen in up to 5% of normal individuals during cholescintigraphy; however, an enterogastric reflux index over 8 ± 6 should be considered abnormal. The reflux index represents the ratio of change in gastric activity over the changes of hepatobiliary activity during a specific period of time. The greatest index (85 ± 7) is found in patients with alkaline gastritis.

In addition to pancreatitis, enterogastric reflux also is commonly seen after pyloroplasty, Billroth I and II anastomosis, partial gastrectomy, post cholecystectomy, and prior gastroplasty; it may also be seen in the normal postprandial period.

Diagnosis: Acute pancreatitis.

CASE 5.8

History: The patient is a 55-year-old man complaining of daily, protracted postprandial vomiting and upper abdominal pain; he was referred for hepatobiliary scan to evaluate the gallbladder and biliary tree.

His right-upper-quadrant ultrasound study showed a normal-appearing gallbladder with no stone, wall thickening, biliary ductal dilatation, or pericholecystic fluid collection. Figure 5.8 A shows the images of his hepatobiliary study.

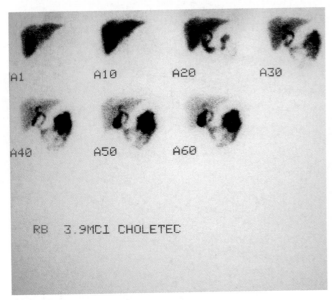

Figure 5.8 A

Figure 5.8 B

Findings: Sequential hepatobiliary images over a period of 60 minutes show essentially normal uptake by the liver. There is normal visualization of the gallbladder and bowel by 40 minutes into the study. There is no evidence of obstruction of the cystic duct or common bile duct.

Discussion: Up to 25% of symptomatic patients with recurrent colic-like pain and no anatomic cause for the pain—such as stone, obstruction, tumor, etc.—are suffering from so-called functional disorder of the gallbladder, which is usually referred to as acalculous cholecystitis, cystic duct syndrome, or gallbladder dyskinesis. In this group of patients,

there is impairment in the contractility of the gallbladder, and the lack of response to cholecystokinin confirms the diagnosis. Figure 5.8 B shows quantitative results of a gallbladder ejection fraction following the infusion of 0.02 μg/kg of CCK over a period of 30 minutes. Calculated ejection fraction is 21% at 30 minutes into the infusion, with normal being over 35%. The patient's operative cholangiogram demonstrated no evidence of filling defect to suggest calculi, and histopathology of the gallbladder revealed evidence of chronic inflammatory changes. The patient's symptoms resolved after cholecystectomy.

It is to be noted that although, in this group of patients, the gallbladder wall appears normal on ultrasound examination and no gross abnormality is identified, on histopathologic examination of the gallbladder, there is evidence of chronic inflammation similar to that in symptomatic patients with chronic calculous cholecystitis. The lack of response to CCK may be due to reduced CCK receptor sites in the gallbladder wall, impaired smooth muscle function as a result of chronic inflammation, or cystic duct dyskinesis.

In cystic duct syndrome, the major pathophysiology resides in the cystic duct itself. The cystic duct is narrowed as a result of chronic inflammation; there is fibrosis, a thickened wall, and occasional ductal kinking. In this syndrome, the bile enters the gallbladder slowly but cannot exit quickly in response to food or CCK infusion. From the functional standpoint in cystic duct syndrome, there is uncoordination between gallbladder contraction and cystic duct relaxation in response to CCK. This uncoordination causes the cystic duct to contract instead of relax. Therefore, in spite of gallbladder contraction, the cystic duct contraction does not allow an increase in the gallbladder ejection fraction. This uncoordination of motility is obviously a dyskinetic abnormality.

Diagnosis of chronic acalculous cholecystitis in the past was a diagnosis of exclusion; however, CCK intervention, cholescintigraphy and calculation of gallbladder ejection fraction can make the diagnosis and may play a major role in the management of a patient with acalculous biliary pain. Lack of response to CCK makes this diagnosis, and more than 90% of these patients benefit from cholecystectomy. However, this diagnosis should be made only in the proper clinical setting. These patients are generally outpatient referrals; they are not acutely ill and have no pain at the time of examination but suffer from chronic, recurrent, colic-type postprandial pain.

For the proper interpretation of CCK cholescintigraphy, one should consider other nongallbladder diseases that demonstrate a poor response to CCK. These include diabetes mellitus, cirrhosis, celiac disease, and obesity and should be considered in the differential diagnosis. Vagotomized patients and the effect of medications that lower gallbladder ejection fraction—such as morphine, atropine, and calcium channel blockers—should also be considered.

Diagnosis: Chronic acalculous cholecystitis—cystic duct syndrome.

CASE 5.9

History: The patient is a 56-year-old male with a 6-month history of midepigastric pain aggravated by food and occasional bilious vomiting. His upper abdominal ultrasound (Fig. 5.9 A) shows a distended gallbladder containing sludge and calculi. The patient is referred for a hepatobiliary scan for further evaluation.

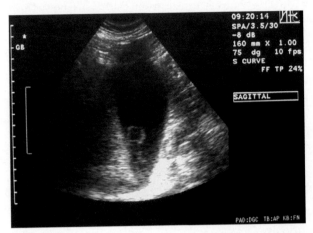

Figure 5.9 A

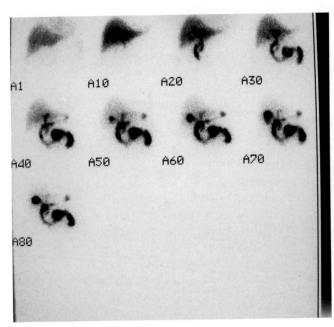

Figure 5.9 B

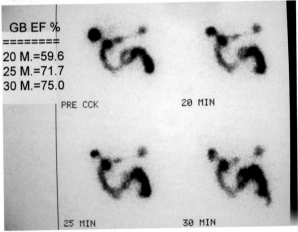

Figure 5.9 C

Findings: Sequential 10-minute images of the abdomen (Fig. 5.9 B) over a period of 90 minutes following the IV injection of 6 mCi of ^{99m}Tc–IDA derivative show normal hepatic uptake with visualization of the bowel and gallbladder at 20 minutes and 50 minutes, respectively, with continuation of gallbladder filling. There is a normal response to CCK (Fig. 5.9 C). Gallbladder ejection fraction is 75% at 30 minutes into the CCK infusion. Trace radioactivity is identified in the left upper quadrant.

Discussion: Patients with typical symptoms of recurrent colic-type pain and demonstration of calculi on ultrasound or other anatomic modality are commonly managed surgically by cholecystectomy. However, there are some patients whose symptoms are not typical of cholecystitis. Clinicians may suspect that the pain and stones are not related. Such patients, therefore, would not benefit from cholecystectomy. A CCK cholescintigram can be used to determine whether the pain and stone are related. A positive response of the gallbladder to CCK and normal gallbladder ejection fraction would make it unlikely that calculous cholecystitis is the cause of the patient's symptoms; usually these patients' symptoms improve with therapy for a nongallbladder disease. This would be in contrast to those who have a low ejection fraction in response to the CCK, which would be consistent with chronic calculous cholecystitis. The infusion of CCK is known to cause contraction of the gallbladder and to relax the sphincter of Oddi. Chronic cholecystitis affects the coordination of these functions, and CCK can be used to confirm or exclude chronic cholecystitis.

It is to be noted that gallstones are common, but most patients with cholelithiasis are asymptomatic and have a normally contractible gallbladder and normal ejection fraction.

Tracer activity identified in the left upper quadrant represents an enterogastric reflux of bile, which is believed to be the etiology of this patient's symptoms.

Diagnosis: Functioning gallbladder, normal response to CCK, enterogastric reflux of bile.

CASE 5.10

History: A 49-year-old patient with abdominal pain and occasional nausea and vomiting had a normal liver function test and ultrasound. A hepatobiliary scan (Fig. 5.10 A) was obtained to evaluate the gallbladder and biliary system.

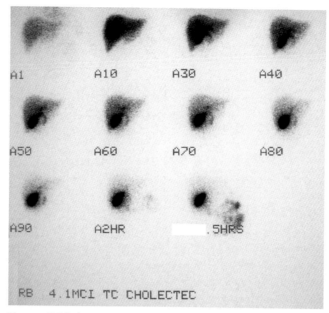

Figure 5.10 A

Findings: There is normal hepatic uptake with visualization of the gallbladder at 30 minutes. There is persistent gallbladder filling and no bowel entry of bile by 90 minutes. Delayed images at 5 hours show trace amount of activity in the loops of small bowel.

Discussion: The pattern of preferential gallbladder filling associated with delayed biliary-to-bowel transit is not an uncommon finding in cholescintigraphy. Most patients exhibiting this finding have a nonspecific chronic cholecystitis; their abnormalities are in and around the area of the sphincter of Oddi.

The existence of Oddi's sphincter in the distal common bile duct and its function are well known. In the fasting state, the normal tonicity of the sphincter prevents the flow of bile into the bowel and reroutes it into the gallbladder, facilitating gallbladder filling. In a disease state, when there is spasm of Oddi's sphincter, or in patients with hypertonicity of this sphincter (a normal variation), there will be preferential gallbladder filling and a delay in bile-to-bowel transit. Spasm of Oddi's sphincter is also called Oddi's dysfunction, papillary stenosis, common bile duct dysfunction, and spasm of the sphincter; it basically acts as a functional obstruction of the distal common bile duct. Spasm of Oddi's sphincter probably represents a sequela of chronic cholecystitis and is a result of repeated subacute bouts of cholecystitis that may have caused mild scarring and fibrotic changes in the area of Oddi's sphincter and the associated spasm.

In patients with preferential gallbladder filling related to sphincter spasm, eventual visualization of the bowel occurs on delayed images up to 24 hours. The prevalence of chronic cholecystitis would be higher in these patients, who have a delay in biliary-to-bowel transit.

In a scan with preferential gallbladder filling, in addition to chronic cholecystitis causing Oddi's spasm syndrome, the effect of narcotic, postvagotomy, or prolonged fasting states as well as distal common bile duct stenosis should be considered.

Morphine, codeine, and other morphine-related drugs have a constrictive effect on Oddi's sphincter, altering the biliary dynamic and producing an obstructive pattern of the distal common bile duct, prolonging biliary-to-bowel transit time, and facilitating early and continuous filling of the gallbladder.

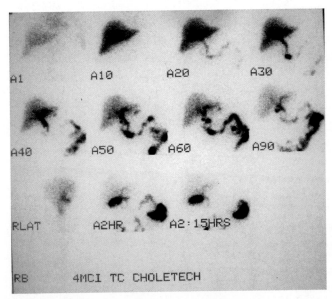

Figure 5.10 B

Filling and emptying of the gallbladder is regulated by the sympathetic–parasympathetic systems and the hormone CCK. In a vagotomized patient, in whom sympathetic–parasympathetic coordination is disrupted, there will be gradual development of gallbladder dilatation, which acts as a low-pressure reservoir, allowing more bile to flow into the gallbladder and leading to preferential gallbladder filling.

Prolonged fasting and TPN administrations result in a decrease in endogeneous CCK production and cause gallbladder distention and stasis and facilitate preferential filling.

Preferential filling of the gallbladder related to the sphincter's dyskinesia is usually not associated with significant activity of pooling in the intra- or extrahepatic biliary tree. This feature can help to distinguish the sphincter's functional abnormality from stenosis of the distal common duct, in which intense pooling of bile proximal to the obstruction occurs.

Contrary to those with preferential gallbladder filling, there is another group of patients in whom, despite normal and early visualization of the common bile duct and bowel, the gall-

bladder is visualized late. Early bowel and delayed gallbladder visualization represents another pattern seen in chronic cholecystitis in which some cystic duct mucosal edema, bile stasis, and debris may be the causative factor. Figure 5.10 B represents the cholescintigram of a 65-year-old male patient complaining of waxing and waning pain over the previous 6 months. Note the normal and early appearance of radioactivity in the bowel but delayed gallbladder visualization by 2 hours.

The other causes of delayed gallbladder visualization include hepatitis, partial biliary stenosis as the result of a pancreatic mass, enlarged node, alcoholic pancreatitis, and surgically altered biliary anatomy.

It is to be noted that the two patterns of cholescintigram described above, preferential gallbladder filling and late gallbladder visualization, effectively exclude acute cholecystitis and total common bile duct obstruction in the majority of clinical situations and play a useful role in patient management.

Diagnosis: Chronic cholecystitis, delayed gallbladder visualization, and sphincter of Oddi spasm.

CASE 5.11

History: Ten days following cholecystectomy for acute cholecystitis, this 50-year-old patient returned with mild fever and complaining of dull right-upper-quadrant pain aggravated by breathing. A hepatobiliary scan was performed to evaluate the integrity of the biliary system and possibility of postcholecystectomy complications (Fig. 5.11 A).

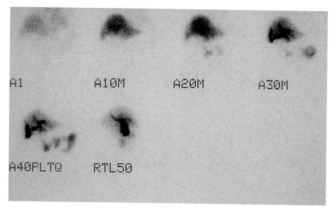

Figure 5.11 A

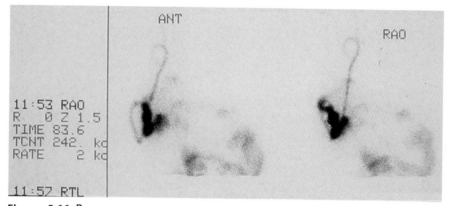

Figure 5.11 B

Findings: There is normal delineation of the liver with visualization of internal hepatic duct and loops of bowel by 20 minutes. However, there is a large collection of activity outlining the perihepatic area around the inferolateral aspect of the right lobe, representing extravasation of bile and consistent with a localized bile leak in this region (biloma).

Discussion: Leak as a postsurgical complication of cholecystectomy is relatively infrequent, averaging approximately 1 for every 500 cases. However, leak appears to be more prevalent in laparoscopic procedures compared with open cholecystectomy.

In any patient following cholecystectomy who complains of unexplained abdominal pain, jaundice, fever, or increased fluid drainage in the draining tube, the possibility of bile leak should be considered. Other complications include retained stone, cystic duct remnant, bile duct strictures or obstruction, pancreatitis, and biliary dyskinesia (Oddi's sphincter spasm).

Recognition of bile leak in cholescintographic examination is quite easy. Identification of activity outside the biliary tree and GI tract is almost diagnostic of bile leak. Bile leak commonly occurs in the subhepatic region, right paracolonic gutter, subcapsular collection, peritoneal cavity, or in a localized walled off area around the liver (biloma) as in this case, where a subhepatic bilious collection was drained percutaneously under ultrasound guidance (Fig. 5.11 B).

Demonstration of bile leak usually requires delayed imaging. If the leak is small, accumulation of extraluminal activity may not be apparent on the early images. Moreover, extraluminal activity persists for hours after the liver parenchyma and biliary tract are no longer visualized. Therefore recognition of a small bile leak becomes easier.

Diagnosis: Bile leak.

CASE 5.12

History: A 36-year-old patient who had had a liver transplant 6 months earlier received an abdominal CT scan following removal of a biliary stent from his left hepatic lobe. The CT scan demonstrated presence of a minimal amount of fluid in the pelvis as well as fluid surrounding the spleen (Fig. 5.12 A). Subsequently the patient was referred for hepatobiliary scan to evaluate the possibility of bile leak (Fig. 5.12 B).

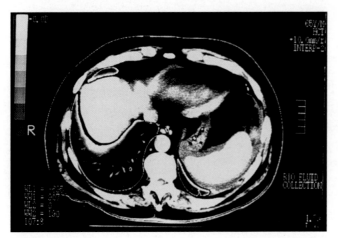

Figure 5.12 A

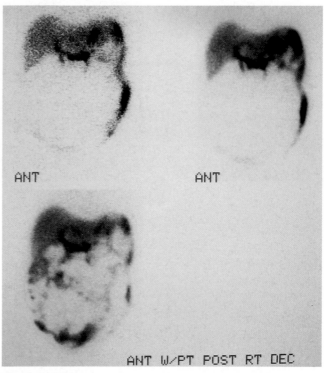

Figure 5.12 B

Findings: Hepatobiliary images of the abdomen in anterior projection show homogeneous uptake by the liver. There is focal uptake projecting over the left lobe and a linear area of uptake in a tubular fashion probably in a surgically altered and mildly dilated biliary duct. Of significance is the appearance of radioactivity in the left paracolonic gutter progressing diffusely within the abdominal cavity and pelvis. These findings are diagnostic for biliary leak.

Discussion: Biliary complication in a patient with liver transplant is not uncommon and occurs in approximately 15% of cases. Bile leak and biliary obstruction are the two major complications. Although the diagnosis of bile leak in transplanted liver is usually made by T-tube cholangiography or percutaneous transhepatic cholangiography, cholescintigraphy as an accurate, noninvasive method can make the diagnosis of leak or obstruction. The major limitation of cholescintigraphy, however, is inability to localize an anatomic origin of the bile leak.

In postsurgical patients such as those who have undergone transplantation, it is not unusual for ultrasound or CT to disclose an intra-abdominal fluid collection that could be due to ascites, hematoma, abscess, seroma, or a collection of bile. The cholescintigram is quite specific and is a physiologic method of identifying the bilious nature of the fluid collection and documenting bile leak, as in this case.

The spread of the bile leak originating from the left upper quadrant to the pelvis and further progression to the right upper quadrant, as in this case, should not be surprising. Spread of intra-abdominal fluid follows a well-defined anatomic boundary (Fig. 5.12 C). The peritoneal cavity is divided into supramesocolic and inframesocolic compartments by the transverse colon and transverse mesocolon. The root of mesentery further divides the inframesocolic compartment into the left and right inframesocolic compartments. Fluid, infectious material, or metastatic dissemination passes through these compartments by a specific anatomically defined pathway. The bile collected in the left upper quadrant and the left inframesocolic space (A) opens directly into the pelvic cavity (B). Although the root of the mesentery and base of the ascending colon in the cecal region defines the inferior border of the right paracolonic gutter (C), this barrier can be breached easily; therefore the leaking bile collected in the pelvis enters into the right paracolonic gutter with further progression into infrahepatic area and Morrison's pouch (D), which medially communicates to the lesser sac (E) through the foramen of Winslow.

In diagnosing bile leak in a patient with a transplanted liver, one should be aware of the type of surgical procedure that was employed in biliary construction during the surgery. Biliary

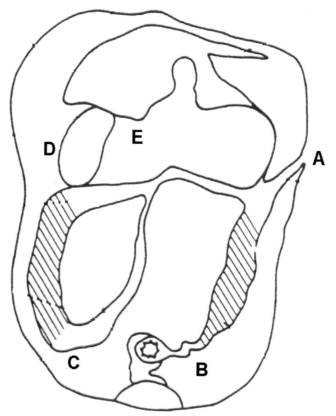

Figure 5.12 (C) Redrawn with permission from Meyers MA. *Dynamic Radiology of the Abdomen: Normal and Pathologic Anatomy.* New York: Springer-Verlag, 1976.

construction is usually performed either as a direct duct-to-duct anastomosis of donor and receiver (choledochocholedocostomy) or as a biliary-enteric anastomosis (Roux-en-Y hepaticojejunostomy). In the latter technique, normally a portion of the Y limb (blind end) is left proximal to the biliary anastomosis, which acts as a reservoir, receiving the bile entering from the hepatic duct. Therefore an accumulation of radioactivity in the blind end of the Y limb should not be confused with bile leak. Activity in the blind end characteristically fluctuates in size and intensity, which helps in differentiating from a more stable pool of activity, as in biloma.

Diagnosis: Bile leak following transplantation.

CASE 5.13

History: Six months following cholecystectomy, this 50-year-old patient returned with biliary colic, mild jaundice, and fatty food intolerance. A hepatobiliary scan (Fig. 5.13) was performed to evaluate the possibility of obstructive jaundice.

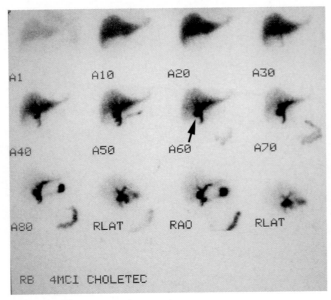

Figure 5.13

Findings: There is prompt uptake by the liver. There is a slow clearance of activity from the biliary ductal system; however, activity in the loops of bowel is identified by 60 minutes. A focus of persistent activity (arrow) appeared at 40 minutes and progressed to increase in size during the study. This activity is located medial to the gallbladder fossa and lateral to the common bile duct. There is enterogastric reflux of the bile.

Discussion: A persistent focus of activity lateral to the common bile duct in a patient with cholecystectomy would be consistent with a cystic duct remnant. The frequency of a cystic duct remnant is not well established; however, if left behind in surgery, it can act as a small gallbladder subject to stone formation, inflammation, and obstruction. Cystic duct remnant is one of the causes of postcholecystectomy syndrome and recurrent cholelithiasis. Visualization of the cystic duct remnant may require delayed views. Also, a focal localization of radioactivity medial to the common bile duct may be due to retention of activity in a duodenal diverticulum, which should be considered in the differential diagnosis.

Diagnosis: Cystic duct remnant.

CASE 5.14

History: Five days following surgery for an abdominal aortic aneurysm, this 58-year-old man was noted to have an elevated bilirubin of 7.2 mg/L, mild fever, and right-upper-quadrant discomfort. A hepatobiliary scan (Fig. 5.14) was performed to evaluate for the possibility of an obstructive jaundice.

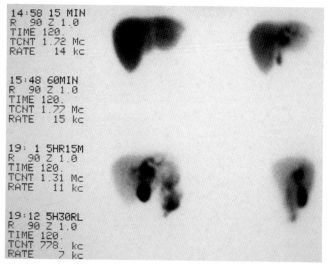

Figure 5.14

Findings: Sequential images over a period of 5.5 hours reveal normal uptake by the liver and marked delay in gallbladder and bowel visualization. The gallbladder is visualized by 60 minutes, and there is slow drainage from the bile duct, causing retention of radioactivity mainly in the left hepatic duct.

Discussion: Discussion of this case revolves around the prolonged retention of liver uptake and slow excretion, which may be due to hepatocellular dysfunction or complete or partial obstruction of the biliary tract.

In case of partial biliary obstruction, the scintigram usually shows progressive accumulation of radioactivity within the biliary tract proximal to the obstruction in addition to delay of bowel visualization and prolonged liver uptake.

The partial stasis and delayed washout produced from the left hepatic duct in this case would be consistent with partial obstruction, which has caused tortuosity and segmental dilatation of the biliary ducts.

Segmental biliary obstruction can be due to cholangitis, or it may be a sequela of hepatic calculi; it can also be congenital. It may also be due to liver tumor, such as hepatoma, metastasis, or cholangiocarcinoma. If the tumor is situated in a strategically located bifurcation area, it may present as a segmental dilatation in the early stage. The left lobe is apt to show segmental dilatation more often than the right, as there is less liver tissue on the left to resist dilatory expansion of a duct proximal to the obstruction. The left hepatic duct is also positioned relatively anteriorly; therefore dilatation is easier to see on the anterior projection of the scan, which is routinely obtained.

On endoscopic retrograde cholangiopancreatography (ERCP), the cause of the partial obstruction in the current case was noted to be cholangitis associated with mild stenosis of the hepatic duct at the bifurcation, complicated by sludge and stasis.

Diagnosis: Partial biliary obstruction.

CASE 5.15*

History: A neonate presented with persistent jaundice and conjugated hyperbilirubinemia. A hepatobiliary scan was performed to rule out biliary atresia (Figs. 5.15 A, 5.15 B, 5.15 C).

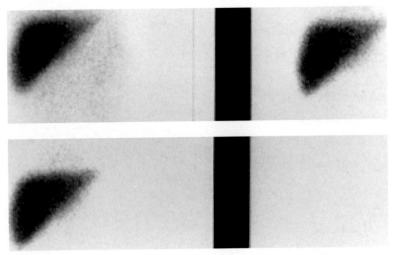

Figure 5.15 A

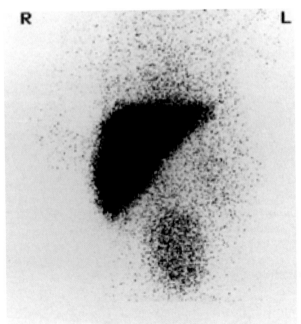

ANT 5 HR DELAY PRIDA

Figure 5.15 B

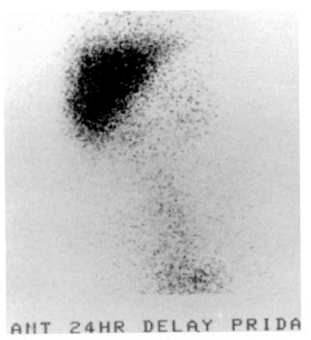

ANT 24HR DELAY PRIDA

Figure 5.15 C

Findings: After the intravenous injection of a ^{99m}Tc iminodiacetic acid derivative (^{99m}Tc IDA), images were taken over the abdomen at 5, 10, and 15 minutes and at 5 and 24 hours. There is prompt hepatic uptake of radiopharmaceutical but no biliary or bowel excretion is noted up to 24 hours after injection.

Discussion: These findings are consistent with biliary atresia. In infants less than 2 months of age, it is important to distinguish biliary atresia from severe neonatal hepatitis. Biliary atresia is treated by the Kasai procedure, wherein a jejunal conduit is anastomosed to a transected hepatic duct at the liver hilus. This procedure is most successful before 60 days of age, with a 90% success rate. At 90 days, this procedure is 17% successful. The success of late surgical intervention is poor and is related to progressive loss of patency of the biliary system involving both the intra- and extrahepatic ducts, ultimately leading to intrahepatic sclerosis at approximately 3 months of age. It is now known that biliary atresia is not a congenital malformation but a progressive, potentially reversible process.

Both biliary atresia and neonatal hepatitis present with jaundice, conjugated hyperbilirubinemia, and pale stools. The differential diagnosis also includes choledochal cyst and alpha$_1$-antitrypsin deficiency.

Patients are pretreated with phenobarbital (recommended dose: 5 mg/kg per day) for 5 to 7 days before scanning to enhance biliary uptake and excretion. The ^{99m}Tc-IDA derivatives are used for diagnosis. In biliary atresia, there is prompt visualization of the liver after injection and absence of bowel activity at 24 hours. In cases of nonobstructive causes of jaundice, imaging is carried out until demonstration of bowel activity or by 24 hours. Serum phenobarbital levels should be checked to confirm adequacy. If any bowel activity is detected, biliary atresia is excluded. The sensitivity of phenobarbital-augmented hepatobiliary imaging in diagnosing neonatal hepatitis and/or biliary atresia is greater than 90%.

Diagnosis: Biliary atresia.

*Courtesy of Susan Passalaqua, MD.

CASE 5.16

History: A 43-year-old man with a history of carcinoma of the tonsil and chronic alcohol abuse presented with clinical hepatomegaly and ascites. A ^{99m}Tc–sulfur colloid liver–spleen scan was performed upon request (Fig. 5.16 A).

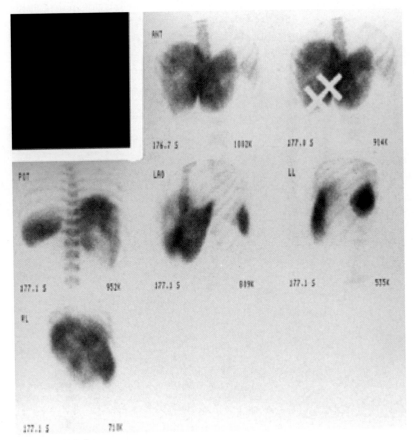

Figure 5.16 A

Findings: There is hepatomegaly with diffusely diminished liver uptake and a heterogeneous, mottled appearance. Extrahepatic distribution of radiocolloid is visualized in the bone marrow of the vertebral bodies, ribs, and sternum (colloid shift). The spleen is not greatly enlarged. The liver appears displaced medially.

Discussion: Hepatomegaly, heterogeneous uptake, and colloid shift are frequent features of alcohol abuse; they are seen in approximately 80% of patients with chronic alcoholic liver disease and may progress to cirrhosis.

Several pathologic processes may diffusely involve the liver and present with a similar scintigraphic appearance. Fatty metamorphosis, cholestasis, hepatitis, leukemic infiltration, lymphomatous involvement of the liver, granulomatous hepatitis, amyloidosis, and chronic passive hepatic congestion are among the better-known entities. However, significant scan abnormality and colloid shift is very uncommon in fatty infiltration of the liver.

In cirrhosis, there is a reduced number of Kupffer's cells per volume of tissue and a decrease in effective blood flow resulting from the intrahepatic shunting that bypasses the Kupffer cells, thus reducing the efficiency of colloid extraction by the liver. This, in turn, causes reduced uptake of radiocolloid by the liver and increased uptake by the spleen and bone marrow, commonly known as colloid shift.

Alteration of the hepatic microcirculation appears to play a more important role than diminution in the number of Kupffer cells. Portal hypertension with or without splenomegaly may

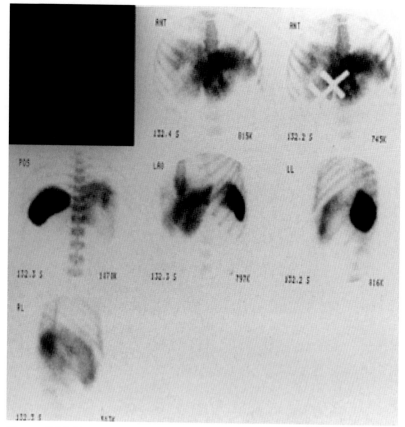

Figure 5.16 B

be a contributing factor in colloid shift, but elimination of portal hypertension by a portocaval shunt procedure does not reverse the scan to normal.

In cirrhosis, the development of regenerating nodules and intrahepatic shunting results in heterogeneous uptake. The scan shows a mottled appearance at this stage, which can be mistaken for multiple small metastases. If a large, dominant hepatic defect is noted, a hepatocellular carcinoma superimposed on cirrhosis should be considered.

On serial scanning of patients with cirrhosis, the degree of colloid redistribution correlates with progress of the disease, and the scan may be used prognostically to predict disease progress. A 3-month follow-up scan (Fig. 5.16 B) of this patient shows further progression of the disease, as suggested by additional increase in colloid shift and atrophy of the right lobe. The medial displacement of the liver on the original scan is due to ascites.

Diagnosis: Hepatic cirrhosis.

CASE 5.17

History: A 57-year-old male on chemotherapy for recently diagnosed renal cell carcinoma was admitted with fever and clinical deterioration. At the time of his initial diagnosis, CT (Fig. 5.17 A) and scintigraphic imaging of the liver (Fig. 5.17 B) were negative for metastasis. Figure 5.17 C shows a follow-up liver–spleen scan.

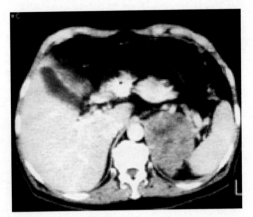

Figure 5.17 A

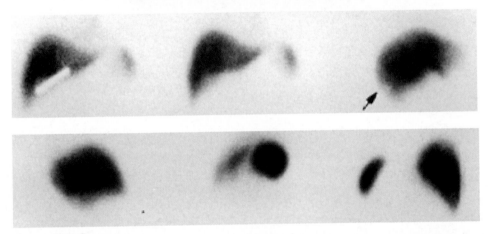

Figure 5.17 B

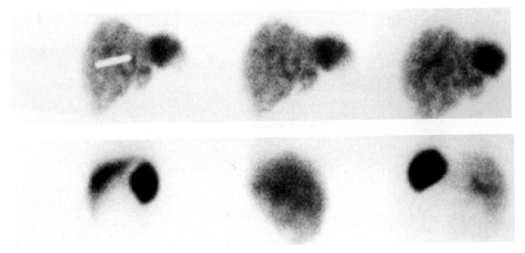

Figure 5.17 C

Findings: Figure 5.17 C shows hepatomegaly with numerous small focal defects distributed uniformly throughout the liver. The scan's appearance has changed dramatically since the study performed 4 weeks earlier. In retrospect, Figure 5.17 B may have shown a small defect posterolaterally (arrow). Two months prior to this admission, CT of the liver was noted to be negative for metastasis; however, a large necrotic mass arising from the left kidney was present (Fig. 5.17 A).

Discussion: The nonspecificity of a focal defect seen on liver scan is well known. The etiology of multiple intrahepatic focal lesions includes four major categories: (a) congenital (polycystic disease), (b) infectious (abscess), (c) degenerative (pseudomass of cirrhosis), and (d) neoplastic (lymphoma and metastasis).

Metastatic disease is by far the most frequent cause of multiple focal defects and was the most widely used single indication for liver scintigraphy in the past.

There are no statistically significant differences in detectability of metastases by CT, scintigraphy, or ultrasonography. A sensitivity of 93% for CT, 86% for scintigraphy, and 82% for ultrasonography has been reported. The specificity of these three diagnostic modalities is 88%, 83%, and 85%, respectively; however, SPECT may increase the sensitivity of the scintigram. In one study, the sensitivity of SPECT is noted to be 94% as compared with 81% for planar images.

Not only are the size and location of the lesion(s) important but the nature of the primary tumor plays a role in the detection of liver metastases. Colorectal carcinoma and renal cell carcinoma, as in the current case, shower the liver with metastases that rapidly generate focal defects. The accuracy of the liver scintigram for these metastatic tumors is generally greater than 90%. Tumor from the lung and breast produce small disseminated metastases, giving the scan a heterogeneous appearance. These lesions may be too small to be detected on scintigraphy and can be easily missed on CT, particularly on non–contrast-enhanced images.

The imaging features of the current case are compatible with disseminated liver metastases or microabscesses. The patient's clinical status deteriorated further. At autopsy, multiple hepatic metastases were present.

Diagnosis: Disseminated liver metastases.

CASE 5.18

History: A 68-year-old man with a past history of resected ileal carcinoid diagnosed during an evaluation for GI bleeding was admitted for assessment of probable tumor recurrence. He complained of only mild abdominal discomfort; his prior symptoms of diarrhea and flushing had resolved with ongoing somatostatin therapy. Urinary excretion of 5-hydroxyindoleacetic acid (HIAA) was normal. Figure 5.18 A shows his abdominal CT and Figure 5.18 B shows a whole-body ^{111}In-octreotide scan.

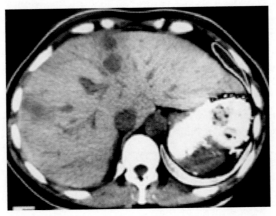

Figure 5.18 A

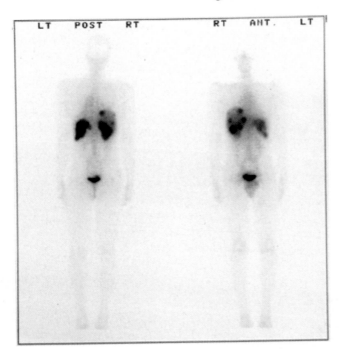

Figure 5.18 B

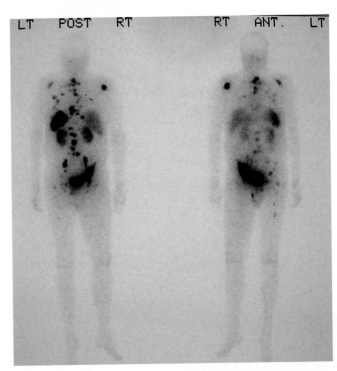

Figure 5.18 C

Findings: The abdominal CT discloses numerous hepatic metastases. The ^{111}In-octreotide images show multiple foci of increased activity throughout the liver. No extrahepatic tumor is identified.

Discussion: Octreotide, a synthetic somatostatin analog, is a peptide of eight amino acids with a high affinity for cell surface somatostatin receptors. Following IV injection, radiolabeled octreotide clears rapidly by renal excretion. At 4 and 24 hours, only 10% and 1%, respectively, of the injected radioactivity remains in the circulation. There is physiologic accumulation in the pituitary, thyroid, liver, gallbladder, bowel, spleen, kidneys, and urinary bladder. The usual dose is 6 mCi, with the highest radiation dose to the spleen and kidneys. Whole-body images are obtained at 4 and 24 hours. Owing to physiologic uptake of ^{111}In-octreotide by the liver, SPECT images of the upper abdomen are required to assess the liver for metastases and to detect pancreatic and duodenal tumor.

There is little evidence to recommend discontinuance of octreotide therapy prior to scintigraphy. Laxatives may facilitate clearance of activity from the bowel, thus enhancing visualization of extrahepatic lesions. Images of the abdomen at 48 hours may be obtained if necessary.

Uptake of radiolabeled octreotide is highly specific for neoplastic and nonneoplastic tissues expressing somatostatin receptors. Most of the tumors are neuroendocrine neoplasms, including carcinoid, islet cell tumors, medullary carcinoma of the thyroid, pheochromocytoma, paraganglioma, neuroblastoma, pituitary adenoma (especially growth hormone–secreting), Merkel cell carcinoma, and small cell carcinoma of the lung. Somatostatin receptors may also be expressed by meningioma, lymphoma, breast carcinoma, and non–small cell lung cancer.

Carcinoid is the most common neuroendocrine tumor of the GI tract and may be found in the stomach, duodenum, distal ileum, appendix, proximal colon, distal colon, and rectum. The most common site of carcinoid is the appendix, followed by the ileum. Rectal carcinoid is usually small; it develops metastases in about 10% of cases and rarely gives rise to carcinoid syndrome.

The carcinoid syndrome consists of flushing, diarrhea, cyanosis, and bronchoconstriction. These symptoms are due to circulating serotonin secreted by the carcinoid tumor and released in the systemic circulation without being inactivated in the liver.

One-third of GI carcinoid tumors metastasize, and they have a tendency to metastasize to the liver with extensive organ involvement. The carcinoid syndrome is seen almost exclusively in patients with liver metastasis. Bone metastases are osteoblastic. Since carcinoid of the bowel grows extraluminally, it infiltrates the bowel wall and lymphatic channels and spreads to the regional and distant lymph nodes.

The majority of carcinoid tumors express a high density of somatostatin receptors and can be detected with a sensitivity of 80% to 100% using octreotide scintigraphy. The primary tumor as well as distant metastases can usually be identified.

Figure 5.18 C shows disseminated soft tissue and nodal metastases from rectal carcinoid in a 60-year-old male. A bulky mass of the carcinoid tissue is also easily identified in the patient's right iliac fossa.

Tumor visualization does not appear to depend on hypersecretion, merely on expression of the somatostatin receptors. In this case (Fig. 5.18 B), there is excellent visualization of the hepatic metastases despite good control of symptoms and normalization of urinary 5-hydroxyindoleacetic acid excretion.

[111]In octreotide scintigraphy is indicated in evaluation of patients with known or suspected neuroendocrine tumors. It has been reported that ^{111}In-octreotide scintigraphy has detected tumor in 28% of patients in whom tumor was not identified using alternative imaging modalities. False-negative scans occurring in patients with neuroendocrine tumor are probably related to the absence of somatostatin receptors or the presence of a subtype of somatostatin receptor with low affinity for octreotide. Small tumors may be difficult to identify, particularly if they are adjacent to regions of physiologic uptake, such as the kidneys or spleen. False-positive scans are infrequent, but they may occur as a result of somatostatin expression by activated lymphocytes in patients with granulomatous and autoimmune disease such as tuberculosis, sarcoidosis, Wegener's granulomatosis, and systemic lupus. Accumulation of ^{111}In octreotide has also been seen in areas of inflammation related to recent surgery, external radiation therapy, and chemotherapy as well as in the nasopharynx and hilar regions in patients with upper respiratory tract infections.

Tumoral uptake of ^{111}In-octreotide is a strong prognostic indicator that a clinical response will occur with institution of somatostatin therapy.

Diagnosis: Metastatic carcinoid tumor.

CASE 5.19

History: A 77-year-old male with a 35-lb weight loss in 3 months had an abdominal CT that demonstrated a 1.9-cm, nonspecific, low-density lesion in his pancreas. Although cystic pancreatic malignancy could not be excluded, pancreatic biopsy was unsuccessful. The patient was subsequently referred for an octreotide scintigram for further evaluation.

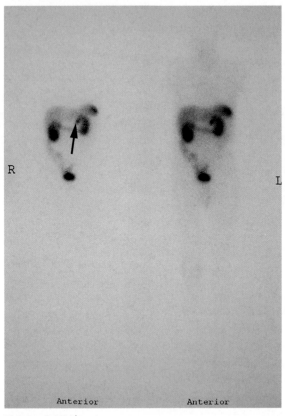

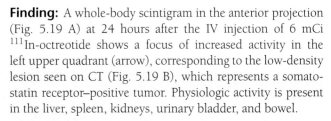

Figure 5.19 A

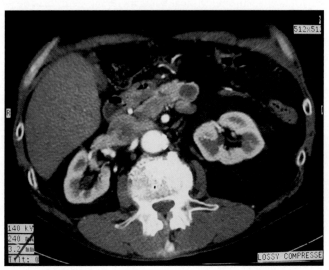

Figure 5.19 B

Finding: A whole-body scintigram in the anterior projection (Fig. 5.19 A) at 24 hours after the IV injection of 6 mCi ^{111}In-octreotide shows a focus of increased activity in the left upper quadrant (arrow), corresponding to the low-density lesion seen on CT (Fig. 5.19 B), which represents a somatostatin receptor–positive tumor. Physiologic activity is present in the liver, spleen, kidneys, urinary bladder, and bowel.

Discussion: In this patient with no specific signs and symptoms related to hormonal secretion by the tumor (flushing, diarrhea, hypoglycemia, etc.), the lesion most likely represents a nonfunctioning pancreatic neuroendocrine tumor.

The neuroendocrine tumor represents a heterogeneous group of clinical and histopathologic entities. The majority of these are well differentiated, very slow growing tumors with a benign behavior to a low-grade malignancy. Or they could be poorly differentiated tumors with a high-grade of malignancy.

Neuroendocrine tumors of the pancreas are relatively rare. They are slow-growing tumors that can be functional such as gastrinoma, insulinoma, vipoma, and others. Or they may be nonfunctional tumors. The nonfunctional tumor represents 10% to 30% of all cases of neuroendocrine lesions of the pancreas. Most neuroendocrine tumors, regardless of their

function, express a high density of somatostatin receptors; therefore, with the exception of insulinoma, they can be detected by octreotide scan with a sensitivity of 80% to 90%. In patients with a space-occupying lesion of the pancreas in whom the diagnosis cannot be made by biopsy or operation, the octreotide scan can help to differentiate a neuroendocrine lesion from nonneuroendocrine tumor.

Although the detection of lesions smaller than 1 cm may be difficult by planar scintigraphy, adding SPECT and particularly combining SPECT-CT (hybrid image) improves the lesion detectability and its localization. The use of ^{18}F-FDG PET for the detection of a nonfunctioning neuroendocrine lesion may be limited. Accumulation of ^{18}F-FDG depends on the metabolic activity and secretional pattern of the tumor.

A recently introduced new somatostatin analog labeled with the positron emitter gallium-68 (^{68}Ga) appears to be a promising agent for the detection of neuroendocrine tumors, particularly metastasis in the bone, liver, and node.

A positive octreotide scan not only helps to narrow the diagnosis but also indicates the feasibility of radiopeptide therapy.

Diagnosis: Nonfunctioning somatostatin receptor–positive pancreatic neuroendocrine mass.

CASE 5.20

History: During the workup for recurrent thrombocytopenia in a 51-year-old man who had undergone splenectomy 6 months earlier, a ^{99m}Tc–sulfur colloid liver–spleen scan was performed (Fig. 5.20 A).

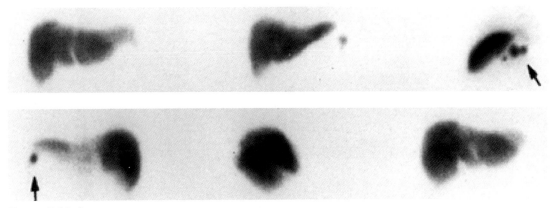

Figure 5.20 A

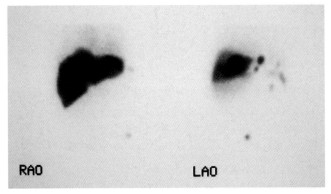

Figure 5.20 B

Findings: The scan shows a normal-appearing liver. There are several areas of focal uptake in the left upper quadrant in the splenic bed (arrow).

Discussion: Focal uptake of the ^{99m}Tc–sulfur colloid in the left upper quadrant in a patient with history of splenectomy may represent an accessory splenic tissue, residual spleen, or splenosis, which would explain this patient's recurrent thrombocytopenia.

Approximately 85% of the injected ^{99m}Tc–sulfur colloid particles are normally phagocytized in the reticular endothelial system of the liver and 5% to 10% localize in the spleen. Therefore splenic visualization on planar imaging may be difficult in conditions where minimally functioning splenic tissue, such as accessory spleen, is present.

The ^{99m}Tc-heat denatured RBC technique is another procedure that is more sensitive than and superior to ^{99m}Tc-sulfur colloid for the detection of an accessory spleen, splenosis, or any active splenic tissue. In heat-denatured RBC procedures,

the mixture of ^{99m}Tc-pertechnetate, stannous pyrophosphate, and the patient's RBCs is heated in a water bath. The RBCs convert to damaged, rigid spherocytes that, upon reinjection, are sequestered in the splenic tissue, allowing visualization of the spleen selectively.

Figure 5.20 B represents a scan of another patient with lymphoma who underwent splenectomy. Splenosis involving the left lobe of the liver and intra-abdominal splenosis in the left upper quadrant is well delineated. In patients with lymphoma following splenectomy, it is not unusual for CT to show an abdominal mass indistinguishable from splenosis left behind after surgery. Using the hybrid SPECT-CT camera, if available, the fused images accurately allow matching of functional and anatomic data and help localize any splenic tissue implanted into liver, thorax, plural space, etc., therefore excluding recurrent malignancy.

Figure 5.20 C represents a CT scan of another patient with vague abdominal pain. A 2-cm mass in the tail of the pancreas

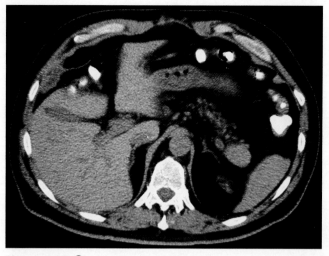

Figure 5.20 C

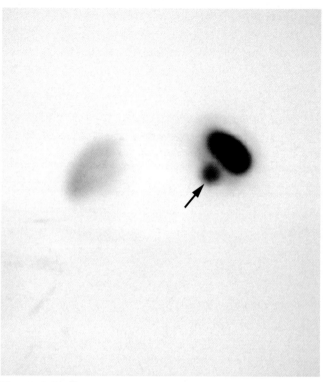

Figure 5.20 D

was detected. The ^{99m}Tc-heated damaged RBC SPECT image (Fig 5.20 D) shows focal uptake (arrow) corresponding to the location of the pancreatic mass, confirming the splenic nature of the lesion and avoiding biopsy.

An accessory spleen may be present in up to 10% of the general population and is usually of little clinical significance except that it may simulate a mass on CT examination. In up to 6% of CT examinations of the abdomen, an accessory spleen is seen. Scintigraphic technique can document the functional nature of the splenic tissue and obviate the need for invasive angiography or even laparotomy in some situations.

Visualization of an accessory spleen in patients with hematologic disorders after splenectomy is of clinical significance. Patients with the two commonly encountered hematologic disorders, spherocytosis and idiopathic thrombocytopenic purpura, often benefit from splenectomy. Thrombocytopenia may,

however, recur as a result of postsplenectomy hypertrophy of an accessory spleen or a splenic remnant requiring repeat surgical intervention.

An accessory spleen is usually located in and around the left upper quadrant in the immediate location of the splenic bed; however, an accessory spleen has been found in the tail of the pancreas, in the mesentery of the small bowel and large bowel, in female adnexa, and even in the scrotum.

It is worth noticing that, in patients following splenectomy, it is not unusual for the left lobe of the liver to extend to the left upper quadrant ("walking liver"); therefore, in a ^{99m}Tc–sulfur colloid scan, a focal uptake may represent a normal activity of the tip of the left lobe and not necessarily residual splenic tissue. This error can be avoided by observing the localization of ^{99m}Tc-HIDA derivative in the left upper quadrant, signifying the presence of liver tissue.

Diagnosis: Accessory spleen and splenules.

CASE 5.21

History: This 39-year-old patient with a history of colorectal cancer metastatic to the liver and spleen is status postchemotherapy. He is not a candidate for resection and is now referred for evaluation of visceral and pulmonary shunting of hepatic artery flow prior to Selective Internal Radiation (SIR) sphere therapy. 3.9-mCi ^{99m}Tc-MAA was injected into the patient's hepatic artery system through a catheter. Images of the abdomen and thorax were obtained in anterior and posterior projection and evaluated quantitatively (Fig. 5.21 A).

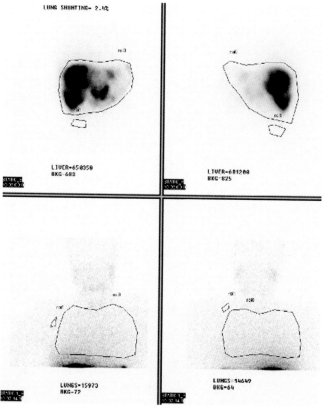

Figure 5.21 A

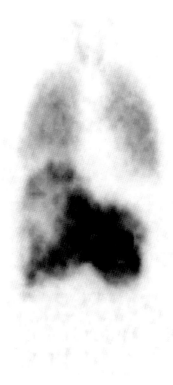

Figure 5.21 B

Finding: Activity is noted primarily within the right lower lobe of the liver. There is no significant pulmonary shunting, which is calculated at 2.4%.

Discussion: Metastatic liver disease has a very poor prognosis. In most patients the disease is inoperable at the time of diagnosis. The patient may get some benefit from hepatic arterial chemotherapy or hepatic artery embolization.

Although most of the liver tumor and metastases receive their blood supply through the hepatic artery, the hepatic artery also supplies the stomach and the duodenum. Therefore intrahepatic artery infusion of a chemotherapeutic agent may result in unwanted infusion into the upper GI tract.

^{99m}Tc-MAA injected directly into the hepatic artery through an inserted catheter is used to predict the distribution of

subsequently administered chemotherapeutic agents or microspheres. The images should be evaluated for the presence of extrahepatic activity, as in the stomach, pancreas, or spleen. Such a finding indicates that the catheter is not optimally positioned. The image should also be assessed for lung activity. Significant lung activity (over 20%) indicates intrahepatic arteriovenous shunting and predicts systemic toxicity following hepatic artery infusion of therapeutic agents. Figure 5.21 B shows a liver–lung image of a patient with liver metastasis following intra-arterial injection of 3 mCi of ^{99m}Tc-MAA. Marked pulmonary uptake identifies the presence of intrahepatic arteriovenous shunting.

The absence of pulmonary activity in Figure 5.21 A allowed delivery of therapeutic dose of 23.6 mCi of yttrium-90

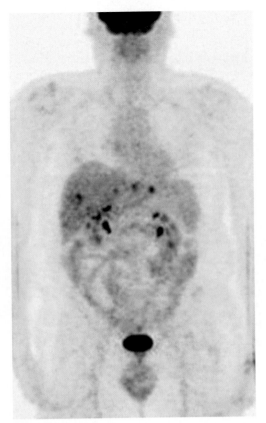

Figure 5.21 C

(^{90}Y)-labeled SIR spheres. A 3-month follow-up PET scan of this patient (Fig. 5.21 C) shows partial improvement, but a sizable tumor burden in the liver and abdomen is still present.

^{90}Y-labeled SIR spheres are used in the palliative treatment of inoperable liver metastases. ^{90}Y is a high-energy (2.29-MeV) pure beta emitter with a half-life of 64 hours. The diameter of the microspheres ranges from 20 to 30 μm, an effective size for microembolization of intravascular tumors. The dual action of radiation and embolization produces ischemic necrosis of the tumor and results in tumor shrinkage. The more vascular the tumor, the more likely it is to receive a greater deposition of microspheres and their associated radiation.

The intrahepatic arterial infusion of ^{90}Y microspheres appears to cause less toxicity than systemic chemotherapy, but significant side effects may be associated with this treatment. Reflux into the GI artery subsequently results in the deposition of particles into the stomach, pancreas, and spleen, which may cause extreme pain and GI toxicity. Hepatic failure and upper GI ulceration is a potential complication. GI bleed may occur. To avoid systemic and pulmonary toxicity, care must be taken to exclude those patients with intratumoral shunting.

Diagnosis: Hepatic arterial infusion in a patient with liver metastases.

CASE 5.22

History: A 42-year-old man with a history of ethanol abuse presents with increasing jaundice, a right pleural effusion, and ascites. He is referred for evaluation of a right-sided pleural effusion (Fig. 5.22).

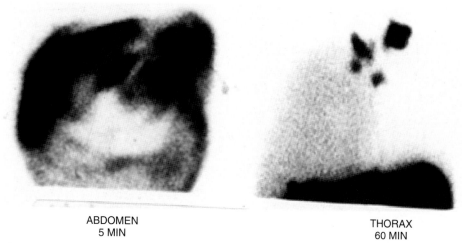

ABDOMEN
5 MIN

THORAX
60 MIN

Figure 5.22

Findings: Figure 5.22 (left) shows a static image of the abdomen 5 minutes following intraperitoneal injection of 5 mCi of ^{99m}Tc–sulfur colloid. Activity is widely dispersed throughout the ascitic fluid surrounding and displacing the bowel centrally, causing an area of void activity (photopenia in the center of the image).

Figure 5.22 (right) shows static images of the thorax 60 minutes following the introduction of ^{99m}Tc-sulfur colloid into the abdomen, delineating the right pleural cavity. A cluster of focal activity is also seen in the cervical thoracic region.

Discussion: The demonstration of unidirectional transdiaphragmatic flow of ascites into the pleural cavity after intraperitoneal injection of ^{99m}Tc-sulfur colloid is diagnostic of hepatic hydrothorax.

The clinical course of cirrhotic patients with or without ascites may become complicated by development of a pleural effusion. The incidence of pleural effusion in cirrhosis is approximately 6%. The passage of fluid occurs through microdefects in the tendinous portion of the diaphragm, which are much more common on the right than the left side. The left diaphragm is thicker and more muscular than the right and resists creation of defects as the result of increased intraabdominal pressure by ascites.

Distinguishing hepatic hydrothorax from other causes of pleural effusion may not be possible all the time. In addition,

ascites may not be completely excluded by physical examination and paracentesis. Ultrasonography may be needed to demonstrate a small amount of free abdominal fluid.

However, in the absence of clinical demonstration of ascites, which is commonly the case in hepatic hydrothorax, demonstration of pleural radioactivity indicates the presence of ascites, because the formation of free peritoneal fluid would be necessary to carry the radiotracer across the diaphragm. In addition, the procedure establishes the ascitic nature of the pleural effusion.

Establishing the diagnosis of hepatic hydrothorax would eliminate extensive investigation for pulmonary or cardiac causes of the pleural effusion. The procedure might also have management implications, as a LaVeen shunt operation may not be effective in these patients. Perhaps a transhepatic jugular intrahepatic portosystemic stent (TIPS) or surgical correction would be more beneficial.

The cluster of activity seen in this case conceivably represents phagocytosis of ^{99m}Tc–sulfur colloid particles by the lymph nodes in the cervicothoracic region. The transpleural absorption of sulfur colloid is known to occur. Radiotracer enters the lymphatic and systemic venous circulation, reaching the organs containing reticuloendothelial system, such as lymph nodes.

Diagnosis: Hepatic hydrothorax.

CASE 5.23

History: One year following LaVeen shunt placement, a 49-year-old man with alcoholic cirrhosis and intractable ascites returns to the nuclear medicine service for evaluation of shunt patency (Fig. 5.23 A).

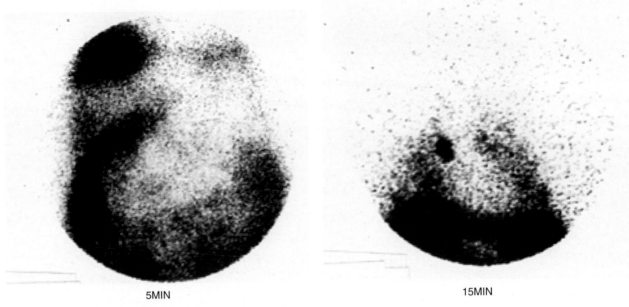

5MIN   15MIN

Figure 5.23 A

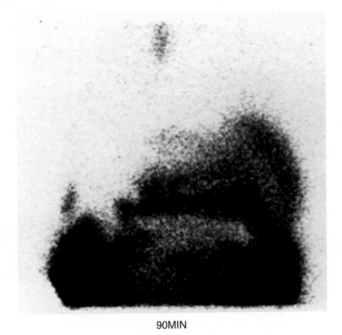

90MIN

Figure 5.23 B

Findings: Static images of the abdomen (Fig. 5.23 A, left) at 5 minutes after intraperitoneal injection of 5 mCi of ^{99m}Tc-MAA show dispersement of radioactivity in the ascitic fluid. The hepatic silhouette and centrally located loops of bowel are seen as areas of photopenia.

Static images of the thorax (Fig. 5.23 A, right) at 15 minutes reveal the presence of radioactivity outlining both lung fields. A focus of activity is seen in the right parasternal region.

Discussion: Visualization of the lung indicates a patent and functioning shunt. Labeled MAA particles have entered the venous circulation through the venous limbs of the shunt and are trapped in the lungs.

Intractable ascites is treated effectively by LaVeen peritoneal venous shunt, which runs along the thoracic wall from the peritoneal cavity to the jugular vein, ending near the right atrium. This shunt has a one-way valve that allows forward flow of ascites from the peritoneal cavity toward the jugular vein and prevents backflow of venous blood. Shunt malfunction occurs in 5% to 8% of cases, and a frequent complication is obstruction. Occlusion usually occurs in the peritoneal limb of the shunt as the result of accumulation of fibrinoid material around its tip. Occlusion at the venous site is less common and occurs as the result of blood clot formation in the lumen around the tip of the shunt.

The scintigraphic procedure of injecting ^{99m}Tc-MAA into the peritoneal cavity followed by imaging of the thorax is a simple and safe method of assessing the patency of the LaVeen shunt. Lung visualization indicates some patency, whereas the lack of activity uptake implies shunt obstruction.

Figure 5.23 B shows the 90-minute image of another patient with a LaVeen shunt. Although dispersement of radioactivity in the abdominal cavity is seen, no activity is present in the thorax, indicating an obstructed shunt.

During the scintigraphic procedure, it is possible to visualize the shunt coursing along the thoracic wall; however, shunt visualization depends on the flow rate of ascites and should not be depended on as a criterion for shunt patency. Lung visualization is the best criterion. In addition, this study can be considered semiquantitative, because the intensity of lung uptake is proportional to the degree of shunt patency and flow rate across the shunt.

The focus of activity in the right parasternal region conceivably represents a small blood clot labeled with MAA. Transperitoneal absorption of MAA has not been reported, and it is very unlikely to occur as early as 15 minutes.

Diagnosis: Patent LaVeen shunt.

CASE 5.24

History: This 50-year-old patient underwent a laparoscopic cholecystectomy 6 weeks earlier; he also has a remote history of splenectomy. The patient had an abdominal CT (Fig. 5.24 A) for reasons not related to the hepatobiliary system. The scan shows a 4-cm area of low attenuation in the lateral aspect of the right lobe, raising the possibility of a subcapsular biloma secondary to postcholecystectomy bile leak. A hepatobiliary scan (Fig. 5.24 B) was performed for further evaluation.

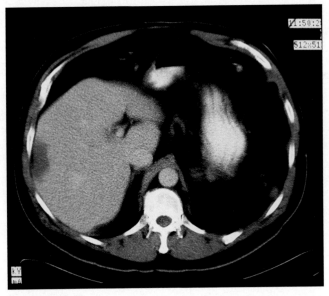

Figure 5.24 A

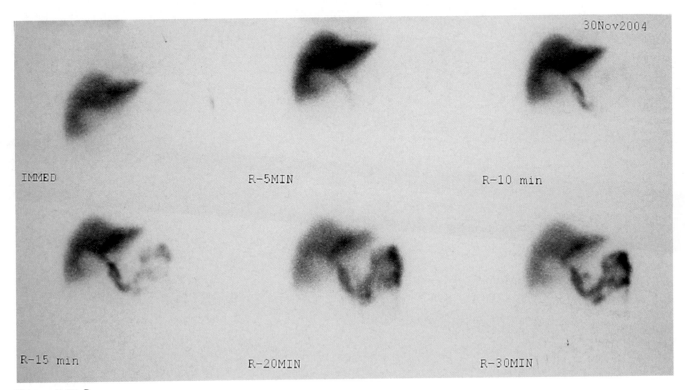

Figure 5.24 B

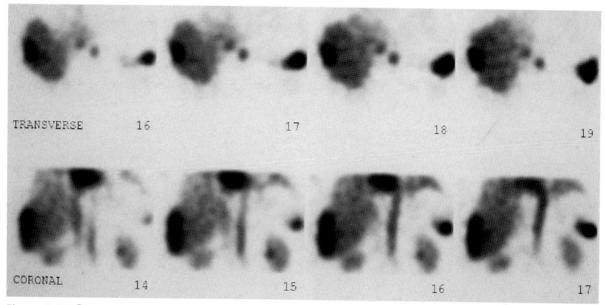

TRANSVERSE   16   17   18   19

CORONAL   14   15   16   17

Figure 5.24 C

Findings: Hepatobiliary scan shows normal visualization of the liver, common bile duct, and loops of bowel by 15 minutes. There is no evidence of extravasation of bile to account for the CT finding.

Discussion: Hepatobiliary scan is an established technique for the diagnosis of bile leak but can also effectively exclude this diagnosis and lead to search for other causes of observed CT abnormality.

Further characterization of this liver lesion was made by a hepatic blood pool scan (Fig. 5.24 C), showing increased blood pool activity congruent with the low attenuation lesion seen on CT and representing a cavernous hemangioma.

Note the presence of focal uptake of blood pool in the left upper quadrant of the splenic bed. In this patient with a history of splenectomy, this activity most likely represents residual splenic tissue or accessory spleen.

Cavernous hemangioma of the liver is a common benign hepatic tumor present in about 5% to 10% of patients and usually presents as a unifocal mass, although it may also be multifocal.

The generally accepted typical appearance of cavernous hemangioma on ultrasound is that of a small (less than 4 cm), well-marginated, echogenic mass usually located in the subcapsular region of the right lobe and often associated with some posterior acoustic shadowing. However, more than 40% of hemangiomas have an atypical appearance on ultrasound and some malignant lesions may appear hyperechoic.

Dynamic enhanced CT is another technique for detecting cavernous hemangioma. It typically shows a hypodense lesion that enhances in a centripetal fashion after administration of IV contrast. However, approximately 24% of hemangiomas do not fulfill the CT criteria and giant hemangioma (those being larger than 4 cm), rarely show complete enhancement, and remain as indeterminate lesions requiring further evaluation.

Hepatic blood pool scintigraphy for detection of cavernous hemangioma consists of a flow study (usually in the projection closer to the known lesion) followed by early (5- to 20-minute) and delayed (1- to 2-hour) planar images often supplemented by SPECT imaging (Fig. 5.24 C).

Both the flow and the delayed images are important. Detection of increased flow despite delayed pooling is not the expected pattern for a cavernous hemangioma. Cavernous hemangiomas are venous structures and do not have an arterial blood supply, so early arterial perfusion is unusual. A substantial number of patients with such a pattern are found to have hepatoma or other neoplasms.

Early (20- to 30-minute) planar images may not provide sufficient time for adequate filling, so delayed (1- to 2-hour), particularly SPECT, imaging may be necessary for visualization.

Lesion diameter is the major limiting factor in detection of hepatic hemangioma by blood pool scintigraphy. Generally, a planar image is able to detect a lesion 3 cm or larger and SPECT is sensitive for a lesion larger than 1.5 cm. Overall, SPECT improves sensitivity for the detection of small cavernous hemangiomas, particularly for multiple or centrally located lesions and for those adjacent to vascular structures. T2-weighted MRI is particularly useful for the characterization of small lesions located near the vascular structures. Furthermore, using a hybrid SPECT-CT camera would allow the functional and anatomic images to be fused in a single view, facilitating localization and characterization of the lesions more accurately.

Characterization of giant cavernous hemangioma may be difficult. A giant cavernous hemangioma is larger than 8 cm in size and has a nonspecific appearance on ultrasound. As a result of fibrosis, hemorrhage, and necrosis, the majority of giant cavernous hemangiomas appear as solid masses with mixed echo patterns indistinguishable from other tumors. However, a delayed ^{99m}Tc–RBC SPECT image in multiple projections and careful examination of the image should help to reveal the nature of the lesion in most cases.

Diagnosis: Cavernous hemangioma.

CASE 5.25

History: On abdominal CT examination of this 70-year-old patient with a history of alcohol abuse and lung cancer, note is made of an area of low attenuation in the anterior segment of the right hepatic lobe (Figure 5.25 A). A planar abdominal blood pool image (Fig. 5.25 B) supplemented by SPECT images (Fig. 5.25 C) were obtained for evaluation of possible cavernous hemangioma of the liver.

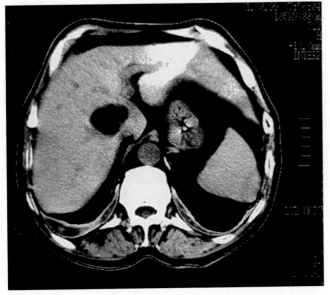

Figure 5.25 A

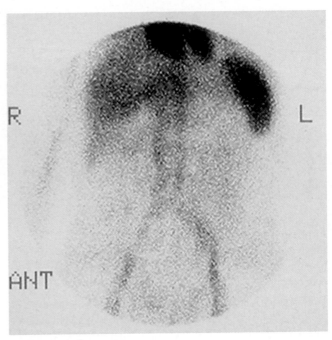

Figure 5.25 B

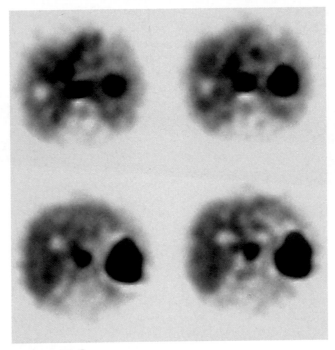

Figure 5.25 C

Findings: A planar image of the abdominal blood pool (Fig. 5.25 B) shows somewhat reduced hepatic blood pool compared with the spleen, perhaps due to early stages of portal hypertension and cirrhosis. However, no focal area of increased or decreased blood pool activity is seen. A normal blood pool in the aorta, inferior vena cava, and iliac vessels is identified. On SPECT images (Fig. 5.25 C), however, a well-defined, rounded area of photopenia corresponding to the location of the liver lesion visualized on CT is easily seen.

Discussion: A low-density lesion on CT examination could represent a cavernous hemangioma; but a metastatic lesion, hepatoma, and infrequently a benign liver lesion may appear similarly. A photopenic area on blood pool images corresponding to a low-attenuation lesion noted on the liver CT excludes the diagnosis of cavernous hemangioma. Cavernous hemangioma is expected to show focally increased uptake on sequential hepatic blood pool images, with an improved detection rate using the SPECT.

The photopenic appearance of the liver lesion on the hepatic blood pool scan may be due to hepatoma with tumor necrosis, abscess, or hepatic cyst. Therefore, on CT examination of patients, particularly with a known primary, if the liver lesion does not have a typical appearance of hepatic cyst, it should be considered indeterminate, requiring further investigation.

The negative blood pool scan for cavernous hemangioma corresponding to the patient's incidental CT finding led to conservative management with follow-up CT and ultrasound examinations at 3 months and 6 months, which show no interval change in the size and configuration of lesion, supporting the presence of a stable cystic liver lesion.

Liver cyst is a congenital anomaly representing a fluid-filled space having an epithelial lining. Therefore other fluid-filled structures—such as abscess, parasitic cyst, and traumatic cyst—are not true cysts. Although they are congenital, it is not known why true liver cysts appear late in life. Their frequency is approximately 2.5% in the general population; however, it reaches 7% in a population over 80 years of age.

Diagnosis: Liver cyst.

CASE 5.26

History: A 30-year-old woman with a past history of esophageal ulcer presented with vague, intermittent abdominal pain and thrombocytopenia. The patient's diagnostic workup included an abdominal CT (Fig. 5.26 A).

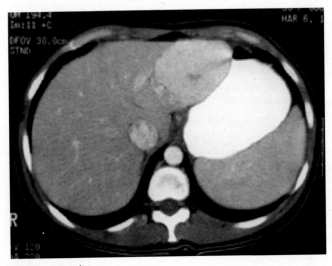

Figure 5.26 A

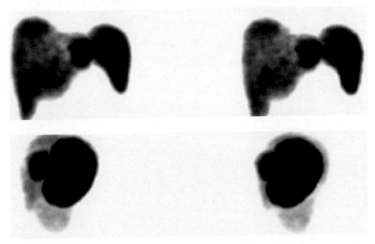

Figure 5.26 B

Findings: The abdominal CT is notable for splenomegaly and a contrast-enhancing, homogeneous, well-demarcated hepatic mass with a small area of central scarring involving the lateral segment of the left lobe.

Discussion: Although CT is the current modality of choice for the detection of liver mass lesions, it does not provide functional information. Ultrasound, scintigraphy, angiography, and MRI each can provide additional clues to the diagnosis.

Scintigraphy using a variety of radionuclides is a powerful tool in the characterization of focal nodular hyperplasia, hepatic adenoma, focal fatty infiltration, cavernous hemangioma, hepatocellular carcinoma, and regenerating nodules.

A ^{99m}Tc–sulfur colloid liver–spleen scan (Fig. 5.26 B) shows a well-defined area of increased uptake in the left lobe corresponding to the mass detected on CT. Correlation of the image's appearance with clinical information is often required to attain a specific diagnosis. Of the clinical information, the patient's

age and gender are important. Although malignant lesions are more frequent in males, benign tumors appear more frequently in females.

For the female who is aged 18 to 40 years, the more common hepatic tumors are cavernous hemangioma, focal nodular hyperplasia, adenoma, and fibrolamellar carcinoma. From the standpoint of image appearance, a mass lesion within the liver generally creates an area of photopenia. An area of radiocolloid accumulation (hot spot) in the liver is an uncommon finding. It is seen most frequently with focal nodular hyperplasia, but cases of hamartoma, hemangioma, and hepatoma have been reported.

Focal nodular hyperplasia appears typically as a solitary solid mass, usually detected incidentally in asymptomatic young women. Histologically, the tumor has a thin capsule with a small central fibrous scar and numerous bile ducts. All the liver's elements, including Kupffer cells, are present. Owing

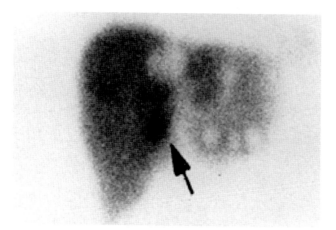

Figure 5.26 C

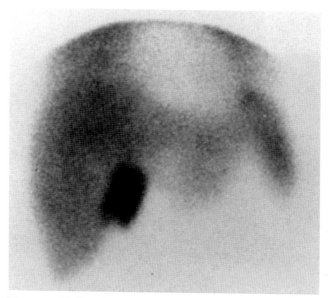

Figure 5.26 D

to the presence of Kupffer cells, 40% to 70% of tumors show a normal or increased uptake of technetium sulfur colloid. Scintigraphy appears to be more specific for characterization of this tumor than CT. A contrast-enhancing lesion with a central area of scarring on CT is highly suggestive of focal nodular hyperplasia; however, increased uptake of ^{99m}Tc–sulfur colloid, seen in 10% of the cases, is quite specific for a focal nodular hyperplasia, assuring a benign mass. Histologic diagnosis of a benign hepatic tumor, compatible with focal nodular hyperplasia, was made by biopsy in this case.

In differential diagnosis of the liver's hot spot on ^{99m}Tc–sulfur colloid scan, the condition causing an alteration in hepatic circulatory dynamic should be considered. This includes obstruction of the superior vena cava and inferior vena cava and hepatovenous occlusive disease (Budd–Chiari syndrome).

A hot spot due to superior vena cava obstruction appears in the region of the quadrate lobe when colloid is injected in the upper extremity. In obstruction of the superior vena cava, the collateral vessels return blood via the internal mammary and left umbilical veins into the quadrate lobe, creating a hot spot in the area of insertion of the left umbilical vein and left main branches of the portal vein. Figure 5.26 C shows a liver–spleen scan of a patient with superior vena cava obstruction secondary to lung cancer, with multiple metastases of the left lobe and a hot spot in the region of the liver's quadrate lobe (arrow).

In obstruction of the inferior vena cava, injection of ^{99m}Tc–sulfur colloid or MAA into a lower extremity vein results in a hot spot in the quadrate lobe. In obstructed inferior vena cava, venous blood returning from the lower extremity reroutes through collateral channels to the left umbilical vein and into the left portal vein. Figure 5.26 D shows a combined liver–lung scan in a patient with obstruction of the inferior vena cava (1). ^{99m}Tc–sulfur colloid had been injected in the upper extremity, visualizing the liver and spleen. ^{99m}Tc-MAA had been injected in the lower extremity, visualizing the lung as well as the quadrate lobe of the liver.

A hot spot due to hepatovenous occlusive disease (Budd–Chiari syndrome) appears in the caudate lobe of the liver, projecting in the midline area of the liver. In Budd–Chiari syndrome, congestion, hemorrhage, and necrosis of the parenchyma occur owing to obstruction of the hepatic veins. The resultant abnormal drainage of the liver causes a marked diffuse decrease in uptake of radiocolloid. However, the caudate lobe, because of its direct drainage to the inferior vena cava, remains intact, hypertrophies, and appears as a zone of increased uptake surrounded by an area of diminished uptake.

Diagnosis: Focal nodular hyperplasia.

CASE 5.27

History: In a 67-year-old man with known squamous cell carcinoma of the lung, CT demonstrated a large 9-cm mass in the left lobe of the liver extending to the hilum that is suggestive of malignancy, either primary or metastatic (Fig. 5.27 A). On a prebiopsy ultrasound to evaluate the feasibility of the epigastric approach (Fig. 5.27 B), the appearance of fatty infiltration was noted. This was further evaluated using ^{99m}Tc–sulfur colloid (Fig. 5.27 C).

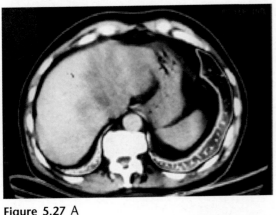

Figure 5.27 A

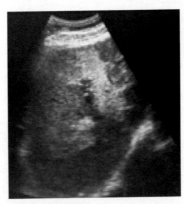

Figure 5.27 B

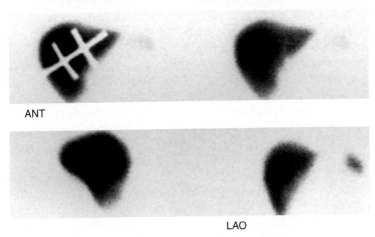

ANT

LAO

Figure 5.27 C

Finding: The liver–spleen scan demonstrates a normal homogeneous distribution of radioactivity throughout the liver with no photopenia to suggest a space-occupying lesion.

Discussion: A normal sulfur colloid liver–spleen scan excludes a space-occupying lesion as the cause of the CT abnormality and helps differentiate hepatic fatty infiltration from a mass lesion. A primary or metastatic lesion appears as an area of photopenia, whereas fatty infiltration has an essentially normal appearance. Fatty infiltration, either diffuse or focal, is characterized pathologically by deposition of the fat droplet in the hepatocyte, sparing the reticuloendothelial system. There is no displacement of the Kupffer cells; therefore a sulfur colloid scan, being a functional image of the Kupffer cells, demonstrates a normal pattern or, at most, may show minimal inhomogeneity of uptake.

The pattern of fatty infiltration of the liver varies depending on the amount of fat deposited, the pattern of distribution, the stage of resolution, and the presence or absence of other intrahepatic disease. Focal fatty infiltration of the liver commonly has a segmental or lobar wedge-shaped configuration. There is no mass effect on adjacent structures. Rapid improvement and changes in the pattern are known to occur on CT.

In a wide cross-section of patients at risk for fatty infiltration (alcohol abuse, diabetes, morbid obesity, hypertriglyceridemia, steroid therapy, parenteral hyperalimentation, malnutrition, cystic fibrosis, jejunal ileal bypass surgery, and carbon tetrachloride exposure) in whom a focal abnormality is discovered on CT or ultrasound, a normal sulfur colloid scan may reveal the abnormality to be related to fatty metamorphosis rather than neoplasm; therefore biopsy can be deferred. However, in patients with a discrete mass detected in a cirrhotic or fatty liver, there should be a very low tolerance for excluding tumor, especially in patients with known primary malignancy. These patients usually require biopsy.

In this patient, due to the history of lung cancer, the clinician decided to perform a CT-guided biopsy of the liver, which revealed fatty metamorphosis without malignancy.

Diagnosis: Fatty metamorphosis of the liver.

CASE 5.28

History: A 79-year-old diabetic patient with end-stage renal disease and ongoing temperature spikes is referred for an ^{111}In-labeled–WBC scan to evaluate the possibility of access infection or other infectious sources (Figs. 5.28 A and 5.28 B).

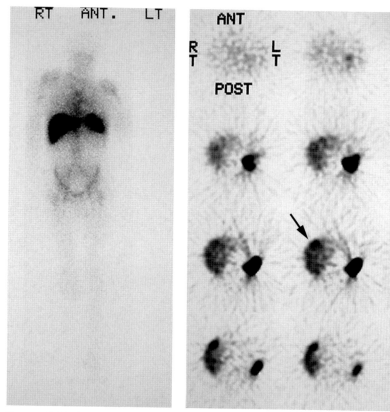

Figure 5.28 A   **Figure 5.28 B**

Finding: A whole-body scan (Fig. 5.28 A) performed 24 hours after injection of autologous WBCs labeled with 418 uCi of ^{111}In-oxime shows a normal distribution of radioactivity in the liver, spleen, and bone marrow. There is a small area of scalloping along the supralateral aspect of the spleen felt to represent an area of infarct. SPECT images of the upper abdomen (Fig. 5.28 B) show a focus of accumulation of radiolabeled WBCs in the anterior segment of the right lobe (arrow) of the liver, most consistent with a liver abscess. This was subsequently evaluated by CT (Fig. 5.28 C) and confirmed by percutaneous drainage.

Discussion: Pyogenic liver abscess is not common these days; however, it is a life-threatening disease. Diabetes mellitus is an important risk factor and is associated with a poor prognosis. Liver abscess may develop following surgery for appendicitis or appendocele abscess. Abscess may be secondary to obstruction of the biliary tract, particularly in elderly patients.

In a patient with fever and hepatic lesions, abnormality may be due to abscess or tumor, particularly in a patient with known primary. Liver abscess as well as tumor present as an area of space-occupying lesion and therefore appear as a photopenic lesion on ^{99m}Tc–sulfur colloid scan, a nonspecific finding. CT appearance of the liver abscess varies and may not be distin-

guishable from other lesions. Differentiation of an abscess from a necrotic tumor may be difficult or impossible. Abscess and noninfected cyst may have the same appearance.

Labeled autologous WBCs with ^{111}In-oxime scintigraphy is extremely useful for imaging most infectious lesions and can differentiate abscess from tumor. If the liver lesion shows accumulation of ^{111}In-labeled WBCs, the abscess is by far the most probable diagnosis. This is due to its high degree of specificity for infectious lesions that have polymorphonuclear infiltration, which is not a feature of hepatic tumor or other noninfected masses. Figure 5.28 D represents an ^{111}In-WBC scan in a patient with polycystic disease. The scan is done to evaluate for evidence of an infected renal cyst. The image shows no evidence of infection; however, an area of photopenia corresponding to a noninfected liver cyst is present. Figure 5.28 E displays a whole-body ^{111}In-WBC scan in a patient with spiking fever and liver metastases. Multiple areas of photopenia are easily identifiable in an enlarged liver, but there is no evidence of liver abscess.

Interpretation of an ^{111}In-WBC scan can be done easily since a normal scan should show distribution of radioactivity in the liver, spleen, and bone marrow. There should be no urinary tract or GI tract activity.

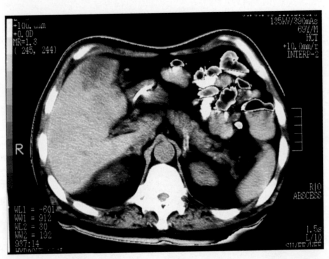

Figure 5.28 C

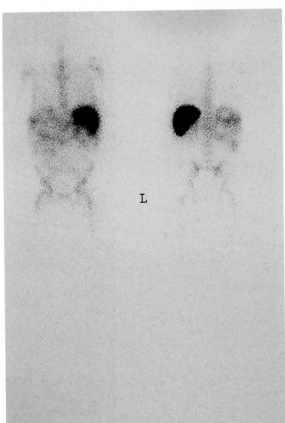

Figure 5.28 E

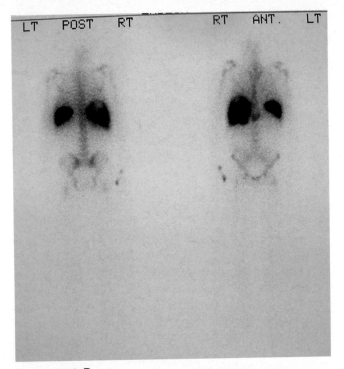

Figure 5.28 D

It is to be noted that because of the physiologic distribution of radioactivity in the liver, spleen, and bone marrow, the localization of pathology in or adjacent to these organs may be difficult. SPECT images are extremely helpful in disclosing the abnormality, which may be obscured on the planar images, as in this case. The integration of scintigraphic and anatomic data (fusion of SPECT and CT image) further improves the lesion's detectability and localization. By careful analysis of the high-quality image, correlation with available anatomic study and utilization of SPECT or SPECT CT, many abdominal infectious processes—such as subphrenic abscess, subhepatic abscess, infected aortic graft, appendocele abscess, infected diverticular disease, psoas abscess, and gallbladder empyema—can be easily identified.

A false-negative scan is not common. The scan may be negative in a few conditions such as chronic encapsulated or nonpyogenic abscess, fungal infection, and infections due to opportunistic organisms (lack of neutrophilic infiltration response). A false-positive scan is also not common. Active bleeding will show activity in the bowel on the early images. Bowel activity on the delayed images may be due to expectorated and swallowed WBCs from the lung and upper airway which usually migrates to the right colon by 24 hours. In patients with a history of splenectomy, the focus of radiolabeled WBCs may be due to an accessory spleen and should not be mistaken for an abscess.

Diagnosis: Liver abscess.

History: A 33-year-old male with Crohn's disease and evidence of stricture in the ileum is referred to assess the inflammatory activity of small bowel disease.

The patient's WBCs were labeled *in vitro* with 13.6 mCi of ^{99m}Tc-HMPAO. One hour following the injection of the labeled blood, a whole-body scan was performed (Fig. 5.29 A).

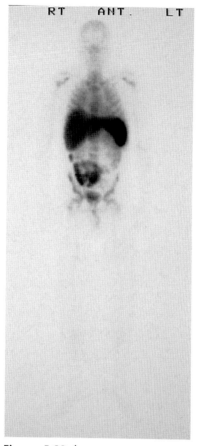

Figure 5.29 A

Finding: Abnormal uptake is present in a long segment of the bowel that courses over the right-mid-lower abdomen extending from the midline. In addition, a focus of abnormal uptake is seen in the right midflank area. There is normal physiologic distribution of activity in the liver, spleen, and bone marrow.

Discussion: Scintigraphic findings of the uptake of radiolabeled WBCs in two segments of small bowel are consistent with active inflammatory disease and the patient's known diagnosis of Crohn's disease.

^{99m}Tc-HMPAO–labeled WBC scintigraphy is an effective technique for identifying the site and extent of inflammatory bowel disease. It reliably localizes the disease to a specific segment and particularly identifies the small bowel.

HMPAO is a lipophilic complex that can penetrate the membranes of WBCs; therefore the ^{99m}Tc-labeled HMPAO enters the cell. Following cell entry, the complex becomes hydrophilic and is trapped inside the cell.

The normal distribution of ^{99m}Tc-HMPAO–labeled WBCs is similar to that of ^{111}In-labeled WBCs, predominantly distributing in the liver, spleen, and bone marrow. Bone marrow activity is prominent in the very early image, as is the lung activity; this is due to margination of labeled granulocytes in the lung and bone marrow. Unlike those of ^{111}In-labeled WBCs, the late images of the ^{99m}Tc-HMPAO WBCs show nonspecific activity in the bowel, kidney, urinary bladder, and gallbladder. This nonspecific activity, which appears on 2- to 4-hour images, is the result of excretion of the hydrophilic complex of the ^{99m}Tc-HMPAO. This nonspecific bowel activity occurring in the late images may cause difficulty in evaluating inflammatory bowel disease. It is to be noted that the localization of ^{99m}Tc-HMPAO-labeled WBCs in the inflamed bowel is extremely rapid. Therefore the scan should be done within the first hour of the injection, before the nonspecific bowel activity appears. However, in doubtful cases, delayed 2- to 4-hour images may be obtained for confirmation. Careful preparation of the patient with voiding of urinary bladder activity before scintigraphy is also necessary in order to avoid a false-negative scan from masking of disease in the pelvis due to the urinary bladder activity.

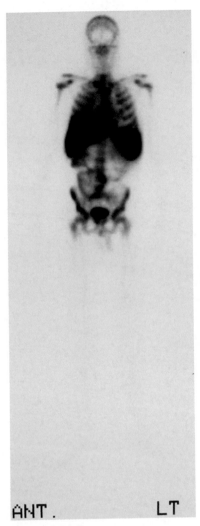

Figure 5.29 B

Scintigraphy with ^{99m}Tc-HMPAO–labeled WBCs is also useful in the follow-up of patients with inflammatory bowel disease to assess disease activity, distinguish fibrosis from active disease or exacerbation, and evaluate the response to treatment.

Figure 5.29 B is a 6-month follow-up showing continuation of the inflammatory process, although with some interval improvement. The bulk of inflammatory bowel has reduced in size and the intensity of activity has decreased.

Crohn's disease and ulcerative colitis can be distinguished from each other by ^{99m}Tc-HMPAO-labeled WBC scintigraphy. Small bowel involvement, skip areas, and rectal sparing are suggestive of Crohn's disease. Ulcerative colitis is usually more pronounced in the left side of the colon, involving the rectum and extending into the rectosigmoid in a continuous pattern with no skip areas.

Although the sensitivity of ^{99m}Tc-HMPAO–labeled WBCs for the detection of inflammatory bowel disease is widely established, there are other abdominal conditions in which the differentiation from inflammatory bowel disease may be difficult. In addition to nonspecific bowel activity, conditions including recently established bowel anastomosis, GI bleeding, radiation enteritis, and graft-versus-host disease may cause a false-positive scan for irritable bowel disease (IBD). An abdominal abscess between the loops of bowel may be interpreted as IBD. Abscess communicating with bowel, as occurs commonly in Crohn's disease, as well as a fistulous formation involving the urinary tract, may be difficult to assess. Obtaining the early images and using hybrid SPECT-CT imaging provides additional anatomic information that may help and allow the correct identification of the involved organs and bowel segment.

Diagnosis: Crohn's disease.

CASE 5.30

History: A 59-year-old man with a history of ventricular tachycardia who had recently undergone placement of an automatic intracardiac defibrillation (AICD) presents with fever of unknown etiology. He had been on long-term antibiotic therapy. An ^{111}In-WBC image (Fig. 5.30) was obtained for the evaluation of possible AICD pocket infection.

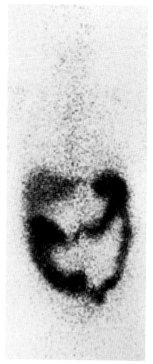

Figure 5.30

Findings: The 24-hour whole-body image of ^{111}In-WBCs shows intense activity in the entire large bowel. There is normal uptake in the liver and spleen.

Discussion: The ^{111}In-labeled WBCs do not normally localize in the bowel, in contrast to ^{67}Ga-citrate, for which the bowel is the major excretory pathway. Therefore colonic localization of ^{111}In-WBCs is abnormal, usually representing a disorder such as inflammatory bowel disease, ischemic colitis, pseudomembranous colitis, or bacterial colitis. Colonic activity also may be produced by multiple enemas. A focal area of increased uptake may also may seen as a result of diverticulitis or bowel fistula.

In the interpretation of bowel activity, one should be aware of the pitfalls and the frequency of false-positive findings. The false-positive cases usually fall into one of two groups. The findings in the first group are due to swallowed WBCs secondary to sinusitis, pharyngitis, a tracheostomy tube, or pulmonary infection. The findings in the second are related to GI bleeding. Clinical correlation and the result of other imaging procedures help to avoid misinterpretation. In general, intense uptake of ^{111}In-WBCs represents a true-positive finding. The false-positive findings are commonly associated with less intense uptake. It may not be possible to distinguish between bowel wall activity due to colitis and intraluminal activity related to swallowing or bleeding. In general, however, activity in the bowel content usually shifts with time, which helps to arrive at a correct diagnosis. For this reason, in the patient suspected of having inflammatory bowel disease, it is helpful to have an early 4-hour image in addition to the routine 24-hour images.

If the scan is done and interpreted properly in appropriate clinical conditions, a sensitivity of 90% and a specificity as high as 95% is expected for ^{111}In-WBC imaging for the detection of abdominal inflammation.

In the current case, further diagnostic workup included stool analysis and sigmoidoscopy, which demonstrated diffuse pseudomembranous colitis due to *Clostridium difficile*. It is interesting that a positive finding is more frequent in pseudomembranous colitis than in ulcerative colitis and Crohn's disease. In addition, when chronic diseases are localized or the area is proximal, the noninvasive scintigram may be helpful in identifying the site of abnormality and directing the invasive techniques, such as colonoscopy, for final diagnosis.

Diagnosis: Pseudomembranous colitis.

SOURCES AND SUGGESTED READING

1. Maurer AH, Parkman HP. Update on gastrointestinal scintigraphy. *Semin Nucl Med* 2006;36:110–118.
2. Urbain JL, Charkes ND. Recent advances in gastric emptying scintigraphy. *Semin Nucl Med* 1995;25:318–325.
3. Nusynowitz ML, Benedetto AR. The lag phase of gastric emptying: clinical, mathematical and in vitro studies. *J Nucl Med* 1994;35(6):1023–1027.
4. Maurer AH. Gastrointestinal bleeding and cine-scintigraphy. *Semin Nucl Med* 1996;26:43–50.
5. Howarth DM. The role of nuclear medicine in the detection of acute gastrointestinal bleeding. *Semin Nucl Med* 2006;36(2):133–146.
6. Levy AD, Hobbs CM. Meckel diverticulum: radiologic features with pathologic correlation. *Radiographics* 2004;24(2):565–587.
7. Ziessman HA. Cholecystokinin cholescintigraphy: clinical indications and proper methodology. *Radiol Clin North Am* 2001;39(5):997–1006.
8. Ziessman HA. Functional hepatobiliary disease: chronic acalculous gallbladder and chronic acalculous biliary disease. *Semin Nucl Med* 2006;36(2):119–132.
9. Rosenberg DJ, Brugge WR, Alavi A. Bile leak following an elective laparoscopic cholecystectomy: the role of hepatobiliary imaging in the diagnosis and management of bile leaks. *J Nucl Med* 1991;32(9):1777–1781.
10. Ramachandran A, Gupta SM, Johns WD. Various presentations of postcholecystectomy bile leak diagnosed by scintigraphy. *Clin Nucl Med* 2001;26(6):495–498.
11. Davis LP, McCarroll K. Correlative imaging of the liver and hepatobiliary system. *Semin Nucl Med* 1994;24(3):208–218.
12. Kinnard MF, Alavi A, Rubin RA, Lichtenstein GR. Nuclear imaging of solid hepatic masses. *Semin Roentgenol* 1995;30(4):375–395.
13. Schillaci O, Filippi L, Danieli R, et al. Single-photon emission computed tomography/computed tomography in abdominal diseases. *Semin Nucl Med* 2007;37(1):48–61.
14. Kwekkeboom DJ, Krenning EP. Somatostatin receptor imaging. *Semin Nucl Med* 2002;32(2):84–91.
15. Schillaci O. Somatostatin receptor imaging in patients with neuroendocrine tumors: not only SPECT? *J Nucl Med* 2007;48(4):498–500.
16. Chintapalli KN, Schinitker JB. Spleen imaging. *Appl Radiol* 1994;23(12):29–37.
17. Phom H, Kumar A, Tripathi M, et al. Comparative evaluation of Tc-99m–heat-denatured RBC and Tc-99m-anti-D IgG opsonized RBC spleen planar and SPECT scintigraphy in the detection of accessory spleen in postsplenectomy patients with chronic idiopathic thrombocytopenic purpura. *Clin Nucl Med* 2004;29(7):403–409.
18. Dancey JE, Shepherd FA, et al. Treatment of nonresectable hepatocellular carcinoma with intrahepatic 90y-microspheres. *J Nucl Med* 2000;41(10):1673–1681.
19. Huynh LT, Kim SY, Murphy TF. The typical appearance of focal nodular hyperplasia in triple-phase CT scan, hepatobiliary scan, and Tc-99m sulfur colloid scan with SPECT. *Clin Nucl Med* 2005;30(11):736–739.
20. Datz FL. Abdominal abscess detection: gallium, [111]In-, and ^{99m}Tc-labeled WBCs, and polyclonal and monoclonal antibodies. *Semin Nucl Med* 1996;26(1):51–64.
21. Peters AM. The utility of [99mTc] HMPAO-WBCs for imaging infection. *Semin Nucl Med* 1994;24(2):110–127.

CHAPTER SIX

RENAL SCINTIGRAPHY

CARLOS CUNHA PEREIRA NETO
AND DOMINIQUE DELBEKE

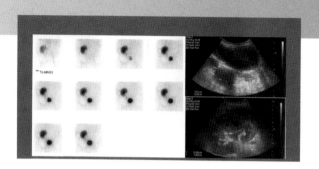

Renal scintigraphy has been used in clinical nephrourology since the early 1960s. It provides functional and anatomic information, both closely related. Structural information, however, is limited. Functional information is quite unique. For example, a radionuclide study can separately measure renal function on each side.

Common indications of renal scintigraphy are assessment of renal perfusion, renal function, renovascular hypertension (RVH), pyelonephritis, urinary tract obstruction, renal transplantation and acute renal failure. Also, radionuclide cystography (RNC) and scrotal scintigraphy have a well-established place in detecting vesicoureteral reflux (VUR) and torsion epididymoorchitis, respectively. In this chapter, renal radiopharmaceuticals and common protocols in nuclear nephrourology are discussed, followed by case presentations. A good review is available (1,2,3,4).

RADIOPHARMACEUTICALS IN RENAL SCINTIGRAPHY

There are many radiopharmaceuticals available for renal scintigraphy. Selection of the radiopharmaceutical depends upon the specific clinical question that is asked. Based on the mechanism of uptake, renal radiopharmaceuticals can be divided into three categories: glomerular, tubular, and cortical agents (5). A basic knowledge about the pharmacokinetics of renal agents is important for correct selection of an agent as well as image interpretation.

Glomerular Agents

These radiopharmaceuticals are filtered by the glomeruli. The two agents commonly used within this category are iodine-125 (^{125}I)-iothalamate and technetium-99m (^{99m}Tc)-diethylenetriamine pentaacetic acid (DTPA).

^{125}I-iothalamate is used only for measurement of ^{125}I-glomerular filtration rate (GFR); it is not useful for imaging owing to the poor imaging quality of ^{125}I.

^{99m}Tc-DTPA is promptly distributed throughout the extracellular fluid space after intravenous injection. It has only 2% to 6% binding to plasma proteins and does not enter the cells. ^{99m}Tc-DTPA has an extraction efficiency of about 20% with each pass through the kidneys, with peak renal activity 3 to 4 minutes postinjection. Overall, approximately 90% of the injected dose is excreted into urine by glomerular filtration in the first 2 hours. ^{99m}Tc-DTPA is used to assess renal blood flow, function, and drainage of the pelvicalyceal systems ureters. Having only glomerular filtration with no tubular reabsorption or secretion, ^{99m}Tc-DTPA is commonly used to measure GFR.

Tubular Agents

Radioiodinated orthoiodohippurate (OIH, hippuran) and ^{99m}Tc-mercaptylacetyltriglycine (^{99m}Tc-MAG3) are cleared from the kidneys mainly by tubular secretion.

^{99m}Tc-MAG3 has replaced ^{131}I-OIH for renal imaging in most institutions. Having optimal imaging properties,

^{99m}Tc-MAG3 provides superior renal functional images with reasonable anatomic evaluation. It has 79% to 90% protein binding in plasma. Renal clearance of MAG3 is 89% by active tubular secretion and 11% glomerular filtration in animal studies (3). It has an extraction efficiency of 50% to 60% with each pass through the kidneys. Although the renal extraction efficiency of ^{99m}Tc-MAG3 is less than ^{131}I-OIH, high blood concentrations of ^{99m}Tc-MAG3 due to significant protein binding compensate for low extraction, and both radiopharmaceuticals have almost identical renal uptake and excretion on time activity curves. ^{99m}Tc-MAG3 is used to measure effective renal plasma flow (ERPF) and assess renal perfusion and function. It is especially recommended for renal scintigraphy of patients with decreased renal function and of infants. The adult recommended dosage is 5 to 10 mCi, intravenously.

Cortical Agents

There are two renal cortical agents available: ^{99m}Tc-dimercaptosuccinic acid (DMSA) and ^{99m}Tc-glucoheptonate (GH). A fraction of injected radiopharmaceuticals are fixed into the normal renal parenchyma, allowing detection of cortical abnormalities such as acute pyelonephritis, scar, infarct, and congenital abnormalities; differential renal function can also be calculated.

^{99m}Tc-Dimercaptosuccinic Acid

Following intravenous administration, ^{99m}Tc-DMSA has 75% serum protein binding within the first 6 hours, with about 5% to 20% urinary excretion in 2 hours and 37% in 24 hours (5,6,7). Because of the slow renal excretion of radiotracer, pelvicalyceal systems are not visualized. ^{99m}Tc-DMSA has 40% to 50% renal cortical localization, and maximum activity is observed 3 to 6 hours postinjection. Cortical uptake is principally in the proximal convoluted tubules. The suggested adult dosage is 2 to 5 mCi administered intravenously. Renal planar and/or single photon emission tomography (SPECT) images are usually obtained 2 to 4 hours after injection.

^{99m}Tc-Glucoheptonate

Following intravenous injection, ^{99m}Tc-GH is excreted by glomerular filtration (80% to 90%) and tubular secretion (10% to 20%). About 25% to 40% of the injected dose is in urine within 1 hour and 70% within 24 hours. Up to 15% of the injected dose is retained in the kidneys by binding to the proximal convoluted tubules. Therefore this radiopharmaceutical is useful for early dynamic functional images (0 to 30 minutes) and delayed cortical imaging (2 to 3 hours). The suggested dose for adults is 10 to 15 mCi administered intravenously.

PROTOCOLS IN RENAL SCINTIGRAPHY

It is important to obtain renal images in a standard manner. The patient should be well hydrated prior to imaging to prevent false-positive studies. In adults, oral hydration with two glasses (500 mL) of water is adequate. Patients should void just prior to the procedure. A large field-of-view camera with a low-energy, high-resolution, parallel-hole collimator is used.

The patient lies supine on the imaging table with the camera under the table viewing the kidneys and bladder. In renal transplant patients, the camera will be over the transplant anteriorly.

After tight bolus injection of radiopharmaceutical (^{99m}Tc-DTPA, ^{99m}Tc-MAG3, or ^{99m}Tc-GH), renal images are obtained in flow phase and sequential functional phase. The flow phase, also called the radionuclide angiogram, evaluates renal perfusion during the first pass of radiotracer through the kidneys. Flow images are acquired 2 to 4 seconds per frame for 60 seconds, starting immediately after injection. It is followed by the sequential functional phase for 30 minutes. Functional images show physiologic radiotracer uptake and excretion. In a normal study, flow to the kidneys is prompt and symmetrical. Maximum renal activity is seen 4 to 6 seconds after peak aortic activity on flow phase. Functional images reveal maximum parenchymal uptake 3 to 5 minutes into the study; excreted activity is in the renal pelves and bladder at the same time. There will be gradual radiotracer washout from renal parenchyma and collecting system as the study progresses. No significant cortical activity should be seen at 30 minutes.

Using scintigraphic data, computer analysis is performed to calculate differential (split) renal uptake and to generate time/activity curves for each kidney. A region of interest (ROI) is drawn around each kidney. A background ROI is placed in curvilinear fashion along the inferolateral aspect or in semilunar fashion along the lateral aspect of each kidney. Background activity is subtracted from the renal activity to eliminate the contribution of overlying soft tissue activity from the total renal count. The renal uptake at 1 to 3 minutes (before activity is excreted into the collecting systems) is used to calculate split renal function. Normally, the relative contribution of each kidney to total renal activity is 45% to 55%.

A normal renal time/activity curve (renogram) has a characteristic configuration. An initial sharp upslope represents sudden appearance of activity within the renal vasculature in the first 30 seconds. The second portion of upslope is less steep and owing to radiotracer accumulation in the renal parenchyma, reaching a peak in 3 to 5 minutes, followed by a downslope due to excretion of radioactivity into the pelvicalyceal system. Using a renogram curve, many indices have been described. Three commonly used indices are the time to peak cortical activity, the ratio of cortical activity at 20 minutes over peak cortical activity, and the percentage of residual renal or cortical activity at 30 minutes. Normally, the ratio of cortical 20-minute activity/peak activity is less than 0.30 on a ^{99m}Tc- MAG3 renogram. Values above 0.30 suggest cortical retention.

Renal Cortical Imaging

^{99m}Tc-DMSA or ^{99m}Tc-GH is used for renal cortical imaging. Planar images with low-energy, high-resolution collimators are obtained 2 to 4 hours after intravenous injection of radiopharmaceutical. Image magnification (e.g., with pinhole collimators) may be needed in children. Standard images are posterior, right posterior oblique, and left posterior oblique views. SPECT with a multihead camera has a higher detection rate for renal lesions than conventional planar or pinhole collimator techniques (8,9). Therefore renal SPECT should be

obtained, if possible, in patients with a clinical suspicion of acute pyelonephritis, especially in children under 3 years of age.

A normal study shows a smooth renal contour with homogeneous cortical activity. Less uptake in the medulla and no activity in the collecting system are expected on high-resolution images (10). With ^{99m}Tc-GH imaging, activity may be seen in the renal pelvis if images are obtained early or an obstruction is present. Flattening of the superolateral aspect of the left kidney due to splenic impression may be observed.

Diuretic Renography

Dilatation of the upper urinary tract (hydronephrosis) is usually detected on renal ultrasound or CT scan and needs further evaluation. Mechanical obstruction will cause gradual deterioration of renal function if it is not treated.

Diuretic radionuclide renography is used to evaluate the presence or absence of obstruction in a dilated system.

In order to standardize the techniques of diuretic renography, the members of the Society for Fetal Urology and the Pediatric Nuclear Medicine Council of the Society of Nuclear Medicine have recommended the "Well-Tempered Diuretic Renogram" (WTDR) protocol for neonates (infants) with hydronephrosis (11). With some modification, this technique can be applied to children. Recently, a panel of experts from the scientific committee of the 9th International Symposium on Radionuclides in Nephrourology published an article entitled "Consensus on Diuresis Renography for Investigating the Dilated Upper Urinary Tract" (12).

The technique is as follows:

1. Adequate hydration: In the WTDR protocol, infants get oral hydration with formula or water ad libitum beginning 2 hours prior to the study. Intravenous hydration with diluted normal saline (NS) solution (D5.3NS or D5.25NS) at a rate of 15 mL/kg over a 30-minute period is started 15 minutes prior to radiopharmaceutical injection and is continued at a rate of 200 mL/kg/24 hour for the duration of the examination. In adults, oral hydration with 500 mL of water or orange juice about 30 to 60 minutes prior to radiopharmaceutical injection is necessary.

2. Bladder catheterization: A full bladder may prevent adequate drainage of upper collecting systems and can cause a false-positive study for obstruction. The bladder is catheterized routinely in the WTDR protocol. In adults and older children, bladder catheterization may not be necessary if there is no evidence of vesicoureteric reflux, neurogenic bladder, or lower tract obstruction.

3. Radiopharmaceuticals: ^{99m}Tc-DTPA and ^{99m}Tc-MAG3 have been commonly used for diuretic renography. Currently, the agent of choice is ^{99m}Tc-MAG3, which provides superior images, especially in neonates, infants, and patients with diminished renal function.

4. Diuretic dosage and timing: Furosemide is given intravenously to induce forced diuresis. The high urinary flow rate induced with furosemide washes out radiopharmaceutical from dilated collecting systems if there is no significant obstruction. A prerequisite to a valid diuretic renogram is

reasonable renal function that can respond to furosemide. The recommended furosemide dosage is 1 mg/kg in infants, 0.5 mg/kg in children, and 40 mg in adults, given intravenously (11,12). It is injected 20 to 30 minutes after radiotracer injection or when the dilated renal pelvis/ureter is full. Then imaging is continued for another 20 to 30 minutes. Functional images, renogram time/activity curves (before and after furosemide injection), and furosemide washout half-time ($T_{1/2}$) are used for interpretation.

Angiotensin-Converting Enzyme Inhibitor Renography (Captopril Renography)

Renovascular hypertension (RVH) affects less than 1% of general hypertensive patients and up to 35% of patients with risk factors for RVH. It is defined as high blood pressure caused by renal hypoperfusion, usually due to renal artery stenosis and activation of the renin-angiotensin-aldosterone system (13,14).

Currently, angiotensin-converting enzyme (ACE) inhibitor renography plays an important role in the noninvasive diagnosis of RVH. The principle of this test is scintigraphic demonstration of physiologic changes due to transient blockage of the activated renin angiotensin system with an ACE inhibitor, such as captopril. Protocols for performance and criteria for interpretation of captopril renography may vary among different nuclear medicine departments. Two protocol/interpretation guidelines are available: (a) a report of the working party group for patient selection and preparation in conjunction with diagnostic criteria of renovascular hypertension with captopril renography, a consensus statement (15,16), and (b) a consensus report on ACE inhibitor renography for detecting RVH by an international panel of experts (17).

In our institution, the following protocol, which is very close to the guidelines of the consensus report on ACE inhibitor renography for detecting RVH, is employed. ^{99m}Tc-MAG3 is routinely used. Patients should be off any ACE inhibitors for 48 hours, and no solid meal is allowed 4 hours prior to the procedure. First, a captopril renogram is obtained. The patient is hydrated with 10 mL/kg of water, orally, if possible. Then an intravenous line is inserted and hydration is continued with normal saline at a rate of 4 mL/min during the entire procedure. Baseline blood pressure (BP) and pulse rate (PR) are recorded. Captopril 50 mg is given orally. Then BP and PR are recorded every 15 minutes for 1 hour. The intravenous infusion rate is increased if there is a significant drop in BP, and a physician is immediately notified. One hour after captopril administration, the patient voids and then lies supine on the imaging table. Renal imaging is started immediately following intravenous administration of ^{99m}Tc-MAG3, 10 mCi, and furosemide, 40 mg (for adults). Flow and functional images are obtained for 30 minutes, and time/activity curves are generated.

If the captopril renogram is abnormal, a baseline (without captopril) study is obtained after 48 hours following the same protocol. Occasionally, ACE inhibitor renography is performed while the patient is on chronic administration of ACE inhibitor, and no additional dose of ACE inhibitor is given prior to the procedure. This procedure is known to be less sensitive than "a true captopril renogram."

In renovascular hypertension, a captopril MAG renogram has a typical appearance consisting of delayed time to peak (T_{max} >5 min) and cortical retention of radiotracer. These findings will markedly improve or normalize on the baseline study. Using ^{99m}Tc-DTPA, the most important finding is a decrease in differential renal function compared to baseline study (17).

Direct Radionuclide Cystography

This procedure is used for the detection and follow-up of vesicoureteral reflux. It is more sensitive and delivers about 100 times less radiation than contrast voiding urethrocystography (VCUG). However, anatomic resolution is poor with the radionuclide cystogram.

The technique is as follows:

^{99m}Tc-sulfur colloid (0.5 to 1.0 mCi) or ^{99m}Tc-pertechnetate (1.0 mCi) is used. The patient voids prior to the procedure. The patient lies supine on the imaging table and, under aseptic conditions, the bladder is catheterized using a Foley catheter (or an infant feeding tube in small children). A gamma camera equipped with a low-energy, high-resolution collimator is placed under the imaging table with the bladder and kidneys in the field of view. The radiotracer is administered through the catheter into the bladder and then flushed with sterile water. The bladder is gradually filled with normal saline by gravity (the bottle of normal saline is 70 to 90 cm above the bladder). Imaging is started at the time of normal saline infusion. The computer monitor is closely watched for vesicoureteral reflux, and the bladder volume at the time of reflux is recorded. Saline infusion is discontinued when the patient feels full with slight discomfort or estimated bladder volume is reached [estimated bladder volume in milliliters = (patient's age + 2) × 30. Infants often urinate around the catheter when the bladder is full; otherwise the bladder is drained via the catheter. In older children, a bedpan is placed under the patient and images are obtained during and after voiding. Normally there is no reflux from the bladder into the ureter renal pelvis.

SCROTAL SCINTIGRAPHY

Scrotal scintigraphy with a blood-flow and blood-pool imaging agent is performed to differentiate testicular torsion from epididymitis/epididymoorchitis. It should be performed urgently when the request is received, because testicular viability is endangered if the surgical treatment for torsion is delayed. Interpretation of nuclear scrotal images is based on expected normal symmetry in the hemiscrotum. Therefore proper positioning of the scrotum under the camera is important.

The patient may be pretreated with sodium or potassium perchlorate orally, 5 to 8 mg/kg, to reduce radiation to the thyroid gland if this does not delay imaging. The radiopharmaceutical agent of choice is ^{99m}Tc-pertechnetate, injected intravenously. The dosage is 15 to 20 mCi for an adult and is adjusted for body weight in children, with the minimum dosage being 5 mCi (18).

The technique is as follows:

The patient lies supine with legs abducted on the imaging table. A scrotal sling or a rolled towel under the scrotum is used to provide support and symmetrical positioning of the scrotum in the center of the field of view. The penis is taped back onto the lower abdomen. A low-energy general-purpose parallel-hole collimator is placed as close as possible to the patient. Image magnification is necessary in children, using a converging collimator. Dynamic anterior flow images are acquired 2 to 5 seconds per frame for 60 seconds, starting immediately after intravenous bolus injection of the radiopharmaceutical, followed by 1- and 5-minute anterior static images, each for 500,000 counts. Another static image is obtained with a thin lead strip over the medial raphe to separate the right from the left hemiscrotum and a lead shield under the scrotum to block background thigh activity. This aids in identifying subtle asymmetrical perfusion within the scrotum.

Dynamic flow images clearly delineate the iliac–femoral arteries. However, small vessels of the scrotum and testes are not usually seen. Injected ^{99m}Tc-pertechnetate is loosely bound into the plasma protein and approximately 75% to 80% of radiopharmaceutical is rapidly diffused into the extravascular space. Therefore static images obtained at 1 and 5 minutes postinjection reveal the distribution of radiopharmaceutical in the extracellular space, which reflects tissue perfusion. This activity is normally symmetrical in the scrotum, with intensity similar or slightly greater than thigh uptake.

Although Doppler color-flow ultrasound becomes the primary imaging modality for evaluation of the scrotum, ultrasound may not differentiate acute epididymitis from early torsion (less than 7 hours after the onset of pain). Moreover, difficulties are often experienced in performing ultrasound on patients with acute scrotal pain. Radionuclide scintigraphy should be of great value in these special situations and may also be used as an adjunct to sonography.

CASE 6.1

History: A 14-year-old boy was brought to the emergency room for acute left scrotal pain of 12 hours' duration. Clinical assessment and laboratory findings were inconclusive. A testicular scintigram (Figs. 6.1 A to 6.1 D) was obtained to assess the vascular integrity of the testicles.

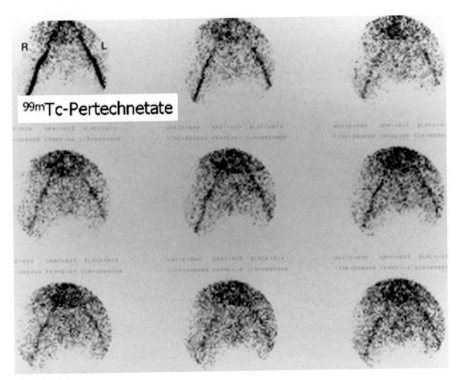

Figure 6.1 A

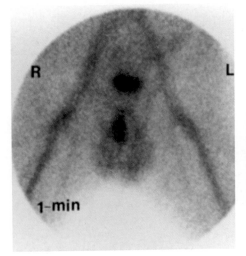

Figure 6.1 B

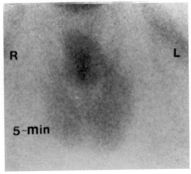

Figure 6.1 C

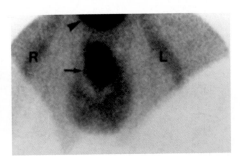

Figure 6.1 D

Findings: On the radionuclide angiogram (Fig. 6.1 A), symmetrical activity is demonstrated in the region of the scrotum. One-minute, 5-minute, and static lead-shielded images (Figs. 6.1 B, 6.1 C and 6.1 D) show homogeneous scrotal activity. No asymmetry or abnormal area of increased or decreased uptake is seen. Normal penile blood pool (arrow) and urinary bladder activity (arrowhead) are easily identified.

Discussion: Symmetrical scrotal activity on the flow study and homogeneous tracer distribution on delayed static images with no area of decreased uptake indicate an intact vascular supply and exclude a left hemiscrotal flow abnormality.

Scrotal scintigraphy, consisting of dynamic blood flow and static blood pool images, is a useful procedure for evaluation of vascularity and perfusion of the scrotum and its contents.

It is to be noted that a normal scrotal scintigram in a patient with acute hemiscrotal pain may represent manual or spontaneous detorsion, torsion of the testicular appendage, referred pain, or even an emotional disorder (19).

Diagnosis: Normal scrotal scintigram.

CASE 6.2

History: A 24-year-old healthy male presented with acute right scrotal pain of approximately 4 hours' duration. There was no history of trauma. Although the clinical impression was that of probable epididymoorchitis, a testicular scintigram was requested to evaluate for acute testicular torsion (Figs. 6.2 A, 6.2 B and 6.2 C)

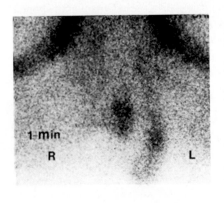

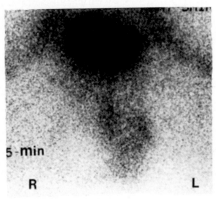

⁹⁹ᵐTc-Pertechnetate

Figure 6.2 A

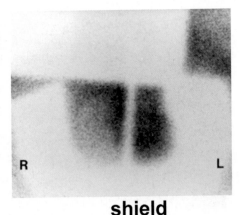

shield

Figure 6.2 B

Figure 6.2 C

Findings: One-minute, 5-minute, and raphe marker/thigh lead shielded static images (Figs. 6.2 A, 6.2 B and 6.2 C) demonstrate a large area of diminished activity within the right hemiscrotum.

Discussion: The testicular scintigram reveals diminished radiopharmaceutical activity in the right hemiscrotum on both flow (not shown) and static images. Common causes of diminished hemiscrotal activity include early torsion, hematocele, hydrocele, and hernia. In the above clinical setting, findings are most consistent with early torsion.

Acute scrotal pain demands prompt evaluation. The main differential considerations are testicular torsion, which needs immediate surgical intervention to salvage the testis, and epididymitis epididymoorchitis, which can be managed medically. The usual clinical presentation is acute testicular pain in a male in his early teens. These patients may also have a low-grade fever, nausea, or vomiting. Urinary symptoms are uncommon and more likely to be encountered in cases of epididymitis or abscess. When the clinical diagnosis is unclear, scrotal scintigraphy has proven to be a safe and sensitive method for differentiating testicular torsion from epididymitis epididymoorchitis and should be performed immediately, if available.

Testicular torsion occurs in 1 in 4,000 males, commonly in adolescents and young adults. Usually an underlying anatomic abnormality predisposes the patient to torsion of the testis, with subsequent testicular ischemia/infarction. The most common anatomic variation occurring in testicular torsion is complete covering of the testes and epididymis by the tunica vaginalis, with absence of the normal uncovered area participating in the scrotal attachment. This leads to the "bell clapper" deformity, where the testicle and epididymis are freely movable on a vascular pedicle. This anatomic variant is frequently bilateral.

The arterial supply to the testis, epididymis, and tunica vaginalis (scrotal contents) is through the testicular artery (which arises from the aorta just below the renal arteries), the deferential artery (a branch of the internal iliac or vesical artery), and the cremasteric artery (a branch of the inferior epigastric artery). These vessels course throughout the spermatic cord. Although anastomosis is present among these arteries, the testicular artery is the major blood supply to the testis. The venous drainage of the scrotal contents is via the paminiform plexus to the internal spermatic veins. The right spermatic vein empties into the inferior vena cava, and the left joins with the left renal vein. Blood supply to the scrotum (scrotal skin and dartos) is from the superficial external pudendal artery (a branch of the femoral artery), the anterior scrotal artery (a branch of the deep external pudendal artery), and the posterior scrotal artery (a branch of the internal pudendal artery).

It is noted that the testis epididymis and the scrotum have separate blood supplies, and there is no anastomosis between these two. Therefore, in testicular torsion, a twist in the spermatic cord disrupts blood flow to and from the testis and endangers the viability of the testis. Scintigraphically, this is seen as an area of decreased activity in the hemiscrotum on flow and static tissue images. Decreased activity may be subtle, especially in the early stage of torsion; therefore a comparison of both the right and left hemiscrotum is very important in order to detect asymmetry, suggesting altered supply on one side. On the other hand, an inflammatory process such as epididymitis causes local hyperemia and is recognized on scintigraphy as an area of increased activity.

Diagnosis: Early right testicular torsion.

CASE 6.3

History: A 41-year-old male with prior left orchialgia presented with a 4-day history of acute left scrotal pain and swelling; he was admitted with a tentative diagnosis of epididymoorchitis. A radionuclide scrotal scintigraphy was obtained (Figs. 6.3 A and 6.3 B).

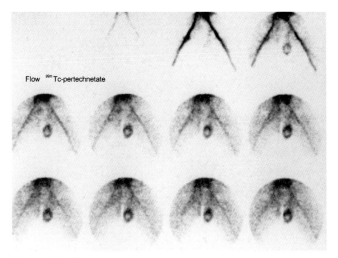

Flow ⁹⁹ᵐTc-pertechnetate

Figure 6.3 A

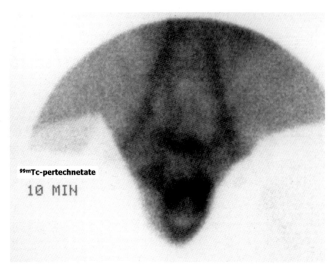

⁹⁹ᵐTc-pertechnetate

10 MIN

Figure 6.3 B

Findings: The symptomatic left hemiscrotum demonstrates a rim of increased activity with a photopenic center on the dynamic flow study (Fig. 6.3 A). Similar findings are also present on the static blood pool image (Fig. 6.3 B).

Discussion: The pattern of a photopenic center with a surrounding rim of activity is not specific and may be seen in late testicular torsion, abscess, hematoma, or tumor. Clinical correlation narrows the differential.

In testicular torsion, the viability of the testis depends on the degree of torsion and the duration of symptoms. It is apparent that an incomplete twist (180 degrees) in the spermatic cord jeopardizes the blood flow to the testis less than a complete twist (360 degrees). Initially, venous flow is obstructed, leading to gradual congestion and edema. This is followed by cessation of arterial flow, and testicular infarction ultimately occurs. The prompt diagnosis of testicular torsion is imperative for salvaging of the involved testicle. Surgical intervention has been successful in approximately 100% of patients with torsion lasting less than 4 hours, as compared with 20% at 10 hours. Hormonal and spermatic function has been preserved in most patients with a duration of torsion between 6 and 12 hours; after 24 hours, viability is rare. Time-dependence of testicular survival dictates that scrotal scintigraphy be performed immediately upon request.

Late testicular torsion (missed torsion) indicates nonviability of the testis. Scintigraphically, this is seen as a photopenic area with a surrounding rim of intense activity (bull's-eye sign) in the symptomatic side of the scrotum (Figs. 6.3 A and 6.3 B).

The photopenic center is the affected testis, and the surrounding rim of increased intensity represents reactive hyperemia in the dartos. Low-grade reactive hyperemia activity in the dartos may be present within 24 hours of torsion, but viability is still possible.

Diagnosis: Late left testicular torsion with acute hemorrhagic necrosis.

CASE 6.4

History: A 22-year-old male presented with acute right scrotal pain; an emergency nuclear scrotal scintigram was obtained (Figs. 6.4 A and 6.4 B).

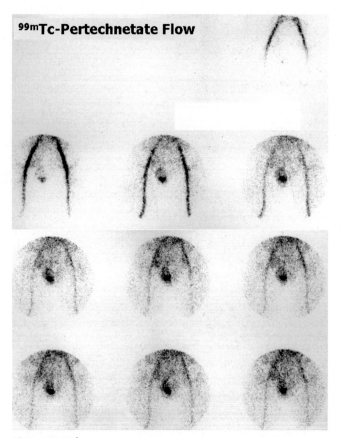

Figure 6.4 A

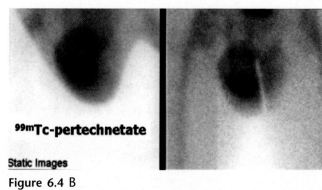

Figure 6.4 B

Findings: The dynamic flow images (Fig. 6.4 A) demonstrate asymmetrical activity in the scrotum, with the symptomatic right hemiscrotum having more activity than the left. Static images also reveal diffuse increased uptake on the right side (Fig. 6.4 B).

Discussion: The increased activity in the right hemiscrotum represents hypervascularity, which is commonly caused by an inflammatory process such as epididymitis/epididymoorchitis. Inflammatory conditions are the most common cause of acute scrotal pain, as they are more frequent than testicular torsion even in patients under 20 years of age. Epididymitis/epididymoorchitis is usually an extension of infection from the lower urinary tract.

An inflammatory process is associated with increased vascularity and hyperperfusion. Inflammation of the epididymis is seen as an area of increased radiopharmaceutical activity in the lateral and superior aspects of the expected location of the testis on blood flow and blood pool images. When inflammation involves the testis (so-called epididymoorchitis), the entire hemiscrotum will show increased activity. The spermatic cord of the symptomatic hemiscrotum may also reveal increased uptake secondary to increased blood flow and vascularity.

Occasionally, spontaneous or manual detorsion causes diffuse hemiscrotal activity and may mimic epididymoorchitis. If epididymal inflammation incites hydrocele formation, it will cause a photopenic area medial to epididymal activity. This pattern may be confused with missed torsion.

Diagnosis: Epididymoorchitis.

CASE 6.5

History: A 3-year-old female presented with a 1-year history of urinary tract infection (UTI). On initial workup, renal ultrasound was normal, and contrast VCUG showed grade III vesicoureteral reflux (VUR) on the right side. She was started on prophylactic antibiotic with no new episode of UTI. One year later, a follow-up radionuclide cystogram (RNC) was obtained (Fig. 6.5 A).

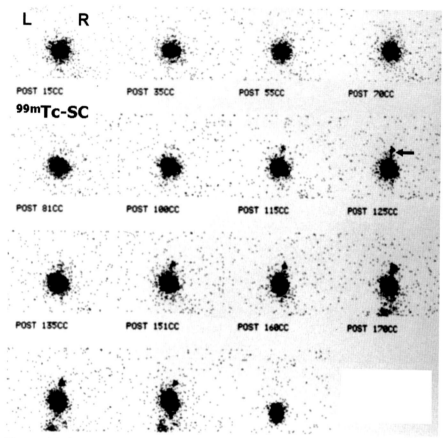

Figure 6.5 A

Findings: Images reveal vesicoureteral reflux on the right side (Fig. 6.5 A), which appears during the middle filling phase at a bladder volume of approximately 115 mL. The reflux reaches into the intrarenal collecting system (arrow) with no evidence of gross dilatation of the ureter or renal pelvis. Low-pressure reflux is seen during bladder filling, and high-pressure reflux is seen during voiding. No residual activity is present in the ureter or renal pelvis on postvoid image. There is no reflux on the left side in this case.

Discussion: After the initial episode of a documented UTI, a child younger than 3 to 5 years of age should have assessment of the upper and lower urinary tract to evaluate for developmental and acquired abnormalities. Renal/bladder ultrasound is the most commonly used modality for evaluation of the upper urinary tract and bladder.

The lower urinary tract is evaluated with contrast VCUG or RNC. A contrast VCUG provides anatomic detail of the lower urinary tract and will disclose the presence or absence of vesicoureteral reflux, paraureteral/bladder diverticulum, or posterior urethral valve. It is recommended for the initial evaluation of the lower urinary tract in children with urinary tract infection, especially boys. Radionuclide cystography is recommended for follow-up of patients with reflux and evaluation of siblings of patients with reflux; it may also be used in initial assessment of girls with UTI.

RNC is more sensitive than contrast VCUG for the detection of reflux, and a volume as little as 0.25 mL can be detected. Continuous imaging during RNC allows detection of intermittent reflux that may be missed with contrast VCUG and delivers 50 to 200 times less radiation. However, diverticula may not be identified, and the urethra cannot be evaluated.

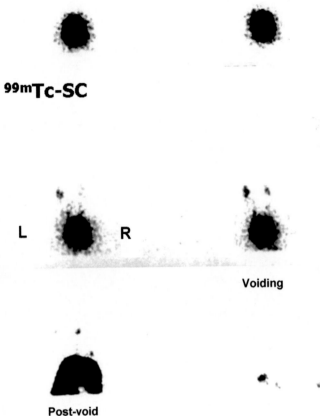

99mTc-SC

L   R

Voiding

Post-void

Figure 6.5 B

The most common abnormality detected in children with UTI is VUR, reported in 29% to 55% of cases. Primary VUR, the most common cause of reflux in children, is due to a short intramural segment of the ureter, causing vesicoureteral incompetence. As children grow, the intramural segment of the ureter lengthens, and reflux often resolves spontaneously by 5 years of age.

Grading VUR is important in the management of patients with reflux. The International Reflux Study (IRS) classification is commonly used for grading and is based on radiographic findings on contrast VCUG. It characterizes reflux as follows: grade I, reflux limited to the ureter; grade II, reflux extending into the ureter and pelvicalyceal system without dilatation; grade III, mild or moderate dilatation of the ureter and renal pelvis but without blunting of fornices; grade IV, moderate dilatation and/or tortuosity of the ureter with moderate dilatation of the pelvicalyceal system and obliteration of sharp angles of fornices but with preservation of papillary

impression; and grade V, severe dilatation and tortuosity of the ureter and pelvicalyceal system with loss of papillary impression in most calyces.

The chance of spontaneous resolution of VUR depends upon the severity of reflux. Resolution occurs in 83% of grade I, 80% of grade II, and 46% of grade III reflux. Grades IV and V reflux require surgical intervention.

Because anatomic detail is suboptimal in radionuclide cystography, the IRS grading system cannot be applied accurately. A good method of conveying the significance of reflux is to describe the extent of reflux (ureter versus ureter and renal pelvis), the presence or absence of gross dilatation in the ureter pelvis if possible, the time of occurrence (filling versus voiding), bladder volume when reflux is first seen, and the presence or absence of residual activity in the collecting system after voiding.

On Figure 6.5 B, significant bilateral VUR is seen in a 4-year-old girl with a history of bilateral grade II VUR.

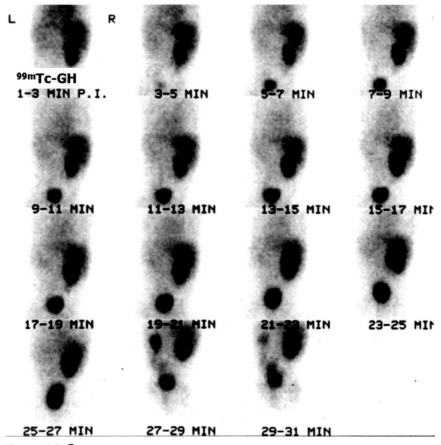

99mTc-GH
1-3 MIN P.I.   3-5 MIN   5-7 MIN   7-9 MIN

9-11 MIN   11-13 MIN   13-15 MIN   15-17 MIN

17-19 MIN   19-21 MIN   21-23 MIN   23-25 MIN

25-27 MIN   27-29 MIN   29-31 MIN

Figure 6.5 C

Another way of diagnosing VUR is with an indirect RNC, as shown in Figure 6.5 C.

The glucoheptonate renogram demonstrates essentially no function in the left kidney. Good function is seen in the right kidney; however, prominent activity in the region of the right renal pelvis raises the possibility of an extrarenal pelvis or nonobstructive hydronephrosis. The last three images show markedly decreased bladder activity with a sudden simultaneous appearance of activity in the left ureter and renal pelvis. Delayed and anterior abdominal/pelvic images (not shown) did not demonstrate an ectopic left kidney. The indirect RNC method does not require bladder catheterization, as bladder filling is physiologic; however, it does require good renal function for excretion of the radiopharmaceutical and the child's cooperation to avoid voiding during bladder filling. Renal uptake and excretion of activity is associated with gradual filling of the bladder. When radioactivity is cleared from the upper collecting system, the patient is asked to void. Any reappearance of activity in the ureter or renal pelvis indicates VUR. Indirect RNC is not commonly used because it is less sensitive than direct RNC for the detection of reflux.

Diagnosis: Right-sided vesicoureteral reflux reaching into the intrarenal collecting system.

CASE 6.6

History: A 10-year-old female with a history of recurrent UTI presented with left flank pain and fever. ^{99m}Tc-DMSA scintigraphy was performed to evaluate the possibility of pyelonephritis (Figs. 6.6 A and 6.6 B).

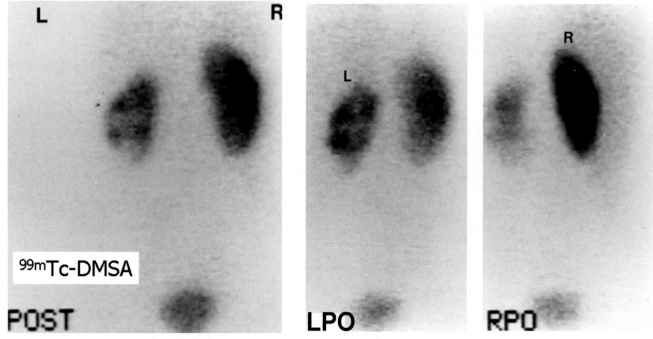

Figure 6.6 A

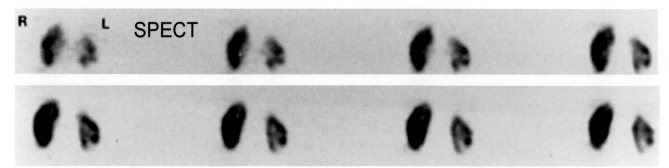

Figure 6.6 B

Findings: ^{99m}Tc-DMSA planar images (Fig. 6.6 A) show normal homogeneous radiotracer uptake in the right renal cortex. The left kidney is small, with multiple photopenic cortical defects. The largest defect is wedge-shaped and located in the lower pole of the left kidney, best seen on the SPECT coronal images (Fig. 6.6 B).

Discussion: Differentiation of pyelonephritis from lower UTI (cystitis) is very important, as clinical and laboratory findings are not often accurate for distinction between these two diagnoses. If there is clinical concern for pyelonephritis, the current imaging modality of choice is renal cortical scintigraphy, as it is more sensitive than ultrasound or CT scan.

Two radiopharmaceuticals are available for renal cortical scintigraphy: ^{99m}Tc-DMSA and ^{99m}Tc-GH. In pyelonephritis, focal ischemia and tubular cell dysfunction cause a decreased or absent cortical radiotracer uptake. Three patterns of decreased/absent cortical uptake have been recognized: single focus, multiple foci, and diffuse involvement. The majority of cases involve the upper or lower poles. The midpoles of the kidneys are usually spared. Acute pyelonephritic changes have no local volume loss, whereas chronic pyelonephritic defects do have associated volume loss. In this case, wedge-shaped cortical defects are strongly suggestive of pyelonephritis. After treatment of the pyelonephritis, follow-up renal cortical imaging 3 to 6 months later is recommended to monitor recovery and evaluate for development of renal cortical scar.

Other causes of cortical photopenic defects are renal cyst, abscess, infarct, postpyelonephritic scar, and tumor (primary or metastatic); ultrasound can differentiate a renal cyst from a solid mass.

^{67}Ga-citrate and ^{111}In-white blood cell (WBC) scintigraphy has been used for detection of acute pyelonephritis. These imaging techniques, however, deliver a higher radiation dose to patients, and the images are obtained 24 hours postinjection; therefore they are less frequently used.

Diagnosis: Pyelonephritis.

CASE 6.7

History: A 72-year-old patient presented with hypertension poorly controlled with medication. A ^{99m}Tc-MAG3 captopril renogram (Figs. 6.7 A and 6.7 B) was performed to evaluate for renovascular hypertension. It was followed by a baseline study 2 days later (Figs. 6.7 C and 6.7 D).

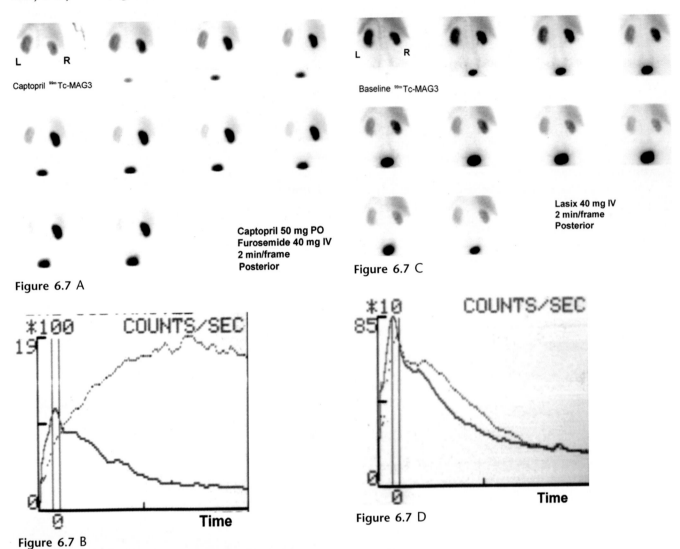

Captopril ^{99m}Tc-MAG3

Captopril 50 mg PO
Furosemide 40 mg IV
2 min/frame
Posterior

Figure 6.7 A

Baseline ^{99m}Tc-MAG3

Lasix 40 mg IV
2 min/frame
Posterior

Figure 6.7 C

Figure 6.7 B

Figure 6.7 D

Findings: On the captopril renogram, the functional images (Fig. 6.7 A) show abnormal progressive radiotracer accumulation within the right kidney, with possible minimal late excretion into the renal pelvis. The left kidney demonstrates diminished radiotracer uptake and normal excretion with activity in the renal pelvis and bladder at approximately 3 to 5 minutes into the study. Captopril renogram time/activity curves with ROI on cortex (Fig. 6.7 B) reflect the same findings. Quantitative parameters from the cortical ROI reveal delayed time to peak activity at >30 minutes, with an elevated ratio of 20-min/peak cortical activity of 0.90 in the right kidney. These parameters are within normal limits for the left kidney. The baseline ^{99m}Tc-MAG3 renogram obtained 2 days later shows marked improvement in the right renal function, as seen on the functional images (Fig. 6.7 C). Renogram curve and quantitative parameters (Fig. 6.7 D) from the cortical ROI are time

to peak, 2.8 minutes; with a 20-min/peak activity ratio of 0.47. No significant change is seen in the left kidney.

The scintigraphic findings are typical for renovascular hypertension on the right side. The captopril ^{99m}Tc-MAG3 renogram reveals a time to peak activity >30 minutes (normal is <3 to 5 minutes) and significant cortical retention. Marked improvement in scintigraphic changes on baseline ^{99m}Tc-MAG3 renogram obtained 2 days later is strongly suggestive of renovascular hypertension. The patient had an aortogram (Fig. 6.7 E), which demonstrates severe stenosis of the proximal right renal artery.

After angioplasty of the right renal artery, the patient again underwent renal scintigraphy, showing normal findings. This is a good example of the reliability of the captopril scintigraphy in predicting a good outcome after invasive treatment (20).

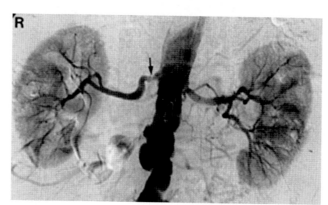

Figure 6.7 E

Hypertension due to renal artery stenosis and renovascular hypertension (RVH) is an uncommon condition occurring in less than 1% of hypertensive patients. Renovascular hypertension is a potentially curable condition with surgical revascularization or renal angioplasty. Two common causes of renal artery stenosis (RAS) are atherosclerosis in older patients and fibromuscular dysplasia in younger patients.

It is important to differentiate between RAS, which is an anatomic lesion without significant physiologic changes, and RVH, which is usually an anatomic narrowing in a renal artery or its branches, causing renal ischemia and hypertension. In an autopsy study of 295 nonselective patients (21), moderate or severe renal artery stenosis due to atheromatous lesion was present in 49% of 256 normotensive patients and in 77% of 39 hypertensive patients. Therefore the presence of anatomic renal artery stenosis in a hypertensive patient does not automatically imply that stenosis is the underlying cause of hypertension.

Captopril renography is a safe, noninvasive screening test that is commonly used for detection of RVH. The principle of this test is scintigraphic demonstration of physiologic changes secondary to transient blockage of activated renin–angiotensin systems with an ACE inhibitor such as captopril in the involved kidney. Significant RAS causes renal ischemia, leading to activation of renin–angiotensin system. As a result, angiotensin I is converted into angiotensin II by ACE. Angiotensin II is a strong vasoconstrictor and also causes sodium retention. In the involved kidney, glomerular filtration pressure and GFR are maintained by the vasoconstrictor effect of angiotensin II on the efferent (postglomerular) arterioles. ACE inhibitors block the conversion of angiotensin I to angiotensin II, with subsequent relaxation of efferent arterioles and a fall in GFR. Therefore administration of ACE inhibitors in a patient with RVH induces a picture of temporary renal failure of varying severity in the involved kidney due to decreased GFR.

On captopril renography, scintigraphic findings of RVH depend on the type of radiopharmaceutical injected and the severity of the condition. Using a glomerular agent such as ^{99m}Tc-DTPA, captopril-induced low GFR in the involved kidney is seen as decreased radiotracer uptake calculated on the 1- to 3-minute image, delayed time to peak activity, and slow or no excretion of activity. Using a tubular agent such as ^{99m}Tc-MAG3, captopril-induced changes are demonstrated as renocortical retention of activity, delayed time to peak activity, and—in severe cases—a decrease in differential uptake. The ratio of 20 minutes/peak cortical activity is a commonly used quantitative parameter to assess the degree of cortical retention. A ratio above 0.3 is abnormal, and a greater than 10% change between the captopril renogram and baseline renogram is considered significant. If the captopril renogram is abnormal, a baseline (without captopril) renogram is indicated.

A pattern of cortical retention is also seen in high-grade obstruction; a renal ultrasound will show hydronephrosis in cases of obstruction.

Overall, captopril renography has a sensitivity and specificity of approximately 90% for the detection of RVH. Sensitivity is reduced in patients with severe renal failure. Captopril renography is suggested in hypertensive patients with a high clinical suspicion for RAS, which may be indicated by the following: (a) abrupt onset of moderate to severe hypertension before age 30 or after age 55; (b) severe hypertension; (c) accelerated or malignant hypertension; (d) refractory hypertension; (e) epigastric bruit; (f) moderate hypertension in a patient with occlusive vascular disease; and (g) renal failure induced by ACE-inhibitor therapy.

Diagnosis: Renovascular hypertension involving the right side.

CASE 6.8

History: A 72-year-old male with hypertension (180/105 mm Hg), abdominal bruit, and occlusive vascular disease was referred for evaluation of RVH. A captopril ^{99m}Tc-MAG3 renogram (Figs. 6.8 A and 6.8 B) and baseline renogram (Figs. 6.8 C and 6.8 D) were obtained. Furosemide was administered at the same time as ^{99m}Tc-MAG3.

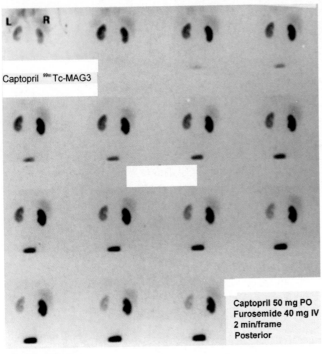

Figure 6.8 A

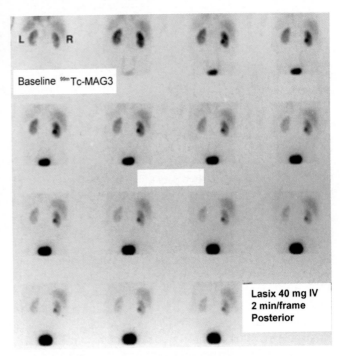

Figure 6.8 C

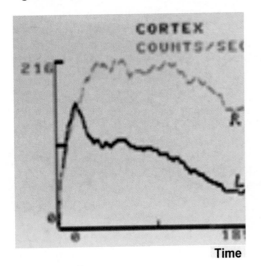

Figure 6.8 B

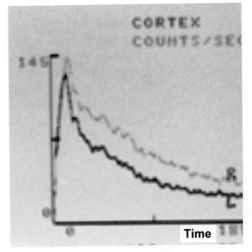

Figure 6.8 D

Findings: The captopril ^{99m}Tc- MAG3 functional images and time activity curve (Figs. 6.8 A and 6.8 B) reveal abnormal radiotracer retention with a 20 min/peak activity ratio of 0.91 (normal <0.3) in the right kidney. The time to peak cortical activity is delayed at 9.3 minutes, and the intrarenal transit time is grossly prolonged, with excreted activity first seen in the right renal pelvis at approximately 7 to 9 minutes (normal is 3 to 5 minutes). Evaluation of the functional images reveals no significant findings in the left kidney except for delayed radiotracer appearance in the renal pelvis at approximately 5 to 7 minutes into the study. However, the shape of the renogram curve suggests slow cortical washout, and 20 min/peak activity is elevated at 0.47, indicating left cortical retention. A subsequent baseline study (Figs. 6.8 C and 6.8 D) performed 3 days later demonstrates normally functioning kidneys and quantitative parameters within normal limits bilaterally.

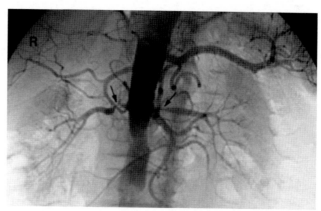

Figure 6.8 E

Discussion: In a patient with moderate hypertension, the presence of abdominal bruit and occlusive vascular disease (cerebrovascular, coronary, or peripheral) is a clinical clue for possible RVH. In this patient, the scintigraphic findings on the captopril renogram in conjunction with normalization of these findings on the subsequent baseline study are highly suggestive of bilateral asymmetrical RVH.

Having a high sensitivity and specificity of approximately 90%, captopril renography is associated with a low incidence of false-positive studies in selected patients with high clinical suspicion for RAS. Glomerulonephropathy and a profound drop in blood pressure after captopril administration are two reported causes of false-positive studies. It is important to note that occlusive diseases of both the large and small renal arteries can cause RVH with the same pathophysiology, and captopril renography does not distinguish between these two.

The patient underwent angiography (Fig. 6.8 E), which revealed significant renal artery stenosis bilaterally, more severe on the right side. The patient had bilateral renal artery balloon angioplasty with stent placement in the left renal artery. Hypertension was subsequently well controlled.

Captopril renography also provides prognostic information regarding blood pressure response to revascularization (by surgery or angioplasty) for renal artery stenosis. If captopril induces renographic changes, there is a high likelihood that hypertension will be cured or improved after revascularization. Absence of renographic changes on a captopril renogram is a predictor of no response following revascularization.

Captopril renography has also been used for the detection of branch renal artery stenosis and renal artery graft stenosis.

Diagnosis: Bilateral renovascular hypertension.

CASE 6.9

History: A 36-year-old male with sepsis developed acute renal failure (ARF), and ^{99m}Tc-MAG3 renal scintigraphy was performed to assess renal vascularity (Figs. 6.9 A, 6.9 B and 6.9 C).

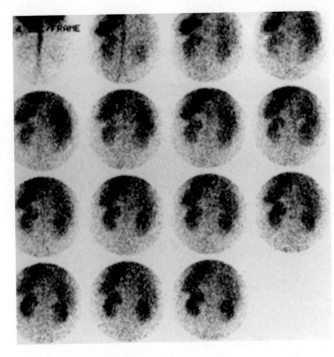

^{99m}Tc-MAG 3 Flow

Figure 6.9 A

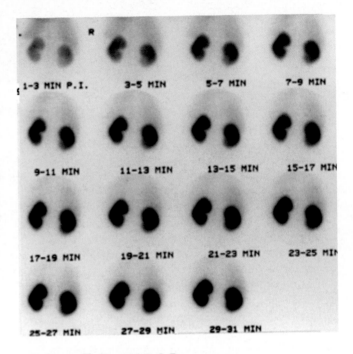

^{99m}Tc-MAG 3 Renogram

Figure 6.9 B

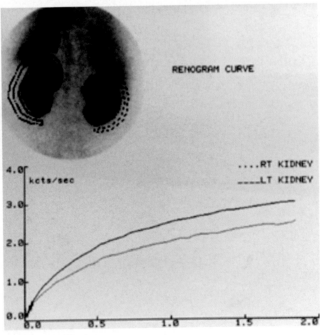

Figure 6.9 C

Findings: On the blood flow images (Fig. 6.9 A), there is rapid symmetrical perfusion of both kidneys. The functional images (Fig. 6.9 B) demonstrate progressive accumulation of ^{99m}Tc-MAG3 in the renal parenchyma. The radiotracer uptake is homogeneous bilaterally. The kidneys are normal in size and shape. There is no excretion of radiotracer into the renal pelves during the 30-minute image. Cardiac blood pool activity disappears in 5 to 7 minutes, and no significant soft tissue background activity is apparent. Renal time/activity curves have an accumulative pattern (Fig. 6.9 C).

Discussion: In this case, there is no gross renal inflow abnormality, and the kidneys are normal in size with no cortical defects; therefore a thromboembolic event is not the cause of acute renal failure.

Renal scintigraphy is occasionally performed to evaluate the vascular integrity of the kidneys in patients with ARF. Although both ^{99m}Tc-DTPA and ^{99m}Tc-MAG3 have been used, ^{99m}Tc-MAG3 is the agent of choice because it produces better images with low background activity.

^{99m}Tc-MAG3 (a tubular agent) will show progressive accumulation of activity in the renal parenchyma due to continuous tubular excretion. Absence of or very low GFR causes radiotracer retention in the renal cortex. However, ^{99m}Tc-DTPA (a glomerular agent) functional images will reveal an initial high renal activity due to blood pool activity. This is then followed by decreased renal activity due to equilibrium of intravascular activity with the extravascular space (it cannot be due to renal excretion if there is no activity in the collecting system).

The accumulative pattern of ^{99m}Tc-MAG3 radiotracer is also seen in high-grade obstruction. All patients with ARF should have a renal ultrasound to assess renal size and evaluate for hydronephrosis, which was not present in this case. Small kidneys suggest chronic renal disease, and hydronephrosis necessitates surgical intervention.

On a normal ^{99m}Tc-MAG3 scintigram, activity is seen in the intrarenal collecting system 3 to 6 minutes into the study. Activity in the renal pelves drains freely into the bladder through the ureters, which are partially visualized on some of the images. Only minimal cortical activity remains on the 30-minute image. Kidney time/activity have a sharp upslope (indicating prompt uptake), with peak activity at approximately 4 minutes. The downslope of the curves can be more gradual when there is focal upper calyceal retention.

Other causes of slow excretion on renography are inadequate hydration of the patient prior to imaging, subcutaneous injection of radiotracer, and various renal pathologic states (22).

Two common causes of ARF are acute tubular necrosis (ATN) and interstitial nephritis. It is reported that ^{67}Ga scintigraphy is helpful in differentiating between the two. The kidneys show intense uptake in interstitial nephritis, while no significant uptake is seen in acute tubular necrosis.

Diagnosis: Acute renal failure.

CASE 6.10

History: A 27-year-old male presented with a history of lower back pain. A furosemide ^{99m}Tc-MAG3 renogram was obtained (Figs. 6.10 A and 6.10 B), as well as a CT scan (Fig. 6.10 C).

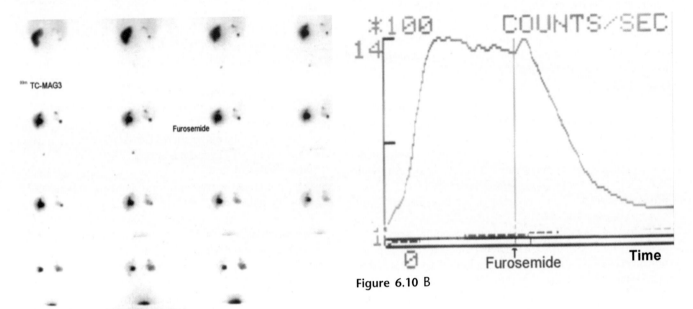

Figure 6.10 A

Figure 6.10 B

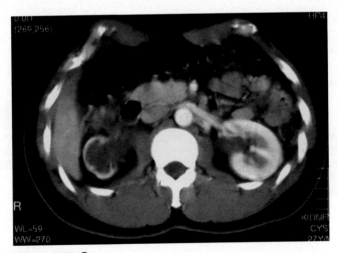

Figure 6.10 C

Findings: On functional images (Fig. 6.10 A), the right kidney has poor radiotracer uptake and excretion, which is confirmed by calculated differential renal uptake of 98% on the left and 2% on the right. The dilated left renal pelvis has a photopenic appearance on 1- to 3-minute images; it fills in with radiotracer gradually. No appreciable drainage is detected on the images or time/activity curve before the administration of furosemide (given 20 minutes after the tracer injection). There is significant radiotracer washout from the left renal pelvis, and calculated washout half-time is 8 minutes. The time/activity curve after furosemide injection also indicates marked tracer clearance (Fig. 6.10 B). A CT scan of the abdomen (Fig. 6.10 C) shows right-sided obstruction of the ureteropelvic junction and an atrophic right renal cortex.

Discussion: There is an obvious retention of excreted radiotracer in the dilated left renal pelvis. This activity diminishes markedly after diuresis induced by furosemide. Findings indicate a dilated nonobstructive system on the left side.

Diuretic renal scintigraphy has a well-established place in assessment of obstruction in hydronephrosis. Pediatric urologists rely on diuretic renograms in the management of patients with hydronephrosis. A nonobstructive hydronephrosis is managed conservatively, whereas an obstructive hydronephrosis requires surgical intervention.

Diuretic (furosemide) is usually injected when maximum radioactivity is apparent in the dilated renal pelvis; imaging is then continued for 20 to 30 minutes. The time/activity curves and washout half-time for dilated systems are used to assess for obstruction. A furosemide washout half-time less than 10 minutes indicates absence of obstruction, between 10 and 20 minutes is indeterminate, and greater than 20 minutes suggests an obstructed system.

Diagnosis: 1. Nonobstructive hydronephrosis on the left side. 2. Atrophic poorly functioning right kidney.

CASE 6.11

History: A middle-aged male presented with a history of right nephrectomy due to a renal carcinoma and a left-sided hydronephrosis on renal ultrasound. A furosemide ^{99m}Tc-MAG3 renogram was obtained (Figs. 6.11 A and 6.11 B) as well as an ultrasound (Fig. 6.11 C).

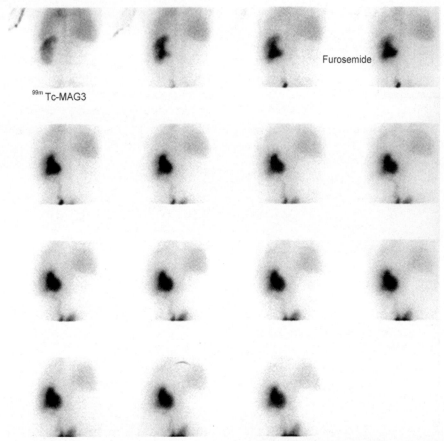

Figure 6.11 A

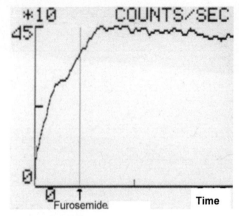

Figure 6.11 B

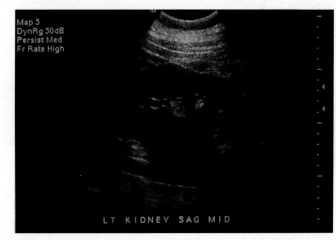

Figure 6.11 C

Findings: Functional images (Fig. 6.11 A) show good radio-tracer uptake by the left kidney; the right kidney is surgically absent. The left kidney has homogeneous cortical uptake with maximum activity on the 3- to 5-minute image. Activity accumulates gradually in the collecting system, without significant washout after intravenous injection of furosemide (given 10

negative result. This furosemide ^{99m}Tc-MAG3 renogram of a 2-year-old boy shows bilateral pelvocaliceal and ureter dilation due to prune-belly syndrome.

Prune-belly syndrome is characterized by absent or deficient abdominal wall musculature, bilateral intra-abdominal testis, and an abnormally dilated urinary tract.

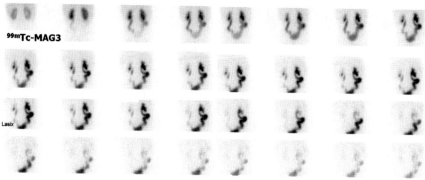

Figure 6.11 D

minutes after the radiotracer injection). The renogram curve for the left kidney (Fig. 6.11 B) reveals an accumulative pattern with no significant washout from the left renal pelvis. An ultrasound (Fig. 6.11 C) shows the dilated collecting system of the left kidney.

Discussion: The left kidney has normal function with a dilated renal pelvis. Significant activity remains in the renal pelvis after furosemide administration. These findings are most consistent with an obstructive hydronephrosis, likely due to obstruction of the ureteropelvic junction.

The main causes of a false-positive diuretic renogram are a huge collecting system, poor response to diuretic (due to renal immaturity in newborns, diminished renal function, or inadequate diuretic dose), full bladder, and dehydration (14). Figure 6.11 D shows an example of a potential cause of a false-

Both the degree of obstruction and the status of renal function constitute important information that is available on diuretic renography. Prolongation of washout half-time and/or decreasing split renal function on sequential studies is indicative of worsening of obstruction and/or deterioration of renal function.

In many cases, visual evaluation of images and quantitative data (e.g., furosemide washout $T_{1/2}$: 10 to 20 minutes) are indeterminate, and obstruction cannot be excluded. To clarify this situation, injection of furosemide 15 minutes prior to radiopharmaceutical administration is suggested, because maximum urine flow occurs 15 to 18 minutes after furosemide injection (14).

Diagnosis: Obstructive hydronephrosis on the right side.

CASE 6.12

History: A 40-year-old diabetic patient presented 1 day after renal transplantation. A baseline ^{99m}Tc-DTPA flow and renogram were obtained (Figs. 6.12 A and 6.12 B). He presented with acute deterioration of renal function 4 weeks later and a ^{99m}Tc-DTPA flow and renogram were again obtained (Figs. 6.12 C and 6.12 D).

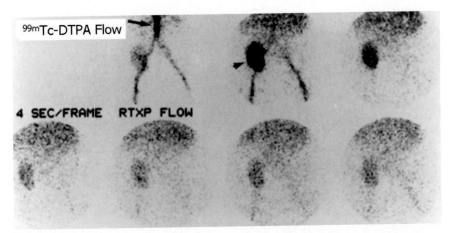

Figure 6.12 A

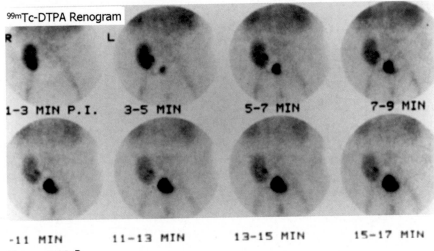

Figure 6.12 B

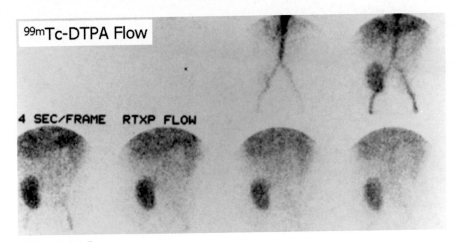

Figure 6.12 C

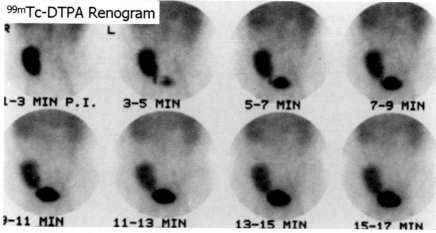

Figure 6.12 D

Findings: On the baseline study, a tight bolus of radiotracer injection is documented by a transient (approximately 4 seconds) presence of activity in the abdominal aorta (arrow) on the first-pass flow study (Fig. 6.12 A). Maximum aortic activity is followed by peak renal activity (arrowhead) in about 4 seconds (normal is 3 to 6 seconds), reflecting good inflow into the allograft. Intense renal activity decreases abruptly, which indicates good outflow from the kidney. Functional images (Fig. 6.12 B) show homogeneous cortical activity within the allograft. Excreted activity is in the renal pelvis and bladder on the 3- to 5-minute image, which is normal. There is good washout of activity from the renal cortex and renal pelvis.

On the study 4 weeks later, the renal flow study demonstrates transient activity within the abdominal aorta (4 to 8 seconds in duration), followed by visualization of the kidney in 4 seconds (Fig. 6.12 C). This indicates injection of a tight bolus of radiotracer and good inflow to the kidney. However, initial renal activity does not wash out promptly on the first-pass study. The sequential renogram images show homogeneous renal uptake and normal excretion into the renal pelvis bladder 3 to 5 minutes into the study (Fig. 6.12 D). No cortical retention is visualized. There is no evidence of obstruction.

Discussion: The baseline study demonstrates a normal transplant renogram. In many renal transplant centers, a baseline radionuclide renogram is obtained 24 to 72 hours after transplantation, and renal function is followed with additional renograms if clinically indicated.

Not having any deleterious effect on an expensive allograft, radionuclide renograms provide visual and quantitative evaluation of renal flow and function. Renal allograft complications that can be evaluated are renal artery or vein thrombosis, acute tubular necrosis, rejection, obstruction in the pelvis/ureter, urine leak, and lymphocele.

Technically, the transplant renogram is obtained very much like a regular radionuclide renogram except for the acquisition of images over the renal allograft above the pelvis anteriorly to avoid attenuation by the pelvis. ^{99m}Tc-MAG3 or ^{99m}Tc-DTPA are usually used for imaging.

On the 4-week posttransplant study, diminished renal perfusion with good renal function is suggestive of early acute rejection in this patient 4 weeks posttransplantation.

Two common complications in the early period of renal transplantation are ATN and acute rejection. ATN typically occurs in cadaveric grafts in the first week of transplantation and resolves spontaneously. Scintigraphically, it is characterized by a good or slight reduction of renal perfusion and prominently decreased renal function. Renal dysfunction resolves within 1 or 2 weeks. Cyclosporine toxicity has a renographic pattern similar to that of ATN.

Acute rejection occurs commonly in the first 3 months after transplantation. Early diagnosis of acute rejection is important, because prompt initiation of therapy will minimize renal damage. Scintigraphically, early acute rejection is characterized by decreased renal perfusion with relatively good renal function. Later on, both renal perfusion and function will deteriorate. In the early stage of acute rejection, visual detection of decreased renal perfusion on the flow study can be difficult. Many perfusion indices have been investigated to detect subtle changes (23). Acute rejection causes a more significant perfusion abnormality than ATN.

^{99m}Tc-sulfur colloid has also been used to differentiate between ATN and acute rejection (20). In acute rejection, there is sulfur colloid uptake within the renal allograft, which does not occur in ATN.

Renal biopsy remains the "gold standard" for the diagnosis of rejection.

Diagnosis: Baseline normal transplant renogram and acute rejection 4 weeks later.

CASE 6.13

History: This 30-year-old male with chronic renal failure received a cadaveric renal transplant in the right pelvic fossa about 1 hour before an emergency radionuclide renogram was obtained. The patient was anuric, and urinary catheter malfunction and hypovolemia were ruled out. The flow phase is displayed in Figure 6.13.

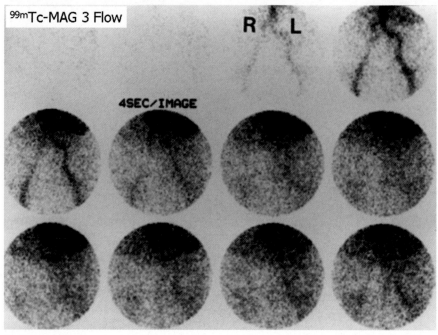

Figure 6.13

Findings: On anterior view of the lower abdomen/pelvis, there is visualization of the distal abdominal aorta and external iliac arteries on radionuclide angiogram (Fig. 6.13). No flow to the transplant kidney is demonstrated.

Discussion: Absence of renal flow in the immediate postoperative period represents a vascular allograft catastrophe, which requires emergency exploration if kidney viability is to be preserved. Usually there is no need for further imaging.

The differential diagnosis of nonvisualized renal allograft includes renal artery occlusion, renal vein thrombosis, and hyperacute rejection. With the modern matching technique, hyperacute rejection is no longer common.

Technical causes such as faulty radiopharmaceutical, camera setup, injection, etc., should always be carefully excluded before sending the patient back to the operating room.

At the reoperation of this patient, a kinked renal vessel was corrected by repositioning the kidney, resulting in a good recovery.

Absence of blood flow associated with photopenia in the region of the transplant bed is an ominous sign and usually represents an infarcted, nonsalvageable kidney, as noted in another, 42-year-old patient after renal transplantation.

Diagnosis: Vascular complication of the transplanted kidney.

CASE 6.14

History: A 49-year-old male presented 2 months after renal transplantation with an increase in serum creatinine. A ^{99m}Tc-MAG3 renogram and ultrasound were obtained (Figs. 6.14 A and 6.14 B)

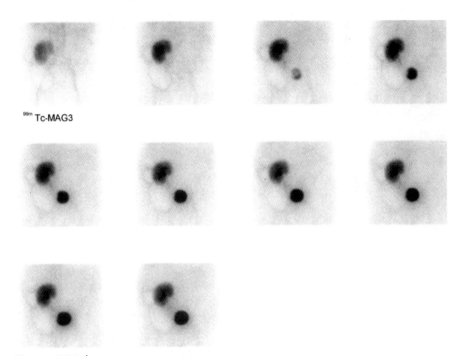

^{99m}Tc-MAG3

Figure 6.14 A

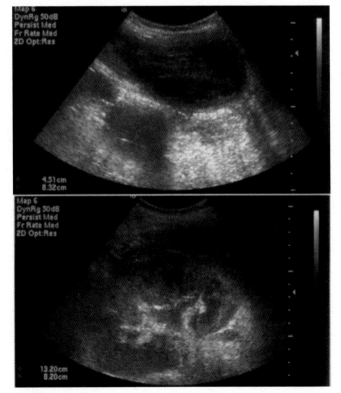

Figure 6.14 B

Findings: Functional images (Fig. 6.14 A) demonstrate radiotracer uptake and excretion by the transplant kidney. Excreted activity is identified in the urinary bladder at 6 to 10 minutes into the study. There is a large photopenic area between the renal transplant and the bladder. This area does not fill in with radiotracer during the study. A renal ultrasound (Fig. 6.14 B) reveals a large fluid collection in this area.

Discussion: A photopenic area around a renal transplant is most likely due to a hematoma, lymphocele, urinoma, or abscess. A hematoma is often seen in the surgical bed within the first few days following surgery. An urinoma defect is characterized by gradual filling in with radiotracer during the procedure. A lymphocele defect does not normally fill in with the radiotracer. In this case, the photopenic area between the bladder and kidney most likely represents a lymphocele.

During exposure of the iliac vessels for renal transplantation, the pelvic lymphatics are damaged, causing leakage and lymphocele formation. Postoperative lymphoceles may develop and present 1 week to 4 months following surgery. They may be asymptomatic or symptomatic, depending on their size and location. A common presentation is deterioration of renal function due to compression and obstruction of the ureter.

Diagnosis: Post–renal transplantation lymphocele.

CASE 6.15

History: A renal transplant patient status post–laparoscopic marsupialization for a pelvic lymphocele had bloody urine and decreased urine output immediately following surgery. A ^{99m}Tc-MAG3 renogram was obtained for further evaluation (Fig. 6.15 A).

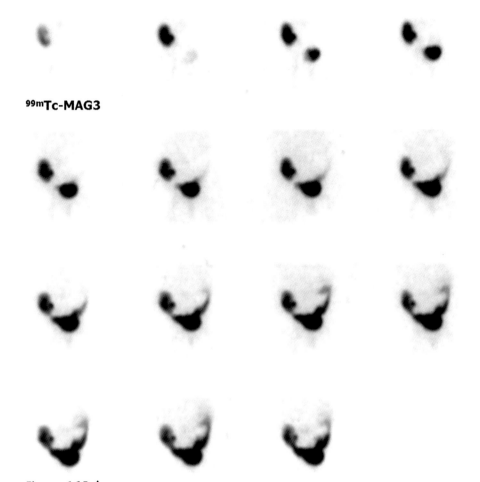

Figure 6.15 A

Findings: Functional images (Fig. 6.15 A) demonstrate good radiotracer uptake and excretion by the renal allograft. Excreted radioactivity is identified in the renal pelvis and bladder 3 to 5 minutes following radiotracer injection. At approximately 10 minutes into the procedure, there is abnormal activity in the superolateral aspect of the bladder on the left. This activity gradually increases in intensity and spreads into the expected location of the left pericolic gutter.

Discussion: On radionuclide renography, the presence of excreted activity outside the urinary tract is strongly suggestive

of a urinary leak. A vesicocolic fistula and vesicoureteral reflux into a nonfunctioning kidney may have a similar appearance. Given the history of recent surgical intervention around the bladder, findings in this case indicate an intraperitoneal leak, most likely from the bladder.

A subsequent contrast cystogram (Fig. 6.15 B) confirms a bladder leak, and a 1.5-cm tear in the bladder was identified on re-exploration.

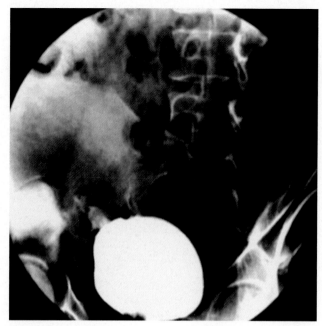

Figure 6.15 B

Urine leak is an infrequent complication in renal transplantation, which typically occurs in the first few days postsurgery and may originate at the level of the bladder, ureter, or renal calyx. It is usually caused by distal ureteral necrosis. A native ureter has a blood supply from several sources along its course; however, the transplant ureter receives blood only from the ureteral artery, a branch of the renal artery or its lower pole branches. Therefore the transplanted distal ureter is at risk for ischemic necrosis and subsequent urine leak.

In renal transplantation, a typical urine leak (urinoma) presents as a perinephric photopenic area that gradually fills in with radioactivity during radionuclide renography.

Diagnosis: Urinary extravasation due to bladder tear.

CASE 6.16

History: A 58-year-old male presented with a history of a renal transplant performed 12 years earlier and increased levels of serum creatinine. A ^{99m}Tc-MAG3 flow study and renogram were obtained (Figs. 6.16 A and 6.16 B)

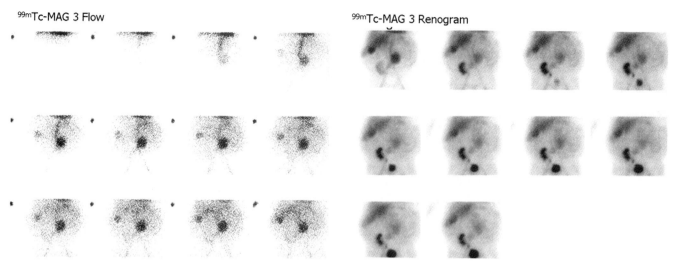

^{99m}Tc-MAG 3 Flow

^{99m}Tc-MAG 3 Renogram

Figure 6.16 A

Figure 6.16 B

Findings: Anterior flow images (Fig. 6.16 A) show decreased flow to the transplanted right pelvic kidney, a focal area of increased flow in the middle abdomen, and a mild area in the right upper abdomen. Functional images (Fig. 6.16 B) show decreased function in the transplanted kidney. They also show the area in the middle abdomen that decreases its intensity over the time, and the focal area of increased uptake in the right upper abdomen, which is likely to be activity within the gallbladder.

Discussion: ^{99m}Tc-MAG3 has an alternative route of excretion through the biliary system. ^{99m}Tc-GH is also a renal imaging agent that has the same excretion path. The visualization of the gallbladder can happen in patients with renal insufficiency. Some drugs—such as penicillin, penicillamine,

acetaminophen, and trimethoprim-sulfamethoxazole—can also increase biliary excretion. In this case, the gallbladder activity is likely due to the patient's renal insufficiency.

The finding in the middle abdomen is due to an abdominal aortic aneurysm that was visualized on an abdominal ultrasound (Fig. 6.16 C). This finding is a good example of the importance of the flow images; these can help with the diagnosis of incidental abdominal findings—such as aneurysms, tumors, and abdominal inflammatory abnormalities—which can increase the blood flow and may not be the aim of the study.

Diagnosis: (a) Gallbladder visualization on ^{99m}Tc-MAG3 renogram due to renal insufficiency. (b) Aneurysm of the aorta.

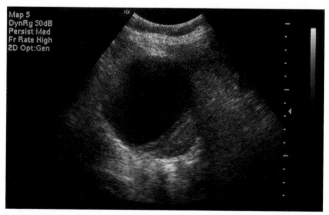

Figure 6.16 C

CASE 6.17

History: In a 40-year-old man with right flank pain, a renal ultrasound (Fig. 6.17 A) reveals an approximately 2.4- by 3.0-cm area of thickened tissue in continuation with the renal cortex and with the same echogenicity extending inward—a pattern suggestive of pseudotumor or prominence of the column of Bertin. A renal cortical scintigram with ^{99m}Tc-DMSA is obtained for further evaluation (Fig. 6.17 B).

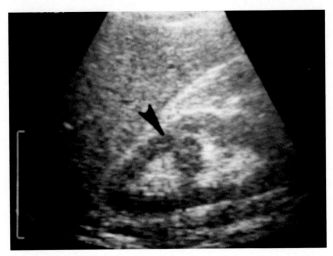

Figure 6.17 A

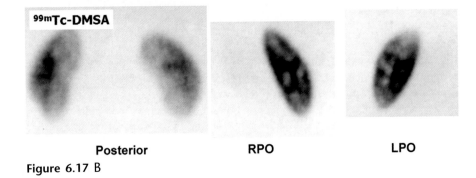

Posterior   RPO   LPO

Figure 6.17 B

Findings: On planar images (Fig. 6.17 B), the kidneys are normal in size, with smooth contours. There is no abnormal photon-deficient focus in the region of the "pseudomass." Mild bilateral heterogeneous uptake within the kidneys is normal and is due to low uptake in the renal pyramids and absence of activity in the collecting systems.

Discussion: Demonstration of ^{99m}Tc-DMSA uptake in the area of the pseudotumor confirms normally functioning renal cortex and represents a hypertrophied column of Bertin.

The column of Bertin is an extension of normal renal cortex between two pyramids, most commonly at the junction of the upper and middle thirds of the kidney. It may be hypertrophied and mimic an intrarenal mass. This normal cortical tissue has radiotracer uptake on ^{99m}Tc-DMSA or ^{99m}Tc-GH on renal scintigraphy. Renal space-occupying lesions such as tumors (primary or metastatic), cysts, or abscesses will show lack of radiotracer uptake on renocortical imaging.

Diagnosis: Prominent column of Bertin.

CASE 6.18

History: This 7-month-old male with UTI was known to have a right-sided duplex system. ^{99m}Tc-MAG3 baseline and post-furosemide renograms were obtained to evaluate the functional status of the kidney (Figs. 6.18 A and 6.18 B).

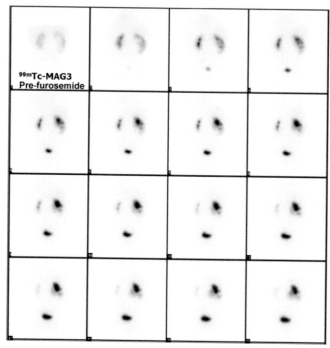

Figure 6.18 A

Figure 6.18 B

Findings: The prefurosemide renographic images (Fig. 6.18 A) demonstrate delayed cortical uptake and excretion of the right upper moiety, suggestive of diminished function. The medially located photopenia represents the dilated renal pelvis, which gradually fills in on the later sequences of the images. The left lower moiety has good cortical uptake and excretion.

The postfurosemide image (Fig. 6.18 B) demonstrates minimal radiotracer washout from the upper moiety, with a calculated washout T$_{1/2}$ of 59 minutes (no obstruction <10 minutes, intermediate 10 to 20 minutes, obstruction over 20 minutes). These findings are consistent with obstruction. Poor response to furosemide due to diminished renal function may have a similar appearance.

Discussion: Early homogeneous cortical radiotracer uptake and subsequent excretion indicate good function of the upper and lower moieties of the left kidney. However, focal radiotracer retention in the upper collecting system is consistent with hydronephrosis.

Although the presence and absence of hydronephrosis can be evaluated by ultrasound, a furosemide renal scintigram plays an important role in evaluating the functional status of the kidney.

Renal duplication is a common anomaly that results from ureteral duplication. In complete duplication, the ureter of the upper moiety has an ectopic insertion into the bladder and is at risk of obstruction and loss of function. The ureter of the lower moiety enters into the bladder at the trigone and is prone to physical ureteral reflux, resulting in scarring and inadequate function (Meyer-Weiger law). In 20% of cases, duplications are bilateral, and an incomplete form is more common than the completed form.

Renal duplication in non-complicated cases is of little clinical significance; however, its presence should be recognized. An unrecognized renal duplication may lead to a serious diagnostic error.

Diagnosis: Left-sided duplication system with an obstructed hydronephrosis of the upper moiety.

History: On a bone scintigram of this 70-year-old female with weight loss, photopenia was noted in the upper pole of the right kidney (Fig. 6.19 A, arrow). The patient was referred for a ^{99m}Tc-MAG3 renogram (Fig. 6.19 B).

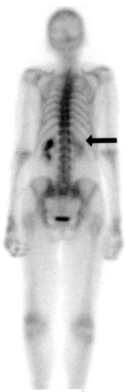

^{99m}Tc-HDP

Figure 6.19 A

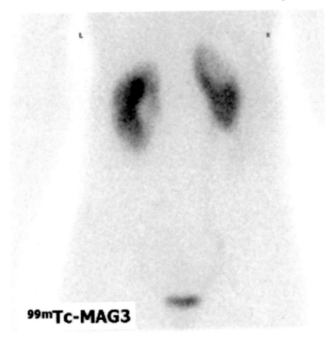

^{99m}Tc-MAG3

Figure 6.19 B

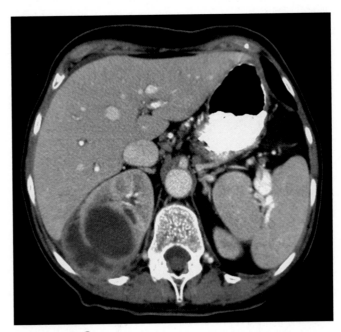

Figure 6.19 C

Findings: Images from a ^{99m}Tc-MAG3 renogram (Fig. 6.19 B) show persistent photopenia in the upper pole of the left kidney. There is abnormal washout of both kidneys, representing moderately poor function (not shown). An abdominal CT (Fig. 6.19 C) shows a large cystic mass in the superior pole of the right kidney (Fig. 6.19 C).

Discussion: Lack of uptake in the upper pole of the right kidney would be consistent with nonfunctioning renal tissue.

Studies with ^{99m}Tc-MAG3 give excellent morphologic images of the kidneys in addition to evaluating their function. Infarcts can be seen as wedge-shaped cortical-based defects. In some cases this technique allows visualization of lesions that are not seen on ultrasound.

This patient had a renal biopsy, followed by nephrectomy. Tissue pathology showed a poorly differentiated carcinoma compatible with a urothelial or bronchogenic origin. A nonfunctioning lower pole could be suggestive of renal duplication, in which the upper pole moiety classically obstructs while the lower moiety refluxes, causing scarring and the development of nonfunctional tissue.

Renal duplication on CT may appear as two distinct groups of renal pelves but is not seen in this case. Instead, CT demonstrates a large cystic mass in the upper pole; it is not consistent with loss of renal tissue secondary to the scarring and atrophy that would be expected to result from reflux.

The other causes of a nonfunctioning upper pole, excluding cyst, could include any space-occupying lesion, a benign tumor (hamartoma), malignant tumor (renal cell carcinoma), metastasis, lymphoma, abscess, hematoma, or postsurgical change. In the absence of fever, history of surgery, or trauma, findings in this patient would be most consistent with a solid tumor of the upper pole of the kidney.

At surgery, a renal cell carcinoma with no evidence of duplication was noted and removed.

The differential diagnosis of a photopenic area within a transplant kidney includes an infectious process (segmental pyelonephritis, abscess), renal cyst, hydrocalyx, vascular problem (localized infarct, traumatic hematoma), benign or malignant (primary or metastatic) tumor and artifact (for example, barium-filled loops of bowel) (24). Anatomic studies (ultrasound, CT scan, or MRI) are needed to narrow the differential diagnosis. Renal ultrasound can easily separate cystic lesions (renal cyst, hydrocalyx) from solid masses. Infiltrative tumors may be isoechoic on ultrasound and difficult to diagnose.

The scintigraphic appearance of all renal space-occupying lesions includes reduced tracer uptake, reflecting the replacement of renal tissue by a pathologic process. This includes all radiopharmaceuticals used for renal imaging, such as ^{99m}Tc-labeled DTPA, GH, DMSA, and ^{99m}Tc-MAG3. The only renal tumor that may concentrate ^{99m}Tc-GH is a nephroblastic nephroma, a tumor of neonates. Although the morphologic evaluation of masses is best achieved by CT and ultrasound, renal imaging is helpful in the study of the functional status of the kidney and the disease process. The diagnostic difficulty of fetal lobulation, dromedary humps, and renal columns of Bertin producing a pseudomass on CT and ultrasound can be resolved easily by renal imaging. Uptake of any renal imaging agents by a renal mass virtually excludes the possibility of malignancy and confirms functional renal tissue. Thus a negative study has a high index value.

Diagnosis: Renal cell carcinoma, upper pole of right kidney.

CASE 6.20

History: A 7-year-old patient presented with an abdominal mass on palpation. The patient had a history of one uncomplicated UTI. At that time, a voiding contrast cystourethrogram was normal. A diuretic renogram was then performed following intravenous injection of ^{99m}Tc-MAG3 (Fig. 6.20).

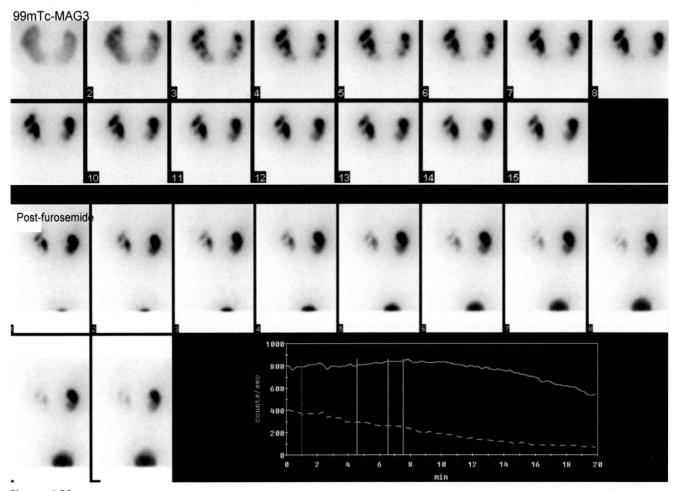

Figure 6.20

Findings: The renogram images (Fig. 6.20) demonstrate parenchymal activity extending across the midline, connecting the two lower poles. There is poor washout of the radiopharmaceutical from the left upper pole and a poor response to furosemide.

Discussion: Functional parenchymal activity is seen to join the lower poles of both kidneys. Often, the kidneys are located more inferiorly than expected. The findings of ectopic kidneys and a conjoined pole are those of a horseshoe kidney. The incidence of horseshoe kidney is 1 in 400. Fusion is most commonly seen between the two lower poles. The tissue connecting the pair may be a fibrous band, functioning renal tissue, or a combination of both. Anterior images are often helpful to demonstrate functioning tissue that may not be apparent on posterior images owing to attenuation by the spine.

The involved kidneys tend to have an abnormal axis with malrotation and an incline of the axis of the inferior poles toward the midline. The axis of the kidneys may also be more anterior than normal. The isthmus is most commonly situated anterior to both the aorta and the inferior vena cava and posterior to the inferior mesenteric artery.

Associated renal abnormalities include ureteropelvic junction (UPJ) obstruction in 30% and ureteral duplication in 10%. Scintigraphy is useful in assessing functional abnormalities, obstruction, and infection. Patients with horseshoe kidney are at increased risk for obstruction, infection, and calculus formation. There is a slightly increased incidence of malignancy when compared with the normal population. Patients are also at risk for traumatic injury to the kidneys secondary to the more inferior location of a horseshoe kidney.

Diagnosis: Horseshoe kidney.

CASE 6.21

History: This 6-year-old girl presented with reduced urine production. A diuretic ^{99m}Tc-MAG3 renal scintigram was obtained (Figs. 6.21 A and 6.21 B).

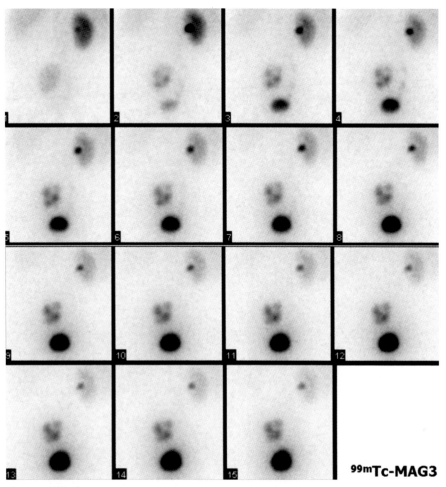

Figure 6.21 A

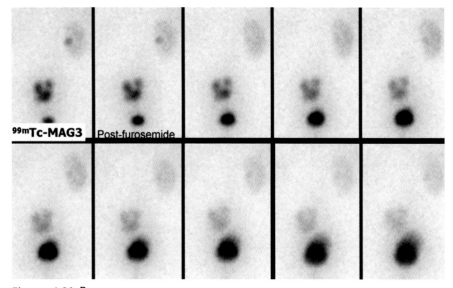

Figure 6.21 B

Findings: The images (Fig. 6.21 A) demonstrate normal location and function of the right kidney. The left kidney is ectopic. It is located within the pelvis on the left. The left renal pelvis is abnormally located. The renal pelvis is oriented anteriorly, indicative of malrotation. There is good function of the left kidney. There is retention of radiopharmaceutical in the collecting system, which cleared promptly after furosemide administration (Fig. 6.21 B). Figure 6.21 C show an abdominal CT showing the right and the pelvic left kidney.

Discussion: The kidneys ascend during fetal life from their origin within the deep pelvis to their expected final position within the abdomen adjacent to the upper lumbar spine. During their ascent, there is a 90-degree inward rotation along the longitudinal axis, such that the hilus is directed medially and slightly anteriorly. If this movement does not occur properly, there is deficient, excessive, or reversed rotation. This case demonstrates failure of the right kidney to achieve the normal ascent into the abdomen, with accompanying reversal of normal rotation. The right renal hilus is directed laterally. In this case, the renal artery is anomalous, arising either from the inferior portion of the aorta or from the right iliac artery. Anomalies of rotation are frequently associated with renal ectopia and renal fusion. In simple renal ectopia, the affected kidney is usually located lower than normal. Abnormal ascent of the kidney into the thorax is rare but has been described. The left kidney is more commonly affected. The kidney is usually located in a diaphragmatic eventration or has moved through a diaphragmatic hernia.

In the case of cross-fused renal ectopia (Fig. 6.21 D, ^{99m}Tc-MAG3 and CT images respectively), the anomalous kidney is located on the opposite side of the abdomen than its origin and is fused with the opposite kidney. The ectopic kidney usually lies lower than the normal kidney. Malrotation of the ectopic kidney is the rule. The ureter of the ectopic kidney usually traverses the ectopic kidney and inserts into the urinary bladder on its site of origin.

Diagnosis: Ectopic right kidney.

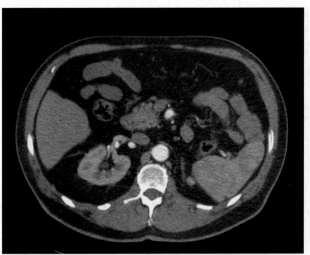

Right kidney

Ectopic left kidney

Figure **6.21** C

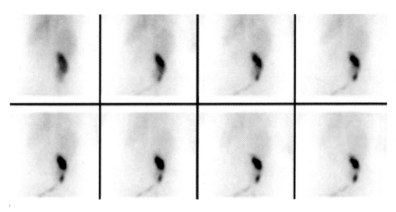

⁹⁹mTc-MAG3

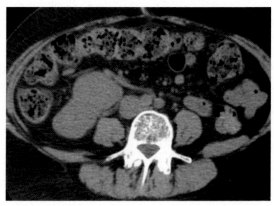

CT

Figure **6.21** D

CASE 6.22

History: A 39-year-old HIV-positive black male presented with a history of chronic renal insufficiency and was referred for a MAG3 renal scintigraphy (Fig. 6.22 A) and ultrasound (Fig. 6.22 B).

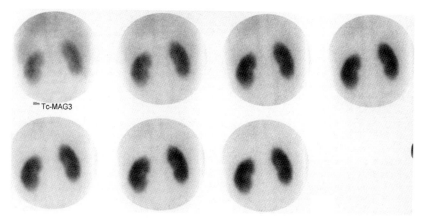

Figure 6.22 A

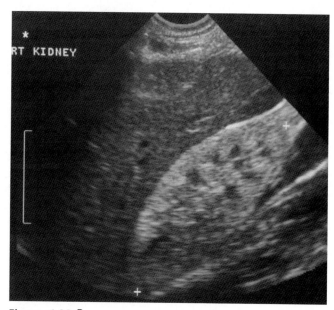

Figure 6.22 B

Findings: ^{99m}Tc-MAG3 scintigraphic images (Fig. 6.22 A) show symmetrically decreased bilateral renal function. Renal ultrasound (Fig. 6.22 B) shows decreased corticomedullary differentiation and increased echogenicity.

Discussion: HIV-associated nephropathy (HIVAN) is an important cause of morbidity and mortality among HIV-infected patients. HIVAN is usually diagnosed when the patient has a significant proteinuria, often but not always in the nephrotic range (>3 g day) (25). This disease affects almost exclusively people of African descent and is the third most common leading cause of end-stage renal disease among African Americans between 20 and 64 years of age (26). Diagnosis is usually made late in the course of HIV infection, but renal involvement can occur early, even during the acute retroviral syndrome prior to HIV antibody seroconversion (25). Pathologic findings of HIVAN involve the glomerular, tubular, and interstitial compartments. Glomerular pathologic findings include focal glomerular sclerosis and collapse of the glomerular tuft. Tubular disease is characterized by tubular dilation. There is also lymphocytic infiltration of the interstitium (24). AIDS mortality rates are stable, but its incidence is still increasing. It has been projected that the burden of renal disease associated with HIV infection will increase exponentially over the coming years (25).

Sonographic findings of HIVAN are increased echogenicity, enlarged kidneys, and loss of corticomedullary differentiation. The findings of MAG3 renal scintigraphy are mainly impaired global renal function, with a good cortical uptake but poor excretion of the radiopharmaceutical. These findings are probably a functional picture of the involvement of the glomerular, tubular, and interstitial compartments.

Diagnosis: AIDS nephropathy.

History: This 50-year-old male received his second renal transplant 2 weeks earlier. Two ^{99m}Tc-MAG3 transplant renograms were obtained 1 week apart (Figs. 6.23 A and 6.23 B).

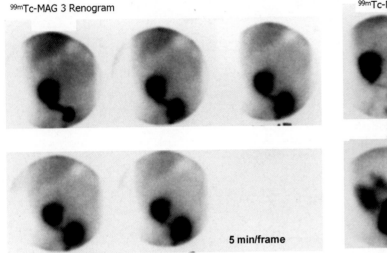

1 week post-transplant

Figure 6.23 A

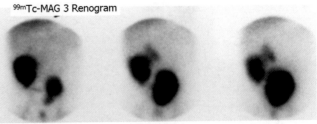

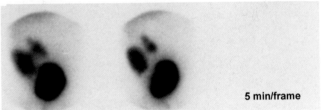

2 weeks post-transplant

Figure 6.23 B

Findings: The initial study (Fig. 6.23 A) demonstrates radiotracer uptake and excretion into the renal collecting system and bladder on the 2- to 7-minute image. Further uptake and excretion are visualized on subsequent images. The follow-up study (Fig. 6.23 B) reveals similar findings. In addition, there is a focus of activity in the superomedial aspect of the most recent allograft on the 7- to 12-minute image, which slightly increases in intensity in the remainder of the study.

Discussion: The differential diagnosis for an area of activity outside the most recent renal allograft is urinoma and reappearance of residual function in the old allograft. Although

^{99m}Tc-MAG3 may accumulate in the gallbladder, it is unlikely in this case, because the above activity is not in the expected location of the gallbladder. Pelvic ultrasound (not shown) is negative for perinephric fluid collection, and an old allograft is present in the superomedial aspect of the most recent transplant. When a patient receives a new renal transplant, immunosuppressive therapy is resumed. If an old transplant is left in place, it will often recover some function and will be visualized on radionuclide renography.

Diagnosis: Residual function in old renal transplant.

CASE 6.24

History: This 6-year-old male presented with severe hypertension and progressively increasing serum creatinine. The patient was known since birth to have cystic changes involving both kidneys, as seen on renal ultrasound (Figs. 6.24 A and 6.24 B). A diuretic ⁹⁹ᵐTc-MAG3 renogram was obtained (Figs. 6.24 C and 6.24 D).

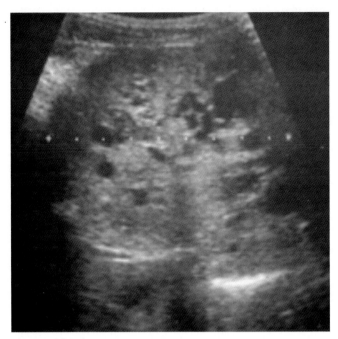

Figure 6.24 A

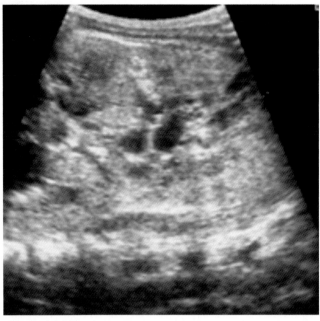

Figure 6.24 B

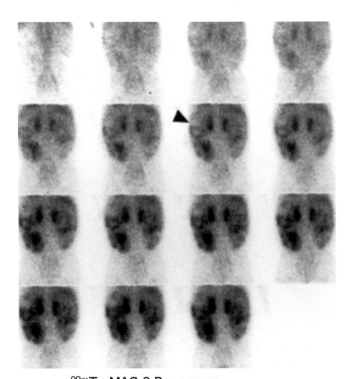

⁹⁹ᵐTc-MAG 3 Renogram

Figure 6.24 C

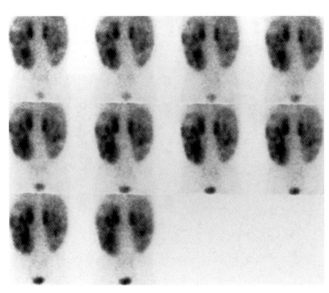

⁹⁹ᵐTc-MAG 3 Renogram post-furosemide

Figure 6.24 D

Findings: The kidneys are normal in position but very large. There is delayed and heterogeneous tracer uptake in the parenchyma of both kidneys, suggesting polycystic kidneys. Slow background clearance and delayed visualization of the bladder indicate overall poor renal function. There is little detectable accumulation in the collecting systems prior to furosemide. Incidentally, photopenic defects are also seen in the liver due to associated polycystic liver disease (Fig. 6.24 C, arrowhead). The diuretic portion of the renogram demonstrates no response to the diuretic infusion at 20 minutes.

Discussion: These findings indicate extremely poor function in a child with autosomal recessive polycystic kidney disease (ARPKD). Most infants with ARPKD expire in the newborn period from pulmonary hypoplasia or renal failure. In less severe cases, affected children have survived into adolescence.

Autosomal recessive polycystic kidney disease is an inherited cystic disorder involving both kidneys. Pathologically, there is medullary ductal ectasia with tubular atrophy. Clinically, there is a progressive loss of the normal concentrating ability of the kidneys and systemic hypertension. The findings associated with ARPKD include hepatic cysts, with associated hepatic dysfunction and fibrosis.

Renal sonography is the method of choice for diagnosis. The sonographic images demonstrate markedly increased echogenicity of the renal parenchyma with both loss of corticomedullary differentiation and nephromegaly (Figs. 6.24 A and 6.24 B). Radionuclide scintigraphy with ^{99m}Tc-MAG3 is utilized to assess renal function. The scintigraphic appearance of the kidneys in patients who survive into childhood is that of nephromegaly with heterogeneous uptake of radionuclide in the renal parenchyma surrounding the cysts. The transit of tracer through the kidneys is delayed. In the case of severe dysfunction, there may be no renal uptake.

Diagnosis: Autosomal recessive polycystic kidney disease.

CASE 6.25

History: A premature female born at 34 weeks' gestation was discovered to have multiple left renal cysts on a prenatal screening sonogram. A diuretic ^{99m}Tc-MAG3 renogram is obtained to evaluate renal function (Figs. 6.25 A and 6.25 B).

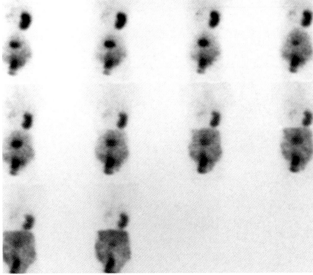

^{99m}Tc-MAG 3 Renogram post-furosemide

Figure 6.25 B

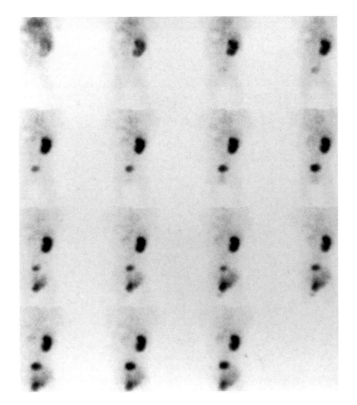

^{99m}Tc-MAG 3 Renogram

Figure 6.25 A

Findings: The renogram demonstrates progressive accumulation of MAG3 in the right renal parenchyma and poor excretion due to immature renal function. The progressively appearing background around the bladder is due to urine accumulation in the diaper. The left kidney has no detectable renal function.

Discussion: Multicystic dysplastic kidney is the most frequent cystic disorder of the kidneys in infants and children. The disorder is nonfamilial and usually unilateral. Bilateral multicystic dysplasia is fatal in the immediate neonatal period. Unilateral renal involvement is variable, with variation in the size of the affected kidney as well as the size of the cysts. The cysts occur in both the cortical and medullary portions of the kidneys. There is no communication between the renal cysts. Figure 6.25 C is a sagittal sonographic image of the left kidney. There is complete lack of corticomedullary differentiation (arrow). A conglomerate mass of large cysts is seen at the lower pole. A second sagittal image (Fig. 6.25 D) demonstrates several smaller noncommunicating cysts (arrow) as well as a central dilated renal collecting system (curved arrow).

The multicystic dysplastic kidney is thought to result from ureteral occlusion before 10 weeks' gestation. There are absent or atretic renal vessels and an atretic ureter. Primitive and dysplastic parenchyma surrounds the multiple cysts.

The most common scintigraphic appearance is absence of uptake of the radiopharmaceutical on the affected side. Computer-enhanced images may be helpful in detecting minimal tracer uptake. Occasionally, patchy tracer uptake is seen in distorted renal parenchyma without the aid of enhancement.

The significant radiographic features of multicystic dysplastic kidney include compensatory hypertrophy of the contralateral kidney. In adults, calcification of the cyst walls may be evident on radiographs. There is a 10% incidence of contralateral renal abnormalities, the most common being obstruction of the ureteropelvic junction.

The right kidney demonstrates immature function. The normal-term infant will have 30% of the glomerular filtration rate/surface area of an adult. There is a dramatic increase in the glomerular filtration rate during the immediate postnatal

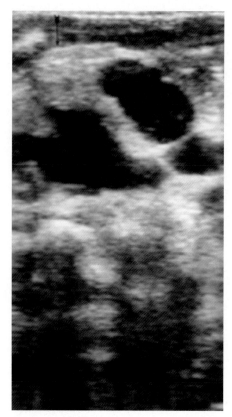

Figure 6.25 C

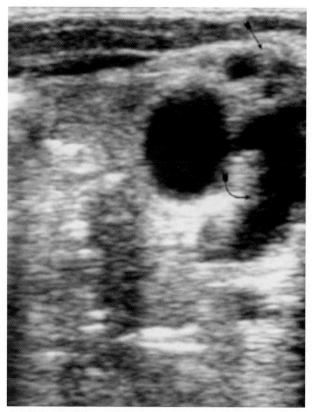

Figure 6.25 D

period, with approximately 50% of the adult corrected value at 2 weeks. The normal adult glomerular filtration rate is attained at anywhere from 6 to 12 months. Premature infants with very low birth weights have, on average, 10% the adult glomerular filtration rate with a slower rise to mature levels.

Sonography is usually the first modality in the evaluation of delayed micturition. In most cases, sonography demonstrates an anatomic cause. Radionuclide scintigraphy is specifically useful in the assessment of renal function. Intravenous urog-

raphy is not the method of choice in evaluating renal function or anomalies owing to poor concentration of contrast material seen with poor renal function in neonates. Overlying bowel gas obscures the already faintly visualized kidneys. Therefore tomography may be the only acceptable way to gather anatomic data, subjecting the infant to high doses of radiation.

Diagnosis: (a) Left multicystic dysplastic kidney. (b) Immature function of the right kidney.

REFERENCES

1. Boubaker A, Prior JO, Meuwly JY, Bischof-Delaloye A. Radionuclide investigations of the urinary tract in the era of multimodality imaging. *J Nucl Med* 2006;47(11):1819–1836.
2. Sandler MP, Coleman RE, Wackers FJT, et al., eds. *Diagnostic Nuclear Medicine*, 4th ed. Baltimore: Lippincott Williams & Wilkins, 2003.
3. Ziessman HA, O'Malley JP, Thrall JH. *Nuclear Medicine: The Requisites,* 3rd ed. St. Louis: Mosby, 2006.
4. Treves S, ed. *Pediatric Nuclear Medicine/PET*, 3rd ed. New York: Springer, 2006.
5. Ponto JA, Chilton HM, Watson NE. Radiopharmaceuticals for genitourinary imaging: glomerular and tubular function, anatomy, urodynamics and testicular imaging. In: Swanson DP, Chilton HM, Thrall JM, eds. *Pharmaceuticals in Medical Imaging*. New York: Macmillan, 1990.
6. Eshima D, Taylor A. Technetium 99m mercaptoacetyltriglycine: update on new Tc-99m renal tubular function agent. *Semin Nucl Med* 1992;22: 61–63.
7. Saha GB. *Fundamentals of Nuclear Pharmacy*, 5th ed. New York: Springer-Verlag, 2004.
8. DeSadeleer C, Bossuyt A, Goes E, Piepsz A. Renal technetium 99m DMSA SPECT in normal volunteers. *J Nucl Med* 1996;37:1346–1349.
9. Yen TC, Chen WP, Chang SL, et al. Technetium 99m DMSA renal SPECT in diagnosing and monitoring pediatric acute pyelonephritis. *J Nucl Med* 1996;37:1349–1353.
10. Major M, Rushton HG. Renal cortical scintigraphy in diagnosis of acute pyelonephritis. *Semin Nucl Med* 1992;22:98–111.
11. Conway JJ. "Well-tempered" diuresis renography: its historical development, physiological and technical pitfalls, and standardized technique protocol. *Semin Nucl Med* 1992;22:74–84.
12. O'Reilly P, Aurell M, Britton K, et al. Consensus on diuresis renography for investigating the dilated upper urinary tract. *J Nucl Med* 1996;37: 1872–1876.
13. Nally JV, Olin W, Lammert GK. Advances in noninvasive screening for renovascular hypertension. *Cleve Clin J Med* 1994;61:328–336.
14. Fine EJ. Interventions in renal scintirenography. *Semin Nucl Med* 1999; 29;128–145.
15. Black HR, Bourgoignie JJ, Pickering T, et al. Report of the working party group for patient selection and preparation. *Am J Hypertens* 1991;4: 745S–746S.
16. Nally JV, Chen C, Fine E, et al. Diagnostic criteria of renovascular hypertension with captopril renography: a consensus statement. *Am J Hypertens* 1991;4:749S–752S.
17. Taylor A, Nally J, Aurell M, et al. Consensus report on ACE inhibitor renography for detecting renovascular hypertension. *J Nucl Med* 1996;37:1876–1882.
18. Chen DC, Holder LE, Melloul M. Radionuclide scrotal imaging: further experience with 210 patients. Part I: Anatomy–pathophysiology and methods. *J Nucl Med* 1983;24:735–742.
19. Chen DCP, Holder LE, Melloul M. Radionuclide scrotal imaging: further experience with 210 new patients. Part 2: Results and discussion. *J Nucl Med* 1983;24:841–853.
20. Meier GH, Sumpio B, Setaro JF, Black HR, Gusberg RJ. Captopril renal scintigraphy: a new standard for predicting outcome after renal revascularization. *J Vasc Surg* 1993;17(2):280–285.
21. Holley KE, Hunt JC, Brown AL, et al. Renal artery stenosis: a clinical–pathologic study in normotensive and hypertensive patients. *Am J Med* 1964;37:14–22.
22. Blue PW, Manier SM, Chantelois RE, et al. Differential diagnosis of prolonged cortical retention of radiotracer in technetium-99m DTPA renal scintigraphy. *Clin Nucl Med* 1987;12:77–83.
23. Dubovsky EV, Russell CD, Erbas B. Radionuclide evaluation of renal transplants. *Semin Nucl Med* 1995;25:49–59.
24. Sanchez FW, Gordon L, Curry N. Photopenic defect within transplant kidney. *Semin Nucl Med* 1984;14:342.
25. Ross MJ, Klotman PE. HIV-associated nephropathy. *AIDS* 2004;18:1089–1099.
26. Olatinwo T, Hewitt RG, Venuto RC. Human immunodeficiency virus–associated nephropathy. *Arch Intern Med* 2004;164:333–336.

CHAPTER SEVEN

MUSCULOSKELETAL SCINTIGRAPHY

M. REZA HABIBIAN AND
CARLOS CUNHA PEREIRA NETO

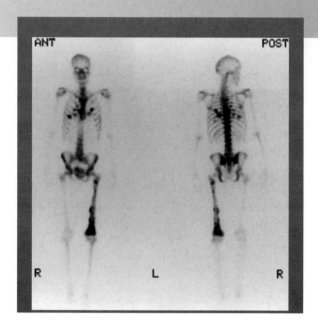

Skeletal scintigraphy, the most frequently performed nuclear medicine procedure second to nuclear cardiology, is an extremely sensitive method for detecting bone abnormalities. The sensitivity of the method relies on its ability to detect functional rather than structural changes, which are more easily visible on conventional radiographs, although not necessarily at an early stage.

All aspects of skeletal scintigraphy are addressed in detail in several major textbooks as well as numerous excellent reviews and scientific articles. This review is limited to only a few common clinical concerns.

RADIOPHARMACEUTICALS

Radiopharmaceuticals available and in use for bone scintigraphy include diphosphonate compounds labeled with ^{99m}Tc-pertechnetate, positron emitter fluorine-18 (^{18}F)-fluoride ion, and ^{18}F-fluorodeoxyglucose (^{18}F-FDG).

Technetium-99m (^{99m}Tc)–labeled diphosphonate is used almost exclusively for conventional bone scanning. ^{18}F-fluoride ion can be used to evaluate a number of benign and malignant bone lesions. ^{18}F-FDG as a tumor imaging agent is of use to evaluate primary and metastatic bone and bone marrow malignancy.

DIPHOSPHONATE COMPOUNDS

Diphosphonate compounds [methylene diphosphonate (MDP), hydroxyethylene diphosphonate (HEDP), and hydroxydiphosphonate (HDP)] labeled with ^{99m}Tc-pertechnetate currently are the agents of choice for bone scanning.

Following the IV injection of 20 to 30 mCi, the radiopharmaceutical distributes uniformly throughout the circulation, slowly clears from the blood, passively diffuses into the extravascular and extracellular space, subsequently binds to the hydroxyapatite crystal of the bone, and allows visualization of the skeleton.

In a normally hydrated patient, 3 hours after the injection of radiopharmaceutical, 30% to 40% of the dose will be associated with bone, 30% to 40% will be excreted by the kidney, 10% to 15% will be distributed in other tissues, and 5% will remain in the blood.

The whole-body radiation dose is 130 mrad per 20-mCi dose, and the target organ (organ receiving the highest radiation dose) is the urinary bladder, with an absorbed dose of 2.6 rad per 20 mCi at 2 hours. Patients should void frequently in order to reduce the radiation to the bladder and ovaries.

^{18}F-FLUORIDE ION

The ^{18}F-fluoride ion localizes in the bone by absorption into the bone surface forming the fluoroapatite by exchanging with hydroxyapatite of the bone.

The mechanism of localization of ^{18}F-fluoride in the bone is similar to that of diphosphonate compound and occurs in proportion to the regional blood flow and the osteoblastic activity of the skeleton, with the highest deposit in the area of high bone turnover and remodeling.

Owing to the smaller size of the fluoride ion as compared to the diphosphonate compound and also not being a protein-bound agent, the clearance of ^{18}F-fluoride from the blood is much faster than diphosphonate and localizes more quickly in the bone, provides a high-contrast image with higher spatial resolution than conventional bone scans as early as 1 hour after the injection of a 5- to 10-mCi dose.

^{18}F-FLUORODEOXYGLUCOSE (^{18}F-FDG)

Uptake of ^{18}F-FDG in the bone lesion represents direct accumulation in the metabolically active cell with a high rate of glycolysis, such as a tumor cell. Therefore the mechanism of ^{18}F-FDG uptake is different from that of diphosphonate and ^{18}F-fluoride, in which bone localization is due to reaction of the bone to the presence of pathology (tumor, infection, trauma, etc.) and their nonspecific uptake occurs in the mineralizing surface of the bone and not inside the cell.

Uptake of ^{18}F-FDG in different tumors varies based on their metabolic activity. Lytic and sclerotic metastatic bony lesions may have a different affinity for ^{18}F-FDG. ^{18}F-FDG has a lower sensitivity in the detection of sclerotic breast and prostate metastases than conventional bone scintigraphy. A sclerotic lesion is less cellular and has a lower rate of glycolysis. However, FDG has the highest sensitivity for the detection of skeletal lymphoma at the earlier stage. Skeletal lymphoma at the earlier stage is confined to the marrow compartment; it is only in the later stage that bone reaction and remodeling occur, allowing their visualization on conventional bone scan.

NORMAL PLANAR BONE SCINTIGRAPHY

In a whole-body conventional radionuclide bone scan, mild to moderate increased activity is normally seen in the base of the skull, external occipital protuberance, paranasal sinuses, thyroid and calcified thyroid cartilage, sternoclavicular and sternomandibular joints, costochondral junctions, sternum, inferior tip of scapula, spinous process of the vertebra, sacroiliac joints, genitalia, and unfused epiphyses.

Although diphosphonates as compared with polyphosphate and pyrophosphates are more stable *in vivo*, have a higher bone uptake, and are more rapidly cleared from the blood, all of these compounds are fairly weak chelating agents and degrade with time, releasing free pertechnetate, which degrades the quality of the images. Therefore freshly prepared radiopharmaceutical should be used.

Image quality is also influenced by the state of the patient's hydration and renal function. The patient should be well hydrated in order to enhance renal excretion. In dialysis patients, the radiopharmaceutical should be injected prior to dialysis and scanning performed after dialysis.

PATHOPHYSIOLOGY OF A POSITIVE BONE SCAN

Meaningful interpretation of a bone scan is enhanced by an understanding of the mechanism of radiopharmaceutical bone uptake.

Uptake of the radiopharmaceutical in the skeleton depends on the regional blood flow, tissue extraction efficiency, and osteoblastic activity of the disease process.

Increased blood flow delivers more radiopharmaceutical to the involved site. Increased vascular permeability and increased extracellular fluid volume associated with lesions enhance tissue extraction.

In areas of osteogenic activity and new bone formation, there is an increase in the amount of the surface area of bone hydroxyapatite crystal available for radiopharmaceutical binding. Diphosphonate compounds are absorbed onto the surface of these crystals.

Formation of new bone or reactive bone as the result of osteoblastic activity is the way that the skeleton responds to the presence of lesions.

When a regional disorder affects bone, the two processes of destruction and repair initiate and coexist in varying proportions depending on the stage of the healing process. Destruction and demineralization begins and is visualized as a radiolucency on x-ray; however, radiolucencies are not detectable unless the bone matrix loses its mineral content by 30% to 50%. This is the stage at which the bone scan is positive, with a normal-appearing x-ray; it is the reason why metastatic foci may be detected up to 18 months before plain film abnormalities become evident.

As the healing process proceeds, the young osteoid gradually matures and mineralizes. X-ray shows mixed bone destruction and formation patterns and scan can demonstrate a considerable amount of uptake. This is the stage at which body x-ray and bone scans are positive.

The final stage of healing of the reactive bone is complete mineralization and appears as a radiodensity on x-ray. Radiodensity seen on x-ray is a manifestation of bone repair and maturity of the reactive bone. This highly mineralized bone metabolically behaves like resting bone and concentration of radioactivity would be normal or near normal. This is the stage at which the x-ray is positive and the scan, as expected, would be normal.

Inasmuch as the positive scan relies on blood flow and increased bone turnover in the lesion, a disease process that has a considerably decreased flow (osteonecrosis) or a destructive process (aggressive tumor, fulminating osteomyelitis, multiple myeloma) that is not accompanied by a significant repair process may appear normal on the scan and be falsely negative.

The finding of a normal scan in the presence of abnormality on conventional radiography also occurs in osteoporosis, benign cortical defect, bone cyst, bone island, multiple exostosis, eosinophilic granuloma, and osteopoikilosis. These lesions are inactive metabolically and are not associated with significant bone turnover.

Stable lesions—for example, metastasis from breast, thyroid, and prostate—that appear as a radiodense lesion on x-ray may be normal on scan. This represents lack of growth and absence of any reactive bone changes in relation to the disease site.

It is to be noted that in diffuse spinal metastases, accumulation of radiopharmaceutical may be so uniform as to give a false-negative impression. However, this circumstance does not represent a true false-negative.

SCINTIGRAPHIC FINDING OF OSSEOUS DISEASE

A large variety of bone lesions belonging to the seven major etiologic categories (congenital, neoplastic, infectious, traumatic, metabolic, vascular, and idiopathic) may lead to similar scintigraphic findings, making the scan quite nonspecific.

The predominant finding in all types of bone abnormalities is areas of increased uptake, which may be focal or diffuse. The photon deficit is also an important sign, and several disease entities may appear as a cold defect.

Inasmuch as bone scan findings are not specific, the scan must be interpreted using all available clinical data and generally should be correlated with radiographs to improve diagnostic specificity.

The full range of bone scan diagnostic capability will be enhanced by imaging the entire skeleton as opposed to a limited anatomic site, the liberal use of single photon emission tomography (SPECT) technology, and application of three-phase bone scanning when indicated.

SPECT is a valuable technique for optimizing the planar bone scan. It increases the image contrast, thus improving lesion detectability and localization; overall, it increases the sensitivity and specificity of the scan. The combination of SPECT and CT data allows formation of a hybrid image that shows both morphologic (CT) and physiologic (SPECT) information in one set of displays, adding further value to the scintigraphic approach.

SPECT is particularly useful in studying regions of bone and joint that have a complex anatomy, such as spine, hips, knees, and temporomandibular joints.

With a SPECT technique, lesion detectability in the lumbosacral region increases by 20% to 50% over the planar images. Localization of the lesion is best determined in the transaxial view, which can be easily analyzed and compared with CT and MR images.

CLINICAL APPLICATION

There are many recognized clinical applications for bone scanning, belongs mainly to the oncologic, infectious, traumatic, and metabolic disorders, which can be divided into the following groups:

1. Search for metastases
2. Detection of primary benign and malignant tumors
3. Evaluation of osteomyelitis
4. Evaluation of vascular disorders

5. Evaluation of trauma
6. Joint prostheses
7. Heterotopic bone formation
8. Metabolic bone disease
9. Arthropathy
10. Musculoskeletal pain of unknown causes

Clinically relevant diagnostic information can also be obtained from nonosseous accumulations of tracer activity.

SEARCH FOR METASTASIS

The most common malignant bone lesions are metastatic, occurring in 30% to 70% of all patients with cancer. The spread of tumor to bone occurs commonly by the hematogeneous route, with the venous system being the main pathway of dissemination. There are several morphologic and functional imaging modalities available for the evaluation of bone metastasis. These include the plain radiograph, bone scintigram, CT, MRI, and ^{18}F-FDG PET imaging.

The sensitivity of radiographs and CT in detecting early metastatic lesions in cortical bone and the bone marrow compartment is low. Considerable cortical destruction is required before the metastase can be detected. CT is also not sensitive for the assessment of early bone marrow infiltration by the tumor.

MRI is an excellent modality for the visualization of bone marrow. Normal marrow has a high T1 signal intensity, which converts to low-intensity signal, indicating the replacement of marrow by tumor cell. However, MRI is less sensitive than CT for the detection of cortical lesions. ^{18}F-FDG PET is an effective method for the assessment of bone metastasis. It can detect lytic, sclerotic, and mixed lesions, although it is more sensitive in detecting lytic lesions than sclerotic metastasis. Using the integrated PET-CT image, both marrow infiltration and sclerotic lesions of metastasis can be characterized in one set of the images. Marrow involvement shows a high uptake of FDG, which can be differentiated from the low uptake of a normal marrow. The reported sensitivity of the FDG PET for the detection of metastasis ranges from 62% to 100%, and specificity ranges from 96% to 100%. It should be noted that false-positive uptake of FDG may occur occasionally. Also, it is difficult to detect calvarial metastasis owing to the high physiologic uptake of FDG in the adjacent brain tissue.

The conventional bone scintigram is by far the most commonly used modality for the detection of bone metastasis. It is widely available, provides visualization of the entire skeleton, has a reported sensitivity of 62% to 100% and specificity of 78% to 100%, and shows evidence of metastatic disease much earlier than radiography can.

Scintigraphic findings of bone metastases include multiple asymmetrical, randomly distributed areas of increased uptake, development of new lesions, increased intensity or size of a lesion over time, a lesion of unusual shape, a photopenic area, and the appearance of a superscan (diffuse increased skeletal uptake and poor renal visualization).

Most bone metastases (over 80%) follow the distribution of red bone marrow and occur in the axial skeleton (spine, pelvis, ribs, sternum) and skull. In the spine, these lesions involve the vertebral body, which may extend posteriorly to the pedicle but rarely into the spinous process. Although destruction of the pedicle, mainly the cortical bone, is an easily appreciated sign of metastasis on plain film, the pedicle is not the primary site of metastases. Destruction of the pedicle occurs only in combination with involvement of the vertebral body.

A significant number of metastases occur in the peripheral skeleton (20% in the extremities and skull); therefore it is important that the bone scan portray the entire skeleton. Moreover, in cancer of the lung, the metastases may be limited to the hands and feet.

The detection of a solitary lesion on bone scan is not unusual and may be seen in 15% of scans. However, when this occurs in patients with known malignancy, it may present a diagnostic problem. In approximately 10% of patients, malignant bone disease presents as a single focus rather than multiple lesions. It has been reported that an overall 10% to 64% of isolated lesions are due to metastasis. With regard to location, 60% to 70% of isolated axial and 40% to 50% of isolated appendiceal or skull lesions are due to metastasis, particularly in those malignancies with a known tendency to metastasize to bone (breast, lung, and prostate).

The detection of rib lesions is common on bone scans; however, only some 10% to 17% of single-rib lesions represent metastases, while 70% to 80% of sternal lesions in patients with breast cancer are due to metastases, particularly when there is an asymmetrical appearance. The sternal lesion may be due to regional lymphatic spread and can be considered as a local recurrence instead of true metastasis.

As a whole, a focus of abnormal activity in a patient with cancer that cannot be explained by conventional radiography can be assumed to be metastatic until proven otherwise. These lesions should be further studied by CT, MRI, PET, or even biopsy.

The detection of new lesions or increasing size or intensity of lesions on the bone scan of a patient with metastases may be due to the flare phenomenon. This worsening appearance is related to the formation of new reactive bone and indeed represents the healing process of a metastatic disease. The true incidence of flare is unknown, but it may be seen in up to 20% of patients within the first 2 or 3 months of treatment. Repeat scanning in 2 to 6 months will show improvement— i.e., decreased intensity. The flare response has been reported in breast, prostate, and small cell carcinoma of the lung, but it may also be seen in other malignancies.

Widespread metastases may represent a pattern characterized as generalized increased bone uptake in association with poor renal visualization (the "absent kidney" sign). This pattern has been called a superscan or "beautiful scan." Superscans are more commonly seen in breast and prostate cancer than in other tumors, but cancer of the lung, stomach, bladder, or colon as well as lymphoma or a malignancy that diffusely involves the marrow, like leukemia, may be associated with a superscan.

The appearance of a superscan is not always representative of a malignancy but may also occur in hyperparathyroidism, osteomalacia, myelofibrosis, mastocytosis, and hypervitaminosis D as well as in patients undergoing dialysis.

The classic picture of a superscan is seen with less frequency when the newer high-resolution cameras are employed. Diffuse metastases will still be seen as a distinct lesion in association with faint visualization of the kidneys.

Metastatic disease may uncommonly appear as a photopenic or cold lesion on bone scan. Lesions that usually generate osteolytic reactions—notably kidney, thyroid, hepatoma, melanoma, Wilms' tumor, uterine cancer, and squamous cell carcinoma of the skin, head, and neck—may manifest as photopenia.

It is to be noted that most of these lesions eventually show some secondary osteoblastic response, at least at their periphery, which will be detected as a hot spot or "doughnut" lesion. A cold defect is inherently more difficult to diagnose; in addition, it may be due to a variety of other causes such as artifact, avascular necrosis (AVN), bone cyst, hemangioma, radiation therapy, osteomyelitis, and a primary tumor of multiple myeloma.

DETECTION OF PRIMARY BENIGN AND MALIGNANT BONE TUMORS

The role of bone scanning in the diagnosis of a primary bone tumor is limited. Bone scan cannot differentiate the malignant from benign bony neoplasm; however, except in the case of osteoid osteoma, increased blood pool activity may favor malignancy.

The bone scan also has limited value in evaluating the local extension of a primary tumor. The scan usually shows enhanced uptake in the area contiguous to the neoplasm, which is related to hyperemia and may give the appearance of more tumor extension than is seen radiographically.

Osteogenic sarcoma appears as an area of intense uptake with or without extension to the adjacent soft tissue, and an extended pattern of uptake may be seen in other bones of the same extremity bearing the tumor. This moderately diffuse uptake is related to hyperemia or may be secondary to alteration in the patient's gait on the involved side. Osteogenic sarcoma can metastasize to the bone and lung. Metastases to the bone have been noted in 16% of patients with or without lung metastases. Although CT remains the procedure of choice for the detection of pulmonary metastases, bone scanning is required for the evaluation of early bone metastases.

Ewing's sarcoma, much like osteogenic sarcoma, may metastasize, and unsuspected metastatic lesions will often be detected on bone scan.

Multiple myeloma is notorious for its association with a negative or photopenic scan. However, the bone scan is frequently positive for rib lesions missed on radiographs. On a lesion-by-lesion basis, radiographs are more sensitive than the bone scan in the detection of myeloma. The scan may fail to show radiographic disease sites in up to 27% of cases. This reflects the predominantly osteopenic nature of the myeloma. In three-fourths of such cases, the scan will demonstrate increased uptake rather than photopenia. Overall sensitivity of the scan is 60%, as compared with 75% for radiographs.

Bone scanning may be useful in the evaluation of benign bone lesions.

Osteoid osteoma characteristically exhibits hyperperfusion, hyperemia, and intense focal uptake. Osteoid osteoma may also appear as a so-called double-density sign, representing diffuse increased uptake with a focal area of more centrally increased uptake possibly representing the tumor nidus. The scan is of special value in the diagnosis of lesions in the spine and pelvis, which are poorly seen on radiographs.

The various types of benign bone lesions—such as aneurysmal bone cyst, fibrous cortical defect, and nonossifying fibroma—are associated with normal or minimal increased uptake unless traumatized.

Osteochondromas and enchondromas show varied uptake, but bone scanning is sometimes useful in detecting malignant degeneration. Fibrous dysplasia is also hot or normal in appearance and does not present as a cold defect. The varying degree of uptake in fibrous dysplasia appears to correlate with the x-ray appearance of ground glass or a cystic pattern: the former appears hot, and the latter may be normal.

EVALUATION OF OSTEOMYELITIS

The three-phase bone scan has a sensitivity and specificity of approximately 90% for the detection of acute osteomyelitis in nonviolated bone with a negative radiograph.

The three-phase scan does not increase the sensitivity of the procedure but helps to differentiate soft tissue infection from bone involvement.

In osteomyelitis, there will be early enhanced arterial flow (first phase), increased blood pool activity (second phase), and intense uptake in the skeletal phase (third phase); however, cellulitis will be positive only in the first two phases.

There will be limitation in the diagnostic ability of the scan when there are preexisting conditions such as diabetic osteopathy, fracture, status postsurgery, areas of orthopedic appliances, and preexisting chronic healed infection. Although sensitivity will still be high, in the 90% range, the specificity will drop significantly to 33% to 54% in patients with these conditions.

The normal healing process of a simple and uncomplicated fracture is associated with osteoblastic activity and increased uptake. Approximately 90% of fractures return to normal by 24 months after the trauma; therefore the healing process may be inseparable from infection during this time. The same applies to the bone scans of patients with previously treated infection, which may take months to return to normal after the infection of the bone is sterilized.

Hip and knee arthroplasty is also associated with increased uptake postoperatively: 6 to 12 months for the hip and occasionally longer than 2 years for the knee.

Differentiation of osteomyelitis from cellulitis in diabetic osteopathy and diabetic foot with or without ulcer presents a special diagnostic dilemma. Although sensitivity is still high, in the range of 85%, specificity is no higher than 54%, and accuracy depends largely on the presence of neuropathy and the site of the suspected lesion. Accuracy is poorest in the transmetatarsal area, where osteomyelitis is uncommon and neuropathy is common. Twenty-four-hour delayed images (four-phase scan) and 24-hour/4-hour uptake ratio of bone and soft tissue improves the accuracy of the diagnosis of osteomyelitis and differentiates osteomyelitis from soft tissue infection in patients with diabetes and/or peripheral vascular disease.

Most of the shortcomings of the bone scan for the detection of osteomyelitis can be overcome by combining skeletal scintigraphy with indium-111 (^{111}In)-white blood cell (WBC) scanning and gallium-67 (^{67}Ga)-citrate scanning.

An increased uptake of ^{111}In-WBCs incongruent with bone scan abnormality will be most consistent with an infectious process of the involved area and indicates that infection is likely to be present. By combining the two procedures (bone scan and ^{111}In-WBC scan), infection can be detected with a sensitivity and specificity of 88% and 85%, respectively, under these circumstances. An accuracy of 95% can be achieved by combining ^{111}In-WBC and ^{99m}Tc–sulfur colloid marrow imaging.

In the diabetic foot, ^{67}Ga-citrate scanning usually is not helpful in evaluating infection because of the high rate of false-positivity due to neuroarthropathy. An ^{111}In-WBC scan has the highest sensitivity, of 87%; but in 31% of cases, the uninfected neuropathic foot may be positive. This is especially true in those cases where there is a rapidly destructive process. ^{67}Ga-citrate, on the other hand, is the preferred method for evaluating spine and disk infection. A negative ^{111}In-WBC scan is usually sufficient to exclude an active infectious process. If the scan is used to follow up a patient treated for osteomyelitis, the patient should be off antibiotics before repeating the scintigram. This would increase the sensitivity of the scan. If ^{67}Ga-citrate activity has normalized after therapy, sterilization has been accomplished.

Acute hematogenous osteomyelitis may appear as a cold area or a photopenic lesion when the scan is performed in the ischemic stages of the disease process. The photopenia is due to the local occlusion of blood vessels and lack of radiopharmaceutical delivery to the site of involvement. Similarly, ^{111}In-WBC scans may also be photopenic.

It is to be noted that uptake of ^{111}In-WBC may occur at the site of an uninfected closed fracture in up to 40% of cases; therefore the presence of uptake does not necessarily mean infection. However, if there is markedly increased uptake of ^{111}In-WBC and the relative intensity at the site of uptake is greater than corresponding bone uptake, a superimposed osteomyelitis should be considered.

For osteomyelitis in a location that appears normal on radiography, MRI gives results similar to those of the three-phase bone scan. MRI is the most sensitive imaging modality for diagnosing osteomyelitis, but in the diabetic foot it suffers drawbacks, as does scintigraphy. MRI cannot reliably distinguish marrow edema from osteomyelitis. There are false-positive results that may reflect occult fractures, osteonecrosis, surgical changes, and neuroarthropathy. Overall, a sensitivity of 90% to 100% and a specificity of 71% to 81% for detecting osteomyelitis in the diabetic foot have been reported for MRI. Bone scan and ^{111}In scan are still needed to evaluate the diabetic foot.

FDG-PET is a useful diagnostic modality for detecting bone infection. Sensitivity and specificity generally exceeds 90%. The high spatial resolution allows differentiation of osteomyelitis from the infection of the soft tissue surrounding the bone. In addition to higher spatial resolution, the rapid accumulation of uptake in the foci of infection allows an earlier diagnosis. However, the expected high uptake of FDG in any cell type with high glycolic activity limits the test's specificity for discriminating infection from inflammation or a tumoral lesion.

EVALUATION OF VASCULAR DISORDERS

Blood flow has a strong influence on the appearance of a bone scan. Therefore a condition that mainly manifests itself by an alteration of the blood flow—such as reflex sympathetic dystrophy (RDS), osteonecrosis, and nonviability of a bone graft—can be assessed by bone scan.

The clinical diagnosis of reflex sympathetic dystrophy can be difficult. The use of bone scan showing characteristic periarticular areas of increased uptake in the involved area, particularly in the upper extremity, is very useful in establishing this diagnosis. Likewise, absence of such findings can be used to exclude this diagnosis. Serial scans usually show a return to normal over many months. Radiographic findings of reflex sympathetic dystrophy include soft tissue swelling, periarticular demineralization, and subperiosteal bone resorption; but the main radiographic finding remains osteopenia, which is seen in over 70% of cases.

The presumed mechanism of uptake is increased blood flow to the bone from loss of vasoconstriction resulting in hyperemia. Hyperemia will cause increased activity on the flow and blood pool images in the three-phase bone scan, with further intensification on the delayed images. The scan finding of reflex sympathetic dystrophy in the foot may appear as diffuse increased uptake throughout the foot, but the juxta-articular accentuation of uptake is still prominent.

Decreased blood flow not only lowers delivery of radiopharmaceutical to the bone but reduces the rate of osteoblastic activity correlating with the reduction of uptake in area of osteonecrosis and aseptic necrosis in the early stages. The mechanisms of osteonecrosis are not fully known; however, there are associated risk factors and causes, such as sickle cell anemia, steroid excess, ETOH abuse, and pancreatitis as well as trauma, idiopathic cases, and caisson disease (decompression illness, which may be seen in divers).

Osteonecrosis due to trauma can easily be explained by a direct interruption of the blood supply; however, 25% of cases have no history of trauma or associated risk factors and remain idiopathic. The hip and knee are the most common locations for the occurrence of osteonecrosis.

In the hip, the osteonecrosis of the femoral head appears as decreased uptake (photopenia), a direct scintigraphic correlation of bone necrosis, which is seen in the first 7 to 10 days following the onset of the disease. There may be a slight diffuse uptake in the intertrochanteric region. As the repair process and revascularization proceed in the second and third week, intertrochanteric uptake intensifies and evolves from a segmental crescent shape into a diffuse heterogenous uptake, masking the photopenic defects.

In adults, the pain of AVN leading to the bone scan often presents during the repair and revascularization phase; therefore, photopenia is not commonly seen in adults. However, SPECT images may still find the central photopenic region. In children, on the other hand, the pain occurs during the avascular phase. Lack of overlying ossification of the acetabulum and of degenerative arthritis in children makes it possible to detect the photopenia more easily. In the diagnosis of AVN, the bone scan is most useful when the x-ray finding is normal or minimal; when the x-ray shows signs of AVN, there is no need for a planar bone scan except for perhaps monitoring the evolution of the process.

Although MRI is the preferred technique for the diagnosis of AVN of the femoral head, bone SPECT, with a sensitivity ranging from 85% to 95%, can be used effectively to identify the AVN.

In the knee, acute osteonecrosis of the femoral condyle characteristically shows increased blood flow and increased blood pool activity corresponding to the articular surface of the medial condyle in association with an intense focal uptake in the same area on the delayed images. This scintigraphic pattern in an elderly patient with intense knee pain will be pathognomonic of spontaneous femoral osteochondrosis. Radiographic examination may show the lucency of the femoral condyle typical of osteonecrosis.

A related disorder is osteochondritis dissecans, commonly seen in teenagers. Its cause has been suggested to be ischemic necrosis, trauma, or even an ossification abnormality. The lesion appears as a positive finding on all three phases of the bone scan; however, the greater intensity and larger area of abnormal radionuclide uptake in the late phase suggests the more likely presence of an unstable and loose fragment, which requires surgical removal or internal fixation of the fragment.

In the evaluation of the bone graft, the vascular status of the bone graft can be evaluated easily by bone scan. A viable graft appears as an area of increased uptake representing integrity of blood supply and osteoblastic activity; the reverse is also true.

EVALUATION OF TRAUMA

Frank fracture results in a positive bone scan within a few hours. In a normal young adult, more than 90% of fractures will show increased uptake within 24 hours following injury. In older patients (over 75 years of age) and in those with osteoporosis, the positive bone scan may be delayed beyond 72 hours. In uncomplicated, well-aligned fractures, increased uptake declines between 3 and 12 months, and over 90% of scans return to normal by 24 months. The process of a healing fracture can be monitored by bone scan even through a cast. Activity of a compound, comminuted, or complicated fracture may remain detectable for years. Persistently increased activity between 3 and 12 months may indicate a reactive nonunion.

An atrophic nonunion is characterized as a photopenic region at the fracture site.

In addition to covert fracture, bone scan is an excellent tool for the detection of stress fractures, shin splints, bone bruises, and sport-related injuries. Stress fracture on three-phase bone scan appears as an area of increased flow and hyperperfusion in association with intense focal fusiform cortical uptake on the delayed skeletal images. Follow-up scans in 6 weeks will show that the hyperperfusion and hyperemia have disappeared, although intense focal skeletal uptake representing bone repair remains for some time. Shin splints are linear and of varying tracer uptake extending over a longer area of the cortex, with normal blood pool and flow images.

A bone bruise appears as a small focus of activity, not fusiform or linear in shape, in association with a normal radiograph. These lesions may be due to repair of interosseous bleeding or elevation of the periosteum secondary to trauma that has not resulted in a fracture.

A variety of occult traumas may be invisible on radiography and are frequently missed on conventional radiograph examination. Hip fractures in the elderly or fractures in the scaphoid and sacrum are among those occult fractures that usually escape detection by radiography but are easily detectable on scintigraphy. The early diagnosis of these injuries for prompt treatment makes scanning a valuable tool. Avulsion injury, sesamoid fracture, and some foot and ankle injuries (such as Lisfranc transmetatarsal injuries) also may escape radiographic detection but are easily detected scintigraphically.

JOINT PROSTHESIS

Bone scanning is a reasonable procedure for the initial evaluation of joint prosthesis complications. Loosening and infection are the two major complications manifesting as pain. In patients with painful arthroplasty, a normal three-phase bone scan can be used as strong evidence against those complications.

Within the first 12 months following hip arthroplasty using a cemented prosthesis, the pattern of uptake is so variable that a bone scan is not reliable for the assessment of hip prostheses during this time unless it is normal. The pattern of uptake will be even more variable if a noncemented prosthesis is used, to the extent that differentiation of normal from abnormal uptake or recognition of infection from loosening will be quite difficult. Knowledge of the type of implant and the age of the implant is important for evaluation.

A normal postprosthetic scan is defined as one in which the periprosthetic uptake is not distinguishable from the presumed normal adjacent bone. In a hip arthroplasty, slightly increased uptake along the acetabular component is normal. Minimal uptake in the region of the greater trochanter is also normal. The tip of the cemented prosthesis shows a mild to moderate degree of uptake within the first 12 months. This is due to preferential stress transferred to the distal prosthesis. In the case of cementless prosthesis, uptake at the stem tip is more prominent and may persist for 24 months.

Abnormal bone scans in hip prostheses show focal increased uptake at the tip of the femoral component of the prosthesis, suggestive of aseptic loosening or diffuse uptake around the stem, which is usually associated with infection. Classically, in the cemented hip prosthesis, the appearance of a loose prosthesis is depicted by a focal three-point uptake; two points of uptake are in the proximal portion (acetabulum–inferior neck), and the third is seen in the distal stem. These three points of focal uptake in a cementless prosthesis within the first 12 to 24 months may be normal and represent a physical mechanical finding instead of pathology.

In the diagnosis of loosening, the probability of loosening increases with the presence of enhanced uptake around the femoral component; seldom does an isolated stem-tip uptake represent loosening. Observation of increased blood flow and blood pool activity at the tip strongly suggests this complication. Serial scans may also be more helpful, as loosening will show more uptake on the follow-up scan, while nonspecific stress-related changes disappear gradually.

The role of the bone scan in the evaluation of a loosening knee prosthesis is limited, owing to the presence of persistent periprosthetic activity for several years. More than 50% of femoral and 75% of tibial components of knee prostheses demonstrate definite increased uptake after 12 months following insertion. Activity of the femoral component decreases by 1 year postoperatively, but activity of the tibial component, in which failure most commonly occurs, persists, and this undermines the value of a single scan for the diagnosis of loosening. However, the presence of intense focal uptake in an asymmetrical distribution should suggest this complication.

The infection rate of hip and knee arthroplasty is low, approximately 1%; it is 3% for revision surgery.

Although the three-phase bone scan has a sensitivity of almost 100% for arthroplasty infection, the specificity, at 18%, is very low. Specificity can be improved by performing ^{67}Ga- or ^{111}In-WBC scanning.

Marked intense uptake of ^{67}Ga- or ^{111}In-WBCs in a pattern incongruent with bone uptake is a diagnostic criterion for establishing the presence of infection.

The overall accuracy of serial ^{67}Ga-WBC bone scan images for orthopedic implant infection is 60% to 80%.

The specificity of combined bone and ^{111}In-WBCs is 85%. The specificity of ^{111}In-WBC scanning can be improved by combining it with ^{99m}Tc–sulfur colloid bone marrow imaging. ^{111}In-WBC scanning and ^{99m}Tc–sulfur colloid bone marrow imaging both reflect the distribution of radioactivity in the reticuloendothelial system of the bone marrow, thus producing congruent images. An infection-stimulating accumulation of WBCs outside the bone marrow would produce an incongruent image. Combined imaging permits distinction of infection from normal marrow displaced by a prosthesis or other entity. For combined WBC and bone marrow imaging, a sensitivity of 90%, specificity of 97%, and accuracy of 97% have been reported.

Combined WBC and bone marrow imaging is an accurate method for diagnosing infectious knee prostheses and provides an accuracy of 95%, similar to 96% to 97% for hip arthroplasty.

HETEROTOPIC BONE FORMATION

Heterotopic bone formation in muscle and soft tissue occurs as a result of trauma, spinal cord injury producing quadriplegia or paraplegia, burn injury and in the soft tissue around the arthroplasty.

A bone scan detects ectopic bone formation as an area of increased blood pool and increased uptake on delayed static images and helps in reaching an early diagnosis prior to radiographic changes.

Bone scanning is also helpful for establishing the maturity of the lesion as a prerequisite for surgical treatment. Premature excision of the lesion may be associated with recurrence, requiring further and more extensive intervention.

Heterotopic bone may take 6 months or longer to mature and can be followed by bone scanning. A steady decrease of uptake on more than two successive examinations followed by a steady-state plateau in uptake is considered a sign of maturity.

METABOLIC BONE DISEASE

Metabolic bone diseases such as renal osteodystrophy, osteomalacia, and primary hyperparathyroidism are characterized by increased bone uptake throughout the skeleton and the appearance of a superscan with faint visualization of the kidneys and, in some cases, prominence of calvarial or mandibular activity. These findings are not specific for any particular metabolic bone disease and represent only an increase in skeletal turnover. In spite of the rather characteristic scan pattern of metabolic bone disease, the main clinical value of this examination lies in the evaluation of focal lesions associated with metabolic bone disease. These include fractures in osteoporosis, pseudofracture in osteomalacia, Brown tumor, and ectopic calcification in hyperparathyroidism.

Precipitation of calcium-phosphate complex in kidney, lung, and stomach in association with hyperparathyroidism, known as metastatic calcification, can be readily seen on bone scans but rarely, and only in extreme cases, on radiographs. In advanced cases of hyperparathyroidism, Brown tumor may occur, which may be detected on bone scan. Focal uptake is also seen in fractures of the vertebrae and cystic changes of hyperparathyroidism. It is to be noted that a mild form of primary hyperparathyroidism is associated with a normal scan and that the feature of metabolic bone disease may be seen only in severe cases.

In osteoporosis, the scan may show relatively low uptake in the skeleton, giving the appearance of a washed-out scan and poor definition of the vertebrae. Vertebral collapse in osteoporosis is associated with an increased plate-like uptake across the vertebrae, which fades out in 6 to 24 months. When multiple vertebral fractures are present, particularly when they show different stages of resolution, osteoporosis is the probable diagnosis. Patients with vertebral fracture commonly have other fractures, and bone scan shows these fractures early, when x-ray is still normal. Fracture of the humerus, scapula, ribs, or pelvis may unexpectedly be detected by scan.

The bone scan in osteomalacia is characterized by generalized increased skeletal uptake (superscan or "beautiful scan") and faint kidney visualization. Focal abnormalities related to pseudofracture are easily seen on bone scan, particularly in the ribs, which are usually missed radiographically. Pseudofractures commonly occur in the acetabulum, femoral neck, pubic rami, and clavicle and are often symmetrical.

The most striking and severe form of generalized uptake in metabolic bone disease is seen in the case of renal osteodystrophy as a result of the combined effect of osteomalacia and secondary hyperparathyroidism. Ectopic calcifications in the lungs, stomach, and kidneys occur commonly in cases of renal osteodystrophy.

Bone scanning is the most sensitive and ideal screening procedure for suspected Paget's disease. In Paget's disease (nicknamed "metabolic madness of the bone"), the bone scan appearances are well known and look like areas of very intense, well-demarcated uptake in the affected portion of the skeleton. This characteristically involves major portions of involved bone, which is often expanded and deformed (osteitis deformans). Common locations are the skull, pelvis, vertebrae, or femurs, but no bone in the skeleton (even the sesamoids) is immune except possibly the fibulas. In Paget's disease of the skull (osteoporosis circumscripta), intense increased uptake is seen at the periphery of the lesion. In the spine, involvement of the vertebral body, posterior element, and spinous process gives the appearance of an inverted triangle, a "Mickey Mouse sign." "Lincoln's sign" or "Blackbeard's sign" of monostotic mandibular Paget's, ivory black vertebra, and the "short pants sign" of the pelvis in upper femoral Paget's have been described.

ARTHROPATHY

MRI has become the imaging modality of choice for the evaluation of joint disease owing to its excellent anatomic resolution, but a radionuclide scan remains the most sensitive test for the detection of early pathologic changes. The radionuclide scan makes an important contribution to the diagnosis and the exclusion of conditions that present with joint pain, such as rheumatoid arthritis, transient osteoporosis, reflex sympathetic dystrophy, septic arthritis, and toxic synovitis. The scan can confirm or exclude the presence of an active inflammatory disease.

In active inflammatory disease of the joint, there will be an increase in uptake on the vascular phase, which correlates with hyperemia, and increase in the soft tissue phase, which correlates with a capillary leak.

Delayed uptake in the absence of this early accumulation indicates a more indolent or inactive process. Delayed uptake represents bone remodeling with or without a significant in-

flammatory reaction. Therefore a positive two-phase joint image is more meaningful in the evaluation of inflammatory joint disease than a three-phase study. In general, the pattern of increased periarticular activity is nonspecific for a given arthropathy, but the pattern of symmetry, location, and appropriate clinical data may limit the differential diagnosis.

Insufficiency fracture complicating rheumatoid arthritis is well documented and has been described in the pelvis, proximal tibia, distal tibia, and fibula. Presentation is insidious swelling and tenderness, usually located near the joint, which may be confused with exacerbation of rheumatoid arthritis. Radiography has a very low sensitivity owing to the presence of associated osteoporosis, but bone scan easily discloses the fracture site by its focal intense uptake.

MUSCULOSKELETAL PAIN OF UNKNOWN CAUSE

Bone scanning makes an important contribution to the diagnosis or exclusion of conditions associated with pain. The extreme sensitivity of the bone scan for the detection of bone lesions makes it an ideal diagnostic procedure for the assessment of painful clinical conditions that may be attributed to the musculoskeletal system.

In addition to metastatic foci, osteomyelitis, and fracture, there are other bone abnormalities that present with pain, and most have a normal initial radiograph.

The cause of chronic low back pain that has a skeletal origin can be diagnosed by bone scanning.

Ten percent of osteoid osteomas—painful lesions—occur in the vertebral column and often escape radiographic detection because of the paucity of reactive sclerosis and difficulty in analyzing the sign of overlying bony structures. Bone scan, on the other hand, demonstrates intense focal uptake, leading to this diagnosis.

Back pain is an early symptom of ankylosing spondylitis. The radiographic changes of ankylosing spondylitis in the early stages may be absent or extremely subtle, but inflammatory changes are detectable on bone scan, in which bilaterally increased activity of the sacroiliac joints (sacroiliitis) as well as focal uptake in the region of the apophyseal joints (apophysiitis) are seen.

The lumbar spine is the most common site of diskitis. The diagnosis of diskitis is difficult and is often delayed owing to nonspecific findings and the late appearance of radiographic signs. Bone scanning in the early stage and within a few days of onset shows a characteristic increase in uptake in two adjacent vertebral bodies.

Overall, the bone scan contributes significantly in the evaluation of patients with low back pain. The three major categories of disease (infection, tumor, and ankylosing spondylitis) can be excluded by normal bone scan. When the scan is positive, SPECT imaging can be used to localize lesions more precisely in these complex bony structures.

One of the major indications for lumbar SPECT in patients with low back pain is the evaluation of spondylolysis. In patients with pars defect and back pain, a negative SPECT excludes spondylolysis as the cause of the pain. A positive SPECT, however, confirms the presence of a painful spondylolysis and predicts a favorable outcome of spinal fusion surgery.

Pain due to facet arthropathy is usually managed by joint injection. SPECT is extremely helpful in localizing the pain-originating facet and identifies the site and the joint level to be blocked.

In the evaluation and management of facet joint syndrome, SPECT images of the spine play an important role. The high negative predictive value of almost 100% makes SPECT especially useful in excluding patients for facet joint injection.

Postoperative lumbar pain is another indication for SPECT scintigraphy. One year after the laminectomy, a normally healed and fused spine usually shows a normal level of uptake. Therefore abnormal uptake beyond the first year of surgery represents a failing fusion and formation of pseudoarthrosis and hypertrophic nonunion, which accounts for patient's pain.

The painful occult fracture of a carpal bone, neck of the femur, and pelvis and a variety of sport-related painful injuries are easily recognizable by bone scan, while x-ray findings are absent or minimal.

The bone scan is of clinical help in diagnosing spontaneous osteonecrosis and painful crisis in a patient with sickle cell disorder.

Transient osteoporosis is a painful, self-limiting condition affecting one or more joints, most commonly the hips. Associated osteoporosis is very difficult to detect radiographically, but the characteristic diffusely increased uptake in the femoral head and neck, which extends into the intertrochanteric region, is seen on bone scan. The cause of transient osteoporosis is not known; many authors believe that this is a mild form of reflex sympathetic dystrophy.

The diagnosis of toxic synovitis is a diagnosis of exclusion after ruling out septic arthritis and Legg-Calvé-Perthes disease. The bone scan is more likely to be normal than abnormal. It may show some increased uptake in the femoral head, but decreased uptake is uncommon.

NONOSSEOUS LESION ON BONE SCAN

Bone scintigraphy can delineate a wide spectrum of nonosseous disorders: neoplastic, inflammatory, ischemic, traumatic, renal excretory as well as artifactual. While the accumulation of bone-seeking radiopharmaceutical in brain, lung, heart, breast, bowel, liver, spleen, skeletal muscle, and kidney can identify important disorders, an area of photopenia may also represent disease. Most of these nonosseous abnormalities are incidental findings seen on scans performed for other reasons.

Nonosseous structures such as the kidney and urinary bladder are normally seen on bone scan. Minimal uptake in the region of the thyroid is commonly seen. Aging frequently leads to the calcification of cartilage and blood vessels; uptake at these sites should not be confused with abnormal soft tissue uptake. Recognition of these abnormalities enhances the diagnostic value of the bone scan.

The mechanism of soft tissue uptake of bone-seeking agents varies: elevated tissue calcium concentration, enhanced regional vascularity, elevated calcium-phosphate products, and the presence of iron deposits are important factors that play a major role.

HEAD

In the central nervous system, uptake of bone-seeking agents can occur in cases of tumor, infection, and cerebral infarction. Generally, any disease process associated with blood–brain barrier breakdown will cause accumulation of the bone-seeking radiopharmaceutical. Activity in the infarcted area may show a wedge-shaped pattern corresponding to the territory of a specific major artery. Meningioma, which usually contains calcification, subdural hematoma, and dural calcification also take up the bone tracer.

THORAX

In the lung, uptake occurs as a result of metastatic calcification due to hyperparathyroidism. The alkaline environment of the alveolar wall enhances calcium-phosphate deposition in metastatic calcification. The high frequency of pulmonary calcification (60%) in patients with long-standing chronic renal failure leads to a pattern of diffuse pulmonary uptake and absence of renal activity on bone scan. Metastatic osteogenic sarcoma, mediastinal neuroblastoma containing dystrophic calcification, and malignant pleural effusion also accumulate bone-seeking radiopharmaceutical. In osteogenic sarcoma, over 90% of patients eventually develop pulmonary metastases, but only 20% to 40% demonstrate uptake of the bone-seeking agent.

Bronchogenic carcinoma and breast cancer may demonstrate uptake of bone-seeking agents. The spectrum of uptake varies from ill defined or barely detectable to an intense, sharply defined lesion. Uptake is apparently related to calcium content, which strongly correlates with uptake; tumor vascularity plays a secondary but important role.

The incidental finding of diffuse myocardial uptake on bone scan is seen in patients with previous infarction and ischemic cardiomyopathy. These patients usually have a low ejection fraction. Patients with unstable angina, amyloidosis, diffuse pericarditis, and recent defibrillation may also demonstrate myocardial uptake.

Following an acute myocardial infarction, ischemic damage to the cellular membrane results in a rapid intracellular influx of calcium, which precipitates following tissue necrosis and appears as an area of avid activity on pyrophosphate scan. A 10% sustained myocardial perfusion is required for delivery of radiopharmaceutical to the infarcted site in order to be seen on images. After 7 to 10 days, the area of infarction is often no longer seen due to cessation of blood flow. Persistent uptake following an infarction correlates with a higher rate of complications and left ventricular aneurysm.

ABDOMEN

Uptake of bone-seeking radiopharmaceutical in the stomach is commonly artifactual and relates to unbound ^{99m}Tc-pertechnetate. In patients with hypercalcemia, metastatic calcification in the stomach is the most common cause of gastric uptake. Bowel visualization is commonly due to urinary diversion surgical procedures but may be due to necrotizing colitis, ischemic bowel disease, and colovesical fistula.

Liver uptake is commonly due to metastatic deposits from the lungs, breast, and GI tract. Changes in regional perfusion, tumor necrosis, and the calcification of liver metastases are implicated as the cause of the uptake.

Diffuse liver uptake is usually artifactual and represents flocculation of the ^{99m}Tc bone-seeking agent secondary to excess aluminum in the ^{99m}Tc generator; it may also be seen in those patients who ingest antacids containing aluminum.

The common cause of splenic uptake is sickle cell disease, which is associated with splenic calcification, splenic infarction, and the deposition of iron, all important factors in localization of bone-seeking agents. Hemosiderosis, Hodgkin's disease, splenic metastasis, and thalassemia are among the uncommon causes of splenic uptake.

The kidneys are normally visualized on bone scan. In as many as 15% of bone scans, an incidental finding of urinary tract abnormality may be noted.

Diffuse, intense bilateral uptake may be due to metastatic calcification, as seen in hyperparathyroidism, nephrocalcinosis, and after the administration of chemotherapeutic agents. However, dehydration is the most common cause. Iron overload and multiple transfusions, acute pyelonephritis, and thalassemia may also be associated with renal uptake. The patterns of obstructive uropathy, ectopic kidney, and horseshoe kidney are easily recognizable.

The most common incidental renal finding on bone scan is an area of decreased uptake or photopenia, representing a space-occupying lesion such as a cyst, primary renal tumor, metastasis, or abscess.

PELVIS

In the region of the pelvis, bladder diverticula, uterine leiomyoma, transplant kidney as an area of increased activity, and urinary bladder mass as an area of photopenia are demonstrable.

SKELETAL MUSCLE

Tissue injury, necrosis, calcification, or ossification of skeletal muscle causes increased uptake of bone radiopharmaceutical. Injury causes calcium influx, inflammation, and edema in the involved region, leading to increased uptake of bone-seeking radiopharmaceutical.

Rhabdomyolysis is a well-known cause of uptake. This condition may follow crush injury, surgical trauma, electrical burn, or alcohol abuse. On bone scintigraphy, the entire muscle is seen, with maximum uptake occurring 48 hours following the injury. Posttraumatic hematoma, myositis ossificans, and heterotropic ossification show uptake.

Most soft tissue sarcomas accumulate ^{99m}Tc radiopharmaceutical bone agents because of calcification and their vascularity. Tumors such as synovial sarcoma are usually positive on three-phase bone scan. Lymphedema of the upper and lower extremity as a result of surgery or blockage and interruption of lymphatic drainage can be visualized scintigraphically as expanded tissue space.

History: A 60-year-old male with resected adenocarcinoma of the rectosigmoid with bladder wall involvement presents for follow-up evaluation and bone scan (Fig. 7.1 A).

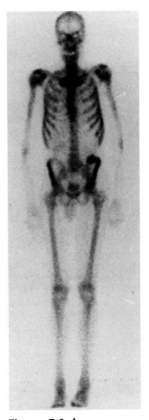

Figure 7.1 A

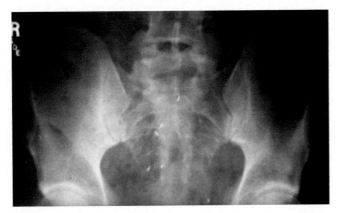

Figure 7.1 B

Findings: Anterior whole-body bone scan shows a single area of markedly increased uptake in the left iliac bone.

Discussion: Correlation with the pelvic radiograph (Fig. 7.1 B) shows that this area of increased uptake corresponds to the sclerotic lesion (arrow) and most likely represents a metastatic focus in this patient with a history of resected malignancy. Note the surgical sutures in the pelvis.

In approximately 10% of cases, metastases initially appear as a single focal uptake, but 10% to 64% of single bone lesions are due to metastases, depending on the primary and the location of the abnormality. Isolated rib lesions represent metastases in less than 10% to 17% of cases, while more than 29% of single spinal lesions are due to metastases.

Identification of a solitary lesion on bone scan requires careful radiographic correlation to exclude a benign disorder. In case of doubt or inconclusive results, a CT, MRI, or biopsy should be obtained, particularly when the result of the scan influences the patient's management.

Metastatic osteosclerotic lesions usually arise from the prostate, stomach, mucinous adenocarcinoma of the colon, bladder adenocarcinoma with involvement of the prostate gland, nasopharyngeal carcinoma, carcinoid, and Hodgkin's disease as well as medulloblastoma. Lung and breast cancer also may be associated with sclerotic metastatic lesions. In the area of bone metastases, there is an increase in osteoid production and new bone formation even before bone destruction occurs. Radiographically, the newly formed bone appears as a sclerotic region that incorporates a significant amount of bone-seeking radiopharmaceutical even up to 15 times more than normal bone and as such appears as a hot spot on the bone scan.

Lytic lesion will also be positive on bone scan, but following successful therapy, a lytic lesion develops a sclerotic appearance and the bone scan appears normal at this time.

The discordance of reparative sclerosis (regression) from active osteoblastic lesion (progression) can be distinguished by serial bone scanning.

Diagnosis: Solitary sclerotic metastasis.

CASE 7.2

History: A 58-year-old male who has had a left upper lobectomy for poorly differentiated adenocarcinoma of the lung presents for a follow-up appointment and a bone scan (Fig. 7.2 A).

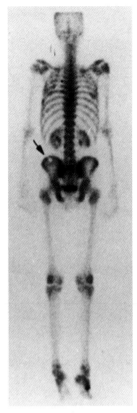

Figure 7.2 A

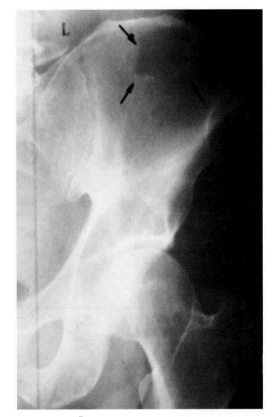

Figure 7.2 B

Findings: A significant finding is a large area of demarcated photopenia in the left iliac bone (Fig. 7.2 A, arrow). Bone scan changes of left thoracotomy are seen on the posterior images of the whole bone scan. Focal uptake is also seen in the right tarsal region.

Discussion: The area of photopenia corresponds to the large lytic lesion (arrows) of the left iliac bone (Fig. 7.2 B) and most likely represents a metastasis in this patient with known lung malignancy.

Pure osteolytic metastases arise from carcinoma of the thyroid, kidney, part of the GI tract, as well as metastases from Ewing's sarcoma and melanoma.

Osteolytic metastases, in spite of their destructive nature, are commonly associated with the formation of reactive bone and present as positive bone scans. Depending on the degree of reactivity, however, they may manifest as areas of normal or decreased uptake.

The scintigraphic degree of uptake is in general unrelated to the degree of lucency on the radiograph. Uptake on bone scan reflects blood flow and metabolic activity, but x-ray lucency represents a net calcium efflux. The positivity of the scan depends largely on the degree of reactive bone process, vascularity, and the size of the lytic lesion.

Extremely aggressive tumors may not be associated with the formation of new bone and therefore appear as cold or photopenic regions. Their sites may be suggested by increased blood pool activity, particularly in a doughnut appearance, which represents reactive vascularity surrounding the lesion.

A cold lesion is due to either focal replacement of the bone by the tumor or occlusion of the blood supply to the involved region. Photopenic metastases are commonly due to carcinoma of the lung or breast. They should be differentiated from the other causes of photopenia, such as multiple myeloma, early osteomyelitis, aseptic necrosis, and bone infarction.

Diagnosis: Solitary photopenic lytic metastasis.

History: A 63-year-old male with bilateral lower extremity weakness and paresthesia and a noncontributory lumbar spine radiograph presents for a bone scan (Fig. 7.3 A).

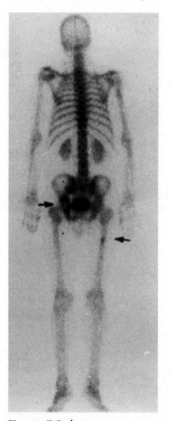

Figure 7.3 A

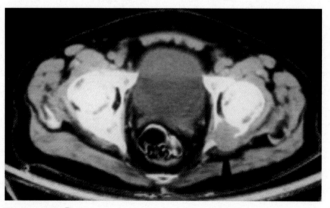

Figure 7.3 B

Findings: Posterior view of the whole-body scan (Fig. 7.3 A) shows an abnormal photopenic region involving the left acetabulum (arrow) surrounded by a halo of increased activity. There is also an increase focal uptake in the proximal right femur (arrow).

Discussion: The unexpected finding of simultaneous hot and cold lesions, although uncommon, should raise the question of a metastatic process in a man of this age group. Involvement of both the axial and appendicular skeleton is in favor of lung metastases. Metastases from the breast and prostate often

metastasize through the vertebral venous plexus and are seen more often in the axial skeleton. Lung tumors, on the other hand, spread both via the venous system and the pulmonary veins to the general arterial circulation and are distributed more randomly throughout the entire skeleton.

The photopenic area correlates with the osteolytic and soft tissue component of the lesion in the posterior aspect of the left acetabulum (arrowhead) seen on the patient's pelvic CT (Fig. 7.3 B) and proved by biopsy to be a metastatic carcinoma of the lung. Although no evidence of extension into the mediastinum

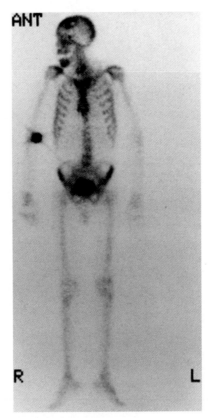

Figure 7.3 C

or beyond was detected by subsequent chest and abdominal CT, this patient was spared a futile surgical procedure as a result of the bone scan.

Lung carcinoma can produce osteoblastic, osteolytic, or mixed lesions or a lesion with a doughnut configuration. Osseous doughnut lesions, however, are more frequent in squamous cell and thyroid carcinoma. Figure 7.3 C shows a calvarial doughnut lesion in a 58-year-old man with squamous cell carcinoma of the esophagus metastasized to the bone and other organs.

A doughnut sign probably indicates osteoblastic reaction along the margin of the large lesions.

Photopenic lesions occur when the blood supply to the area is compromised or there is a lack of reactive new bone formation. The presence of soft tissue involvement in the region of the left acetabulum in this patient suggests compromise of the nutrient vessel, with subsequent bone infarction being responsible for the photopenia.

Photopenic lesions may be seen in a variety of diseases, not only in metastasis but in posttraumatic conditions, aseptic necrosis, sickle cell disease, multiple myeloma, eosinophilic granuloma, Legg-Calvé-Perthes disease, hemangioma, and giant cell tumor.

Some of the cold lesions may accumulate other tracers, such as ^{67}Ga-citrate. Accumulation of gallium in the cold lesion of multiple myeloma is usually associated with a fulminating course.

It should be noted that any abnormality on bone scan suggestive of metastasis even in a typical pattern must still be correlated with radiograph. A plain radiograph not only helps to exclude the benign bone lesions but quite often defines the feature of a specific disease process.

Diagnosis: Hot and cold metastases of the lung.

CASE 7.4

History: This 57-year-old male recently diagnosed with lung cancer complained of excruciating pain of the right shoulder. His x-ray was negative. A bone scintigraph was obtained (Fig 7.4 A).

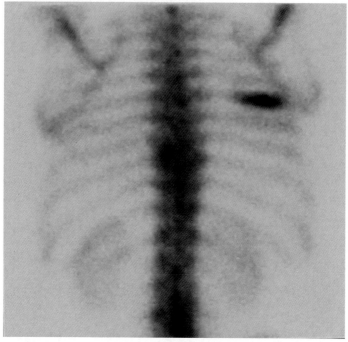

Figure 7.4 A

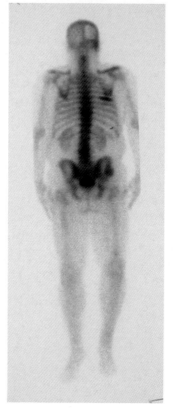

Figure 7.4 B

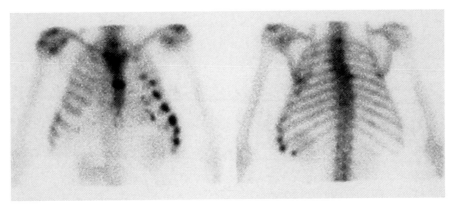

Figure 7.4 C

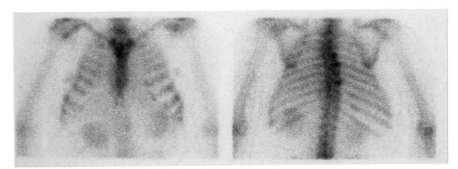

Figure 7.4 D

Findings: Posterior images of the thorax showed a solitary area of increased uptake along the posterior aspect of the right sixth rib. There is a suspicious lesion probably in the pedicle of the tenth dorsal vertebra on the left. There is normal renal uptake.

Solitary bone abnormality is not rare and may be encountered in 15% of bone scan studies. The etiology may be benign, commonly trauma, or could be malignant, frequently metastasis. However, the location of the lesion has a bearing on the probability of metastasis.

A solitary lesion in the spine, pelvis, or sternum associated with a negative radiograph most likely represents a metastasis, and further evaluation and follow-up is warranted.

Solitary rib lesions, on the other hand, commonly represent a benign process even in patients with cancer. Approximately 10% to 17% of these lesions are due to metastasis.

Rib lesions with an elongated appearance, as in this case, most probably represent an early stage of a destructive malignant process not yet detectable on radiography. Patients later develop further metastasis in the brain and the right ilium (Fig 7.4 B). Note the photopenia of the right calvarium, a bone flap resulting from a craniotomy for the removal of a right-occipital-lobe metastatic lesion.

Rib lesions are probably traumatic if they are aligned and the uptake is focal as opposed to linear.

Fig 7.4 C shows multiple focal lesions aligned in the anterolateral aspect of chest wall on the left, most consistent with multiple rib fractures. Uptake due to rib fracture decreases in 3 to 6 months. The annual follow-up bone scan of this patient for other reasons (Fig 7.4 D) shows a marked improvement of the fractures.

Rib fracture may occur with trivial trauma or even by coughing; therefore the history may not be contributory.

Diagnosis: Metastatic rib lesions. Rib fractures.

CASE 7.5

History: A 72-year-old male initially presented with left shoulder pain and was diagnosed with stage II prostate carcinoma with widespread bony metastases (Fig. 7.5 A). Some $5\frac{1}{2}$ months later, following the commencement of hormonal therapy, he returned for follow-up, and a second bone scan was obtained (Fig. 7.5 B).

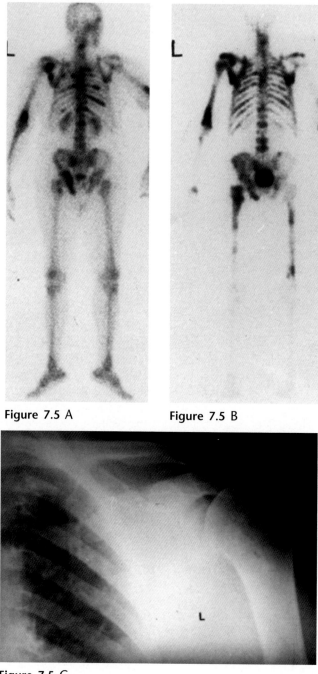

Figure 7.5 A

Figure 7.5 B

Figure 7.5 C

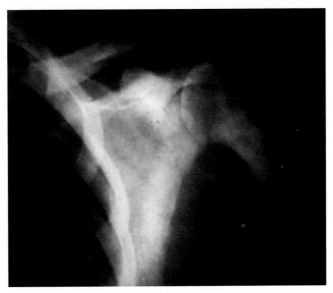

Figure 7.5 D

Findings: On posterior view of the initial scintigram (Fig. 7.5 A), in addition to the abnormal uptake in the left scapula and humeral head, disseminated metastases are seen throughout the skeleton. The left scapular uptake corresponds with the sclerotic changes noted on radiography (Fig. 7.5 C). Follow-up scan (Fig. 7.5 B) shows a further increase in the intensity and the number of lesions. There has been a further increase in the sclerotic appearance of the lesions of the scapula and humeral head (Fig. 7.5 D).

Discussion: Radiographic assessment of response of metastatic lesions to therapy is difficult. Development of a sclerotic appearance in a lytic lesion with no evidence of new lesions has been considered a sign of healing; however, changes in osteoblastic lesions are unpredictable.

Temporal changes and increased sclerosis on serial radiographs may be a part of the healing process and a favorable response to therapy or could be due to further osteoblastic tumor deposition and disease progression. Distinction of healing reaction and progressing disease is possible by comparison of sequential bone scans, which will reveal the nature of the sclerosis. The presence of active neoplasia in the sclerotic region appears as increased uptake, while healing sclerosis will be associated with decreasing or normal uptake on serial scans.

The concordance of increased uptake and increased sclerosis in this case represents disease progression.

An increase in the intensity of tracer uptake and/or the appearance of new lesions may occur after the initiation of therapy for metastases. This has been referred to as the flare phenomenon and indicates a successful response to therapy. Therefore the scintigraphic phenomenon of flare should be considered in evaluating an area of increased uptake on scans obtained during the first 6 months of therapy and should not be confused with further metastases.

The flare phenomenon usually occurs within the first 3 months of treatment and reverts to normal by 6 months. It has been reported to occur in 5% to 10% of patients with breast or prostate carcinoma and has also been reported in lung metastases and skeletal lymphoma.

In patients with interval clinical improvement and worsening scan appearance, the flare phenomenon should be suggested and a follow-up scan should be obtained in 6 months. The 6-month scan will show marked improvement from the pretreatment scan in the case of flare. Continued deterioration of scan appearance would indicate progressing disease.

Diagnosis: Progressing skeletal metastases.

CASE 7.6

History: A 63-year-old male is admitted for workup of progressive weakness, lethargy, and weight loss. The level of prostate-specific antigen is elevated. The patient is referred for a bone scan to rule out metastases (Fig. 7.6 A).

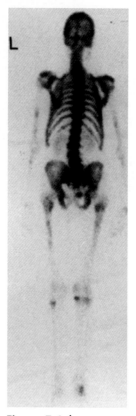

Figure 7.6 A

Findings: The posterior view of the whole-body scan (Fig. 7.6 A) shows diffuse symmetrical uptake throughout the skeleton. There is faint visualization of the kidneys and a high ratio of bone to soft tissue activity.

Discussion: The appearance of symmetrical homogeneous uptake with enhanced visualization of bone relative to the soft tissue uptake and faint or absent renal activity has been referred to as a superscan and is seen in various conditions including metastatic disease, metabolic bone disease, hematologic disorders, and some other entities.

The superscan appearance, although not common, may be mistaken for a normal scan. The majority of such scans represent diffuse metastatic disease, as in this case, which was proven by biopsy to be an adenocarcinoma of the prostate.

Superscan abnormalities of metastatic disease most likely start with the typical pattern of multiple disseminated, focal, hot lesions which coalesce as the disease progresses and eventually appear as homogeneous uptake—a pattern associated with a poor prognosis.

Lack of kidney visualization is due to the fact that a significant portion of radiopharmaceutical localizes to disseminated bone lesions and only minimal activity is available for excretion. Technically, image intensity adjustment also contributes

to the suppression of renal visualization (reduced renal sign) and enhances the appearance of a superscan.

The pattern of superscan due to metastasis usually represents a diffuse uptake in the axial skeleton and in proximal portion of large bones containing red marrow. This pattern is different in distribution from that seen in metabolic bone disease or myeloproliferative disease.

The most common causes of a metastatic superscan are prostate and breast carcinomas; however, other malignancies—including stomach, colon, lung, lymphoma, transient cell carcinoma of the bladder, and nasopharyngeal carcinoma—have been reported as the etiology of a superscan.

Metabolic disorders such as hyperparathyroidism cause diffuse reactive bone formation and as such can produce the diffuse symmetrical uptake of a superscan with faint visualization of the kidneys. In the superscan of hyperparathyroidism (Fig. 7.6 B) due to a large parathyroid adenoma (Fig. 7.6 C), the prominent activity of the appendicular skeleton, skull, mandible, and sternum (bowtie sternum) may help to differentiate the scan from diffuse metastasis, in which the main area of abnormality is in the axial skeleton and marrow compartment.

Other metabolic bone diseases that can lead to a superscan appearance include osteomalacia, renal ostedistrophy,

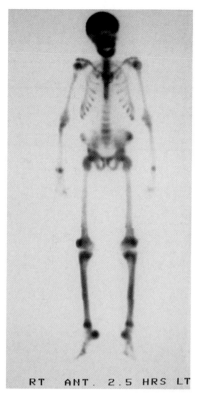

Figure 7.6 B

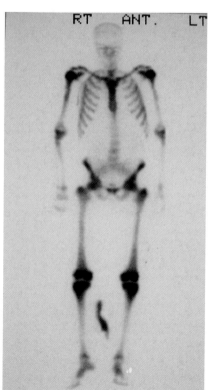

Figure 7.6 C

RT   ANT.   LT

Figure 7.6 D

hypervitaminosis D, Paget's disease, and osteopetrosis. Clinical history, radiography, and laboratory findings help to arrive at the correct diagnosis.

Superscan appearance may be due to a variety of hematologic disorders, such as myeloproliferative disease, aplastic anemia, lymphoma, and mastocytosis. Figure 7.6 D represents the superscan of a 67-year-old patient with myelofibrosis.

Note the diffusely increased activity of the bony structures, particularly around the joint area. Renal activity is not visualized.

The mechanism of increased bony uptake in hematologic disorders, including myelofibrosis, is not clear.

It is known, however, that myelofibrosis as one of the clinical entities of myeloproliferative disease is associated with

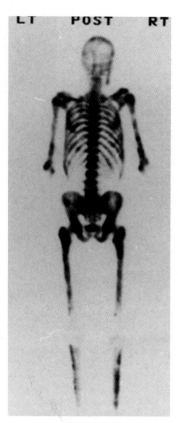

LT   POST   RT

Figure 7.6 E

increased blood flow and extension of the bone surfaces of the marrow cavity, and both of these are considered to be important factors for uptake of bone radiopharmaceutical.

Increased bone surface of the marrow cavity occurs as the result of extension of marrow into the normal inactive trabecular bone, altering the compact bone to spongiosa, which microscopically has a larger bone surface than compact bone. This process initiates to compensate for loss of the hematopoietic marrow cavity to other areas, such as spleen and posterior mediastinum, resulting in extramedullary hematopoiesis.

Superscan may be seen rarely in fibrous dysplasia, hyperthyroidism, or artificially secondary to elevation of traces of aluminum in ^{99m}Tc-labeled bone radiopharmaceutical products.

In a superscan, although there is usually faint to absent kidney visualization, the spectrum of renal visualization depends on the degree of reactive bone formation as well as renal function.

Absence of renal activity cannot be used as a criterion for superscan. For example, in growing children, there is intense epiphyseal uptake and the kidneys may not be visualized. This appearance should not be confused with a superscan. The classic appearance of the superscan is not as common these days as in the past. This is due to improved resolution and improvements in instrumentation technology. Most disseminated metastases are still discernible as multiple focal discrete abnormalities throughout the skeleton with reduced renal uptake, but they are less likely to be mistaken for a normal appearance. Figure 7.6 E represents a superscan pattern of another patient with disseminated metastatic prostate carcinoma in which multiple focal abnormalities are seen. Minimal bladder activity suggests that some renal function is present.

Diagnosis: Superscan.

History: A 71-year-old indigent man was brought to the hospital for right ankle pain after a minor fall. Radiographic examination of the ankle shows no evidence of fracture but demonstrates osteoblastic lesions in the calcaneus (Fig. 7.7 A), leading to the performance of a bone scan (Fig. 7.7 B).

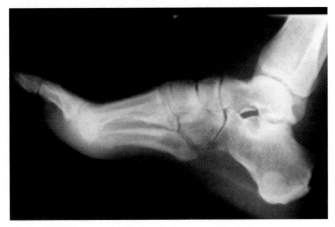

Figure 7.7 A

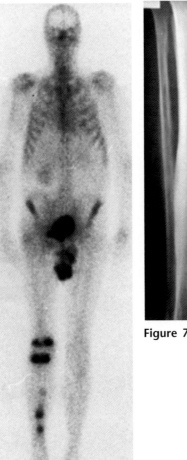

Figure 7.7 B

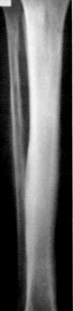

Figure 7.7 C

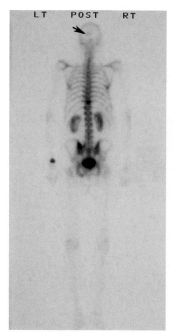

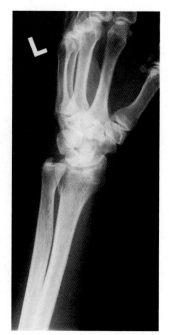

Figure 7.7 D   **Figure 7.7** E

Findings: There are several foci of abnormal uptake involving the distal right lower extremity around the knee, midtibia, and ankle. Radiography of the right leg (Fig. 7.7 C) shows a thickened and deformed midtibia with periosteal new bone formation.

Discussion: Although multiple foci of uptake located in one extremity could be related to fracture or multifocal osteomyelitis, correlative radiography suggests a metastatic process that proved, on further workup, to be prostatic in origin.

Lesions limited to the distal extremity are not a usual feature of the metastatic process and are less common than the axial skeletal metastasis. However, they do occur with an overall frequency of 11.1%, in which bone of the forearm, leg, and foot does not account for more than 4.9% of the lesions.

Metastases to the long bones usually occur in the medullary cavity of the diaphysis and metaphysis, producing a diffuse bone sclerosis. However, they do occur in the cortex of the bone as well.

Cortical bone metastases are not as rare as previously believed. The majority originate from the lung. The dissemination is via pulmonary veins into the systemic arterial circulation reaching the appendicular skeleton.

Cortical metastasis creates lytic cortical lesions (cookie-bite lesions) that affect the integrity of the bone. Bones with cortical metastasis are more prone to pathologic fracture than those with medullary metastasis. Some of these lesions are asymptomatic and located in the end of the extremities; they are easily missed if the entire skeleton is not included in the routine imaging studies.

Figure 7.7 D shows the bone scan of a 65-year-old patient with lung cancer. Note the abnormal uptake in the calvarium (arrow) and distal right radius, representing metastatic lung disease. The right radial metastasis resulted in the pathologic fracture in less than 2 weeks from the original scan (Fig. 7.7 E).

The increased bone density and sclerosis of the midtibia (Fig. 7.7 C) represent simultaneous osteoblastic activity by tumor cells and the host response attempting to heal the lesions. As much as a positive spot on bone scan reflects metabolic activity and formation of new reactive bone, the pattern of dissemination of a new spot along the large area of bone sclerosis (Fig. 7.7 B) suggests that some healing process has already occurred and the scan portrays a different stage of the disease process, a mixture of healed and active foci.

Note that both the lytic lesion of the radius (Fig. 7.7 E) and the sclerotic lesion of the tibia (Fig. 7.7 C) are associated with uptake indicating that the scintigraphic degree of uptake is generally not related to the degree of lucency on the radiograph and that a positive scan is mainly a reflection of blood flow of increased metabolic activity.

It is well known that completely healed lesions manifest as a dense sclerotic abnormality on x-ray and are not associated with abnormal uptake. These should not be considered as false-negative scans, but scintigraphy simply reflects stability and lack of activity of the process.

Blastic lesions associated with a low metabolic rate can produce false-negative scans, but false-negative scans are more often due to purely lytic lesions with minimal reactive bone formation, such as may occur with multiple myeloma and with highly anaplastic, or rapidly progressing tumors. Overall, the rate of false-negative scans is not more than 1% to 8%.

Any patient with an x-ray abnormality suggestive of or suspicious for metastatic disease, as in this patient with calcaneal lesions, should have a radionuclide bone scan to identify additional lesions. The scan should routinely include the extremities.

Diagnosis: Appendicular skeletal metastasis of the prostate to the tibia and the lung to the radius.

CASE 7.8

History: A 73-year-old man with past history of prostate carcinoma and bilateral orchiectomy is referred for a bone scan for evaluation of possible bony metastases (Fig. 7.8 A). Figure 7.8 B represents his concurrent abdominal radiograph.

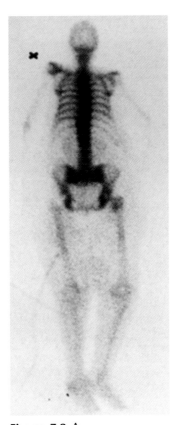

Figure 7.8 A

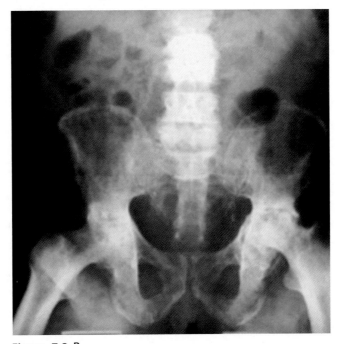

Figure 7.8 B

Findings: There is homogeneous uptake throughout the axial skeleton with no discrete focal area of increased or decreased uptake, and the kidneys are faintly visualized. A urinary bladder catheter is faintly seen.

Discussion: Distribution of axial skeletal uptake is so uniform that the scan appears normal and may give a false impression if interpreted blindly and without radiographic correlation.

Hyperparathyroidism secondary to chronic renal disease may be considered, but lack of abnormal calvarial and long-bone uptake as well as visualization of the kidneys, although faint, does not suggest renal osteodystrophy or superscan of metabolic cause.

The so-called superscan due to diffuse metastases could be responsible, particularly in correlation with the radiograph (Fig. 7.8 B) demonstrating multiple diffuse osteoblastic lesions in the spine and pelvis. A normal-appearing scan is known to occur in a uniformly disseminated metastatic process in which no focal preferential uptake occurs to stand out as a hot lesion. Correlation with the radiograph, however, discloses the true nature of the process and helps to avoid a false-negative interpretation. The mild abnormality or basically normal-appearing scan is probably related to the indolent course of the patient's disease.

It is to be noted that the appearance of normal uptake corresponding to sclerotic disease, as in this case, may actually represent healed metastases and be a sign of inactivity. This evaluation requires the availability of serial scans and radiographs. A single set of scans and radiographs represents only a single point of static information over the curve of a dynamic process.

The false-negative scan is not a common occurrence. Only 1% to 8% of scans are false-negatives, and these are usually due to lytic lesions, rapid destruction, or slow expansion. The false-negative scan also occurs in instances of blastic lesions associated with a slow bone turnover. In the case of cancer of the prostate, as in this patient, it is conceivable that the metastases are androgen-dependent tumors that show an undulant course secondary to orchiectomy.

It is general knowledge that skeletal scintigraphy is the most sensitive technique for the detection of bone lesions, but there are entities that, despite abnormal radiographs, appear normal on the scan.

Benign entities such as bone cyst, benign cortical defects, multiple exostosis, histiocytosis X, bone island, and osteopoikilosis have been associated with a normal scan. Multiple myeloma and purely destructive metastases are among those lesions that may be positive on the radiograph and negative on the scan. Most of these lesions have a characteristic pattern on radiography that can be easily recognized, and this emphasizes the value of plain radiographs in the meaningful evaluation of bone scintigrams.

Diagnosis: Indolent prostatic osteoblastic metastases, false-negative scan.

History: A 48-year-old male drug addict complained of low back pain and was referred for a bone scan (Fig. 7.9 A).

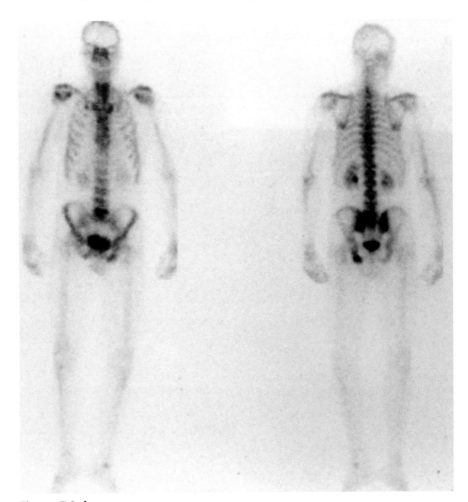

Figure 7.9 A

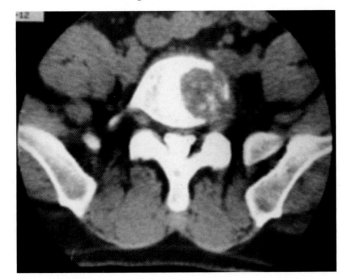

Figure 7.9 B

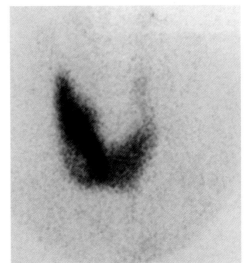

Figure 7.9 C

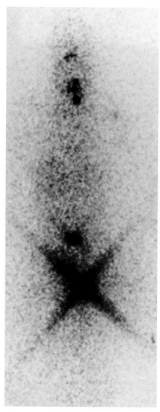

Figure 7.9 D

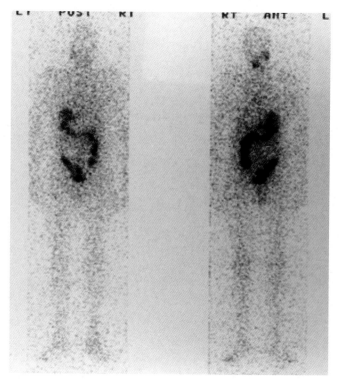

Figure 7.9 E

Findings: Significant abnormalities on the bone scan are increased uptake involving the fifth lumbar vertebra as well as the left ischium.

Discussion: Abnormal uptake, particularly in the pelvis, although not specific, could be due to metastases or be related to a multifocal infectious process in this patient with a history of drug addiction and no history of trauma to the pelvis.

On prebiopsy guided CT (Fig. 7.9 B), a large destructive process involving the fifth lumbar vertebra corresponding to the abnormal bone uptake is seen; it proved to be a metastatic follicular carcinoma of the thyroid.

Thyroid carcinoma occasionally metastasizes to the bone. The type that metastasizes most frequently is follicular and the most frequent sites are the spine and the flat bones of the pelvis, skull, scapula, and ribs. Most of the lesions are lytic on radiography and usually have a low rate of mineralization, which may make the scan less sensitive for their detection. However, the bone scan in metastatic thyroid carcinoma is more often positive than negative. There may be photopenia surrounded by increased activity. Bone scanning can detect metastases from a variety of thyroid cancers regardless of their function and their ability to take up iodine-131 (^{131}I). This includes medullary

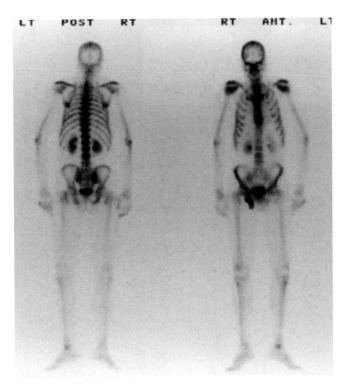

Figure 7.9 F

carcinoma of the thyroid. Combining an ^{131}I scan and a bone scan not only increases confidence in recognition of the lesion but allows evaluation of the lesion's functional status while also providing an opportunity for therapy.

The patient's thyroid scan (Fig. 7.9 C) reveals a cold nodule in the right lobe as the primary site of the tumor. A whole-body ^{131}I scan following thyroidectomy (Fig. 7.9 D) indeed demonstrates accumulation of radioiodine in the fifth lumbar lesions providing the opportunity for radioactive iodine therapy, which was subsequently initiated. There is minimal residual postoperative thyroid tissue in the neck. (Note that a detail of the pelvis and functional status of the left ischial lesion is not available owing to significant urinary bladder activity. Also note the star-pattern artifact related to the collimator's septal penetration).

Although it is generally believed that bone metastases from thyroid carcinoma indicate a low survival rate and the response of bone metastases to treatment with radioactive iodine is poor, this patient's ^{131}I scan (Fig. 7.9 E) and bone scan (Fig. 7.9 F) were negative 6 years following the initiation of therapy. There may still be minimal residual tissue in the neck.

Diagnosis: Metastatic thyroid carcinoma to the bone, treated.

History: A 28-year-old male with a 3-month history of knee pain at rest and no history of trauma was referred for a bone scan (Fig. 7.10 A).

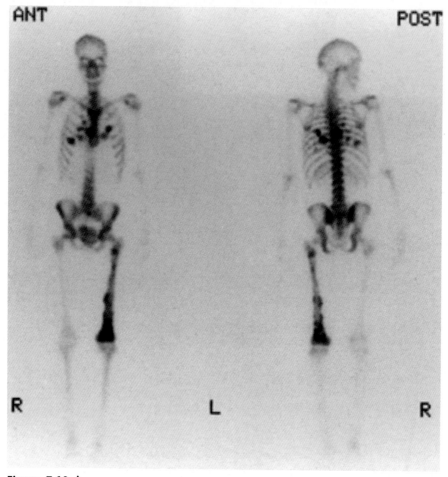

Figure 7.10 A

Findings: There is grossly increased uptake in the distal left femur with abnormal but less intense uptake proximally over virtually the entire left femur. In addition, there are multiple focal areas of increased uptake projected over both hemithoraxes.

Discussion: Focal uptake in both hemithoraxes in correlation with a chest radiograph done on the same day (Fig. 7.10 B) demonstrates the intraparenchymal locations of the lesions.

The constellation of findings in this patient is most consistent with a primary bone neoplasm with metastasis to the lung.

A high-grade osteogenic sarcoma was diagnosed by biopsy.

Conventional osteosarcoma is the most frequent type of osteosarcoma and represents the second most common primary tumor of the bone (next to multiple myeloma), with the knee, distal femur, and proximal tibia being the most commonly

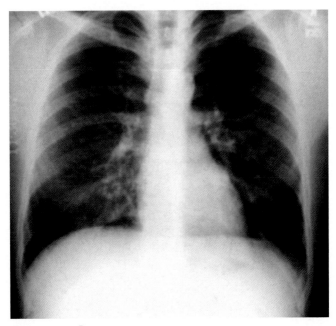

Figure 7.10 B

affected sites. The incidence is highest in the second decade of life. The tumor metastasizes by the hematogeneous route to the lung, bone, liver, and kidney.

It is generally believed that pulmonary metastases precede osseous metastases and that therefore bone scanning may not be helpful for further evaluation. However, advances in adjunctive chemotherapy have modified the natural course of this disease, and it has been reported that 16% of patients treated with chemotherapy develop bone metastases before or without pulmonary metastases. In addition, up to 10% of patients with osteosarcoma have skeletal metastases at the time of presentation. Therefore bone scan plays an important role in the evaluation and follow-up of patients with osteogenic sarcoma for the detection of skip metastases and distant osseous metastases as well as evaluation of the primary tumor.

Osteogenic sarcoma generally demonstrates intense uptake of bone-seeking radiopharmaceutical, to such an extent that the primary lesion occasionally appears larger than the actual site. This false extension is related to the hyperemia, medullary reactive bone, and periosteal reaction in the adjacent area of tumor. CT and MRI are invaluable in the evaluation of this tumor, particularly in demonstration of tumor extension with the bone marrow.

The mechanism of uptake in pulmonary metastases of osteosarcoma is not quite clear; however, it appears to be related more to the process of active ossification than calcification in the lesion. Uptake in pulmonary metastases should be differentiated from overlying rib lesions. SPECT images of the thorax should be employed in cases of doubt.

Diagnosis: Osteogenic sarcoma with pulmonary metastasis.

History: A 48-year-old man with a lung mass (Fig. 7.11 A) and the diagnosis of a small cell anaplastic carcinoma was referred for a bone scan (Fig. 7.11 B).

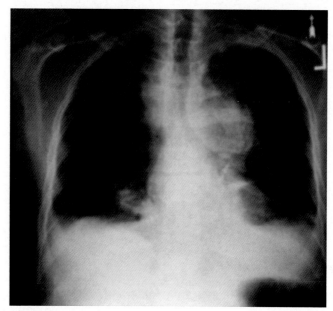

Figure 7.11 A

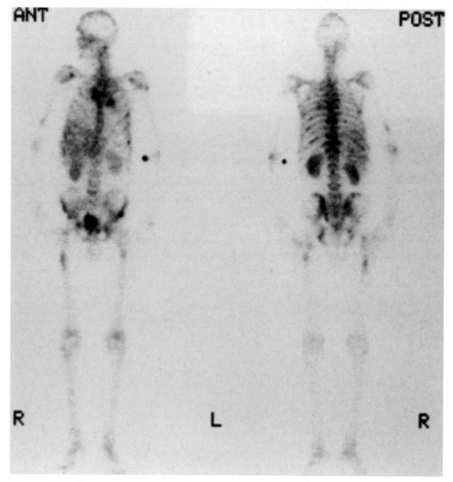

Figure 7.11 B

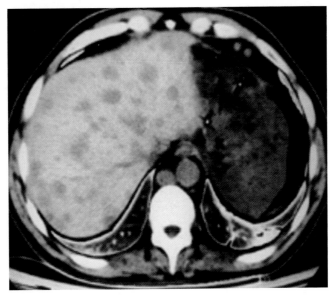

Figure 7.11 C

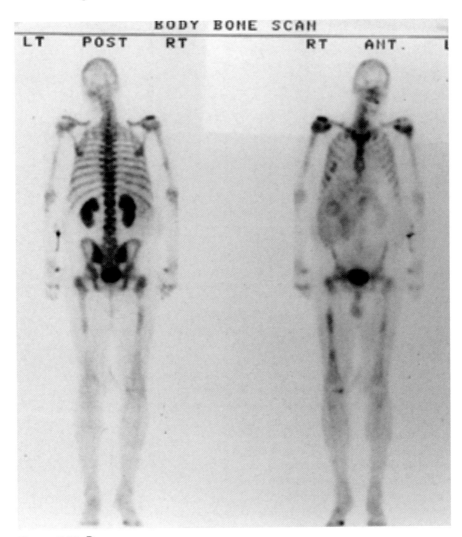

Figure 7.11 D

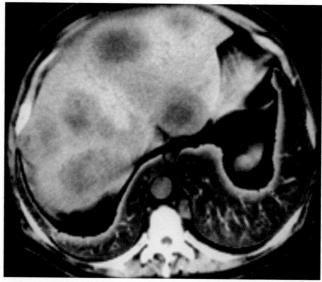

Figure 7.11 E

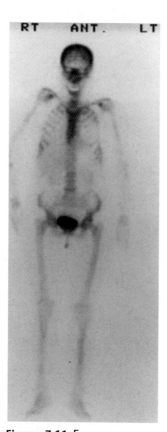

Figure 7.11 F

Findings: There are disseminated abnormal foci of uptake in the axial and appendicular skeleton. There is increased tracer activity in the thorax corresponding to the location and configuration of a large hilar mass. There are no calcifications and the overlying bone structures appear intact. In addition, there is heterogeneous scattered uptake in the liver.

Discussion: The scan findings are essentially diagnostic for disseminated skeletal and liver metastases.

Soft tissue accumulation of bone-seeking radiopharmaceutical is known to occur in benign tumors, primary and metastatic lesions, and inflammatory disease. This case demonstrates accumulation of radiopharmaceutical in both the primary tumors of the lung and hepatic metastases in addition to the disseminated osseous involvement.

A number of primary and secondary liver malignancies have been shown to take up the bone-seeking radiopharmaceutical.

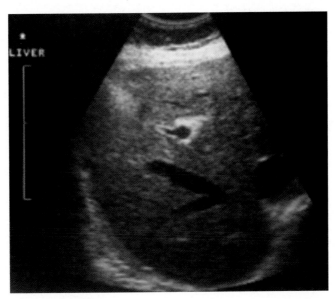

Figure 7.11 G

Hepatoma, hepatoblastoma, cholangiocarcinoma, and a variety of metastases from the lung, breast, esophagus, stomach, colon, and prostate as well as melanoma, lymphoma, and others have demonstrated the ability to localize diphosphonate compounds.

Of these tumors, metastases from the colon and lungs are more often associated with liver uptake. Approximately half of colon metastases to the liver and 15% of lung metastases to the liver are visualized on bone scan. When they are visualized on bone scan, they usually represent advanced disease.

The mechanism of uptake is not clear. Increased blood perfusion, hypercalcemia, and necrosis with or without calcification have been postulated. Deposition of calcium in dead or dying tissue is a well-known phenomenon that can occur without any abnormality in calcium metabolism. However, detection of calcification by x-ray or CT is variable. Figure 7.11 C is the patient's corresponding noncontrasted abdominal CT, which shows no calcification in or around the numerous visualized liver metastases. It is possible that diphosphonate may accumulate in metastases before the calcification appears on x-ray or CT.

It is to be noted that liver uptake secondary to metastases is scattered and inhomogeneous instead of being diffuse and intense. Figure 7.11 D portrays the anterior and posterior whole-body bone scan of another patient, a 64-year-old male with squamous cell carcinoma of the lung with skeletal and liver metastases. Note the hepatomegaly and the appearance of doughnut lesions in the liver, which correlates with the necrotic tumor seen in the liver on CT (Fig. 7.11 E). Also note the intense diffuse renal uptake secondary to chemotherapy.

Visualization of the liver on bone scan is not a usual or common finding. When it is seen, residual activity from previous liver scan should be considered.

High serum aluminum (dialysis treatment, Maalox or other aluminum-containing product) or high concentrations of aluminum, ion in ^{99m}Tc-generated eluate (which results in the flocculation of diphosphonate compounds and the subsequent phagocytosis by Kupffer cells) results in hepatic visualization on bone scan.

Hepatic uptake due to intervenous iron therapy occurs and is probably related to the formation of an iron–colloid complex that is taken up by the Kupffer cells.

Hepatic necrosis secondary to viral hepatitis, hepatic toxic agents, hepatic venous occlusive disease, and hepatic hypoxia and ischemia secondary to respiratory failure or prolonged hypotension are recognized as causes of hepatic visualization on bone scan. In most of these cases, despite marked abnormality in liver function tests, ultrasound and CT are normal. Scan visualization of the liver in these conditions usually signifies a grave prognosis.

Diffuse liver uptake of radiopharmaceutical due to artifactual causes is usually mild, but hepatic necrosis is usually associated with intense diffuse uptake.

Figure 7.11 F shows faint liver uptake in this 64-year-old female who habitually used Maalox for her presumed indigestion. Note the photopenic region over the left anterior thorax, which is secondary to an artificial breast (the patient has had a left mastectomy).

The presence of faint right-upper-quadrant uptake on a bone scan should suggest an additional study, such as an ultrasound or CT, to further delineate its anatomic cause. Figure 7.11 G represents the ultrasound image of this patient and shows normal liver architecture.

Diagnosis: Lung metastases to bone and liver.

CASE 7.12

History: A 55-year-old male was referred for bone scan (Fig. 7.12 A) because of left calf pain and low-grade fever suspicious for osteomyelitis. There was no history of trauma, and blood culture was negative. Past history includes abdominal aortic aneurysm (AAA) repair.

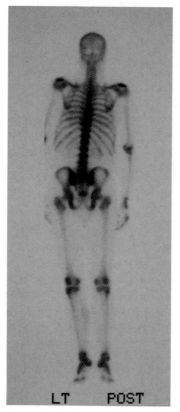

Figure 7.12 A

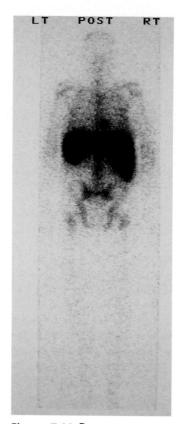

Figure 7.12 B

Findings: Posterior images of the whole-body bone scan are remarkable for increased soft tissue uptake in the symptomatic left calf. There is diminished left renal activity. The underlying bone appears normal.

Discussion: Several entities can cause accumulation of a bone-seeking agent in soft tissue and skeletal muscle, in particular trauma, neoplastic disease, localized vascular disorder, and infectious processes.

The mechanism of muscle uptake includes increased perfusion, muscle necrosis with or without calcification, hypercalcemia, precipitation of calcification in soft tissue, and sometimes this occurs artifactually owing to faulty preparation of the radiopharmaceutical.

Benign and malignant soft tissue masses accumulate the bone agent. Tumoral calcinosis, a benign, painless, commonly periarticular mass; myositis ossificans, a benign process of bone formation within the muscle bundles; and soft tissue sarcoma, a malignant neoplasm of mesenchymal origin, all avidly take up the bone-seeking agent. Most of the soft tissue sarcomas accumulate radiopharmaceutical because of their vascularity, calcification, or both.

Trauma to muscle or muscle injury as the result of unaccustomed physical activity and rabdomyolysis shows increased uptake of bone agent. Trauma can also cause the formation of hematomas. In an organizing hematoma, hemosiderin and calcium precipitate in combination with hyperemia, contributing

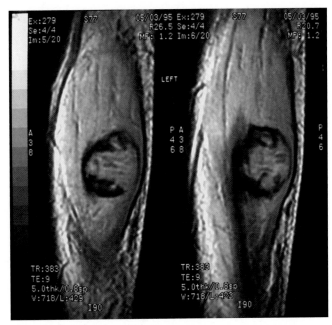

Figure 7.12 C

to increased uptake. If not completely resolved, the hematoma progresses and moves into the lamellar bone within the muscles, forming myositis ossificans.

Vascular calcification within the soft tissue, thrombophlebitis, chronic venous insufficiency, and lymphedema are the well-known causes of the soft tissue uptake. These local circulatory abnormalities cause expansion of the extracellular space and interstitial edema. There will be slow clearance of the radiopharmaceutical from the expanded extracellular space, enhancing the visualization of soft tissue uptake.

Local inflammation, cellulitis, and the sites of soft tissue abscess also show increased uptake. Although the cavity of abscess is avascular and deprived of the entry of radiopharmaceutical, it may be photopenic and hyperemic, and altered capillary permeability of the abscess site results in increased uptake.

Formation of the abscess causes the infiltration of surrounding tissue with WBCs, mainly granulocytes. ^{111}In-labeled WBC is an effective tool in including or excluding the abscess.

Figure 7.12 B is the posterior image of the patient's ^{111}In-WBC scan, revealing no accumulation of WBCs in the region of the left calf, excluding the abscess as the cause of bone scan abnormality.

A small focus of ^{111}In-WBC accumulation in the right posteroinferior mediastinum corresponds to the large known osteophytes.

Diminished renal activity noted on bone scan is due to involvement of the left renal artery by known AAA.

Further workup including MRI (Fig. 7.12 C) shows the presence of a well-circumscribed mass in the left gastrocnemius muscle with no invasion of bone. The tumor was diagnosed as a malignant fibrous histocytoma.

Evaluation of the soft tissue uptake should be an integral part of any bone scan interpretation. Recognition of the extraskeletal uptake enhances the diagnostic value of the bone scan.

Diagnosis: Malignant fibrous histocytoma.

CASE 7.13

History: A 68-year-old male with mild chronic pain over the right hip was referred for a bone scan (Fig. 7.13 A).

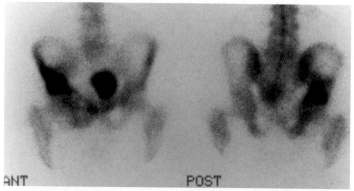

Figure 7.13 A

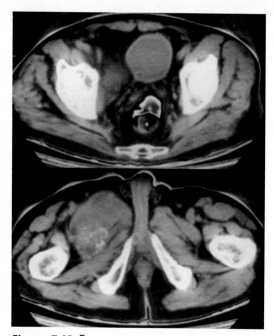

Figure 7.13 B

Findings: Spot images of the pelvis in the anterior and posterior projections show abnormal uptake involving the right supra-acetabular region. The urinary bladder appears displaced to the left.

Discussion: The right acetabular abnormality associated with displacement of the urinary bladder suggests either a pelvic mass with involvement of the adjacent bone or a bone lesion extending medially to the pelvis. A pelvic CT (Fig. 7.13 B) discloses the nature of the process as a lobulated mass showing scattered calcification consistent with the diagnosis of chondrosarcoma.

Skeletal scintigraphy is invariably abnormal in chondrosarcoma and delineates the lesion and the extent of the tumor better than plain radiographs. However, the extent of the tumor is usually exaggerated owing to hyperemia and edema of the tissue adjacent to the tumor. CT and MRI are the procedures of choice in the staging and evaluating the extent of tumor extension into the bone marrow and the soft tissue.

Chondrosarcoma is the third most common bone tumor following multiple myeloma and osteogenic sarcoma. The usual sites of involvement are flat bones, the limb girdles, and the proximal portion of long tubular bone. Most chondrosarcomas are low-grade and have indolent courses. Chondrosarcomas that occur at a site with a large potential space, such as the pelvis, as in the current case, may grow immense yet not be detected clinically.

Peripheral or surface chondrosarcomas, which usually arise from an underlying benign lesion such as osteochondroma and as such are called secondary chondrosarcomas, manifest as peripheral masses, allowing earlier diagnosis.

Diagnosis: Chondrosarcoma of the pelvis.

CASE 7.14

History: A 20-year-old male with a palpable, painless mass in the lower left thigh was referred for a bone scan (Fig. 7.14 A). Figure 7.14 B represents his correlative radiograph.

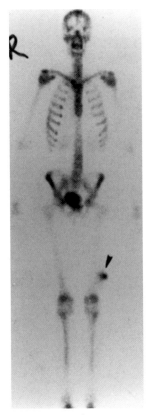

Figure 7.14 A

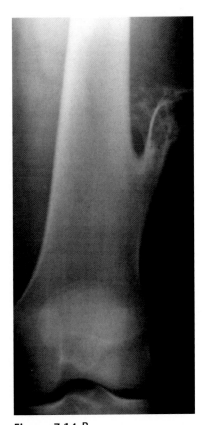

Figure 7.14 B

Findings: The bone scan shows a focal area of markedly increased uptake arising from the distal left femur and extending outward. This corresponds to the pedunculated osseous excrescence seen on the radiograph (Fig. 7.14 B).

Discussion: The radiographic appearance of a pedunculated tumor-like osseous structure is characteristic of a solitary osteochondroma or exostosis. This tumor may be solitary or multiple, as in the case of multiple hereditary exostosis.

Solitary steochondroma is the most common benign tumor. It may occur in any bone that develops by endochondral ossification. The distal femur, proximal tibia, fibula (around the knee), and proximal humeri are the preferential sites of its occurrence.

Osteochondroma in children usually shows a marked increased uptake as the enchondral growth continues. Since the growth of osteocartilaginous exostosis ceases with fusion of the epiphyseal plate, uptake of this lesion also wanes at the time of closure of the adjacent epiphysis. Increased uptake beyond this age and after the complete closure of the epiphysis suggests a complication such as fracture or malignant transformation to a chondrosarcoma. The incidence of malignant transformation is approximately 1%, but it is considerably higher (perhaps as high as 20%) in cases of multiple hereditary exostosis. Malignant transformation may be signaled by pain, swelling, or the development of a soft tissue mass. A normal bone scan excludes malignant transformation. However, reactivation of a previously quiescent exostosis, shown by uptake of radiopharmaceutical, is a significant finding that may suggest malignant transformation. CT has been used to measure the thickness of the cartilage cap and is considered suggestive of malignancy if it is greater than 1 cm; however, this is not a reliable index. In the current case, the partial fusion of the epiphysis seen on x-ray, along with some epiphyseal uptake, suggests the diagnosis of a benign active exostosis.

Diagnosis: Solitary osteochondroma.

CASE 7.15

History: A 21-year-old male with left thigh pain for 18 months and an abnormal radiograph (Fig. 7.15 A) was referred for a bone scan (Fig. 7.15 B) for further evaluation.

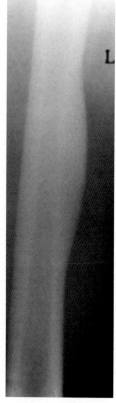

Figure 7.15 A

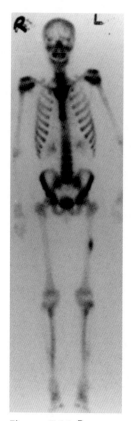

Figure 7.15 B

Findings: There is intense focal cortical uptake in the lateral aspect of the midfemur corresponding to the thickened cortical bone noted on the radiograph. The remainder of the skeleton is unremarkable.

Discussion: The finding of a single focal cortical uptake in the long bone is not specific. Stress fracture, infection, single metastasis, as well as a cortically located benign lesion should be considered. These are not distinguishable from each other by bone scan, but history, clinical findings, and radiographic correlation help to arrive at a proper diagnosis, which, in this case, is an osteoid osteoma.

An osteoid osteoma typically appears as a cortical lesion on x-ray. There is a sclerotic region containing a small (less than 1-cm) lucency representing a nidus. Intermittent night pain relieved by aspirin and possibly local tenderness are typical clinical presentations.

In the classic presentation and typical x-ray appearance of osteoid osteoma in the long bone, a bone scan has relatively less value than in cases of atypical presentation and lesions occurring in the spine and small bones. It is to be noted that in 30% to 50% of cases, the history is atypical and x-rays have a varied radiographic appearance. It is often a confusing

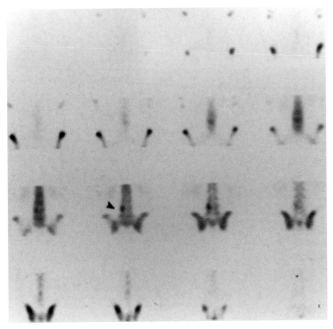

Figure 7.15 C

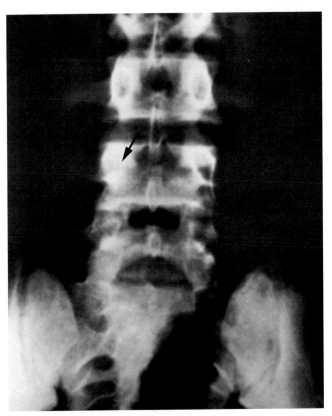

Figure 7.15 D

picture of pain in a young adult, which leads to the bone scan and the diagnosis of osteoid osteoma. Moreover, an intramedullary, subperiosteal or intra-articularly located ostoid osteoma has an entirely different appearance. In the case of intra-articular osteoid osteoma of the hip, the pain is usually referred to the knee and the paucity of reactive sclerosis makes the diagnosis quite difficult radiographically. However, regardless of its location and clinical presentation, the lesion of osteoid osteoma appears as an area of intense uptake during all phases of a three-phase bone scan, which makes the scintigram an invaluable procedure for evaluating a young patient with skeletal pain of undetermined etiology.

In the diagnosis of osteoid osteoma by bone scan, it is important to obtain a high-resolution image using a pinhole or converging collimator. This high-resolution scan may disclose an area of diffuse increased uptake with a superimposed second focus of more avid uptake representing the nidus of the lesion. This has been called a double-density sign.

The double-density sign can be used to suggest the diagnosis of an osteoid osteoma and is also helpful for an accurate preoperative localization of the nidus.

Osteoid osteoma is a common lesion. It occurs predominantly in the young male (10 to 30 years of age), and the usual locations are the femur and tibia, but it can occur in almost any bone.

The spine is involved in approximately 6% of the cases. Lesions occur in the posterior elements, and a painful scoliosis is its usual manifestation.

Radiographic evaluation of spinal osteoid osteoma is difficult. CT may show an area of sclerosis within the posterior elements. A SPECT image can be used to better advantage over the planar for evaluation of complex osseous structures of the vertebrae and localization of osteoid osteoma.

Figure 7.15 C is a SPECT image of a 17-year-old with a 1-year history of low back pain. There is focal intense uptake (arrowhead) involving the right pedicle of the fourth lumbar vertebra. This was recognized on a radiograph obtained afterward (Fig. 7.15 D), which shows the sclerotic lesion of the osteoid osteoma (arrow).

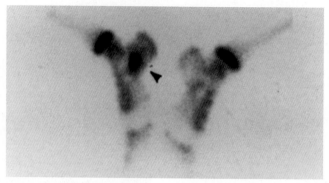

Figure 7.15 E

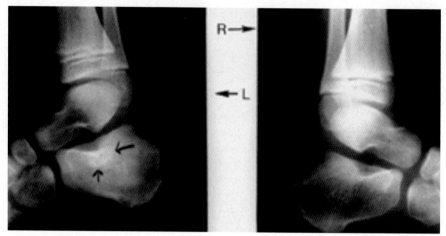

Figure 7.15 F

Occurrence of osteoid osteoma in the calvarium, mandible, scapula, and ribs has been reported. Occurrence in the hands and feet is extremely rare and may appear as an area of lucency surrounded by sclerosis. These lesions sometimes appear as areas of punctuate increased density with a radiolucent center indistinguishable from Brodi's abscess, chondroblastoma, osteoblastoma, stress fracture, and osteochondritis dissecans. A bone scan shows nonspecific intense uptake. CT is most helpful for diagnosis, clearly showing the nidus and surrounding sclerosis.

Figures 7.15 E and 7.15 F shows the scan and radiograph of a 7-year-old boy with left ankle pain for over 2 months and no fever or history of trauma. Surgical exploration and subsequent excision revealed calcaneus osteoid osteoma.

Diagnosis: Osteoid osteoma of the femur, spine, and calcaneus.

History: A 35-year-old man with right knee pain aggravated by exercise was referred for a bone scan (Fig. 7.16 A).

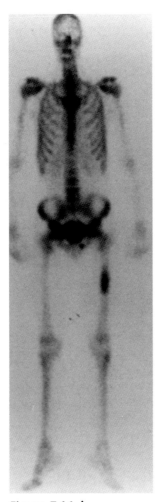

Figure 7.16 A

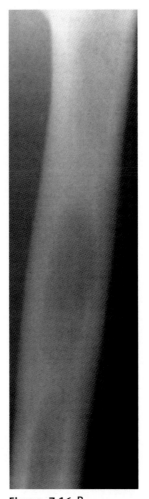

Figure 7.16 B

Findings: There is marked intense uptake in the medullary portion of the mid-left femur. There is also a small focus of uptake in the left pubic ramus (urine contamination). Otherwise the scan is unremarkable.

Discussion: A single oblong uptake in the left femur corresponding to the lesion recognized on the radiograph obtained following bone scan (Fig. 7.16 B) is most consistent with fibrous dysplasia.

Mono-ostotic fibrous dysplasia of a long bone typically produces a well-defined radiolucent area in the medullary canal; this may vary radiographically from a complete lucent cyst-like lesion to a homogeneous ground-glass density. Density variation depends on the relative balance of the fibrous and osseous components of the lesion in the medullary canal. There may

be local bone expansion and deformity and development of an irregular band of sclerosis that crosses the cyst-like lesions and gives a multiloculated cystic appearance to the lesion.

The lesions of fibrous dysplasia are vascular and have some degree of bone remodeling providing the basis for a positive bone scan.

The scintigraphic appearance of fibrous dysplasia varies from markedly increased uptake to an area of mild abnormality. Lesions with a radiographic ground-glass appearance have a tendency to show more uptake than those with cystic changes that have less uptake or may even be normal. However, they do not appear as a cold defect.

Figure 7.16 C shows increased uptake in the right iliac bone due to fibrous dysplasia and as an incidental finding in

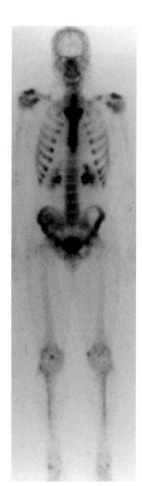

Figure 7.16 C

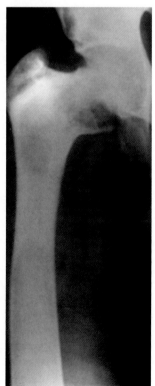

Figure 7.16 D

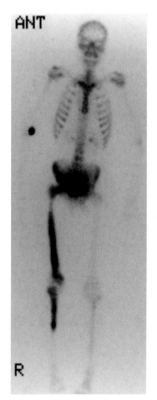

Figure 7.16 E

Figure 7.16 F

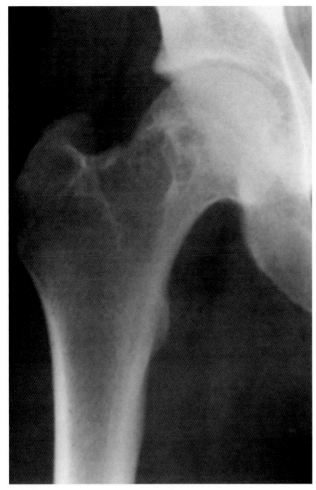

Figure 7.16 G

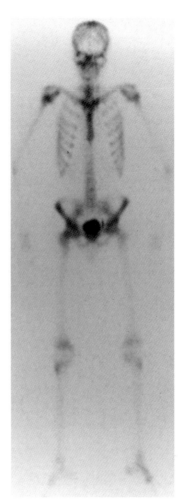

Figure 7.16 H

this 28-year-old male referred for a bone scan to rule out a stress fracture. Note the ring-like appearance of the lesion, which corresponds to the cyst-like lesion on the radiograph (Fig. 7.16 D).

Mono-ostotic fibrous dysplasia accounts for 70% of all cases. It usually occurs in early childhood and becomes quiescent at puberty. Fibrous dysplasia is one of the benign bone lesions that have the potential for malignant transformation to osteosarcoma, fibrosarcoma, or chondrosarcoma. The sarcomatous degeneration may develop during the second to fourth decades of life. A history of previous radiation to the area may play a role. The scintigraphic appearance of fibrous dysplasia does not warrant the suggestion of malignant transformation or even changing the initial radiographic diagnosis.

The diagnosis of fibrous dysplasia is usually made radiographically, and its features are sufficiently characteristic to render a definite diagnosis. A bone scan, however, is useful in detecting the unexpected cases or demonstration of polyostotic cases. Polyostotic fibrous dysplasia accounts for 30% of cases. The incidence of pathologic fracture, "shepherd's crook deformity," and craniofacial involvement is more common in the polyostotic than the mono-ostotic form.

Figure 7.16 E shows the scintigram of another patient with polyostotic fibrous dysplasia. Note the marked intensity of up-

take in the proximal left tibia and in the bowed and deformed (shepherd's crook deformity) left femur (Fig. 7.16 F).

A scintigraphically silent area of fibrous dysplasia may occur in both cystic and ground-glass lesions. These lesions, despite marked radiographic changes, may show normal or very minimal uptake. Figure 7.16 G shows a lesion of fibrous dysplasia in the neck of the right femur. However, the bone scan (Fig. 7.16 H) is minimally abnormal, showing slight asymmetry of uptake, with the right hip being slightly more active than the left.

Craniofacial fibrous dysplasia tends to have more sclerotic changes than do peripheral lesions. When the base of the skull is involved, there is sclerosis with a ground-glass appearance, and the paranasal sinuses are often opaque owing to bone invasion. Involvement of the facial bone causes marked sclerosis, bone thickening with obliteration of the sinuses and orbits, and creates leontiasis ossea. Lesions of craniofacial fibrous dysplasia are positive on all phases of a three-phase bone scan. The pattern of markedly increased uptake can be confused with Paget's disease or meningioma producing hyperostosis of the frontal and sphenoid bones. The patient's age and abnormal biochemistry of Paget's as well as predilection for the occipital bone in Paget's may help to differentiate Paget's from fibrous dysplasia. Neurofibromatosis and osteoblastic

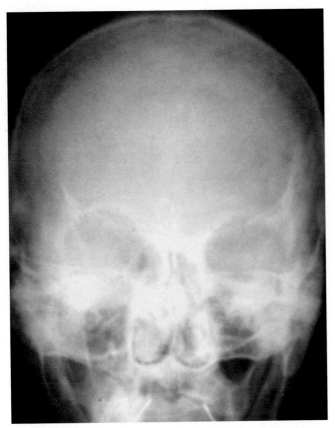

Figure 7.16 I

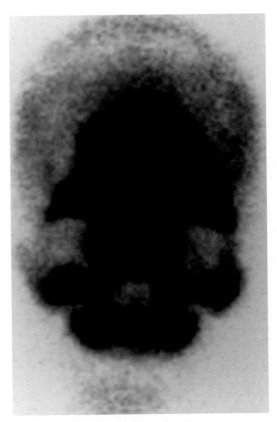

Figure 7.16 J

metastases may also mimic facial fibrous dysplasia. Skull x-ray and CT will help to rule out most of these lesions.

Figures 7.16 I and 7.16 J shows the scan and skull radiograph of a 38-year-old Asian woman with known craniofacial fibrous dysplasia. Note the marked radiographic sclerosis and intense uptake of radioactivity of the sphenoid and frontal bones. Although approximately one-third of patients with craniofacial fibrous dysplasia have at least one other area of skeletal involvement, this patient's fibrous dysplasia was limited to the craniofacial area.

Diagnosis: Fibrous dysplasia.

CASE 7.17

History: A lesion in the proximal right fibula (Fig. 7.17 A) of this 50-year-old male was incidentally noted and a bone scan (Fig. 7.17 B) obtained.

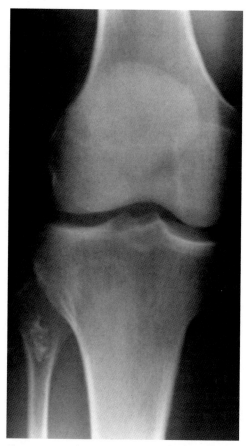

Figure 7.17 A

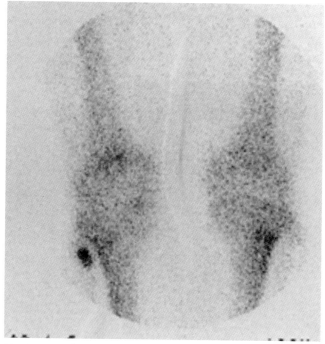

Figure 7.17 B

Findings: There is an area of mild activity corresponding to the spotty calcified lesion in the proximal fibula.

Discussion: The incidental finding of an amorphus intramedullary calcification limited to the head of the fibula in this patient would be typical for an enchondroma; however, it should be differentiated from a medullary bone infarction, in which serpentine distribution of calcification is usually seen. Although infarction may be idiopathic, it usually occurs as a result of sickle cell disease, collagen vascular disease, trauma, infection, or steroid use, and the clinical presentation is different.

A solitary enchondroma is seen mostly in the second to fifth decades of life and usually occurs as an incidental finding. The site of origin in long bone is usually metaphyseal, extending down the shaft of the bone.

Benign enchondroma shows normal or slightly increased uptake of the bone-seeking agent. Malignant transformation to chondrosarcoma may occur but is more frequent in patients with multiple enchondromatosis, in which it may be as high as 50%.

Diagnosis: Solitary benign enchondroma.

CASE 7.18

History: A radiodense lesion in the right femoral neck (Fig. 7.18 A) of this 35-year-old male was incidentally noted and a bone scan (Fig. 7.18 B) obtained.

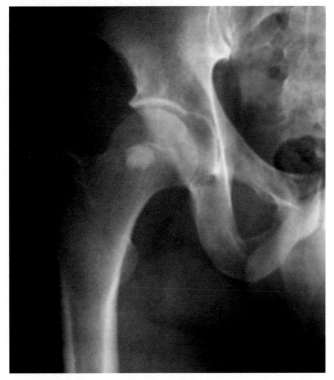

Figure 7.18 A

Figure 7.18 B

Findings: There is minimally increased uptake corresponding to the right femoral sclerotic lesion.

Discussion: The incidental finding of a well-circumscribed, sharply marginated, dense lesion in the femur of an asymptomatic young male would be typical for a bone island (insula compacta) but still occasionally must be differentiated from an osteoblastic metastasis.

From the standpoint of histology, a bone island is a nodule of cortical bone within the cancellous or medullary bone. As such, on a CT examination a bone island has the same density as cortical bone, which, in combination with normal or minimal bone uptake and a sharply marginated lesion in an asymptomatic patient should allow its differentiation from a osteoblastic lesion.

Bone islands may appear as nodules with spiculated margins; they can occur in any bone (except the skull) but are seen mostly in the pelvis, proximal femur, and humerus. Characteristically they are not associated with increased uptake. Their metabolic activity is either normal or mildly increased. Therefore they occasionally appear as focal areas of increased uptake.

Bone islands develop after puberty and have the capacity to grow and increase in size over a prolonged period of observation.

Diagnosis: Bone island.

History: A 43-year-old man with a penetrating wound to the right leg and the question of a hairline fracture on the proximal tibia (Fig. 7.19 A, arrowhead) is referred for a bone scan (Figs. 7.19 B, 7.19 C and 7.19 D).

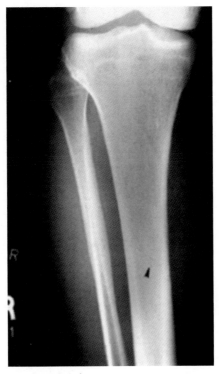

Figure 7.19 A

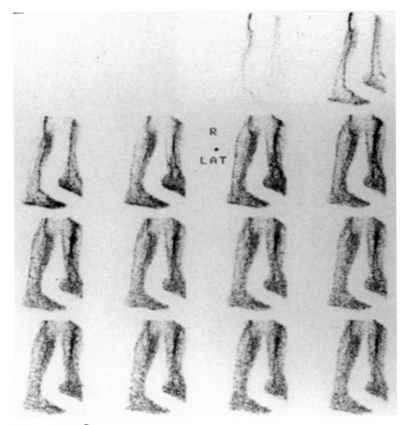

Figure 7.19 B

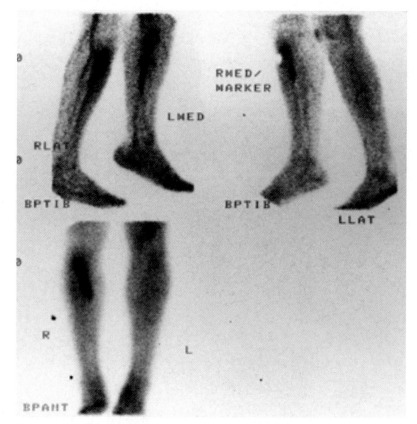

Figure 7.19 C

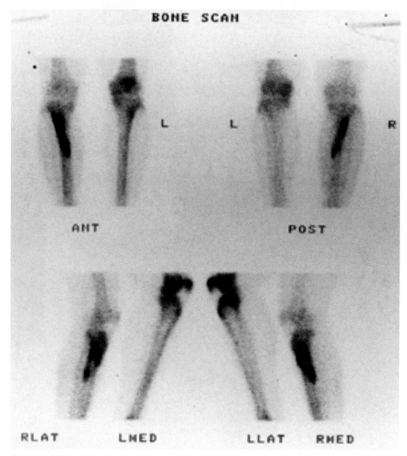

Figure 7.19 D

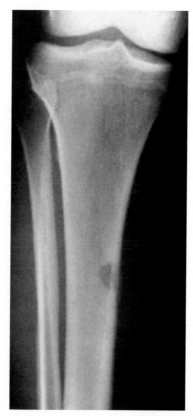

Figure 7.19 E

Findings: There is a positive three-phase bone scan in the region of the proximal right tibia. Abnormal uptake includes a central area of photopenia.

Discussion: A positive three-phase bone scan in the setting of trauma and penetrating wound would be compatible with acute fracture, osteomyelitis, or a combination of fracture complicated by osteomyelitis.

Photopenia in the region of a traumatized bone may be a sign of an atrophic nonunion, which is a late complication of fracture and can be excluded clinically and on the basis of history of recent trauma.

Osteomyelitis occasionally appears as an area of photopenia. This is most often seen in the very early stage of the disease and probably is the etiology of the positive bone scan in this case. Photopenia is due to disruption of the blood supply due to thrombosis of the vessels induced by the infectious process.

The patient's clinical course and subsequent radiographic finding (Fig. 7.19 E) of a developing lytic lesion with minimal periosteal reaction confirm the diagnosis of posttraumatic osteomyelitis.

A three-phase bone scan is the routine nuclear medicine procedure for the diagnosis of osteomyelitis. In individuals who have a normal radiograph and no other lesions that increase bone turnover, the finding of a positive three-phase bone scan is quite reliable for the detection of osteomyelitis. A sensitivity of 94% and a specificity of 95% have been reported. Commonly the scan shows abnormality 10 to 14 days prior to the development of radiographic signs.

The three-phase bone scan does not increase the sensitivity but improves the specificity by excluding cellulitis or arthritis; however, specificity is significantly reduced when bone remodeling is present. The specificity can be improved by using ^{67}Ga- or ^{111}In-WBC scanning.

Diagnosis: Osteomyelitis, right tibia.

History: A 37-year-old quadriplegic patient with a right foot ulcer is referred for a bone scan (Fig. 7.20 A). His radiograph (Fig. 7.20 B) was reported to show osteopenia with no soft tissue gas or focal bone abnormality.

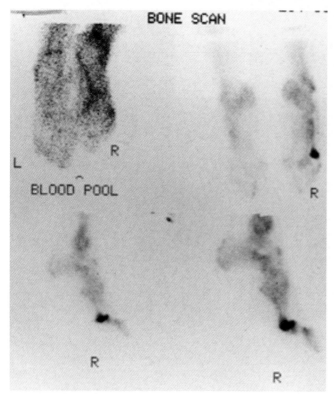

Figure 7.20 A

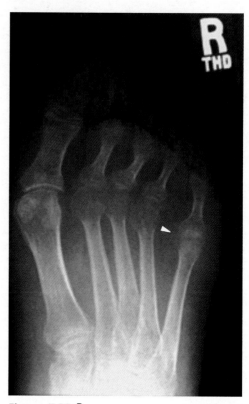

Figure 7.20 B

Findings: The two-phase image reveals soft tissue and skeletal uptake in the head of the fifth metatarsal bone, more pronounced on the skeletal phase than the blood pool image.

Discussion: Intense focal skeletal uptake increasing over time would be indicative of a focal bone process. In retrospect, this correlates with the erosive changes (arrowhead) of the fifth metatarsal head (Fig. 7.20 B) and proved positive for osteomyelitis by culture, leading to amputation (Fig. 7.20 C).

The diagnosis of pedal osteomyelitis by a three-phase bone scan even in a nondiabetic patient is difficult. Although this type of scan is quite sensitive and generally permits much earlier detection than does a radiograph, it has limited specificity. Sensitivity and specificity are lower in the foot than in the long bone. This is due to the frequent presence of degenerative changes, arthritis, skin ulcer, edema, and vascular insufficiency.

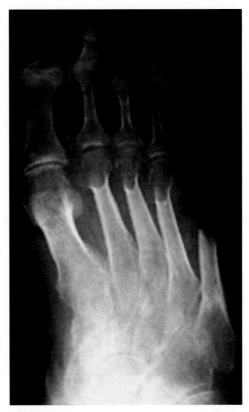

Figure 7.20 C

Small bones, relatively low counts, and inherent poor resolution add to the difficulty in the detection and differentiation of bone from soft tissue uptake.

Patients with edema or ulcer usually have positive vascular and blood pool images, and this can be misleading in the assessment of pedal osteomyelitis.

Overall, the contribution of the early blood flow and blood pool images in the detection of pedal osteomyelitis is less relevant than it is for the long bone. On the contrary, delayed static images, even up to 24 hours, are a more reasonable approach for the evaluation of pedal osteomyelitis.

Bone uptake in osteomyelitis is usually prolonged, and uptake continues beyond the 4 hours. The pattern of increasing uptake with time, even as early as 2 to 4 hours, should suggest osteomyelitis. Delayed 24-hour (four-phase bone scan) or combined bone scan and ^{111}In-WBC images may further strengthen the diagnosis. By using a 24 hours - 4 hour uptake ratio in the lesion and in the adjacent normal bone, a specificity of 92%, and an accuracy of 85% can be expected.

Diagnosis: Pedal osteomyelitis.

CASE 7.21

History: A 51-year-old patient with the complex presentation of type 2 diabetes mellitus, urinary tract infection, fever, and end-stage renal disease (on hemodialysis) is noted to have a nonhealing wound on his right foot, requiring radiography (Fig. 7.21 A) and bone scan (Fig. 7.21 B) for the decision on medical versus surgical management.

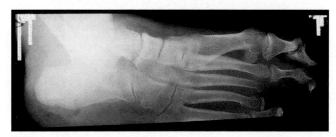

Figure 7.21 A

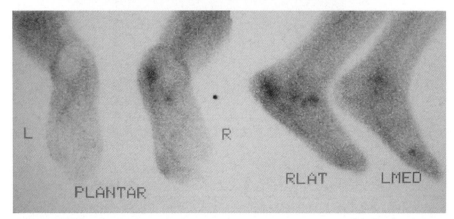

Figure 7.21 B

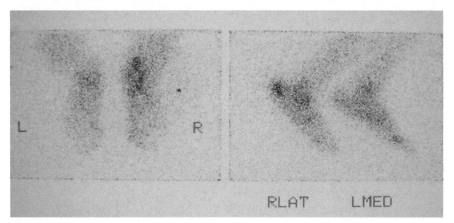

Figure 7.21 C

Findings: Radiograph of the right foot (Fig. 7.21 A) shows bone erosion on the plantar aspect of the right calcaneous in the area of skin ulceration. Bone scan (Fig. 7.21 B) is positive for increased uptake in the right calcaneous.

Discussion: Increased uptake of the calcaneous adjacent to the skin ulceration in correlation with bony erosion noted on the radiograph of this diabetic patient is most consistent with the diagnosis of osteomyelitis. However, nonspecificity of bone scan finding, particularly in the foot of a diabetic patient,

and the paucity of x-ray findings in this complex patient required further evaluation with ^{111}In-WBC scan (Fig. 7.21 C), confirming the presence of the osteomyelitis. The scan is positive, showing increased localization of labeled WBCs in the calcaneous.

Nonspecificity of bone scan finding for the diagnosis of osteomyelitis can be improved significantly by a sequential bone and ^{111}In-WBC scan. This technique is quite accurate in detecting even subtle infection.

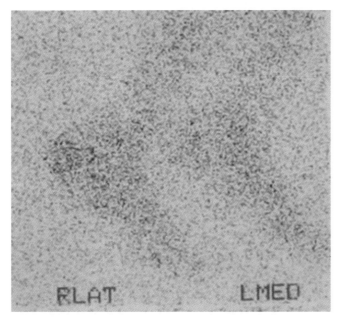

Figure 7.21 D

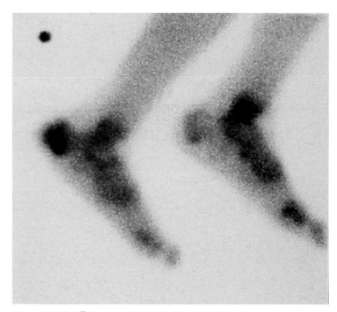

Figure 7.21 E

Although detection of osteomyelitis by ^{111}In-WBC scan in rich, marrow-containing skeleton such as the spine may be difficult, acute or chronic complications of osteomyelitis in a non-marrow-containing area such as peripheral bone is easily recognizable.

The activity of osteomyelitis also can be evaluated with a ^{111}In-WBC scan.

A 3-month follow-up ^{111}In-WBC (Fig. 7.21 D) and bone scan (Fig. 7.21 E) after completion of 4 weeks of therapy shows continuation of the positive bone scan, but the ^{111}In-WBC has reverted to a negative examination.

The ^{111}In-WBC scan has a negative predictive value of 92% and can be used to monitor the efficacy of treatment in non-marrow-containing bone.

Bone scanning is of no clinical value for follow-up or monitoring the response to the therapy. Bone scan uptake is mainly a reflection of the repair process of bone in response to the insult (i.e. infection, trauma, etc.), whereby the healing process occurs over a period of at least 6 months.

Diagnosis: Osteomyelitis of calcaneous, interval improvement.

CASE 7.22

History: A 55-year-old patient with poorly controlled diabetes presented with a history of a swollen right foot. The initial radiograph (Fig. 7.22 A) was negative, and a bone scan (Fig. 7.22 B) was obtained to evaluate for osteomyelitis.

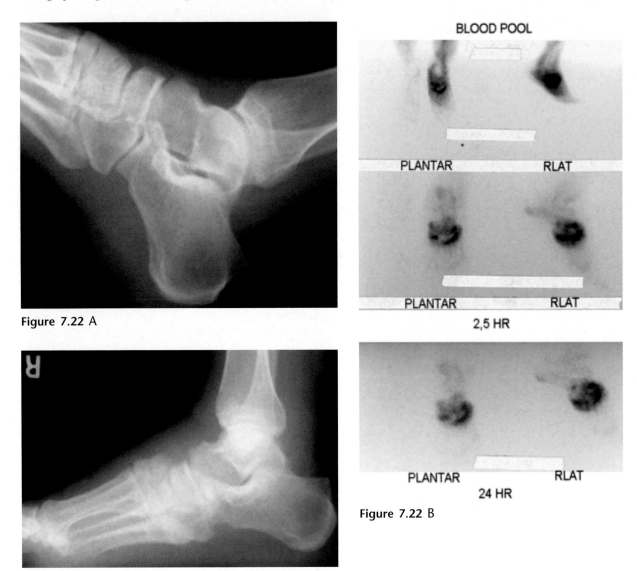

Figure 7.22 A

Figure 7.22 C

Figure 7.22 B

Findings: Plantar and lateral projections of the blood pool and skeletal phase images at 2.5 and 24 hours reveal moderately increased, diffuse soft tissue uptake and increased skeletal uptake in the course of the intertarsal joints of the right foot.

Discussion: Increased uptake following the course of intertarsal and the tarsometatarsal joints would be suggestive of arthropathy, probably Charcot joints, in a diabetic patient.

A radiograph obtained the same day (Fig. 7.22 C) reveals marked destruction of the tarsal bone and subluxation of the talonavicular joint, which developed over a period of 2 weeks; this was felt to represent a rapidly progressing neuropathic osteoarthropathy.

Three-phase bone scanning is extremely sensitive in the detection of early Charcot's osteoarthropathy but cannot

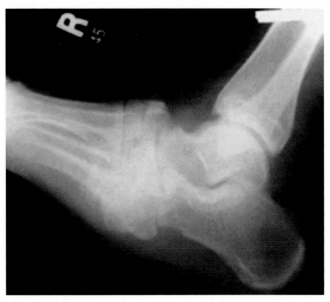

Figure 7.22 D

differentiate between neuropathic osteoarthropathy and osteomyelitis. Exclusion of osteomyelitis in a diabetic foot is better achieved by ^{111}In-WBC imaging. A negative ^{111}In-WBC scan is usually sufficient to exclude osteomyelitis. However, a positive scan is not specific and may occur in up to 31% of patients with Charcot joints without infection, particularly in those with rapidly progressive destruction. MRI is extremely useful in equivocal cases, but unfortunately false-positives occur in neuropathic osteoarthropathy, microfracture, and osteonecrosis, all common features of Charcot joints.

Abnormalities of Charcot joints are commonly located in the midfoot and hindfoot, as in this case, but a forefoot abnormality may represent infection or a combination of infection and neuroarthropathy.

In most cases, osteomyelitis of a diabetic foot (over 90%) originates from the spread of infection from an adjacent pedal ulcer, which was not present in this patient.

Such ulcers may occur at the site of pressure under the metatarsal head, at the tips of the toes, and near the calcaneus, corresponding to the frequent sites of osteomyelitis.

Bone scan accuracy in the detection of osteomyelitis in diabetic feet depends on the site of abnormality. In tarsometatarsal joints, osteomyelitis is uncommon, while neuroarthropathy is common.

In this patient, despite treatment with multiple courses of antibiotics, no improvement was noted, and the clinical course was more compatible with Charcot joint, which was managed accordingly.

A 6-month follow-up radiograph (Fig. 7.22 D) reveals changes of a stable midfoot Charcot joint.

Diagnosis: Charcot joints.

CASE 7.23

History: A 64-year-old paraplegic patient with bilateral buttock decubitus and paroxysmal spiking temperatures had both a bone scan and ^{111}In-WBC scan for evaluation of possible osteomyelitis.

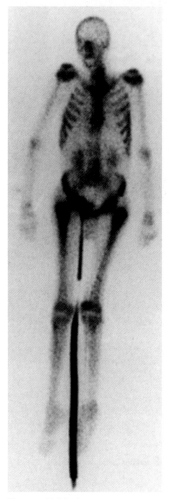

Figure 7.23 A

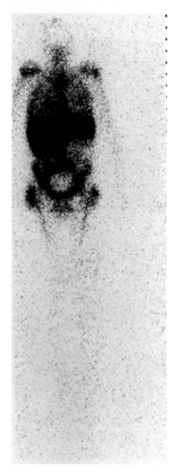

Figure 7.23 B

Findings: On the anterior whole-body scan (Fig. 7.23 A), increased uptake in the area of both femoral greater trochanters is noted, right greater than the left. The flow and blood pool images (not shown) demonstrate increased flow and soft tissue uptake. The anterior whole-body ^{111}In-WBC image (Fig. 7.23 B), is remarkable for increased localization of ^{111}In-WBCs in the general area of bone abnormality.

Discussion: A positive three-phase bone scan in the trochanteric region of this patient with decubitus ulcer would be most consistent with spread of infection to the bone and represent osteomyelitis. The diagnosis can be further substantiated by ^{111}In-WBC images. Since WBCs do not usually accumulate at the site of increased bone turnover but migrate to areas of infection, a positive ^{111}In-WBC scan would be confirmatory evidence for osteomyelitis.

The ^{111}In-WBCs are normally confined to the liver, spleen, and active marrow of the axial skeleton, proximal femurs, and humerus (marrow-containing bone). There will be faint visual-ization of activity in the non-marrow-containing appendicular skeleton.

^{111}In-WBC localization outside the liver, spleen, and bone marrow compartment by definition represents an abnormality such as infection. In order to avoid a false-positive, only uptake that is definitely greater than that in bone marrow or similar to that in the liver or spleen, and particularly focal lesions, should be considered as a positive sign of infection. Fortunately, the ^{111}In-WBC scan yields images that are easily interpretable for abnormal focal uptake.

In the interpretation of ^{111}In-WBC images for osteomyelitis, the uptake of ^{111}In-WBCs should be compared with that in the bone, in both intensity and distribution. When the distribution of bone and ^{111}In-WBC activity is incongruent, especially when the intensity of ^{111}In-WBC exceeds the bone uptake, osteomyelitis, in all likelihood, is present.

In this case, incongruity in the shape and distribution of two tracers is seen, particularly in the area of the right greater

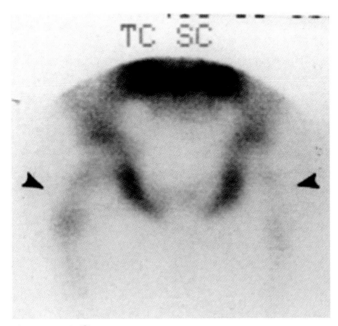

Figure 7.23 C

trochanter, as the uptake of ^{111}In-WBC appears to be more global, extending laterally even into the soft tissues.

By combining bone and ^{111}In-WBC scanning, a sensitivity of almost 90% and a specificity of 95% has been reported. It should be noted that false-positive cases have occurred in the absence of infection with the incongruency pattern. These are usually related to asymmetrical marrow distribution. Since ^{111}In-labeled WBCs distribute in the active bone marrow and distribution of hematopoietic marrow can vary significantly from one patient to another, bone marrow imaging as a supplement to ^{111}In-WBC scans can distinguish normal marrow from infection.

Figure 7.23 C represents static images of the anterior pelvic bone marrow, showing no uptake of ^{99m}Tc–sulfur colloid in the greater trochanteric region (arrows), thus further indicating that ^{111}In-WBC localization is due to infection.

The three-phase bone scan remains the procedure of choice for the evaluation of osteomyelitis; in complicated cases, however, it should be combined with leukocyte and bone marrow imaging.

In the case of suspected osteomyelitis of marrow-containing skeleton, perhaps the ^{111}In-WBC and marrow study would be sufficient for diagnosing osteomyelitis. The accuracy of WBC and marrow imaging has been excellent, reportedly ranging from 89% to 98%. In peripherally located lesions, however, owing to lack of anatomic landmarks and difficulty in differentiating soft tissue from bone uptake, combining the bone scan and WBC image provides both the anatomic landmark and the specificity required for the detection of osteomyelitis. Bone marrow images would still be helpful in the evaluation of pedal osteomyelitis when a Charcot joint is present.

Diagnosis: Osteomyelitis of the greater trochanter (combined bone, WBC, and marrow imaging).

CASE 7.24

History: A 53-year-old male with low back pain and a radiograph suggestive of erosion and disk space narrowing at the L4 level (Fig. 7.24 A) underwent bone scanning (Fig. 7.24 B).

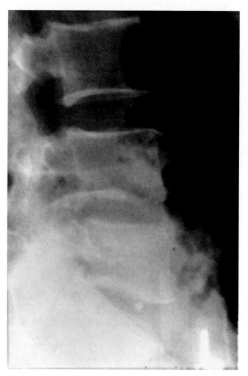

Figure 7.24 A

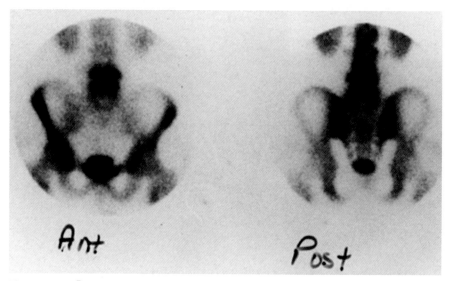

Figure 7.24 B

Findings: Delayed spot images of the lumbar spine and pelvis in the anterior and posterior projections reveals abnormal uptake in two endplates adjacent to the L4-L5 intervertebral space.

Discussion: The finding of increased uptake in the two adjacent vertebrae is characteristic although not specific for an inflammatory process of the intervertebral disk space, which was proved by direct biopsy with cultures of *Staphylococcus aureus* in this patient. The same pattern may be seen in post-diskectomy patients without infection; however, this is easily excluded by history.

The diagnosis of diskitis is often delayed owing to non-specific symptoms and the late appearance of radiographic findings.

Although the focus of infection in diskitis is the vertebral endplate, enzymes produced by bacteria destroy the disk faster than the endplate. Therefore disk narrowing is the earliest sign.

The bone scan is usually positive within a week of symptoms. The diagnosis can be confirmed by a positive ^{67}Ga-citrate scan. The ^{111}In-WBCs have not been found to be very useful for diagnosing vertebral osteomyelitis and diskitis.

Diskitis may be complicated by spread to the soft tissues, with paravertebral abscesses. In paravertebral abscesses, bone scan and ^{67}Ga-citrate abnormalities extend to the paravertebral region and produce a butterfly appearance instead of a simple horizontal endplate pattern.

The endplate appearance is related to the special vascular anatomy of the spine. The vertebral endplates have a rich arterial supply. There are numerous vertical anastomoses on the surface of the vertebrae. These vertical vessels connect the supply of the inferior and superior endplates of the same vertebra and cross the disk space, connecting the two endplates adjacent to a single intervertebral disk.

Spinal osteomyelitis and diskitis are most common in patients with cancer, urinary tract infection, diabetes, drug abuse, and bacterial endocarditis.

Although the lumbar spine is the most common site, there is a much higher incidence of cervical diskitis among intravenous drug abusers.

Untreated diskitis and associated paravertebral and dural abscess may lead to cord compression and paralysis. Patients with cervical diskitis, diabetes, and rheumatoid arthritis are at high risk for this complication. Early diagnosis is necessary to reduce morbidity. Bone scan and ^{67}Ga-citrate scan are helpful for early diagnosis. A normal bone and gallium scan virtually exclude the diagnosis.

Diagnosis: Lumbar diskitis.

History: A 64-year-old male diabetic with urosepsis and fever who had experienced low back pain for a week is referred for a bone scan to evaluate the possibility of osteomyelitis (Fig. 7.25 A).

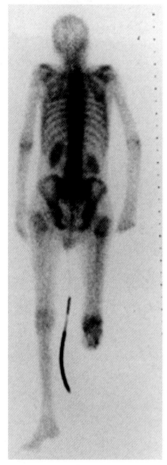

Figure 7.25 A

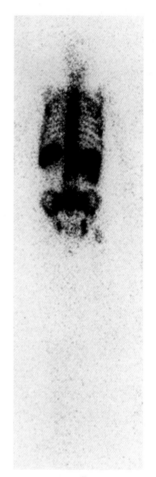

Figure 7.25 B

Findings: The whole-body images show abnormal uptake involving the fourth lumbar vertebra. The flow and blood pool studies (not shown) demonstrate increased flow and soft tissue uptake. There is below-the-knee amputation on the right in this diabetic patient.

Discussion: The positive three-phase bone scan of the L4 vertebra with the pertinent history is most consistent with vertebral osteomyelitis.

Inasmuch as the three-phase bone scan is not specific, the patient was further studied with ^{111}In-WBC imaging (Fig. 7.25 B). A posterior whole-body image shows photopenia in the area of L4, corresponding to the region of abnormal bony uptake.

Osteomyelitis is known to cause photopenia on ^{111}In-WBC imaging, and 14% of osteomyelitis may appear as a cold defect. The cause and significance of a cold defect on a ^{111}In-WBC scan is similar to that on a bone scan; in 75% of cases, it usually signifies pathology. Fracture, AVN, solid tumor, radiation therapy, leukemia, prosthesis, myelofibrosis, advanced age, and Paget's are among the other causes of photopenia on ^{111}In-WBC scan; they can be excluded by history, laboratory findings, and other diagnostic imaging procedures.

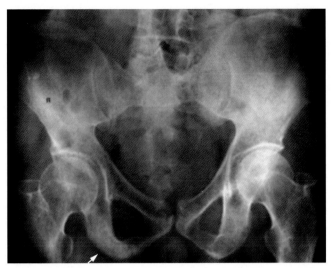

Figure 7.25 C

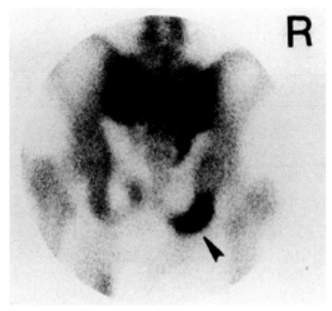

Figure 7.25 D

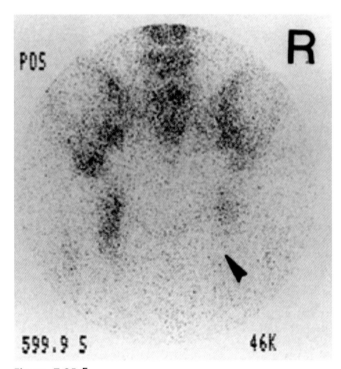

Figure 7.25 E

Figures 7.25 C, 7.25 D, and 7.25 E represent the radiograph, bone scan, and ^{111}In-WBC images of a patient being evaluated for osteomyelitis. Note the radiographic changes of Paget's involving the right ischium (arrow). Bone scintigraphy (Fig. 7.25 D) is positive in the right ischium (arrowhead). On the ^{111}In-WBC scan (Fig. 7.25 E), there is photopenia (arrowhead) corresponding to the Pagetic region and dichotomy of the bone

and ^{111}In-WBC scan. Photopenia is most likely to be seen in the sclerotic phase of Paget's disease.

In Paget's, there is loss of marrow component through displacement of abnormal proliferating and sclerotic tissue. This appears to be the underlying mechanism for the lack of ^{111}In-WBC uptake in Paget's disease.

Diagnosis: Spinal osteomyelitis. Pelvic Paget's disease.

History: Six years following a left total hip arthroplasty for a complex fracture of the femur, this 72-year-old patient complained of severe hip pain and difficulty in walking. He was referred for a sequential bone Indium-111 white blood cell and bone marrow study (Figs. 7.26 A, B, C) in order to evaluate infection versus aseptic loosening of the prosthesis. The plain radiograph finding (not shown) was consistent with the loosening of both the femoral and acetabular components of the prosthesis.

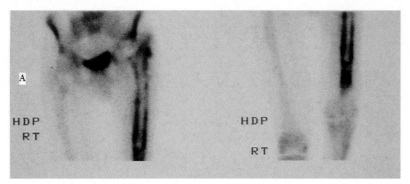

Figure 7.26 A

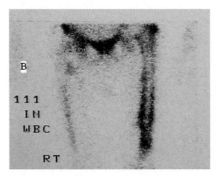

Figure 7.26 B

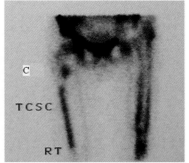

Figure 7.26 C

Findings: The anterior bone scintigram (Fig. 7.26 A) shows diffuse periprosthetic uptake, similar in distribution to that in the ^{111}In-WBC image (Fig. 7.26 B), which is congruent with the uptake of ^{99m}Tc–sulfur colloid bone marrow images (Fig. 7.26 C).

Discussion: Identification of the presence of infection depends on the demonstration of incongruent WBC and colloid marrow images. The congruency of uptake in this case excludes infection as the cause of a loosening and failing prosthesis.

In evaluating joint prosthesis complications, the plain radiograph finding is not sensitive or specific. The use of CT and MRI is limited owing to artifact emanating from the prosthetic implant. Bone scintigraphy is helpful only if the result of the exam is normal, excluding the related hardware and prosthetic complications. The combination of an ^{111}In-WBC scan and colloid bone marrow scintigram is the modality of choice for diagnosing prosthetic joint infections and has an accuracy rate around 90%.

WBC images are obtained 24 hours after injection of mixed autologous WBCs labeled with 500 mCi of ^{111}In-oxime. WBCs can also be labeled with ^{99m}Tc-HMPAO (hexamethylpropyleneamine oxime) and scanning can be done as early as 1 to 4 hours thereafter. The distribution of ^{99m}Tc-HMPAO is similar to that of ^{111}In-WBC except for a variable amount of activity in

GI, genitourinary (GU), and gallbladder on later images. However, this would not affect the test's accuracy in the evaluation of peripheral bone infection.

HMPAO is a lipophilic complex that can penetrate the cell membrane and enters the blood cells. In the cell, the complex becomes hydrophilic and trapped within the cells. There are reports indicating that ^{99m}Tc-HMPAO has greater sensitivity and specificity than ^{111}In-WBC, even when the scan is prolonged up to 24 hours. The superior resolution of ^{99m}Tc-HMPAO and high image quality are potential advantages over the ^{111}In-WBC scan.

Figures 7.26 D and 7.26 E represent the bone and ^{99m}Tc-HMPAO of a patient with a painful right knee prosthesis. Note the improved quality and image resolution of ^{99m}Tc-HMPAO (Fig. 7.26 E) and incongruency in the distribution of labeled WBCs and bone uptake, supporting the clinician's diagnosis of infection. No bone marrow images were obtained; however, the course of the patient's disease and the results of joint aspiration confirmed the diagnosis.

^{18}F-FDG PET is a promising agent that has been used to evaluate painful joint prostheses. In PET images, in addition to infection, the periprosthetic activity may occur as the result of bone marrow uptake. Interpretation of ^{18}F-FDG images combined with colloid bone marrow images improves the

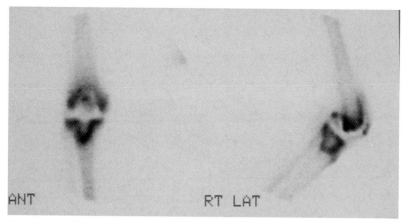

Figure 7.26 D

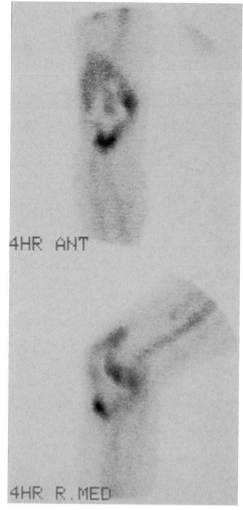

Figure 7.26 E

specificity. An accuracy rate of 58% to 91.9% has been reported by different authors for the detection of bone infections with PET images. Therefore the procedure has not been recommended as a suitable replacement for WBC marrow imaging.

In evaluation of prosthetic infection, note should be made that 30% of infection occurs in the first 3 months and 30% within the first year after surgery. Aseptic loosening is a late complication, with 50% of failures occurring 10 years or more after the surgery.

Diagnosis: Aseptic loosening of femoral prosthesis. Knee prosthetic infection.

History: A 58-year-old male patient presents with right groin pain and a temperature of 102° to 103°F. His pelvic radiograph CT and MRI have been unrevealing. He is referred for a ¹¹¹In-WBC scan for further evaluation (Fig. 7.27 A).

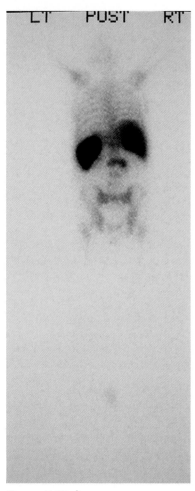

Figure 7.27 A

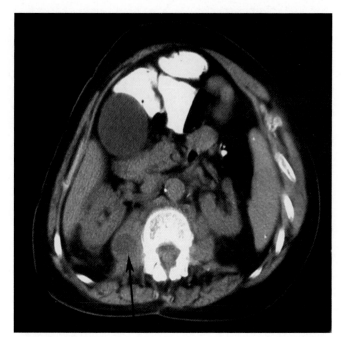

Figure 7.27 B

Findings: Posterior whole-body images obtained 24 hours after injection of the autologous WBCs labeled with 600 mCi of ¹¹¹In-oxime is remarkable for the presence of a crescentic focus of increased uptake in the mid-upper abdomen posteriorly that projects over and crosses the spine. Physiologic activity is identified in the liver, spleen, and bone marrow.

Discussion: Accumulation of ¹¹¹In-WBC localized in what appears to be the superior portion of the retroperitoneal space is most consistent with an infectious process in this area.

Pancreatitis, phlegmon, and paraspinal abscesses are among the most frequent differentials. Bleeding of the duodenal ulcer, retroperitoneal hematoma, and artifact may represent the same pattern, although the possibility is remote and their clinical presentation quite different.

Reexamination of the upper abdomen by CT in the lateral decubitus position (Fig 7.27 B) shows a hypodense area within the right psoas muscle (arrow). The abscess was drained percutaneously under CT guidance.

Psoas abscess is rare, but its frequency is rising. Clinical diagnosis is difficult. Symptoms are not specific and may be misleading. The psoas muscle originates from the lateral border of the lumbar vertebrae and inserts in the lesser trochanter of the femur. Therefore the patient's pain is commonly referred to the buttock and groin area.

Predisposing factors in developing psoas abscess are diabetes, intravenous drug use, psoas hematoma, spinal osteomyelitis, and Pott's disease (tuberculosis of spine).

CT is the most effective method for the diagnosis of psoas abscess. However, for the feverish patient with no localizing signs or misleading symptoms, an ¹¹¹In-WBC image could be of great diagnostic value.

Not uncommonly, a focus of abnormality in unexpected regions will be identified that redirects the clinician's attention and alters the patient's management.

Diagnosis: Psoas abscess.

CASE 7.28

History: A 21-year-old male military recruit complained of discomfort in his right lower leg during 2 weeks of physical training. His initial radiograph is negative, and he is referred for a bone scan (Fig. 7.28 A).

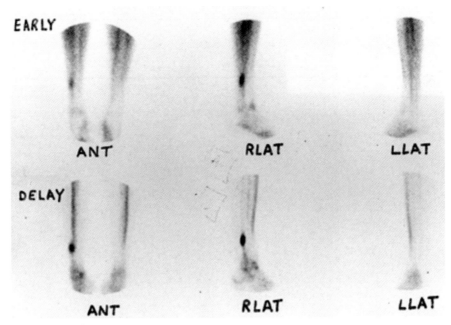

Figure 7.28 A

Findings: A blood pool and delayed skeletal images of the legs show focal fusiform uptake involving the distal fibula on the right on both blood pool and skeletal phase images.

Discussion: The localized area of increased skeletal uptake associated with increased blood pool activity favors an acute or subacute stress fracture in the clinical context of trauma in a military recruit. The radiograph obtained 2 weeks later (Fig. 7.28 B) shows focal periosteal changes (arrow) confirming stress fracture as the cause of the scan abnormality.

Bone scan is the procedure of choice for evaluating a stress fracture. It demonstrates the subtle alterations in bone physiology before anatomic radiographic changes occur.

In a stress fracture, typically the bone scan shows a dense, focal, fusiform, cortical hyperconcentration at the site of fracture. There is increased blood flow and blood pool activity. The initial radiograph is frequently normal.

A bone scan, particularly a three-phase study, is helpful in differentiating a stress fracture from shin splints, the other common cause of pain in the athlete. Shin splits are not associated with hyperperfusion or hyperemia, and abnormal uptake of shin splints appears as linear activity extending over a longer portion of the bone.

Healing of the stress fracture occurs gradually over a period of at least 6 months. Abnormal bone uptake becomes less intense and fades first in the angiographic and blood pool phase and subsequently in the skeletal phase. The skeletal phase uptake decreases gradually and becomes more diffuse, with an appearance more similar to that of a shin splint. However, correlation with the radiograph at this stage shows signs of the healing process, such as periosteal changes, endosteal bone or callus formation, or sclerotic changes.

Figure 7.28 C shows delayed images of the right and left lower leg of a 20-year-old soldier with a past history of a right

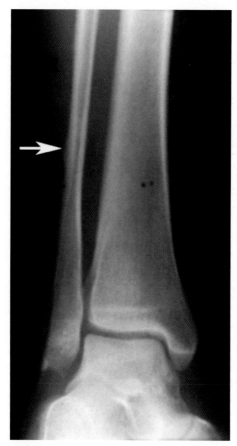

Figure 7.28 B

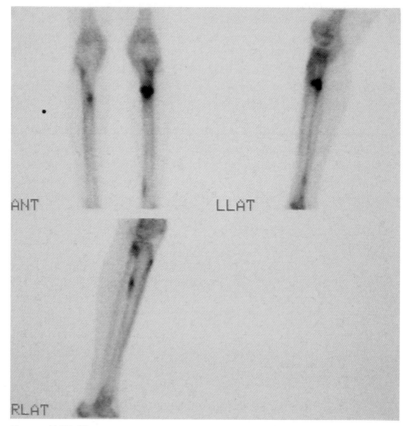

Figure 7.28 C

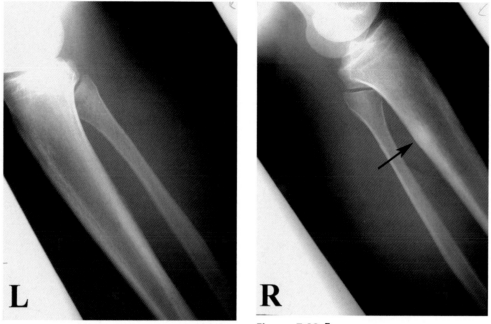

Figure 7.28 D

Figure 7.28 E

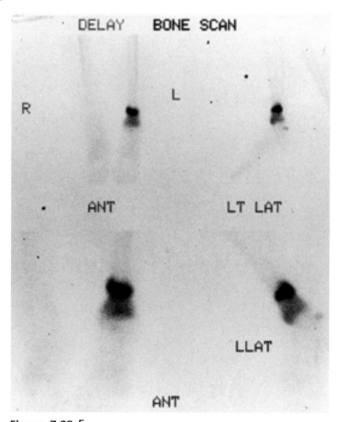

Figure 7.28 F

proximal tibial stress fracture who was referred for evaluation of pain along the left leg. On the left there is focal hyper-concentration of activity with no corresponding radiographic abnormality (Fig. 7.28 D), which is most consistent with the occurrence of an acute stress fracture. On the right and at the site of the previous fracture, activity is less intense and appears linear and mottled; it might be mistaken for a periosteal stress injury. Radiographic correlation (Fig. 7.28 E) shows cor-

responding sclerotic cortical thickening (arrow), representing the evolution and healing process of the stress fracture.

In the diagnosis of a stress fracture, the radiograph, with a sensitivity of less than 15%, is of little use; however, follow-up radiography within 1 or 2 weeks is helpful and usually shows diagnostic signs of the fracture, although this appears only in about 50% of the cases.

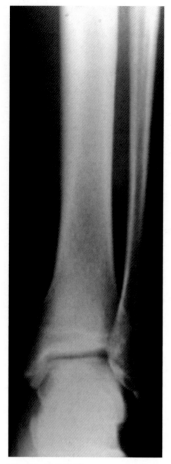

Figure 7.28 G

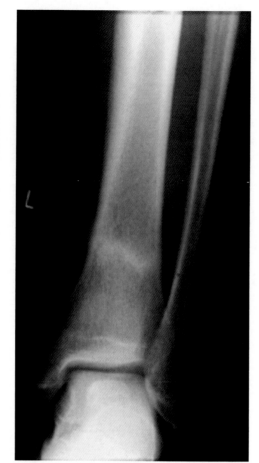

Figure 7.28 H

The radiograph and scintigraphic appearance of the stress fracture within a dense cortical bone and trabecular cancellous bone is different. The known intense fusiform uptake in the long axis parallel to the shaft of the cortical bone seen in a stress fracture of compact cortical bone is not a scintigraphic feature of cancellous bone stress fractures. The pattern of abnormal uptake in cancellous bone varies depending on the location, severity of the fracture, and the time course of injury.

Cancellous bone includes the calcaneous, distal tibia, proximal tibia, femoral neck, and pelvis.

Figure 7.28 F shows abnormal uptake as a band of marked intense uptake horizontally oriented within the cancellous bone of the distal tibia in this 36-year-old runner with a history of shin splints who had experienced new pain in the shin and left ankle area for a week. No abnormalities are noted on the accompanying radiograph (Fig. 7.28 G).

Radiographic detection of such a stress fracture within the cancellous bone is quite difficult, requiring at least 50% density changes before radiographic signs become visible. The patient's cancellous bone stress fractures after progressions and during evolution become apparent (Fig. 7.28 H) as a sclerotic area, revealing the region of the injury within the cancellous bone.

Stress fractures occur most commonly in runners, military recruits, and other athletes. The most frequent sites of stress fractures in runners are the metatarsal shaft, tibia, and pubic symphysis; however, any other osseous structures—such as the spine, femoral neck, sacroiliac joints, and even the upper extremity—may be involved. A stress fracture of the fibula, a non-weight-bearing bone, occurs more often in ballet dancers, gymnasts, and acrobats.

In the tibia, the most common location of a stress fracture is within the compact bone in the proximal and midtibial cortex anteriorly (in ballet dancers) and posteriorly (in runners).

A distal tibial cancellous stress fracture is not a usual feature; however, it may be seen in the long distance runner and occurs as a result of repetitious compressive forces on the bone. These athletes, despite experiencing pain, continue their exercise regimen, which produces increasingly significant abnormalities.

Diagnosis: Stress fractures.

History: A 23-year-old female runner complained of having had pain along the shaft of the tibia bilaterally for 2 weeks. Because her radiograph showed no abnormality, she was referred for a bone scan (Fig. 7.29 A).

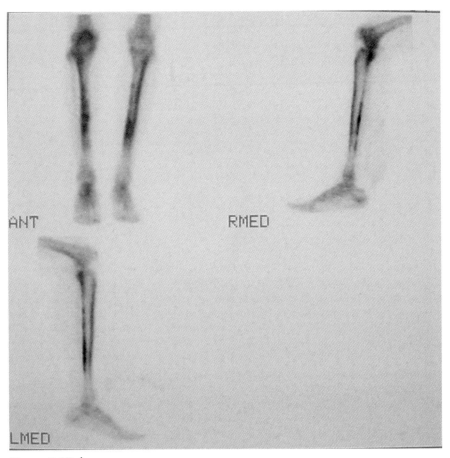

Figure 7.29 A

Findings: Anterior and lateral delayed bone scan images of the leg show dense, linear uptake along the anterolateral and posteromedial border of the tibia (double-stripe sign), bilaterally corresponding to the line of muscle attachment.

Discussion: The findings are most consistent with a bilateral shin splint stress injury. This is referred to as a periosteal stress reaction, a lesser injury than a true stress fracture.

The classic entity of shin splints has been specifically characterized as pain along the posteromedial border of the tibia related to the origin of the soleus muscle. The appearance of a shin splint is a linear area of varying intensity along the medial and dorsal aspect of the mid- and distal third of the tibial cortex. There are no flow abnormalities, and blood pool images are normal. Radiography is normal for both bone and soft tissue. The classic picture is not invariably present. The scintigraphic findings can vary depending on the location of the lesion and evolution of the process. Scans may show an area of varying uptake in the anterolateral border or posteromedial aspect of the tibia. When both borders are involved, the scintigraph will show the double-stripe sign as in this case. Recognition of linear and cortical uptake of shin splints requires high-resolution and often lateral images.

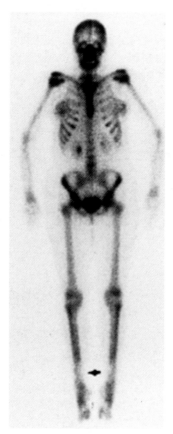

Figure 7.29 B

Scan abnormalities of shin splints will revert to normal in approximately 3 months, as compared with the stress fracture, which requires more than 6 months for complete healing.

It is to be noted that not only shin splints but anterior compartment syndrome, posterior compartment syndrome, and anterior tibial tendonitis are distinct entities associated with shin pain and no image abnormality. In anterior compartment syndrome, however, decreased symmetrical uptake may be seen in the region of the distal tibia (arrow, Fig. 7.29 B).

Other entities may appear as increased linear cortical activity similar to the shin splint, such as hypertrophic pulmonary osteoarthropathy, chronic venous insufficiency, and diaphyseal dysplasia. However, the x-ray findings and different clinical presentations allow their differentiation.

It also should be noted that there are several controversial detailed studies regarding the scintigraphic interpretation and classification of stress fractures and shin splints. However, the following generalizations can be made:

1. A positive three-phase bone scan disclosing an intense focal oval or fusiform uptake is most consistent with the diagnosis of a stress fracture.
2. Mild to minimal increased uptake of a focal nature not associated with increased flow or blood pool abnormality that remains normal on x-ray most likely represents a periosteal stress reaction.
3. The specific tibial location and linear shape of activity of varying intensity associated with normal flow, blood pool image, and radiography is highly accurate for the scintigraphic diagnosis of shin splint.
4. There are lesions that do not have the fusiform appearance of a true stress fracture or linear pattern of shin splints. Their radiography is also normal. These lesions have been called bone bruises and represent minimal interosseous bleeding and periosteal elevation as the result of trauma.

Diagnosis: Shin splint.

CASE 7.30

History: A 59-year-old man complained of pain in the left knee, which gives way. He is referred for a bone scan (Fig. 7.30 A).

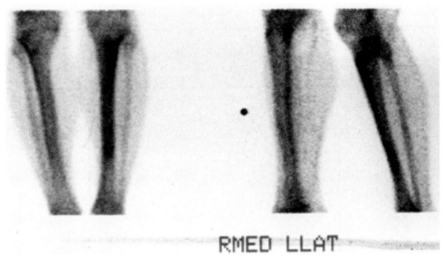

Figure 7.30 A

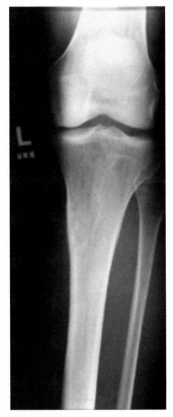

Figure 7.30 B

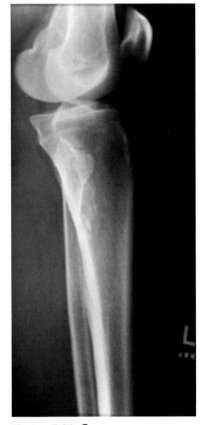

Figure 7.30 C

Findings: Spot images of the leg in the anterior and lateral projections disclose mild longitudinally oriented diffuse uptake along the lateral cortical margin of the mid- and proximal left tibia.

Discussion: The subsequently obtained radiographs (Figs. 7.30 B and 7.30 C) in the posteroanterior and lateral projections reveal longitudinally oriented rarefication intermixed with sclerosis in the proximal and distal left tibia corresponding to the area of scintigraphic abnormality. There is sclerosis of the posteromedial metaphyseal portion of the tibia. On subsequent CT and MRI evaluation, the lesion was diagnosed as a longitudinal stress fracture superimposed on a healed fibrous cortical defect.

The diagnosis of longitudinal stress fracture is difficult because of atypical imaging features in which the fracture line is oriented longitudinally to the shaft of the bone. Longitudinal stress fractures have been reported to occur mainly in the tibia, but the femur may also be affected. Initial radiographic findings may vary from normal to marked periosteal reaction and endosteal bone formation. Follow-up x-ray may show the vertical lucent line. Scintigraphy is always positive and usually shows a pattern of diffuse uptake along the shaft of the bone. CT is the procedure of choice for the diagnosis of longitudinal stress fracture by showing the vertically oriented fracture line as well as endosteal and periosteal bone formation.

Diagnosis: Longitudinal stress fracture superimposed on a healed fibrous cortical defect.

CASE 7.31

History: A 60-year-old man involved in a motor vehicle accident was released from the emergency department following a negative radiographic examination of the left hip (Fig. 7.31 A). The patient returned the next day complaining of difficulty walking and left hip pain aggravated by walking. A bone scan was obtained approximately 36 hours from the time of injury (Fig. 7.31 B).

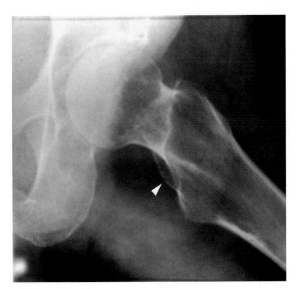

Figure 7.31 A

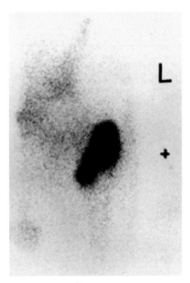

Figure 7.31 B

Findings: Selected magnification views of the left hip reveal markedly increased uptake in the intertrochanteric region, most consistent with a nondisplaced fracture.

Discussion: Traumatic, occult, and nondisplaced fractures of the hip, especially in older patients, are not uncommon. Their radiographic findings are often subtle and overlooked. In the proper clinical setting, a positive bone scan confirms the diagnosis.

In this case, subtle cortical breaks (arrow in Fig. 7.31 A) seen retrospectively indicate the traumatic injury of the left hip.

Although radiographic detection is difficult, these occult fractures usually become positive within hours of the injury, and their obvious radiographic signs become apparent between 7 and 10 days.

Scintigraphic detection of occult hip fractures requires high-quality images. Catheterization or shielding of radioactivity in the urinary bladder enhances visualization of the hip region. Multiple projections and high-resolution images are useful. Delayed images, which allow soft tissue clearance and improve the ratio of bone to the soft tissue uptake, enhance lesion detectability. Even a 24-hour delayed image may be necessary to detect lesions when they are not well seen on initial scintigrams.

In a properly done three-phase, high-resolution bone scan, an occult fracture of the hip can be detected with a sensitivity and specificity of approximately 95% within the first 24 hours of injury.

False-negative scans even in elderly and osteoporotic patients are not common. At worst, the result will be uncertain or equivocal rather than normal, leading to further delayed studies up to 24 hours or repeat imaging at 72 hours.

False-negative scans may result from the disruption of the blood supply as the result of a displaced fracture or increased interarticular pressure secondary to hematoma causing reduced perfusion of the femoral head.

Fracture of the greater trochanter may be mistaken for a femoral fracture. Fracture of the trochanter, which is not a true hip fracture, usually causes abnormal uptake in the region of the greater trochanter extending into the intertrochanter region and mimicking an intertrochanteric fracture. This pattern is believed to result from the so-called recruitment phenomenon, in which blood flow to the area of fracture causes increased metabolic activity in the adjacent normal bone. Careful analysis of the scan in this situation shows the intertrochanteric region activity to be much less than the uptake in the true intertrochanteric fracture, in which intense homogeneous uptake extends from the lateral to the medial aspect of the bone.

Traumatic fractures proceed from an acute stage, showing abnormal diffuse uptake, to a subacute stage, associated with more localized intense uptake of activity, to a healing stage in which uptake gradually decreases and fades. It is to be noted that the scan remains positive well beyond the time of clinical and radiographic improvement. Depending on the site and severity of injury, an uncomplicated fracture returns to normal after 6 months to 3 years. Bone scintigraphy is an important adjunct to the early diagnosis of hip fracture regardless of the patient's age and should be employed as soon as the patient seeks medical advice.

Diagnosis: Hip fracture.

CASE 7.32

History: A 24-year-old active-duty soldier complained of an insidious onset of pain in the area of the first metatarsophalangeal joint of the right foot, which was aggravated by exercise. The result of his radiograph (Figs. 7.32 A and 7.32 B) was not conclusive, and he was referred for a bone scan (Fig. 7.32 C).

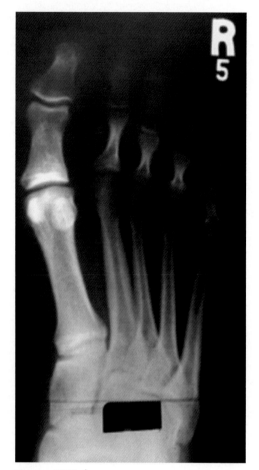

Figure 7.32 A

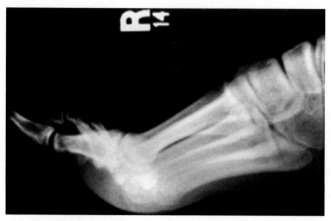

Figure 7.32 B

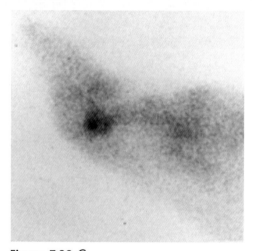

Figure 7.32 C

Findings: Delayed magnification views of the right forefoot in the medial projection show a focus of increased uptake in the area of the great toe sesamoid bone.

Discussion: Foot fractures are relatively common. They have the potential for long-term disability. These very disabling injuries pose a radiographic diagnostic challenge. The subtle, often unrecognizable fracture includes fracture of the great toe sesamoid bone (Fig. 7.32 C), fracture of the diaphysis of the fifth metatarsal bone (Jones fracture), stress fracture of the tarsal and navicular bones (Fig. 7.32 D), and fracture of the talar bone and os trigonum.

Three-phase, magnification, high-resolution bone scans are helpful in locating sites of injury, leading to further diagnostic tests for confirmation.

Painful sesamoid bones may result from trauma, infection, or ischemic or arthritic changes.

Trauma may cause acute fracture, stress fracture, or dislocation, or it may precipitate an inflammatory process termed sesamoiditis.

The metatarsal sesamoid joints are affected by common arthritides similar to those seen in other synovial joints.

Osteomyelitis and septic arthritis can affect the sesamoid bone and joints as well.

Ischemic necrosis may occur as a result of crush fracture or postinfection infarction, causing interruption of the blood supply. Fragmentation, irregularity, mottling, flattening, collapse, and bone sclerosis occur radiographically but usually late (6 to 12 months) after the onset of pain.

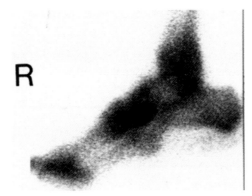

Figure 7.32 D

All of these painful conditions are associated with nonspecific increased uptake of the bone-seeking radiopharmaceutical. However, a diagnosis is usually established by a combination of the clinical, laboratory, and imaging findings, including radiography, scintigraphy, CT, and MRI.

The radiographic diagnosis of sesamoid bone injury is quite difficult and is usually delayed for months despite persistent symptoms. Detection of sesamoid bone fractures is challenging owing to the fact that the bipartite sesamoid is a common finding, which may be seen in up to 30% of individuals, and differentiation from fracture is difficult. Comparison radiographs are of limited help, since the bipartite variant is unilateral in up to 50% to 75% of cases.

A bipartite sesamoid bone has a normal appearance on bone scan. Increased tracer uptake, as in this case and in the proper clinical setting, would indicate a complication such as fracture, infection, or infarction. Stress fracture may be differentiated from acute fracture by the gradual onset of the process and a lesser degree of abnormality in the intensity of uptake than in the case of an acute fracture.

The diagnosis of sesamoid stress fracture is important from the standpoint of patient management. Although most stress fractures are healed by curtailing physical activity and further immobilization, healing of the stress fracture of a sesamoid bone requires a prolonged period of immobilization; surgical excision has been advocated for this injury.

Figure 7.32 D is a lateral magnification view of the right foot of a 31-year-old female active-duty soldier who complained of tarsotarsal pain over a period of 3 months aggravated by movement and no response to nonsteroidal anti-inflammatory drugs (NSAIDs). The bone scan shows marked intense uptake in the region of the tarsal navicular bone, consistent with a stress fracture.

Routine radiographs often do not demonstrate a navicular fracture. If bone scan is positive, a CT scan should be obtained. There is a high rate of delayed union, nonunion, and refracture of the navicular bone due to its delicate blood supply.

Diagnosis: Stress fracture of the great toe sesamoid bone. Stress fracture of the tarsal navicular bone.

History: One week following a motor vehicle accident and an initially reported negative radiograph of the pelvis (Fig. 7.33 A), this 23-year-old man received a bone scan (Fig. 7.33 B) for evaluation of low back pain aggravated by walking.

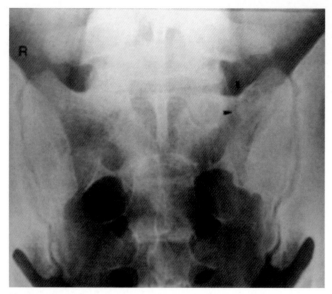

Figure 7.33 A

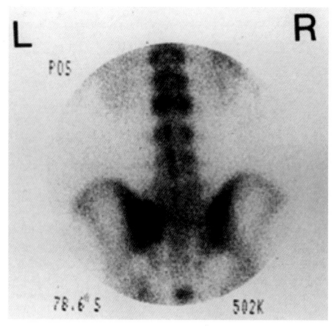

Figure 7.33 B

Findings: Selected posterior images of the pelvis show transverse uptake across the second lumbar vertebra and linear, vertical uptake in the sacral ala on the left.

Discussion: The scintigraphic finding is most consistent with fractures of the lumbar vertebra and sacrum.

The bone scan has limited utility in the workup of the acutely traumatized patient; however, in an appropriate clinical setting, bone scanning will localize the injury and direct further diagnostic study for confirmation.

Identification of an occult sacral injury on a plain radiograph is difficult. The findings are usually quite subtle and may easily be overlooked. Minor density changes in the sacrum may be the only clue to the presence of a fracture. This sign is seen in retrospect in Figure 7.33 A (arrows).

The vertical sacral alar fracture usually results from severely transmitted force to the pelvis from the lower extremity, similar to the vertebral fracture, and commonly occurs following a fall from height or a severe motor vehicle accident. The vertical pelvic injury is almost always unstable. Because the sacrum and sacroiliac joints form the posterior weight-bearing part of the pelvic ring, early detection of injury in this region is important in order to reduce morbidity and mortality.

Isolated sacral injuries are unusual; frequently other fractures are present which can easily be detected by a bone scan.

As in other parts of the skeleton with complex anatomy, SPECT can detect a subtle abnormality in the sacrum; it is preferred over the planar image and should be used when available.

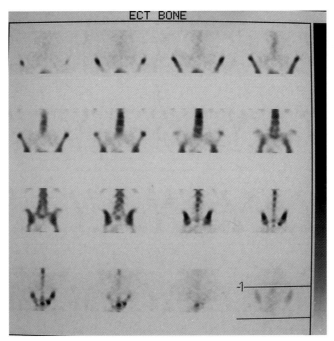

Figure 7.33 C

Figure 7.33 C represents a coronal SPECT image of a 48-year-old female who fell and struck the ground. The patient had persistent pain in the sacral area. Radiography and CT examination were not contributory. SPECT demonstrates a focus of abnormal uptake in the second segment of the sacrum as well as in the left sacral ala, representing fracture and explaining the patient's pain.

It is to be noted that for obtaining the optimum SPECT result of the pelvis, the patient's position should be quite symmetrical and the bladder free from residual urine. The patient should void just prior to the examination and, if possible, a drainage catheter should be in place during the examination.

The most subtle fractures of the sacrum are insufficiency fractures, usually seen in the pelvis of osteoporotic patients or following radiotherapy to the pelvis or in association with steroid therapy. These patients present with low back pain, and radiographic detection of their fracture is extremely difficult. However, radionuclide bone scanning readily identifies the fracture. The classic scintigraphic appearance of a sacral insufficiency fracture is an H (or butterfly) pattern ("Honda sign"). This is produced by the two vertical bands of sacral alar uptake connected by a horizontal component.

Diagnosis: Sacral and vertebral fracture.

CASE 7.34

History: A 67-year-old smoker with multiple medical problems including coronary artery disease (CAD), peripheral vascular disease (PVD), steroid-dependent chronic obstructive pulmonary disease (COPD), and elevated prostate-specific antigen (PSA) presents with back pain and is referred for bone scan (Fig. 7.34 A) to rule out skeletal metastasis.

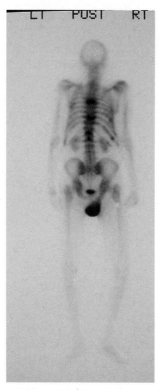

Figure 7.34 A

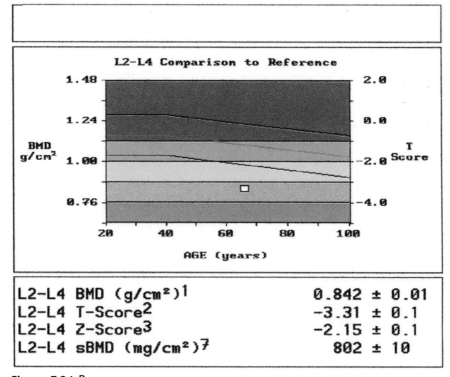

L2-L4 BMD (g/cm²)[1]	0.842 ± 0.01
L2-L4 T-Score[2]	-3.31 ± 0.1
L2-L4 Z-Score[3]	-2.15 ± 0.1
L2-L4 sBMD (mg/cm²)[7]	802 ± 10

Figure 7.34 B

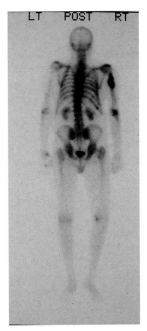

LT   POST   RT

Figure 7.34 C

Findings: Posterior images of the whole-body bone scan show a band-like increased uptake involving the sixth and tenth thoracic vertebrae. There is abnormal activity in the first lumbar vertebra and focal increased activity in the posterolateral aspect of the right ninth and eleventh ribs.

Discussion: The linear, plate-like increased uptake at multiple levels of the dorsal vertebrae is the common appearance of osteoporotic compression deformity, particularly in patients with no history of known significant trauma.

Detection of an osteoporotic compressed vertebra at clinical examination is difficult. It may be asymptomatic or show minor symptoms. Diagnosis depends heavily on radiographic examination.

Vertebral deformity and reduced height of the vertebrae occurs as the result of osteoporosis, but unless there is increased activity on the bone scan, it cannot be assumed that the deformity is due to fracture.

Acute vertebral fracture as the result of osteoporosis shows the typical pattern of linear uptake on bone scan within 48 hours of fracture and fades within 6 to 18 months. Therefore a negative scan in a severely deformed vertebra suggests an old injury.

Although most osteoporotic patients are postmenopausal women, renal failure, hyperparathyroidism, and exogenous steroid use are also well-recognized causes of osteopenia. Corticosteroid-induced osteopenia mainly involves the trabecular bones and vertebra. Prolonged use of steroid may occur in patients with rheumatoid arthritis, COPD, asthma, and inflammatory bowel disease; assessment of bone mass density is extremely important in these patients.

Bone mass densitometry (BMD) measurement by DEXA is currently the procedure of choice for the diagnosis of osteoporosis, prediction of future fracture risk, and monitoring of the efficacy of therapy.

Figure 7.34 B represents the patient's posteroanterior dual energy x-ray absorptiometry (DEXA) scan, revealing markedly reduced bone mass density (BMD). A T-score of L2-L4 (− 3.31) is the diagnostic criteria for osteoporosis, which predicts an approximately 10 times increased risk of fracture as that in a young adult.

The World Health Organization has established criteria for BMD based on the standard deviation from BMD (T-score) obtained from young healthy individuals of the same gender, race, and age, as follows.

Osteoporosis: T-score less than or equal to −2.5
Osteopenia: T-score between −1 and −2.5
Normal: T-score above or equal to −1

Figure 7.34 C is a 6-month follow-up scan of the patient. Posterior images of the thorax show an interval of decreased uptake in the T6 and T10 vertebrae. There is improvement in the healing fracture of the right ninth and eleventh ribs. The first lumbar vertebra appears essentially normal, perhaps as a reflection of the healing and stabilization of the older bony insult. There is, however, an interval development of a fracture involving the shaft of the right humerus as a result of the mild trauma in this osteoporotic patient, as predicted.

There is some controversy concerning the validity of DEXA measurements in patients that have been injected with ^{99m}Tc bone and cardiac agents preceding the DEXA. Although the effect is measurable, it is unlikely that it would significantly affect the result of dual x-ray absorptionmetry scans.

Therefore, when required, the performance of a DEXA and bone scan on the same day should be allowed. This not only makes the procedure more convenient for the patient but also saves time.

Diagnosis: Osteoporosis and vertebral fractures.

CASE 7.35

History: A 23-year-old man who had injured his left foot approximately 13 months earlier is referred for a bone scan (Figs. 7.35 A, 7.35 B and 7.35 C). His concurrent radiograph is shown in Figure 7.35 D.

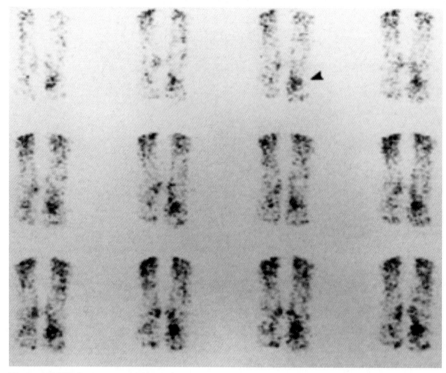

Figure 7.35 A

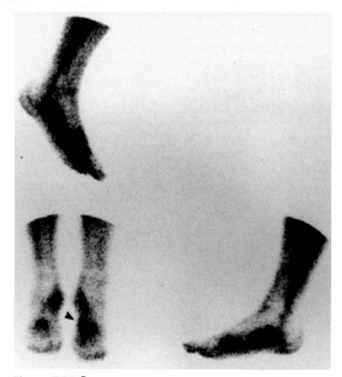

Figure 7.35 B

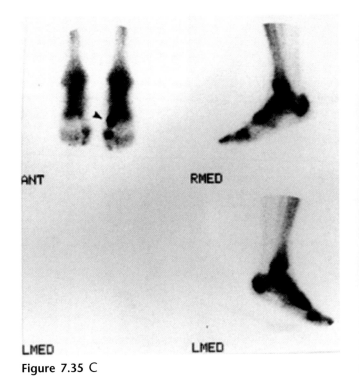

Figure 7.35 C

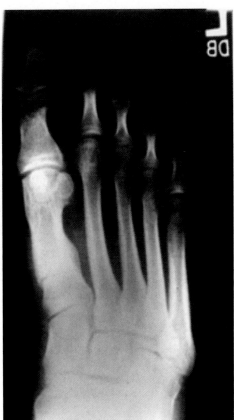

Figure 7.35 D

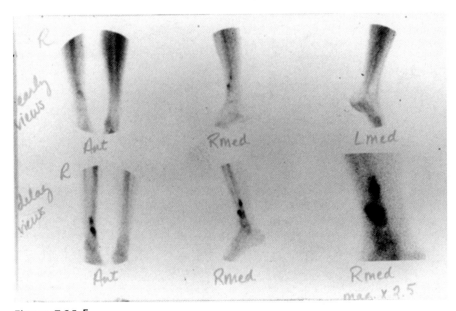

Figure 7.35 E

Findings: Radiographically, there is evidence of old fracture with eburnation along the fracture line involving the proximal shaft of the first metatarsal bone.

Scintigraphically, the three-phase bone scan is positive (arrowheads), showing increased flow (Fig. 7.35 A), increased soft tissue uptake (Fig. 7.35 B), and increased skeletal uptake (Fig. 7.35 C) in the region of the fracture.

Discussion: The healing process of a fracture is associated with a positive three-phase bone scan.

Repair at the fracture site usually begins within 24 hours following injury; however, the rate of healing varies according to location, age of the patient, method of reduction, and degree of bone remodeling. Most of these fractures heal by 6 to 8 months. Fractures that seem to take too long to heal properly

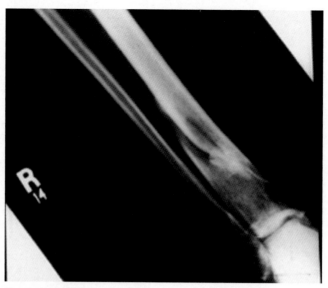

Figure 7.35 F

and beyond the expected time frame of 6 to 8 months are referred to as having a delayed union or in some instances nonunion.

The distinction between a delayed union and nonunion is difficult, both clinically and scintigraphically. However, scintigraphy is useful in differentiating the two types of nonunion, reactive and atrophic.

Reactive nonunion is associated with increased tracer uptake at the fracture site, as in this case. Differentiation of a reactive nonunion from normal healing of an extensive fracture is not possible by scan alone, but the history of injury 13 months earlier would indicate the abnormal process of a nonunion.

In atrophic nonunion, on the other hand, there will be decreased uptake or even a photopenic region at the fracture site. Figure 7.35 E shows a two-phase bone scan of the leg of a 30-year-old woman with an atrophic nonunion corresponding to the site of a fracture of the distal right tibia (Fig. 7.35 F). Note the photopenic region outlined by minimal uptake on both sides of the fracture line. This pattern represents inability of the bone ends to develop a proper healing process.

Diagnosis: Reactive nonunion and atrophic nonunion fracture.

CASE 7.36

History: A 71-year-old man complained of pain in the left hip after a fall from bed the night before. The initial radiograph (Fig. 7.36 A) shows no evidence of fracture. The patient was therefore referred for a bone scan (Fig. 7.36 B).

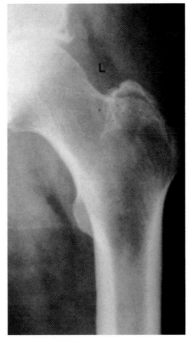

Figure 7.36 A

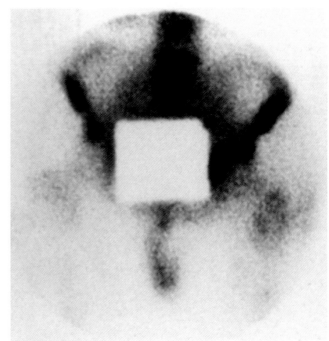

Figure 7.36 B

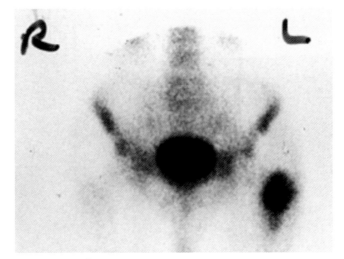

Figure 7.36 C

Findings: There is asymmetry with minimally increased diffuse uptake in the left intertrochanteric region as compared with the right.

Discussion: Although no obvious fracture line is seen on the radiograph, a close inspection discloses the presence of a large area of radiolucency within the intertrochanteric region, which roughly corresponds to the area of abnormal uptake seen on the bone scan. The bone scan, although abnormal, is not classic for a typical fracture. Acute fracture classically appears as an area of intense uptake at the site of fracture, as early as 6 hours. In elderly and osteoporotic patients, the detection of fracture may be delayed by 72 hours or even longer. This does not mean, however, that the scan should be postponed for 72 hours after the trauma; even in the elderly, the majority of fractures are detectable as soon as the patient presents for evaluation. When the clinical suspicion of fracture is high and the initial scan is negative, a repeat scan beyond 72 hours following injury is appropriate. Figure 7.36 C shows the scan done 1 week following the trauma, which discloses marked intense uptake in the left intertrochanteric region.

The constellation of history and findings on initial scan, radiograph, and repeat scan is most compatible with a fracture superimposed on a large lytic lesion, which subsequently proved to be a single metastasis from lung cancer: a pathologic fracture. Detection of a hip fracture, particularly in the elderly, requires an image without interference from bladder activity, which can be accomplished by shielding the bladder or by catheterization.

The most common complication of osseous metastasis is pathologic fracture. Identification of a pathologic fracture depends on demonstration of a fracture through a preexisting lesion, such as a cyst, fibrous dysplasia, giant cell tumor, or metastasis, commonly an osteolytic one. Development of markedly increased uptake in a preexisting osseous lesion should suggest this complication. The sequelae of pathologic fracture depend on its site and are the same as for nonpathologic fracture. For example, fracture of the hip can cause osteonecrosis and, in the vertebrae, can result in a compression deformity, which may compromise the spinal canal and neural foramen. Differentiation of pathologic from nonpathologic fracture of the spine can be very difficult. In the nonpathologic case, there is a tendency for anterior wedging; but in pathologic fracture, there is a greater degree of collapse, causing vertebra plana.

Diagnosis: Pathologic fracture, left intertrochanteric region.

History: A 3-month-old female presented for a bone scan (Fig. 7.37) after her parents described a 2-day history of right knee swelling and decreased range of motion. The patient's parents deny any previous injury. Plain films of the right knee are normal.

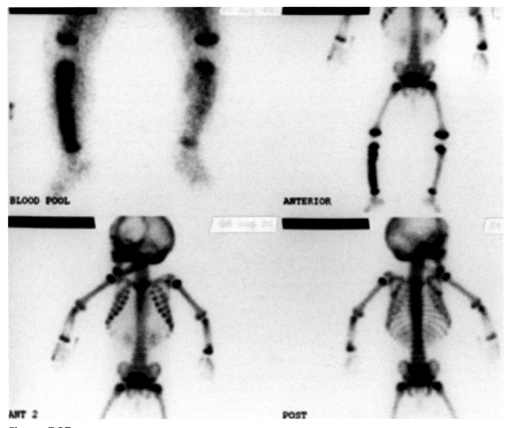

Figure 7.37

Findings: The bone scan demonstrates diffuse increased activity within the entire right tibia on all three phases of the bone scan. Additionally, there is increased activity in the region of the left distal radial and ulnar physis as compared with the right.

Discussion: The finding of two separate regions of increased radiopharmaceutical uptake in this patient suggests nonaccidental trauma or possibly a multifocal infection. The finding of diffuse increased activity involving the right tibia suggests nonaccidental trauma. In nonaccidental trauma, diffuse radiopharmaceutical uptake in long bones is thought to occur secondary to cellular proliferation along the entire periosteum. This finding is seen prior to the plain radiographic findings of fracture. A subsequent skeletal survey performed 8 days after the bone scan demonstrates periosteal elevation of the distal left ulna and right tibial diaphysis, indicative of healing fractures at the sites of the previous bone scan abnormalities.

The role of bone scintigraphy is complementary to the skeletal survey in cases of nonaccidental trauma. Bone scintigraphy can detect 25% to 50% additional skeletal injuries when inter-

preted by a radiologist experienced in its use. The main pitfalls with bone scintigraphy as compared with the radiographic bone survey is that scintigraphy cannot detect healed fractures or be used to determine the age of fractures. Scintigraphy is also less sensitive in detecting epiphyseal lesions.

The most common fracture in nonaccidental trauma is spiral fracture of the femur. Spiral fractures of the femur and humerus are more commonly seen than those of the tibia, fibula, radius, or ulna. Fractures of the femur or humeri are often bilateral and are the result of direct or torsional forces. Diaphyseal fractures are usually seen in older children.

Metaphyseal injuries are virtually pathognomonic of nonaccidental trauma. These fractures commonly involve the knee, ankle, and wrist. Metaphyseal fractures are thought to occur secondary to indirect shearing forces during shaking, twisting, or pulling. The result is a fracture through the metaphyseal spongiosa with separation of the epiphysis. Metaphyseal injuries are more common in younger children.

Rib fractures are seen in infants less than 1 year of age. The injury is thought to occur secondary to squeezing of the chest by the caretaker. The rib fractures are typically multiple, bilateral, and located either posteriorly or at the midaxillary region. Fractures of the sternum and scapulae, when present,

*Courtesy of Susan Passalaqua, MD.

are specific for nonaccidental trauma. Fractures of the clavicle are not specific for nonaccidental trauma because of the relatively common incidence of fracture of the clavicle during birth.

Skull fractures found in cases of nonaccidental trauma are usually linear and involve the parietal bone. Depressed skull fractures and sutural diastasis are uncommon. Bone scintigraphy is relatively insensitive for skull fractures. Children with positive radiographic or scintigraphic bone surveys are usually referred for head CT to exclude intracranial injury and fractures of cranial vault.

The most common scintigraphic finding on bone scans of children having suffered nonaccidental trauma is increased uptake of radiopharmaceutical in the affected osseous structures. The findings are typically multifocal and occur in the above mentioned areas. Careful positioning of the child is important to demonstrate subtle asymmetry of uptake in the metaphyseal regions in cases of metaphyseal fracture.

Uncommonly, important extraosseous pathology associated with nonaccidental trauma may be detected on bone scintigraphy. Renal injuries may be detected on the initial blood pool images in cases of pedicle avulsion or laceration. The delayed images may demonstrate abnormal increased uptake within the abdomen in the case of intestinal hematomas or increased uptake in the soft tissues if there is a hematoma or an area of rhabdomyolysis.

Most cases of physical abuse occur in children under the age of 5. Risk factors include prematurity, congenital defects, and physical or intellectual deficiencies. Caretaker risk factors include alcohol or drug addiction, intellectual inadequacy, illness, poverty, social isolation, and a history of being abused. It is not uncommon for the radiologist to be the first person to suggest abuse to the primary physician if the typical fractures seen in nonaccidental trauma are incidentally found on a radiographic examination completed for another purpose.

Diagnosis: Nonaccidental trauma.

CASE 7.38

History: A 68-year-old man with an abnormal electrocardiogram and markedly elevated creatine phosphokinase was admitted with the presumed diagnosis of subendocardial infarction. His ^{99m}Tc-pyrophosphate myocardial scan is normal. A whole-body scan was obtained with the same injection of radiopharmaceutical to evaluate for skeletal muscle injury (Fig. 7.38 A).

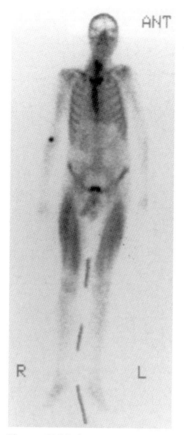

Figure 7.38 A

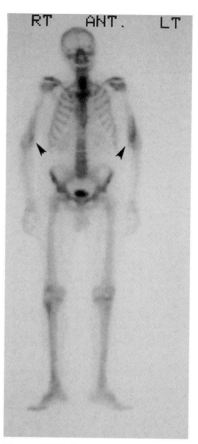

Figure 7.38 B

Findings: Anterior whole-body images show generalized soft tissue uptake as well as relatively reduced renal uptake. There is markedly increased uptake in both thighs bilaterally in a distribution corresponding to skeletal muscle.

Discussion: The symmetrical, diffuse muscle uptake of the thighs is consistent with rhabdomyolysis.

Bone scanning is invariably positive during the acute phases of the disease. The amount of uptake is proportional to the extent of muscle necrosis, and the extent of the disease can be estimated by bone scan. Scan abnormality disappears as healing occurs; therefore, muscular recovery can be evaluated.

The most intense abnormality appears within 24 to 48 hours of the injury, gradually disappearing over a week. This is basically the same time and course known to occur in the study of myocardial infarction with ^{99m}Tc-pyrophosphate (PYP).

The mechanism of uptake in rhabdomyolysis is probably similar to the accumulation of ^{99m}Tc-PYP in infarcted myocardium. Calcium deposits within the muscle as the result of ischemia and muscle damage have been postulated as the mechanism of a positive bone scan. Occasionally, conventional radiography may be positive for calcium deposits, but only when there is an obvious muscle injury.

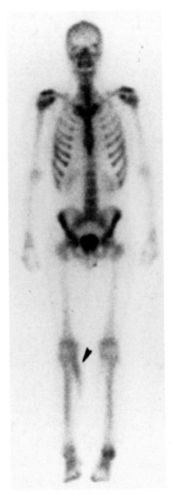

Figure 7.38 C

Injury to skeletal muscle results in myogloblinuria, hypocalcemia, and elevated creatine phosphokinase; oliguria and renal failure may occur.

Although a scan done with pyrophosphate usually has a higher soft tissue background, reduced renal uptake—as in this case—and the extent of soft tissue uptake despite some urinary bladder uptake indicate moderate impairment of renal function as well.

Rhabdomyolysis is muscle necrosis, which may occur as a focal or a more generalized process, as in this case.

In the generalized form, rhabdomyolysis occurs in different conditions such as generalized seizure, hyperthermia, shock, chemical toxins, viral infections, and sepsis.

Focal rhabdomyolysis is usually seen as a result of local trauma, vigorous physical exertion, or even after an extensive number of push-ups. Figure 7.38 B shows focal rhabdomyolysis of both arms (arrowheads) in a patient complaining of pain 24 hours following weight-lifting. Figure 7.38 C shows focal rhabdomyolysis (arrowhead) in the right calf muscle in this 23-year-old runner 24 hours after he had to withdraw from running owing to severe right leg pain.

Focal rhabdomyolysis also occurs in alcoholic patients following a period of unconsciousness and immobility on a hard surface, which results in prolonged, unrelieved pressure on the muscle. Pressure on muscles for a long period of time interferes with blood supply and causes necrosis. Even 2 hours of muscle compression can result in myoglobinuria.

Diagnosis: Rhabdomyolysis.

History: A 46-year-old man with a painful swollen right knee presents for a bone scan (Fig. 7.39 A). His concurrent radiograph is shown in Figure 7.39 B.

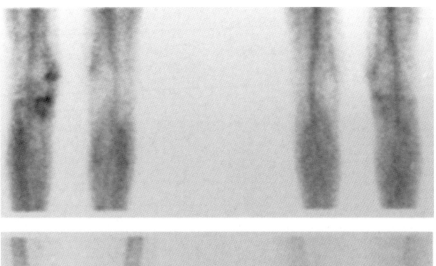
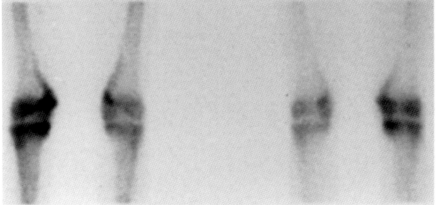

Figure 7.39 A

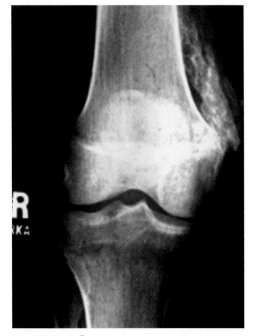

Figure 7.39 B

Findings: Blood pool and delayed static images of the knee show increased uptake in an area adjacent to the medial condyle of the right femur corresponding partially to soft tissue ossification present medial to the femoral condyle (Fig. 7.39 B). There is increased uptake in the knee joint, more pronounced in the medial compartment.

Discussion: Bone-seeking radiopharmaceutical is known to accumulate in ectopic ossification. Subtle changes in the rate of bone formation are detected by bone scan even if radiographs are normal.

Soft tissue ossification occurs in a number of conditions, of which myositis ossificans is the best known. Myositis ossificans presents in one of two patterns.

In the focal form, the disease appears as a localized process that develops in a single muscle or group of muscles. The second form is a familial condition known as myositis ossificans progressiva, in which widespread ossification occurs in many muscles.

Focal myositis ossificans is a nonmalignant focus of heterotopic bone formation in muscle and soft tissue which, in 60% of cases, is related to direct trauma. The other causes are total joint replacement and spinal cord injury. It is also seen in patients who have been comatose for an extended length of time. Third-degree burns and hemophilia may be complicated by myositis ossificans.

The radiographic appearance of heterotopic ossification is different from soft tissue calcification. In ossification, some degree of skeletal organization is seen, which extends along the anatomic plane of the muscle; whereas in calcification, it appears as amorphous flocculant calcification with no organization, usually occurring outside the anatomic plane.

The three-phase bone scan usually shows hyperperfusion, increased blood pool, and increased tracer uptake on the delayed images.

The progression, maturation, and stabilization of heterotopic ossification can be evaluated by bone scan. Maturity of the heterotopic ossification must be established in order to time surgical resection of lesion properly.

A distinctness in the outline of heterotopic ossification has been considered as a radiographic sign of stabilization; however, radiographic evidence of maturation and stabilization precedes the scan finding, which remains abnormal for a varying period of time. Repeated bone scans are used to follow the progression of the lesion. A normal scan or a steady decline in radionuclide uptake on more than two successive scans at 6-month intervals is a better indication of stability. Stability usually occurs after 2 years.

In this case, although the radiograph is more compatible with stability, the bone scan indicates activity of the process and indicates that surgery should be postponed.

It is to be noted that ^{67}Ga-citrate commonly localizes in the lesion of myositis ossificans and should not be confused with infection.

Diagnosis: Myositis ossificans.

History: On a chest radiograph of this 69-year-old male with chronic renal failure, incidental note is made of increased density over the left shoulder (Fig. 7.40 A). The patient was referred for a bone scan for evaluation of renal-related bone disease (Fig. 7.40 B).

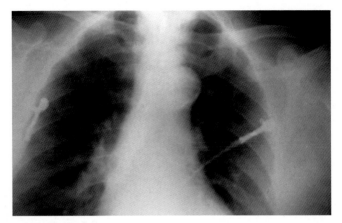

Figure 7.40 A

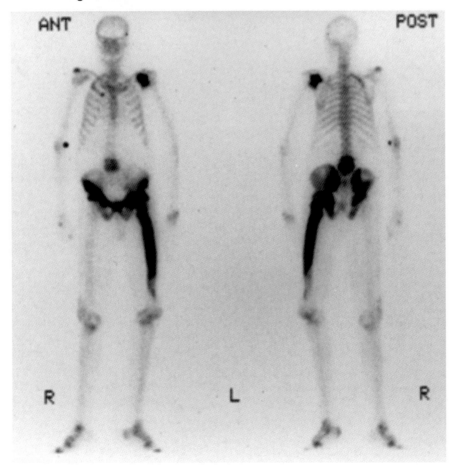

Figure 7.40 B

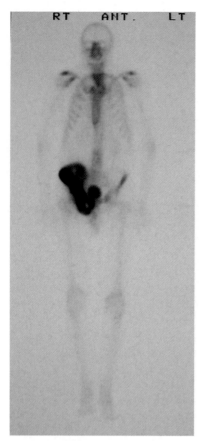

Figure 7.40 C

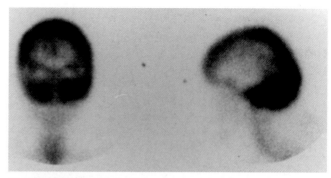

Figure 7.40 D

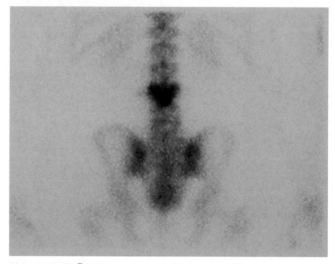

Figure 7.40 E

Findings: Anterior and posterior whole-body images show abnormal intense uptake in the articular surface of the left shoulder, second right rib, fourth and fifth lumbar vertebrae, major portion of the pelvis, left hip, and along the course of the left femur, ending abruptly at the distal diaphysis. There is absence of renal visualization and urinary bladder activity consistent with the patient's renal failure.

Discussion: The bone scan findings are virtually diagnostic of polyostotic Paget's disease. Note the characteristic scan findings of an enlarged and deformed femur with an area of uptake that localizes at the metaphyseal side of the hip and distally, being well demarcated from adjacent bone. The pattern and distribution of polyostotic Paget's on bone scan is sufficiently characteristic to allow the diagnosis. In questionable cases, further radiographic correlation may be needed.

The radiographic characteristics of Paget's disease depend on the phase of the process.

In the mixed phase, usually coarse, thick trabeculae and enlarged bone with cortical thickening are seen.

On bone scan, increased uptake in the anatomically preserved individual bone becomes easily recognizable; uptake is intense and evenly distributed throughout the affected bone.

On Figure 7.40 C, note the marked increased uptake delineating the entire right hemipelvis with clear demarcation of abnormal from normal bone.

In osteoporosis circumscripta of the skull, activity is more intense at the advancing margin of the lesion than in the central area of lytic bone (Fig. 7.40 D)

Approximately 10% to 20% of patients with Paget's are asymptomatic and are diagnosed incidentally through unrelated imaging. It is well known that more Paget's lesions can be detected on bone scan than on a radiograph (probably about 16% more). Not only the greater scan sensitivity, especially at early stage, but also the inherent difficulty of radiographic evaluation of the scapula, clavicle, ribs, and spine contribute to the risk of overlooking lesions in this area.

Figure 7.40 E is a posterior image of the bone scan of a 65-year-old man with an elevated PSA and a negative x-ray being evaluated for bone metastasis. The image is significant for abnormal uptake in the third lumbar vertebra in a pattern known as the "Mickey Mouse sign," representing the involvement of both the posterior element and spinous process of the vertebra. The Mickey Mouse sign has a fairly high positive predictive value (82%) for Paget's disease.

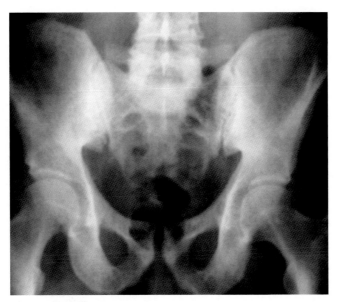

Figure 7.40 F

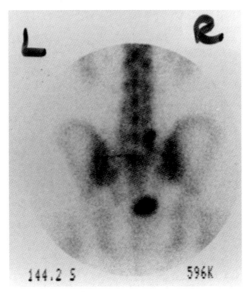

Figure 7.40 G

Paget's disease is generally polyostotic, but in 20% of cases it appears as a solitary lesion that is difficult to differentiate from metastasis, trauma, or infection. The common sites in descending order are pelvis, femur, lumbar and thoracic vertebrae, tibia, scapula, humerus, and ribs; however, any bone in the body, including the calcaneus and patella, may be involved.

Occasionally, intense uptake in a deformed pagetic bone may be mistaken for changes of fibrous dysplasia. The patient's age, normal laboratory findings, and x-ray characteristics of fibrous dysplasia allow for the differentiation.

A small number of Paget's lesions are visualized on radiography but not seen on scan. This often happens in cases of burnout disease. In pagetic bone, the uptake correlates with activity of the disease; therefore, in burnout Paget's with no further formation of new reactive bone, there will be no increased uptake. Figure 7.40 F and 7.40 G represent a radiograph and scan of a patient with burnout Paget's of the pelvic bone.

Diagnosis: Paget's disease.

History: As part of a workup for pelvic osteomyelitis in this 52-year-old male with end-stage renal disease, a bone scan (Fig. 7.41 A) was obtained. The scan is correlated with subsequently obtained chest (Fig. 7.41 B) and pelvic (Fig. 7.41 C) radiographs.

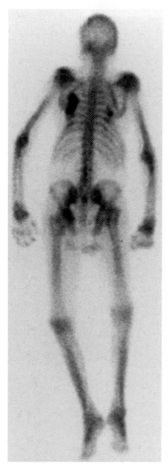

Figure 7.41 A

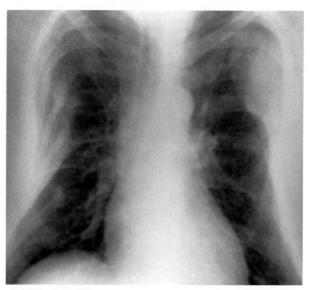

Figure 7.41 B

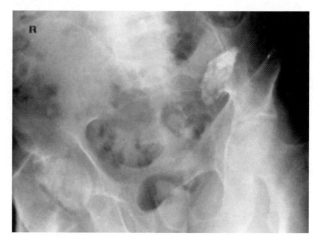

Figure 7.41 C

Findings: The posterior total bone scan is remarkable for increased uptake in the axillary margins of multiple ribs in the bell-shaped thorax, more pronounced on the left than the right. There is absence of renal uptake and urinary bladder activity consistent with the patient's end-stage renal disease. There is an asymmetrical appearance with foreshortening of the right hip as compared with the left.

The abnormal rib uptake and bell-shaped thorax correlate with the chest radiograph, which reveals evidence of bilateral multiple rib fractures and bulky callus formation. The pelvic radiograph shows a deformed pelvis with a fracture in the right intertrochanteric region and rotation of the head fragment, correlating with the scan appearance. There is severe loss of bone density.

Discussion: Prolonged chronic renal disease has a profound effect on the metabolism of bone and interferes with the normal physiologic mechanism of bone formation and bone resorption. Renal tubular disease such as vitamin D–resistant rickets and renal tubular acidosis may induce osteomalacia but rarely causes secondary hyperparathyroidism. Hyperparathyroidism is more commonly seen in chronic glomerular disease, in which osteomalacia and soft tissue calcification also occur.

Traditionally, the combination of hyperparathyroidism, osteomalacia, osteoporosis, and soft tissue calcification of renal disease has been referred to as renal osteodystrophy.

The scintigraphic appearance of renal osteodystrophy is a well-recognized pattern of metabolic bone disease. There is generally good skeletal uptake in a diffuse pattern. Renal

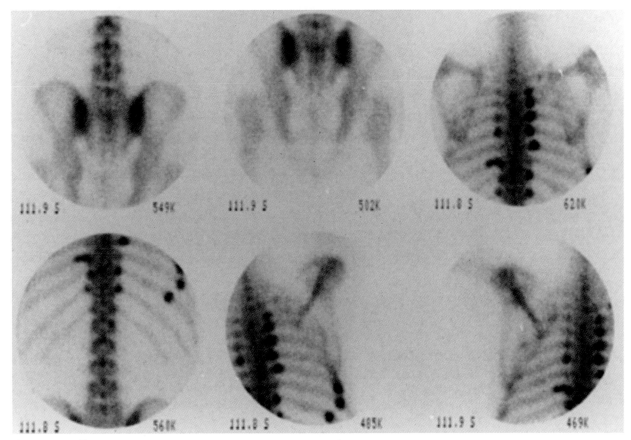

Figure 7.41 D

activity may be faint or not visualized. Despite renal failure, there is a high ratio of bone to soft tissue uptake. Prominent calvarial and mandibular activity may be seen in those cases associated with hyperparathyroidism. On occasion, soft tissue calcification may be detected in lung, stomach, and kidney.

The mechanism of increased uptake in renal osteodystrophy is controversial. In chronic renal disease, there is failure to convert vitamin D to the active form. This reduces calcium absorption from the gut, causing reduced phosphate clearance from the kidney. Hyperphosphatemia and hypocalcemia cause increased secretion of parathormone, leading to the picture of hyperparathyroidism.

In cases of associated hyperparathyroidism, increased bone resorption and osteoblastic activity explain the cause of intense uptake, but in osteomalacia, there is slow bone turnover. However, in osteomalacia, there is an increased amount of osteoid and immature collagen, which may indeed bind the radiopharmaceutical and be responsible for the elevated uptake.

Bone scan is not routinely used for the evaluation of metabolic bone disease except for focal lesions, such as fracture in osteoporosis and pseudofracture in osteomalacia.

Pseudofractures or Looser zones are often apparent early in the disease; they are usually symmetrical and frequently seen in the scapula, medial aspect of the femoral neck, pubic rami, ribs, and clavicle. Looser's sign has been considered as unequivocal radiographic evidence of osteomalacia in a patient with renal failure. Bone scans are capable of showing more pseudofractures than radiographs; one report indicates 75% versus 58%. These appear as focal areas of increased uptake. Figure 7.41 D shows multiple pseudofractures in a 48-year-old male with end-stage renal disease secondary to adult polycystic disease.

It is to be noted that in dialysis patients, there is a special form of osteomalacia, iatrogenic in origin, caused by aluminum deposits in the skeleton. Aluminum is present not only in the dialysis fluid but is also used orally as a phosphate binding agent, which causes elevation of the serum aluminum.

A technical note: In dialysis patients, dialysis should begin immediately after administration of radiopharmaceutical, with scanning following dialysis. This improves the ratio of bone to soft tissue and improves the quality of the scan.

Although the bone scan is quite sensitive, it may be falsely negative in the case of osteomalacia and fracture. The right hip fracture in this patient is not associated with detectably increased uptake. Osteomalacia is known to be associated with delayed bone healing. In osteomalacia of renal osteodystrophy, organic matrix is poorly calcified. Despite a normal bone matrix, calcification does not occur or proceeds very slowly.

Note the presence of an amorphous, elliptical, calcified density projecting in the left iliac fossa (Fig. 7.41 C), which represents a nonfunctional calcified transplant kidney and might be taken for a cartilaginous tumor by a novice interpreter.

Diagnosis: Renal osteodystrophy.

CASE 7.42

History: A 68-year-old male who had had end-stage renal disease for 9 years was being evaluated for possible hip fracture. On a plain radiograph (Fig. 7.42 A), a lytic lesion (arrowheads) was incidentally noted in the left supra-acetabular region. The patient was therefore referred for bone scan for further evaluation (Fig. 7.42 B).

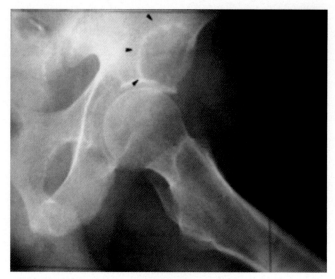

Figure 7.42 A

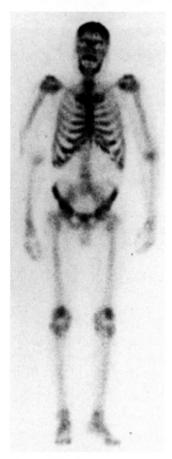

Figure 7.42 B

Findings: An anterior whole-body bone scan shows mild enhanced uptake in the skeleton with prominence of the calvarium and costal cartilage. There is absence of renal visualization and urinary bladder activity. The left supra-acetabular region shows no area of increased uptake or photopenia.

Discussion: The scan appearance is that of a well-recognized metabolic bone disease which is commonly seen in renal osteodystrophy.

Lesions of multiple myeloma, purely destructive metastatic lesions, simple bone cysts, and histiocytosis X are well-known lytic lesions detected on x-ray that remain undetected on bone scan. Although clinical and other ancillary findings would help to arrive at a reasonable diagnosis, definitive diagnosis usually requires bone biopsy, which, in this case, demonstrated amyloid deposition.

Amyloidomas may be encountered as a complication of long-term hemodialysis. The lesions appear as well-defined juxta-articular lytic lesions without matrix calcification which may be indistinguishable from the changes of multiple myeloma or metastases, although neither of these lesions is associated with a juxta-articular predilection.

Multiple myeloma and rheumatoid arthritis are the most common predisposing causes of amyloidosis. There is usually deposition of amyloid material within the soft tissue about the hips and shoulders. This is usually associated with some increased uptake of bone-seeking radiopharmaceutical within the soft tissue. Osseous deposition of amyloid also occurs.

In the case of chronic renal failure and hemodialysis, a special form of amyloidoma may be seen; it is due to beta II microglobulin, a low-molecular-weight serum protein that is not filtered by the standard dialysis membrane.

The few cases of amyloidoma that have been studied by bone scan have shown no associated increased uptake.

In patients with chronic renal failure and lytic bone lesions, the development of brown tumor should also be considered.

Brown tumors or osteoclastomas are subject to fracture and may cause expansion of the cortex. Brown tumors do not typically occur in juxta-articular regions. The scintigraphic portrait of an osteoclastoma, if it is large enough to be resolved, is generally that of a region of photopenia. It may have a narrow zone of rim activity. Pathologic fractures through brown tumors, however, will induce an intense uptake.

Diagnosis: Amyloidoma of renal osteodystrophy.

History: A 54-year-old man with left shoulder pain and tenderness of the left wrist who had a normal radiograph (Fig. 7.43 A) was referred from the rheumatology clinic for a bone scan (Fig. 7.43 B).

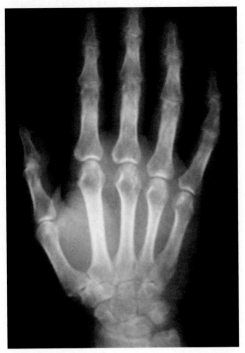

Figure 7.43 A

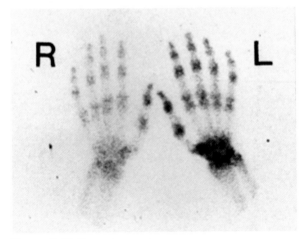

Figure 7.43 B

Findings: The scan of both hands and wrists shows increased uptake in the carpal, metacarpophalangeal, and interphalangeal joints of the left hand as compared with the normal-appearing right hand.

Discussion: Characteristic periarticular hot spots have been recognized as the scintigraphic sign of reflex sympathetic dystrophy (RSD). The absence of such a finding is useful in excluding that diagnosis.

"Sudeck's atrophy," "shoulder–hand syndrome," and "complex regional pain syndrome" are also used to designate RSD, but the last term is more familiar to many clinicians.

The classic bone-scan findings in RSD of the upper extremity are increased blood flow, increased blood pool, and increased periarticular uptake on the delayed scan. The sensitivity and specificity of delayed images have been reported at 96% and 97%, with a negative predictive value of 99%. It is to be noted that in 15% to 20% of cases, the scan may show decreased flow or decreased periarticular uptake, depending on the severity and duration of the process (stage I, hyperemic; stage II, dystrophic; stage III, atrophic).

Findings on bone scintigraphy are more sensitive and specific for RSD than those on plain radiographs. On plain

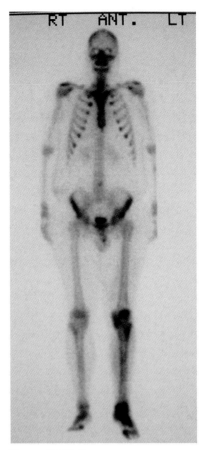

Figure 7.43 C

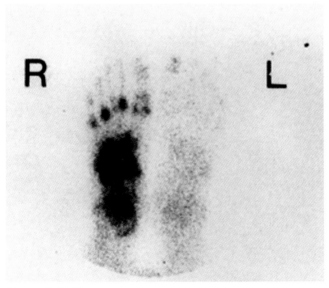

Figure 7.43 D

radiography, patchy osteopenia is seen in approximately 50% of patients; however, patchy osteopenia may be seen in association with disuse or immobilization. As the disease progresses, diffuse osteopenia and a ground-glass appearance become evident.

The signs of RSD on MRI include periarticular marrow edema, soft tissue swelling, and joint effusion.

The characteristic scan findings of RSD of the upper extremity also applies to the lower extremity, in which the abnormality is periarticular and more pronounced distally than proximally.

Figure 7.43 C is a total-body bone scan of a 25-year-old male with paresthesia and pain of the left lower extremity, aggravated by walking.

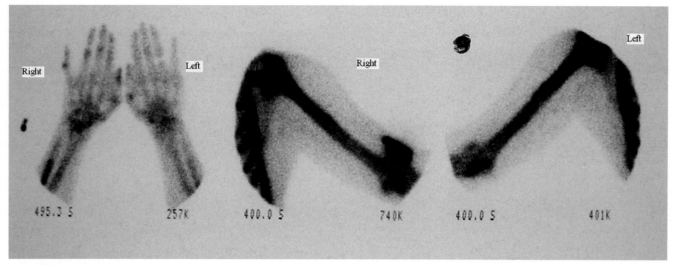

Figure 7.43 E

Note the generalized uptake over the symptomatic left leg as compared with the right. Increased activity is more pronounced around the ankle than in the knee joint. This pattern is most consistent with the diagnosis of RSD and perhaps represents stage II of the clinical course.

Figure 7.43 D shows periarticular increased uptake of reflex sympathetic dystrophy in the right foot as compared with the left. The pattern and distribution of uptake are specific enough to make the diagnosis of RSD of the right foot.

The scan sensitivity for the RSD of the lower extremity is 100%, specificity 80%, positive predictive value 54%, and negative predictive value of 100%.

The lower specificity of the scan for the foot reflects the fact that more abnormality such as infection and diabetic arthropathy are present in the foot than in the hand.

The cause of RSD is not known. Trauma, although minor, can be considered as the most common precipitating factor in the development of RSD. Previous fracture, soft tissue trauma, peripheral nerve injury, myocardial infarction, calcified tendonitis, cardiovascular disease, and cervical spine disease have all been associated with RSD.

In Figure 7.43 E, note the sequelae of soft tissue injury in the right elbow and changes of RSD in the right hand.

The pathogenesis of RSD is also not clear. It is believed that the syndrome begins with a nerve injury, either to the peripheral nerve as the result of trauma or to the central nerve from a cerebrovascular accident. Such an event leads to abnormal autonomic vasodilatation and increased blood flow. Such increased blood flow is due to loss of sympathetic vasoconstriction, which opens the vascular bed and increases the blood flow. Hyperemia of sinovitis, which is a histologic feature of RSD, is responsible for increased soft tissue uptake and may enhance prearticular uptake on the delayed image. Although increased flow and blood pool are features of RSD, they are not highly sensitive in the diagnosis. Increased uptake on the delayed images in the recognized pattern is the characteristic finding.

The mechanism of vasodilatation may be neurogenically mediated (release of neuropeptide at the ends of the nerve fibers) instead of sympathetically mediated. However, regardless of the mechanism, with vasodilation increased bone uptake occurs as a result of the combination of increased blood flow and increased bone turnover.

Diagnosis: Reflex sympathetic dystrophy.

CASE 7.44

History: A 65-year-old man with a history of prostate cancer complained of pain over the left hip area, aggravated by walking. A scan was performed for evaluation of possible metastatic disease (Fig. 7.44 A).

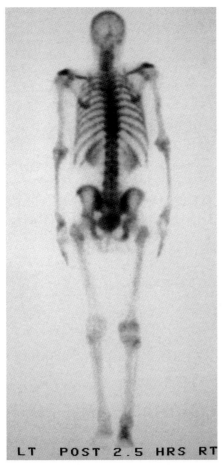

Figure 7.44 A

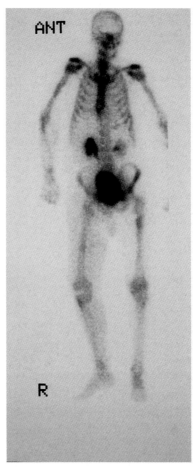

Figure 7.44 B

Findings: The posterior whole-body image is remarkable for the asymmetrical appearance of the lower extremities, with a generalized decreased uptake over the symptomatic left side. There are no scintigraphic findings of metastasis.

Discussion: Uniappendicular increased or decreased uptake (asymmetry) of the lower extremity is not a common presentation on bone scan. However, asymmetry due to increased uptake is more prevalent than decreased uptake and is usually due to conditions such as lymphedema, venous stasis, thrombophlebitis, cellulitis postrevascularization, and a few other uncommon entities.

Disease processes affecting the blood flow to regional bone, the bone's metabolic activity, or the rate of bone turnover—as well as conditions that result in alteration of the mechanical stress on the bones of either the right or left limb—can cause uniappendicular asymmetrical uptake. Of these causes, blood flow is the dominant factor. Increased or decreased flow parallels bone uptake.

In the case of Figure 7.44 A, further investigation with lower extremity arterial Doppler and segmental pressure revealed

iliofemoral obstructive vascular disease and required revascularization, resulting in a marked improvement in the patient's claudication.

Figure 7.44 B is the anterior projection of a whole-body scan of a patient with a history of a left cerebral cerebrovascular accident (CVA) and prostate cancer. Note the right-sided hydroureters and marked increase in the size of the soft tumor of the right leg, which is due to venous stasis and deep venous thrombosis. This process is secondary to the pelvic prostate cancer mass affecting both the drainage of the right ureter and the return of flow to the right femoral vein. Note the faint activity in the left cranium, representing the residual of the patient's CVA.

Figure 7.44 C represents another patient with an asymmetrical appearance of the lower extremity on bone scan. This is a 63-year-old man with a history of recurrent colon carcinoma. Five months following a complicated back surgery resulting in paralysis of the right lower extremity, a bone scan was obtained for the detection of suspected metastasis.

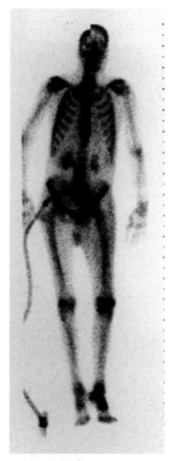

Figure 7.44 C

Note the increased uptake in the L5 region, in the area of surgical intervention. Also note abnormal uptake about the hip and knee and more pronounced in the ankle joints of the left side. Also note the markedly reduced soft tissue mass of the right lower extremity, which is consistent with the paralyzed limb.

In a paralyzed limb, despite commonly developing bone demineralization and osteoporosis, the uptake of radiopharmaceutical is maintained (as seen in Fig. 7.44 C) and may even appear increased. This is due to preservation of bone blood flow. Unlike the skeletal muscle, blood flow to the bone is not severely affected by paralyzed limbs and immobilization. In a paralyzed limb, the arterial flow to the skin and muscles is reduced owing to less metabolic demand. Blood diversion occurs from the soft tissue to the osseous tissue, enhancing the uptake of bone-seeking radiopharmaceutical.

It is only in cases of long-standing paralysis and severe disuse osteoporosis that uptake of radiopharmaceutical may be subnormal. Patients with long-standing paralysis and severe osteoporosis have decreased osteogenesis and decreased bone resorption (reduced metabolic activity). Lack of uptake of radiopharmaceutical indicates that all compensatory efforts for osteogenesis have been exhausted.

Nerve injury and paralysis may result not only in disuse osteoporosis but also in reflex sympathetic dystrophy, of which bone demineralization is also a feature.

The increased uptake around the hip, knee, and ankle of the left lower extremity seen in Figure 7.44 C is a recognized pattern of RSD as a result of nerve damage secondary to the patient's back surgery.

Diagnosis: Uniappendicular abnormal uptake of (a) vascular occlusive disease, (b) RSD, (c) paralyzed limb.

CASE 7.45

History: A 47-year-old man who has undergone kidney transplantation complains of right hip pain. Findings on plain radiography (Fig. 7.45 A) were suggestive of AVN, and the patient was referred for a bone scan (Fig. 7.45 B).

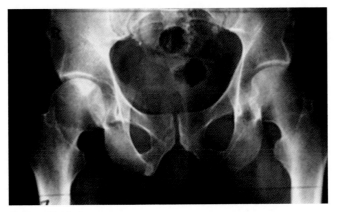

Figure 7.45 A

Figure 7.45 B

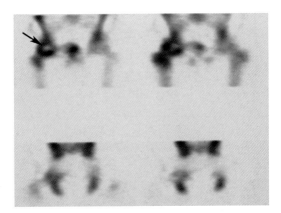

Figure 7.45 C

Findings: Anterior and posterior static spot images of the pelvis show markedly increased uptake in a plate-like fashion in the right femoral head. There is visualization of the transplanted kidney in the right iliac fossa.

Discussion: The scan findings are consistent with the changes of AVN of the right hip. There is a high incidence of osteonecrosis in renal transplant recipients partially because of the use of steroid. The other common causes of osteonecrosis include fracture, dislocation, slipped epiphysis, sickle cell disease, alcohol, collagen vascular disease such as lupus erythematosus, and rheumatoid arthritis. Idiopathic osteonecrosis is seen in different sites; various forms of this are known eponymically, such as Legg-Calvé-Perthes disease in the capital femoral epiphysis, Kohler's disease in the tarsonavicular bone, Freiberg's disease in the head of the second metatarsal bone, Kienbock's disease in the lunate, and Osgood-Schlatter's disease in the tibial tuberosity.

Osteonecrosis of the femoral head can be studied by plain radiography, radionuclide bone scan, CT, and MRI. MRI appears to be more effective than CT and scintigraphy, but bone scanning is more sensitive than radiography in detecting early disease.

The radiographic changes of AVN, such as the crescent sign, occur late; when they are detected, most hips progress to collapse within 6 to 24 months.

The earliest scintigraphic finding of femoral head AVN is a photon deficit, which can be detected to better advantage by SPECT images (Fig. 7.45 C, arrow, right hip).

The photon deficit is generally seen within 7 to 10 days after initiation of the events and is a direct scintigraphic translation of bone necrosis.

Subsequently, over a period of weeks to months, increased bone uptake appears in the femoral metaphysis. Eventually the zone of increased activity advances from the metaphysis to the femoral head, obscuring the originally detected photopenia and becoming indistinguishable from other causes of increased uptake around the hip joint.

At this stage the planar bone scintigram cannot distinguish the AVN from the other causes of increased uptake, such as osteoarthritis, but SPECT may still show the central photopenia covered by overlying activity. Increased uptake represents the revascularization and repair process.

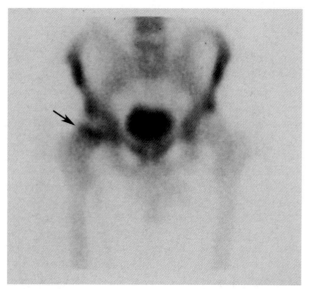

Figure 7.45 D

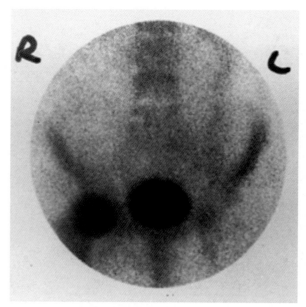

Figure 7.45 E

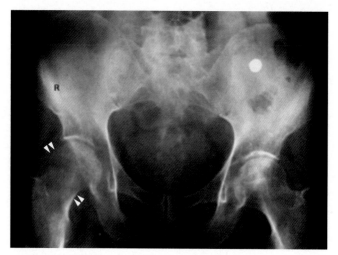

Figure 7.45 F

The sensitivity of SPECT for detection of femoral head AVN ranges from 85% to 95% as compared to 55% to 78% of planar images.

Increased uptake in the metaphyseal zone has been postulated to be due to hyperemia. After occlusion of capsular artery early in AVN, there will be establishment of rich collaterals through the medial circumflex artery reaching near the metaphysis and causing hyperemia of the metaphysis (Fig. 7.45 D, arrow). It has been suggested that when photopenia is not detected, the recognition of metaphyseal hyperemia may be helpful in establishing the early diagnosis of AVN. However extra care should be taken not to confuse the activity of the unfused growth plate or a subcapital fracture with metaphyseal hyperemia of AVN.

Although bone scan is less specific than MRI for detection of AVN, scintigraphy can provide information that sheds light on the etiologic diagnosis of the painful hip before changes appear on x-ray examination. The early sign of photopenia of AVN, the pattern of stress fracture of the femoral neck and pubic rami, and the scintigraphic signs of transient migratory osteoporosis and its typical distribution (Fig. 7.45 E) are sufficient to allow the diagnosis and explain the cause of a painful hip.

Figure 7.45 E is the pelvic scintigram of a patient with intermittent right hip pain due to idiopathic regional migratory osteoporosis. Note the markedly increased uptake in the region of the right femoral head. There is minimal demineralization (arrowheads, Figure 7.45 F) of the right hip. The cause of this disorder is unknown. It is believed to be a variant of RSD. The disease is self-limiting. Radiography and scan return to normal within 2 to 6 months, but recurrence is frequent in the other joints.

Diagnosis: Avascular necrosis of the femoral head.

CASE 7.46

History: A 33-year-old male with insidious onset of right foot pain and discomfort, worsening over a period of 2 months, was referred for a bone scan (Fig. 7.46 A). His concurrent right foot radiograph is seen in Figure 7.46 B.

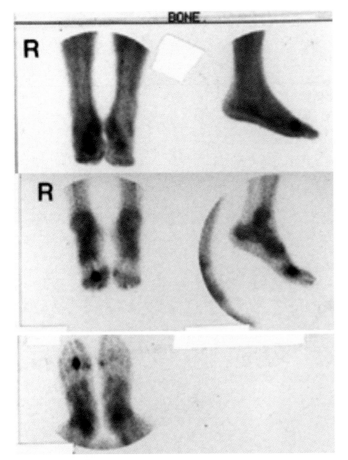

Figure 7.46 A

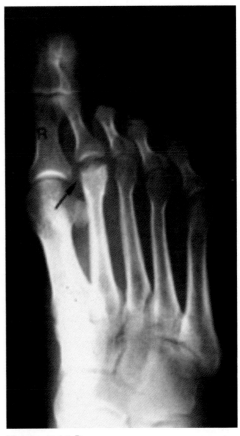

Figure 7.46 B

Findings: On the radiograph, there is flattening and sclerosis (arrow) of the second metatarsal head. The bone scan shows increased blood pool and focal increased uptake corresponding to the radiograph abnormality.

Discussion: Flattening and sclerosis of the head of the second metatarsal bone is consistent with osteonecrosis of the bone and is known as Freiberg's disease. The bone scan is typically positive, showing an increased blood pool representing hyperemia and increased uptake on the delayed image due to osteonecrosis in evolution.

As with any other AVN, the high-resolution scan in the early stage of the disease might reveal photopenia; but since patients tend to present late in the course, increased uptake is the most common finding.

Freiberg's disease is most common in young girls. The second metatarsal bone is the most frequent site. This bone is the longest metatarsal bone and is subject to the greatest weight-bearing stress and trauma. In 10% of cases, it is bilateral.

Stress fracture, osteomyelitis, and other painful conditions of the foot can be excluded by the presentation, history, and clinical findings as well as radiographic findings.

Diagnosis: Freiberg's disease.

History: A 64-year-old male with right renal cell carcinoma presented for a bone scan (Fig. 7.47 A) for evaluation of possible bone metastasis.

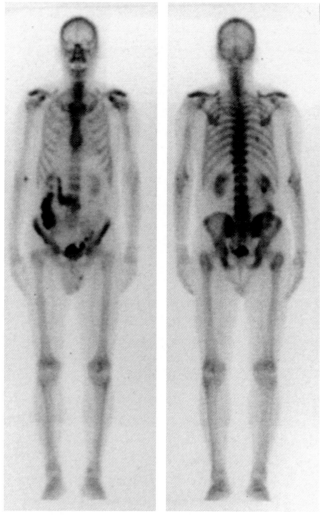

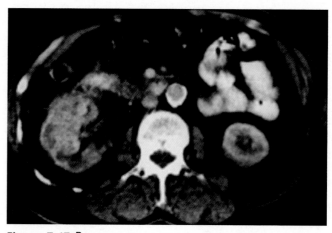

Figure 7.47 B

Figure 7.47 A

Findings: Anterior and posterior whole-body images show evidence of an old rib fracture on the right. A significant finding, however, is accumulation of radiopharmaceutical in the large bowel.

Discussion: Bone-seeking radiopharmaceutical is excreted in the urine; therefore, communication between the genitourinary system and the intestine would cause bowel visualization on the bone scintigram.

Vesicocolic, ureterocolic, vesicorectal, and ureteroenteric fistulas and urinary diversions all have been associated with bowel visualization on bone scan.

In this case, a large renal mass is noted on the CT (Fig. 7.47 B) abutting the right colon and duodenum. Bowel activity represents the result of direct bowel invasion and access of urine leak or bleeding into the intestinal lumen.

The diagnosis of vesicoenteric fistula is difficult. Often a variety of tests—such as barium enema, cystogram, and cystoscopy—are done without success. Bone scanning, as a noninvasive procedure, may be quite helpful in defining the fistula when there is a high index of clinical suspicion.

In the evaluation of bowel visualization, the possibility of faulty radiopharmaceutical, the presence of free ^{99m}Tc-pertechnetate, and residual activity from another radionuclide study should be considered.

Diagnosis: Renocolonic communication.

CASE 7.48

History: As part of an evaluation for a malignant lung mass in this 56-year-old male, a bone scan was obtained to rule out metastases (Fig. 7.48 A).

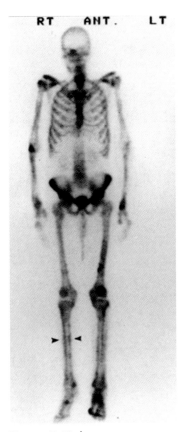

Figure 7.48 A

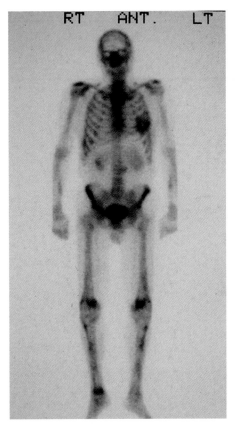

Figure 7.48 B

Findings: An anterior whole-body scan shows no evidence of bony metastases. However, there is diffuse cortical uptake in the shafts of the femur, tibia, radius, and ulna bilaterally.

Discussion: A number of conditions can be associated with increased periosteal or cortical uptake of radiotracer in bone scintigraphy.

Secondary hypertrophic osteoarthropathy (HPO) and shin splint injury are by far the most common causes.

Other conditions—such as primary hypertrophic osteoarthropathy (pachydermoperiostitis), long-standing vascular insufficiency, thyroid acropachy, fluorosis, hypervitaminosis A, and other conditions that manifest primarily by periosteal thickening—show a similar pattern on bone scan.

The pathogenesis of HPO is not well known. Eighty percent of HPOs are secondary to bronchogenic carcinoma and 4% to 12% of patients with bronchogenic carcinoma may develop pulmonary osteoarthropathy. Other intrathoracic conditions—such as tumors of the pleura and mediastinum, suppurative lung conditions (abscess, bronchiectasis), as well as cystic fibrosis—can cause HPO. Of extrathoracic conditions, biliary cirrhosis, Crohn's disease, and ulcerative colitis may demonstrate the changes of HPO.

Although arthritis is the presenting clinical feature of HPO, there are no radiographic findings of joint erosion or cartilaginous destruction.

The radionuclide appearance of HPO varies. The usual presentation includes bilateral and equal involvement of the appendicular skeleton. Diffusely increased cortical uptake in long bones covered by periosteum will give the appearance of a parallel track (arrowheads, Fig. 7.48 A). Periarticular zones are usually spared owing to lack of periosteal coverage. Joint erosion and cartilaginous destruction are not seen unless synovitis is present. HPO can also appear as a patchy deposition of tracer activity in the long bones. Figure 7.48 B shows long bone patchy uptake of HPO in another patient, a 57-year-old male with a metastatic lesion of unknown origin, probably from the kidney, superimposed and intermixed with pleural thickening secondary to previous chronic suppurative pleuropulmonary lesions. Note abnormal uptake in the involved area of the left chest wall.

The signs and symptoms of HPO are reversible, and the scan returns to a normal pattern within 1 to 6 months following removal of the cause, but radiographic resolution lags the scan by several years.

Diagnosis: Hypertrophic osteoarthropathy.

History: A 22-year-old female with sickle cell disease and 3 days of pain in the legs, worse on the right than the left, with a negative radiograph presents for a bone and bone marrow scan for evaluation of possible osteomyelitis versus infarction versus sickle cell crisis (Figs. 7.49 A, 7.49 B and 7.49 C).

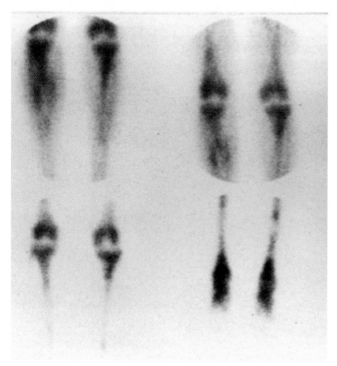

Figure 7.49 A

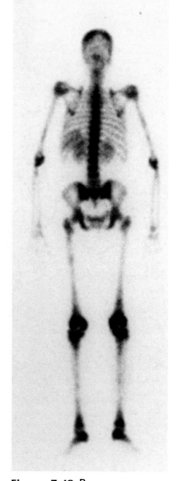

Figure 7.49 B

Findings: There is increased soft tissue uptake in the right leg (Fig. 7.49 A). There is a photopenia in the tibias bilaterally. There is increased uptake in the calvarium in an enlarged metaphysis around the knee, in the distal tibia, and in the spleen (Fig. 7.49 B). On bone marrow scan (Fig. 7.49 C), there is visualization of the liver but not the spleen. There is bilateral tibial photopenia corresponding to the bone scan abnormality in this region.

Discussion: Distribution of uptake is consistent with patient's history of sickle cell disease.

Increased soft tissue uptake in the right leg is suggestive of cellulitis.

Painful crisis is a well-known feature of sickle cell disease and is the result of vaso-occlusive disease secondary to sickling. The vaso-occlusion causes reduced blood flow; if it is severe enough, infarction occurs.

Painful crisis of sickle cell disease is not associated with radiographic or scintigraphic abnormalities; however, in os-

teomyelitis or infarction, there will be detectable alterations in the appearance of the bone scan and the bone marrow scintigram.

Differentiation of infarction from osteomyelitis by scintigraphic criteria is improved by knowledge of the time from the onset of symptoms to the time of scan performance. The interval between the onset of pain and scintigraphy can be divided into three periods:

1. In the first period, from 1 to 3 days, infarction appears as areas of reduced bone marrow activity on sulfur-colloid scan. The bone scan may be normal or show reduced uptake. In osteomyelitis, however, one typically expects to see increased uptake on bone scan while the bone marrow appears photopenic. The exception would be fulminating osteomyelitis, particularly in children, which may appear photopenic on bone scan.

2. In the second period, from 4 to 6 days, infarction appears as photopenia on marrow scan but normal or increased

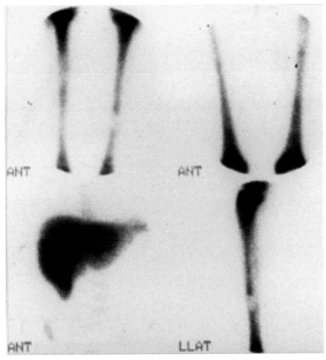

Figure 7.49 C

activity on bone scan. Osteomyelitis definitely shows increased bone uptake but remains as an area of reduced marrow uptake.

3. In the third period, beyond 7 days, the bone scan will be positive in infarction and marrow uptake will be suppressed. The positive scan is due to the healing process of the infarcted area; its uptake cannot be differentiated from uptake of osteomyelitis during this period. Although repopulation of the marrow may occur, repopulation is unusual and the marrow scan continues to show photopenia in adults with large infarctions.

In the current case, the presence of photopenia in both bone and bone marrow images in the first 3 days of symptoms would be most consistent with multiple infarction, whether old or new, in association with sickle cell crisis. The distinction of old and new infarct requires a prior bone marrow scan for comparison, although old infarction may show some calcification on the radiograph.

Splenic uptake of bone-seeking radiopharmaceutical is known to occur commonly in sickle cell disease but also in hemosiderosis, Hodgkin's disease, thalassemia major, glucose-6-dehydrogenase deficiency, splenic metastases from lung and breast cancer, acute myelogenous leukemia, chronic lymphocytic leukemia, and severe combined immunodeficiency disease.

Splenic uptake of bone-seeking agents in sickle cell disease persists and future scans will also show increased uptake. Absence of splenic visualization on ^{99m}Tc–sulfur-colloid scanning in patients with sickle cell disease is also common (Fig. 7.49 C, bottom). Nonvisualization of a noninfarcted but anatomically present spleen on a ^{99m}Tc–sulfur-colloid scan is termed functional asplenia.

The mechanism of splenic uptake may be related to splenomegaly, with anemia predisposing the tissue to hypoxia and microthrombus with infarction and calcification. Calcification may be at the cellular level and not visible on radiography. Excessive amounts of iron compound in tissue with an affinity for uptake also play a role.

In patients with increased uptake in the left upper quadrant, in addition to hematologic disorders, other causes such as metastatic calcification to the stomach, left renal hydronephrosis, lesions of the left adrenal gland, subcapsular hematoma, and splenic artery calcification should be considered.

Diagnosis: Sickle cell disease, marrow infarction, functional asplenia.

History: A 55-year-old male with low back pain and elevated calcium (14.5 mg/mL) and alkaline phosphatase presented for a bone scan (Fig. 7.50).

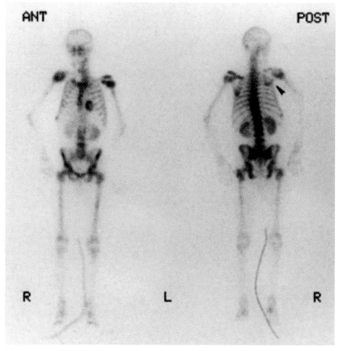

Figure 7.50

Findings: The total-body bone scan is remarkable for an area of increased uptake in the left thorax anteriorly, in a doughnut pattern consistent with myocardial uptake.

Discussion: ^{99m}Tc bone-seeking radiopharmaceuticals, principally ^{99m}Tc-pyrophosphate, are known to concentrate in areas of acute myocardial necrosis and have been used to diagnose myocardial infarction. This test is very sensitive but not specific. Not only transmural but also subendocardial infarction as well as acute myocardial necrosis due to DC cardioversion will show increased uptake. The mechanism of uptake in acute myocardial necrosis is felt to be due to the influx of calcium ions in and around the zone of myocardial damage in an area where some coronary blood flow still is present.

In the absence of infarction and acute myocardial damage, localization of radiopharmaceutical may also occur in angina pectoris (stable and unstable), atherosclerotic heart disease, and congestive cardiomyopathy. It has been postulated that the same mechanism and similar exchange of calcium ions occurs in chronic ischemia as it does in acute events leading to myocardial uptake.

Hypercalcemia is known to cause metastatic visceral calcification and uptake of bone-seeking agents. Conditions causing calcification are extensive bony malignancy, multiple myeloma, metastatic bone disease, sarcoidosis, milk–alkali syndrome (in patients with peptic ulcer disease and high intake of milk and alkaline products), hypervitaminosis D, and, most commonly, hypercalcemia associated with chronic renal failure.

The most common sites of involvement are lung, stomach, and kidney. These organs excrete acid and have an alkaline tissue environment suitable for the deposition of calcium and uptake of the bone-seeking agent.

Myocardial calcification secondary to renal failure is much less common; if myocardial uptake is seen, it is usually associated with uptake in other organs, particularly lung and stomach.

Visualization of the kidneys and activity in the urinary catheter in this patient does not suggest renal failure as the cause of hypercalcemia. In this case, myocardial uptake is most likely due to known atherosclerotic heart disease and chronic myocardial ischemia.

It is to be noted that cardiac uptake of bone-seeking radiopharmaceutical may be due to dystrophic calcification of a valve, coronary artery, ventricular aneurysm, or pericarditis. Doxorubicin (Adriamycin) cardiac toxicity, cardiac amyloidosis of chronic renal failure, Chagas' disease, and viral myocarditis are also known to cause generalized diffuse uptake in the myocardium.

Incidentally, note the small, high position of the right scapula (arrowhead). This patient was known to have a variant of Sprengel's deformity.

Diagnosis: Myocardial uptake of the bone-seeking agent is probably due to atherosclerotic heart disease.

History: A 67-year-old man with a history of prostate cancer and back pain needed a bone scan (Fig. 7.51) to assess for metastatic disease.

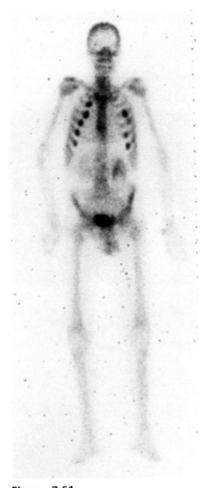

Figure 7.51

Findings: There is intense focal uptake in multiple costochondral junctions bilaterally.

Discussion: The striking pattern of uptake is a characteristic of multiple fractures sustained during CPR a month earlier.

Diagnosis: CPR-induced rib fracture.

History: A 50-year-old male with bowel carcinoid presented for a bone scan (Fig. 7.52) for evaluation of possible metastases.

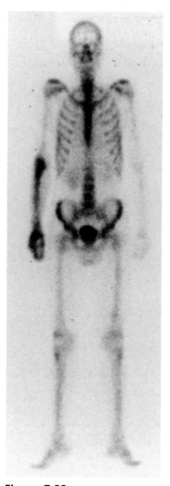

Figure 7.52

Findings: The scan is remarkable for diffusely increased uptake in the right forearm and hand.

Discussion: Diffuse uptake limited to the forearm and hand may be due to reflex sympathetic dystrophy. These patients are symptomatic and the shoulder-hand distribution is usually present.

The identical pattern may be seen if radiopharmaceutical is unintentionally injected into the brachial artery, as in this case. The intra-arterial injection in the antecubital fossa allows more radiopharmaceutical uptake in the bone and joint below the elbow. This pattern is known as a "gauntlet" image.

Diagnosis: Intra-arterial injection.

History: A 60-year-old man who had undergone mandibular bone grafting was referred for a bone scan to evaluate graft viability (Fig. 7.53).

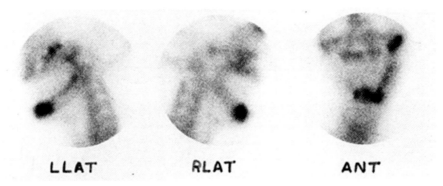

LLAT   RLAT   ANT

Figure 7.53

Findings: The static images of the left mandibular graft demonstrate radionuclide uptake throughout the length of the graft.

Discussion: Because bone scanning reflects the vascularity and metabolic activity of bone, it can be used as an effective tool to assess the viability of vascularized bone grafts.

Bone graft healing or nonunion can be predicted by bone scan 2 to 6 weeks before there is radiographic evidence.

Vascularized and viable grafted bone appears as an area of increased blood flow, blood pool, and delayed skeletal uptake on a three-phase bone scan. In grafted bone with a normal healing process and successful clinical outcome, there will be increased uptake of radiopharmaceutical within 1 to 2 weeks of surgery. Activity persists with no significant change over the first 8 weeks and eventually becomes equal to that of the surrounding bone.

A bone graft with vascular occlusion will show a decreased concentration of radiopharmaceutical on all three phases of the scan.

It is to be noted that infection will also appear positive on a three-phase bone scan.

Diagnosis: Vascularized viable mandibular graft.

SOURCES AND SUGGESTED READING

1. Even-Sapir E. Imaging of malignant bone involvement by morphological, scintigraphic and hybrid modalities. *J Nucl Med* 2005;46:1356–1367.
2. Roodman GD. Mechanisms of bone metastasis. *N Engl J Med* 2004; 350:1655–1664.
3. Buckley O, O'Keeffe S, Geoghegan T, et al. [99m]Tc bone scintigraphy superscan: a review. *Nucl Med Commun* 2007;28:421–527.
4. Taoka T, Mayr NA, Lee HJ, et al. Factors influencing visualization of vertebral metastasis on MR imaging versus bone scintigraphy. *AJR* 2001;176:1525–1530.
5. Sarikaya I, Sarikaya A, Holder LE. The role of single photon emission computed tomography in bone imaging. *Semin Nucl Med* 2001;31:3–13.
6. Horger M, Bares R. The role of single photon emission computed tomography/computed tomography in benign and malignant bone disease. *Semin Nucl Med* 2006;36:286–294.
7. Cook GJR, Fogelman I. The role of positron emission tomography in skeletal disease. *Semin Nucl Med* 2001;31:50–61.
8. Brown ML. Bone scintigraphy in benign and malignant tumor. *Radiol Clinic North Am* 1993;31:731–738.
9. Hartshorne MF. Benign bone scans. *Appl Radiol* 1993;22:22–33.
10. Gates GF. SPECT bone scanning of the spine. *Semin Nucl Med* 1998;28:78–94.
11. Prandini N, Lazzeri E, Rossi B, et al. Nuclear medicine imaging of bone infections. *Nucl Med Commun* 2006;27:633–644.
12. Morrison WB, Ledermann HP. Workup of the diabetic foot. *Radiol Clin North Am* 2002;40:1171–1192.
13. Love C, Marwin SE, Tomas MB, et al. Diagnosing infection in the failed joint replacement: a comparison of coincidence detection ^{18}F-FDG and ^{111}In-labeled leukocyte/^{99m}Tc-sulfur colloid marrow imaging. *J Nucl Med* 2004;45:1886–1871.
14. Wolf G, Aigner RM, et al. Localization and diagnosis of septic endoprosthesis infection by using ^{99m}Tc-HMPAO labeled leukocytes. *Nucl Med Commun* 2003;24:23–28.
15. Anderson MW, Greenspan A. Stress fractures. *Radiology* 1996;199:1–12.
16. Holder LE. Bone scintigraphy in skeletal trauma. *Radiol Clin North Am* 1993;31:739–781.
17. Etchebehere ECSC, Etchebehere M, et al. Orthopedic pathology of the lower extremities: a scingraphic evaluation of the thigh, knee and leg. *Semin Nucl Med* 1998;28:41–61.
18. Spitz DJ, Newberg AH. Imaging of stress fractures in the athlete. *Radiol Clin North Am* 2002:40:313–331.
19. Groshar D, Gorenberg M, Ben-Haim S, et al. Lower extremity scintigraphy: the foot and ankle. *Semin Nucl Med* 1998;28:62–71.
20. Hodges DS, D'Alessio T, Lenchik L. Practical approach to dual x-ray absorptiometry interpretation. *Contemp Diagn Radiol.* 2006;29:1–6.
21. Lentle BC, Prior JC. Osteoporosis: what a clinician expects to learn from a patient's bone density examination. *Radiology* 2003;228:620–628.
22. Lonergan GY, Baker AM, et al. Child abuse: radiographic-pathologic correlation. *Radiographics* 2003;23:811–845.
23. Ryan PJ, Fogelman I. Bone scintigraphy in metabolic bone disease. *Semin Nucl Med* 1997;27:291–305.
24. Fernandez-Ulloa M, Klostermeier TT, Lancaster KT. Orthopaedic nuclear medicine: the pelvis and the hip. *Semin Nucl Med* 1998;28:25–40.
25. Belran J, Herman LJ, Burke JM, et al. Femoral head avascular necrosis: MR imaging with clinical-pathological and radionuclide correlation. *Radiology* 1988;166:215–222.
26. Mankin HJ. Non-traumatic necrosis of bone (osteonecrosis). *N Engl J Med* 1992;326:1473–1479.
27. Fournier RS, Holder LE. Reflex sympathetic dystrophy: diagnostic controversies. *Semin Nucl Med* 1998;28:116–123.
28. Intenzo CM, Kim SM, Capuzzi DM. The role of nuclear medicine in the evaluation of complex regional pain syndrome type I. *Clin Nucl Med* 2005;30:400–407.
29. Peller P, Ho VB, Kransdorf MJ. Extraosseous ^{99m}Tc-MDP uptake: a pathophysiologic approach. *Radiographics* 1993;13:269–292.
30. Love C, Din AS, Tomas MB. Radionuclide bone imaging: an illustrative review. *Radiographics* 2003;23:341–358.

CHAPTER EIGHT

ONCOLOGIC IMAGING

DOMINIQUE DELBEKE
AND WILLIAM H. MARTIN

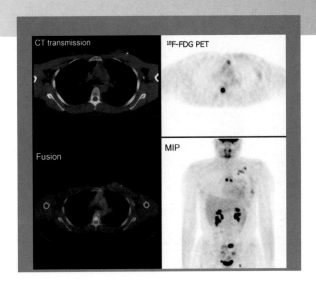

Some scintigraphic techniques used for oncologic imaging—such as technetium 99-m (^{99m}Tc)-diphosphonate bone imaging for primary and metastatic disease, ^{99m}Tc–sulfur colloid liver/spleen imaging for hepatic masses, ^{99m}Tc-pertechnetate and iodine-123 (^{123}I)-iodide for thyroid masses, and ^{99m}Tc-diethylene triamine pentaacetic acid (DTPA) and ^{99m}Tc-mercaptylacetyltriglycine (^{99m}Tc-MAG3) for renal masses—are discussed in other chapters. Some nuclear medicine techniques offer relatively high specificity for tumor in general or for specific types of tumors. ^{131}I-iodide and ^{123}I-iodide imaging for metastatic thyroid carcinoma offer high specificity in the proper clinical context and are addressed in Chapter 1. Other agents that offer relatively high specificity include ^{131}I-metaidobenzoguanidine (MIBG) or ^{123}I-metaiodibenguanidine for neuroendocrine tumors, ^{111}In-octreotide for tumor expressing somatostatin receptor (SSR), and radiolabeled monoclonal antibodies for tumors expressing a specific antigen. Gallium-67 (^{67}Ga) citrate, thallium-201 (^{201}Tl) chloride, ^{99m}Tc-sestamibi, and monoclonal antibodies have been used as an important complement to cross-sectional imaging but have been largely replaced by ^{18}F-fluorodeoxyglucose (FDG)-positron emission tomography (PET), which became the imaging modality of choice for oncologic imaging.

^{18}F-FDG IMAGING

^{18}F-FDG is an analog of glucose and behaves as a tracer of glucose metabolism. Therefore the distribution of ^{18}F-FDG is not limited to malignant tissue. ^{18}F-FDG enters into cells by the same transport mechanism as glucose and is then intracellularly phosphorylated by a hexokinase into ^{18}F-FDG-6-phosphate (^{18}F-FDG-6-P). In tissues with a low concentration of glucose-6–phosphatase—such as the brain, the myocardium, and most malignant cells—^{18}F-FDG-6-P does not enter into further enzymatic pathways and accumulates intracellularly proportional to the glycolytic rate. Some tissues—such as liver, kidney, intestine, muscle, and some malignant cells—have varying degrees of glucose-6-phosphatase activity and do not accumulate ^{18}F-FDG-6-P to the same extent. To interpret ^{18}F-FDG images, one must be familiar with the normal distribution of ^{18}F-FDG, physiologic variations, and benign conditions associated with ^{18}F-FDG accumulation (1,2).

The cortex of the brain uses glucose as its only substrate; therefore ^{18}F-FDG accumulation is normally high. The myocardium, on the other hand, can use various substrates according to substrate availability and hormonal status. In the fasting state, the myocardium utilizes free fatty acids; but after a glucose load, it favors glucose. When the thorax is evaluated with ^{18}F-FDG to assess the presence of malignant lesions, a 12-hour fast is recommended to avoid artifacts due to myocardial activity. For evaluation of coronary artery disease, a glucose load with or without insulin supplementation is usually given to promote myocardial uptake of ^{18}F-FDG. Unlike glucose, ^{18}F-FDG is excreted by the kidneys, and focal ureteral accumulation should not be mistaken for metastasis. Concentration of ^{18}F-FDG in the renal collecting system may obscure the evaluation of that region. This can be minimized by maintaining good hydration and by the administration of loop diuretics. For adequate visualization of the pelvis, irrigation of the bladder via a urinary catheter can be useful.

At rest, skeletal muscle uptake of ^{18}F-FDG is low, but after exercise, significant accumulation of ^{18}F-FDG in selected muscle groups may be misleading. For example, in the evaluation of head and neck cancer, uptake in the muscles of mastication or laryngeal muscles may mimic metastases. Therefore it is important for the patient to avoid chewing or talking during the distribution phase following ^{18}F-FDG injection. Hyperventilation may induce uptake in the diaphragm, and anxiety-induced muscle uptake is often seen in the trapezius and paraspinal muscles. Muscle relaxants such as benzodiazepines may be helpful in anxious patients.

Another source of misinterpretation is uptake in the gastrointestinal (GI) tract. There is usually uptake in the lymphoid tissue of Waldeyer's ring, and prominent uptake in the cecum of many patients may also be related to abundant lymphoid tissue in the intestinal wall. The wall of the stomach is often faintly seen and can be used as an anatomic landmark; similarly, esophageal activity is often seen.

Physiologic thymic uptake may be present in children and in patients after chemotherapy. Its typical smooth, symmetrical "V" shape usually allows differentiation from residual lymphoma. Marked diffuse bone marrow uptake is often seen after chemotherapy, especially if colony-stimulating factors were administered concurrently, and may compromise evaluation of the marrow for malignant involvement. Marrow uptake returns to normal 4 to 6 weeks after completion of chemotherapy.

^{18}F-FDG is taken up by activated macrophages at sites of inflammation, and the uptake may often be sufficient to resemble malignant lesions when there is granulomatous inflammation, as with tuberculosis, sarcoidosis, fungal infections, and aspergillosis.

In order to avoid misinterpretation of ^{18}F-FDG images, it is critical to standardize the environment of the patient during the uptake period, to examine the patient for postoperative site, drainage tubes, stoma, etc., and to time ^{18}F-FDG imaging appropriately after invasive procedures and therapies. Although ^{18}F-FDG shares some of the limitations of other tumor imaging agents—such as ^{67}Ga, ^{201}Tl, and ^{99m}Tc-sestamibi—the relatively high ratio of tumor-to-nontumor activity observed in most malignant lesions accounts for the reported high sensitivity and specificity of ^{18}F-FDG imaging and the intrinsic characteristics of PET imaging.

Evaluation of PET images can be performed visually or semiquantitatively using the standard uptake value (SUV) or the lesion-to-background ratio (L/B). The SUV is the activity in the lesion in microcuries per milliliter corrected for the patient's weight and the dose of ^{18}F-FDG administered. The SUV may be more accurate when measured relative to body surface area or lean body mass than body weight. Although semiquantitative assessment offers a more objective estimation of the metabolic activity of the lesions, visual analysis is adequate for clinical purposes in most instances. The average SUV of normal liver parenchyma and blood pool is approximately 2.0 and can be used as a visual reference. The SUV depends on accurate calibration of the positron emission tomography (PET) system, accurate soft tissue attenuation correction, and reconstruction algorithms among other factors. With PET/CT, attenuation correction is performed using CT-transmission maps acquired just before acquisition of the emission data; this procedure can be compromised by imperfect registration of the transmission and emission scans due to patient motion. The SUV is also dependent on factors that are difficult to control in the clinical environment, such as the patient's plasma glucose and insulin levels, fasting state, dose infiltration, recent physical activity, and uptake time of ^{18}F-FDG. In addition, there is inter- and intraobserver variability in identification of the lesion and slice with highest uptake and in drawing contours around the regions of interest. Therefore comparison of SUVs between two studies in the same patients for assessing response to therapy requires rigorous quality control, especially if performed on different PET systems or using different protocols and variation between institutions (3,4).

INDICATIONS

It is well established that neoplastic cells demonstrate increased metabolic activity. This is due in part to an increased density of glucose transporter proteins and increased intracellular glycolytic enzyme levels. Although variations in uptake are known to exist among tumor types, elevated uptake of ^{18}F-FDG has been demonstrated in most malignant primary tumors. Therefore the most common indications for ^{18}F-FDG imaging are as follows:

1. Differentiation of benign from malignant lesions
2. Staging and restaging malignant lesions
3. Detection of malignant recurrence
4. Monitoring of response to therapy

Following are the specific instances in which ^{18}F-FDG imaging is most useful:

1. Rising serum tumor markers in the absence of a known source
2. Equivocal lesions on conventional imaging
3. Differentiation of posttherapy changes from residual or recurrent tumor
4. Preoperative staging of patients contemplated for curative resection

SOMATOSTATIN RECEPTOR (SSR) IMAGING

Somatostatin is a peptide hormone widely distributed throughout the central nervous system (CNS) and GI tract, including the pancreas. It interacts with its target cells via specific cell-surface SSRs, of which there are five subtypes (5). A wide variety of neoplasms also express high-affinity SSRs, most importantly the neuroendocrine tumors of the amine uptake precursor decarboxylation group, such as pituitary adenomas, carcinoid tumors, pancreatic islet cell tumors, pheochromocytomas, paragangliomas, medullary carcinoma of the thyroid, and small cell carcinomas of the lung. Activated lymphocytes

and some lymphomas may also express SSRs. The high density of the type II SSRs on tumor cells allows their visualization with ^{111}In-labeled octreotide, a somatostatin analog that is cleared rapidly from the circulation by the kidneys and has relatively minor hepatic activity, thus allowing identification of hepatic metastases.

Following the intravenous injection of 6 mCi of ^{111}In-octreotide, planar whole-body images are acquired using a medium-energy collimator at 4 and 24 hours postinjection. SPECT images are required to assess the liver for metastases, and SPECT of the pelvis or thorax is required if clinically suspicious. Bowel activity at 24 hours can usually be differentiated from tumor by the absence of activity in that location on the early images; 48-hour images may sometimes be necessary. Liver, spleen, kidney, bladder, and bowel activity is virtually always seen, and thyroid and gallbladder activity is often seen. One must be careful not to mistake gallbladder activity for hepatic metastasis. Interfering activity may be seen in the lungs following radiotherapy and bleomycin therapy as well as with concurrent viral or bacterial infections.

The presence of SSRs on tumor cells correlates well with the success of pharmacologic nonradioactive somatostatin therapy. In imaging of growth hormone–secreting tumors, it is often advised to judge prospectively the potential success of parenteral octreotide therapy for effective growth hormone suppression and tumor regression. ^{111}In-octreotide scintigraphy may be used to successfully differentiate adenocarcinoma of the pancreas from an islet cell tumor, and SSR imaging is the most accurate modality for the detection of these typically small islet cell neoplasms. Owing to the frequent absence of type II receptors on the cells of insulinomas, the sensitivity of SSR scintigraphy for the detection of insulinoma is only 50%. The success rate in the detection of paraganglioma and metastatic pheochromocytoma is high, and SSR scintigraphy is likely the most sensitive and specific indicator of carcinoid tumor extent. Various other tumors—such as medullary carcinoma of the thyroid, Merkel cell tumors, small cell lung cancer (SCLC), and lymphomas—have been imaged successfully. In general, ^{111}In-octreotide imaging is preferable to MIBG scintigraphy in neuroendocrine tumors with the exception of benign pheochromocytoma.

^{131}I- AND ^{123}I-META-IODOBENZYLGUANIDINE (MIBG) IMAGING

MIBG is a guanethidine analog that acts as a norepinephrine analog localizing in pheochromocytoma and paraganglioma via the normal norepinephrine uptake mechanism (6). The agent can be radiolabeled with ^{131}I or ^{123}I, and tumor uptake is not inhibited by adrenergic blocking drugs other than labetalol. ^{123}I-MIBG is commercially available outside the United States, whereas ^{131}I-MIBG is used in the United States to image patients with suspected pheochromocytoma and paraganglioma as well as a number of other neuroendocrine neoplasms. Because of the undesirable dosimetry associated with ^{131}I, the injected dose is restricted to 0.5 to 1.0 mCi, yielding a poor-count image unsuitable for SPECT imaging. ^{123}I-MIBG imaging results in improved resolution, less noise, and statistics suitable for SPECT imaging without the 48- to 72-hour delay necessary for ^{131}I-MIBG. Physiologic liver, spleen, bladder, and salivary gland activity is routinely observed, but distinct normal adrenal tissue is only rarely identified except when using ^{123}I-MIBG. This technique is not used for screening but more for localization of a tumor suspected to be present due to elevated catecholamine levels. Since pheochromocytoma is bilateral in 10%, extra-adrenal in 10%, and malignant in at least 10% of patients, routine preoperative imaging with ^{131}I-MIBG has been recommended and should be the first step in the evaluation of patients suspected to have recurrent or metastatic pheochromocytoma/paraganglioma. Owing to relatively poor sensitivity, radiolabeled MIBG is not used clinically to image medullary carcinoma of the thyroid and carcinoid tumors. Conventional imaging techniques are highly accurate in the detection of the primary focus of neuroblastoma and most metastases, but MIBG scintigraphy exhibits unique benefits in detecting skeletal metastases and differentiating a posttreatment scarring/healing mass versus persistent, viable tumor. Sensitivity for the detection of metastases is 88%, but it rises to 98% with SPECT utilizing ^{123}I-MIBG.

MONOCLONAL ANTIBODY IMAGING

With the advent of hybridoma cell culture technology in the 1970s, it became possible to produce large quantities of homogenous murine monoclonal antibodies to a specific antigen expressed by tumor cells (7). The ideal antigen should be specific for one or several malignancies and be consistently expressed in high density in every patient with tumor and in every tumor deposit in each patient. However, because the extent of antigen expression is correlated with the degree of tumor cell differentiation, antigen expression for a specific tumor and even for a specific patient at different sites or times is heterogenous or mosaic. Furthermore, most tumor-associated antigens are not truly specific and are often expressed by various benign tissues, albeit at a lower density.

The first two monoclonal antibodies to become commercially available in the United States were (a) satumomab pendetide (OncoScint), an ^{111}In-labeled whole murine IgG antibody directed against an antigen, TAG 72, expressed by 83% of colon and 97% of ovarian carcinomas, and (b) nofetumomab (Verluma), a ^{99m}Tc-labeled murine Fab-fragment directed against a cell-surface glycoprotein expressed by most lung cancers, both small cell (SCLC) and non–small cell (NSCLC). OncoScint and Verluma have been largely replaced by PET and are no longer commercially available.

Capromab pendetide (ProstaScint) is an FDA-approved ^{111}In-labeled murine IgG antibody that reacts with a cytoplasmic antigen found in both benign and malignant prostatic cells but not with prostate-specific antigen (PSA) or prostatic acid phosphatase. Concurrent ^{99m}Tc-RBC imaging is often utilized to differentiate retained vascular activity from pathologic nodal activity. Fused SPECT/CT images are more useful. Although the images are difficult to interpret, preliminary results indicate that their sensitivity for the detection of pelvic nodal

metastases preoperatively and in postprostatectomy patients is much higher than those of CT. ProstaScint scintigraphy is still utilized because of the limitations of ^{18}F-FDG PET for the evaluation of prostate cancer.

Two monoclonal antibodies have also been approved by the FDA for radioimmunotherapy of low-grade or transformed low-grade lymphoma: (a)^{131}I-tositumomab (Bexxar) and (b) yttrium-90 (^{90}Y)-ibritumomab tiuxetan (Zevalin). Discussion related to these agents is beyond the scope of this book.

Whole antibodies are larger molecules that require delayed imaging at 72 to 96 hours because of the slow clearance of background activity; they are thus labeled with ^{111}In. Liver, spleen, and marrow activity are considerable, to the extent that hepatic metastases appear photopenic and are extremely difficult to detect. Antibody fragments, on the other hand, are smaller molecules that can be imaged at 4 and 12 hours owing to rapid renal clearance; therefore they are usually labeled with ^{99m}Tc. Significant interfering renal and GI tract activity is often present, although hepatic and marrow activity is less intense.

Because the murine fragments are less antigenic than the whole antibodies, they less frequently result in the formation of human antimouse antibody (HAMA). This immune response is detectable to a variable degree within the first 2 to 3 months following exposure. It is dose-related but may resolve over the ensuing months. The presence of HAMA may result in interference with radioimmunoassays (serum tumor markers, for instance) and alteration of subsequently administered monoclonal antibody biodistribution. Although adverse reactions such as fever, chills, rash, flushing, and angioedema occur in 3% to 4% of patients, they do not increase in frequency or severity in the presence of HAMA. Anaphylactic reactions are rare, but patients are advised to remain in the department for 1 hour after the infusion.

The clinical promise and projected benefits of radioimmunoscintigraphy have yet to be realized, but further developments in molecular biology and immunology are expected to advance this technology.

INTEGRATED PET/CT AND SPECT/CT IMAGING

A summary of literature regarding the performance of ^{18}F-FDG PET in various malignancies was published in 2001 (8). Although numerous studies have shown that the sensitivity and specificity of ^{18}F-FDG imaging is superior to that of CT in many clinical settings, the inability of ^{18}F-FDG imaging to provide anatomic localization remains a significant impairment in maximizing its clinical utility. Because ^{18}F-FDG is not limited to malignant tissue, the interpreter must be familiar with the normal pattern and physiologic variations of ^{18}F-FDG distribution and with pertinent clinical data to avoid misinterpretations. Limitations of anatomic imaging with CT are well known and related to size criteria to differentiate benign from malignant lymph nodes, difficulty differentiating posttherapy changes from tumor recurrence, and difficulty differentiating nonopacified loops of bowel from metastases in the abdomen and pelvis.

Close correlation of ^{18}F-FDG studies with conventional CT scans helps to minimize these difficulties. Interpretation has traditionally been accomplished by visually comparing corresponding ^{18}F-FDG and CT images. The interpreting physician visually integrates the two image sets in order to precisely locate a region of increased uptake on the CT scan. To aid in image interpretation, computer software has been developed to coregister the ^{18}F-FDG PET emission images with the high-resolution anatomic images provided by CT. An alternative approach that has gained wider acceptance is the hardware approach to image fusion using multimodality imaging with integrated PET/CT and SPECT/CT imaging systems. Design innovations continue to be developed.

Integrated PET/CT and SPECT/CT Systems

The fusion of anatomic and molecular images (PET or SPECT and CT) obtained with integrated PET/CT or SPECT/CT systems, sequentially in time but without moving the patient from the imaging table, allows optimal coregistration of anatomic and molecular images leading to accurate attenuation correction and precise anatomic localization of lesions with increased metabolism. The fusion images provided by these systems allow the most accurate interpretation of both PET/CT and SPECT/CT studies in oncology. Fusion ^{18}F-FDG PET/CT imaging is also a promising tool for optimizing radiation therapy.

Published data regarding the incremental value of integrated PET/CT or SPECT/CT images compared to PET or SPECT alone, or PET or SPECT correlated with a CT obtained at a different time, conclude the following: (a) improvement of lesion detection on both CT and PET or SPECT images, (b) improvement of the localization of foci of uptake resulting in better differentiation of physiologic from pathologic uptake, and (c) precise localization of the malignant foci—for example, in the skeleton versus soft tissue or liver versus adjacent bowel or node. PET/CT and SPECT/CT fusion images affect the clinical management by (a) guiding further procedures, (b) excluding the need of further procedures, and (c) changing both inter- and intramodality therapy. PET/CT fusion images have the potential to provide important information to guide the biopsy of a mass to active regions of the tumor and provide better maps than CT alone to modulate field and dose of radiation therapy (9).

Technical issues regarding optimal protocols and technical and clinical expertise regarding performance and interpretation of PET/CT and SPECT/CT imaging have been discussed (10). Procedure guidelines for tumor imaging using ^{18}F-FDG PET/CT and for SPECT/CT imaging have also been published and list numerous sources of false-positive and false-negative findings (3,11). This new, powerful technology provides more accurate interpretation of both CT and PET or SPECT images and therefore more optimal patient care.

CASE 8.1

History: A 44-year-old female with a poorly differentiated carcinoma involving the left nasal cavity was treated with chemotherapy. A posttreatment gadolinium (Gd)-enhanced MRI demonstrated a poorly defined soft tissue density in the anterior ethmoid sinuses with peripheral enhancement (Fig. 8.1 A). ¹⁸F-FDG PET/CT imaging was performed to differentiate residual viable tumor from posttreatment scarring (Fig. 8.1 B).

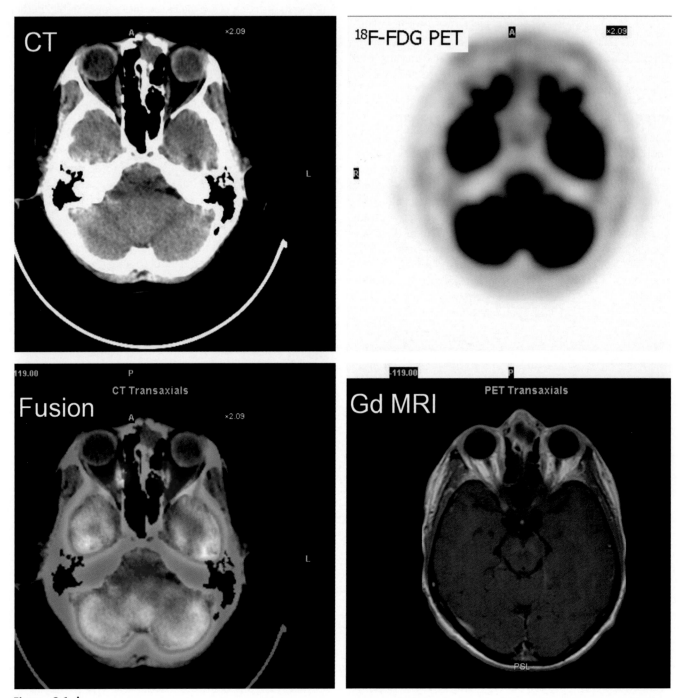

Figure 8.1 A

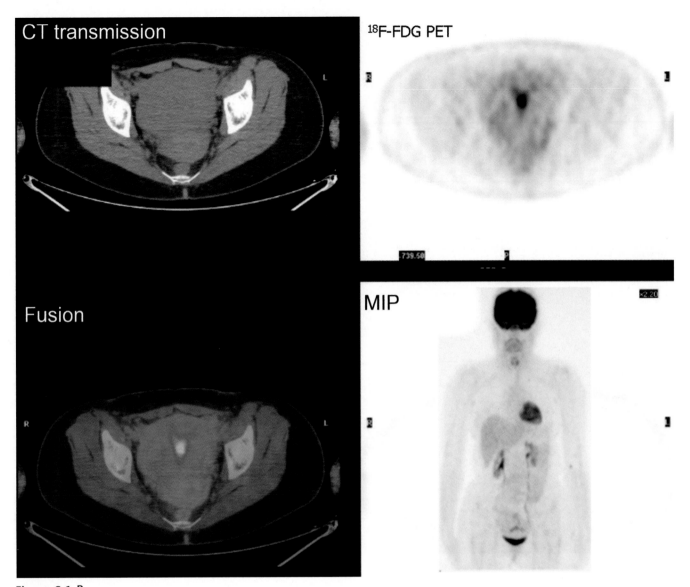

Figure 8.1 B

Findings: The ^{18}F-FDG PET/CT scan demonstrates no ^{18}F-FDG-avidity in the uptake within the ethmoid sinuses (Fig. 8.1 A). However, mildly increased activity is identified in the endometrial cavity (Fig. 8.1 B).

Discussion: The absence of ^{18}F-FDG activity in the lesion seen on MRI is indicative of a good response to therapy and associated with a good outcome.

It is essential to be fully familiar with the normal patterns and variations of ^{18}F-FDG biodistribution as well as the numerous benign conditions that accumulate ^{18}F-FDG and can mimic neoplasm. ^{18}F-FDG uptake in the endometrial cavity can be variable, and it may occur especially in menstruating women. During normal menstruation, approximately 40 mL of blood and an additional 35 mL of serous fluid are excreted

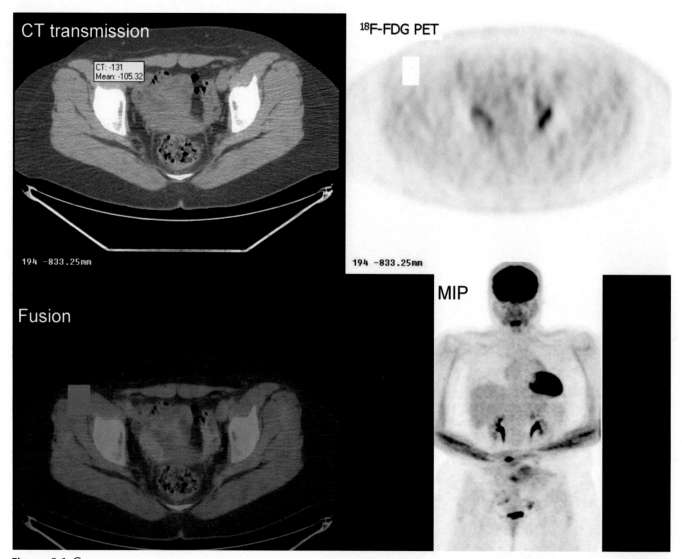

Figure 8.1 C

into the uterine cavity. This, associated with the inflammatory process due to the necrotic endometrial epithelium from the sudden reduction of estrogen and progesterone levels at the end of the secretory phase of the menstrual cycle, can result in physiologic uterine accumulation. Focal activity in the pelvis can be misinterpreted as a malignant lesion; but the mild degree of uptake and the correct identification of the uterus on the CT transmission images, accompanied by pertinent history, leads to a correct impression of physiologic uptake related to menstruation.

Physiologic uptake in the ovaries has also been reported in premenopausal women, as illustrated in Figure 8.1 C. In postmenopausal females, however, ^{18}F-FDG uptake in the reproductive organs is associated with a higher incidence of malignancies and warrants further workup (12).

Diagnosis: (a) No abnormal uptake of ^{18}F-FDG in the neck indicative of a good response to therapy. (b) Physiologic uptake in the endometrial cavity due to menstruation.

CASE 8.2

History: One year after undergoing resection of a melanoma of the right ear, a 54-year-old male presented with a palpable lymph node in the left neck. ^{18}F-FDG PET/CT imaging (Figs. 8.2 A and 8.2 B) was performed for restaging.

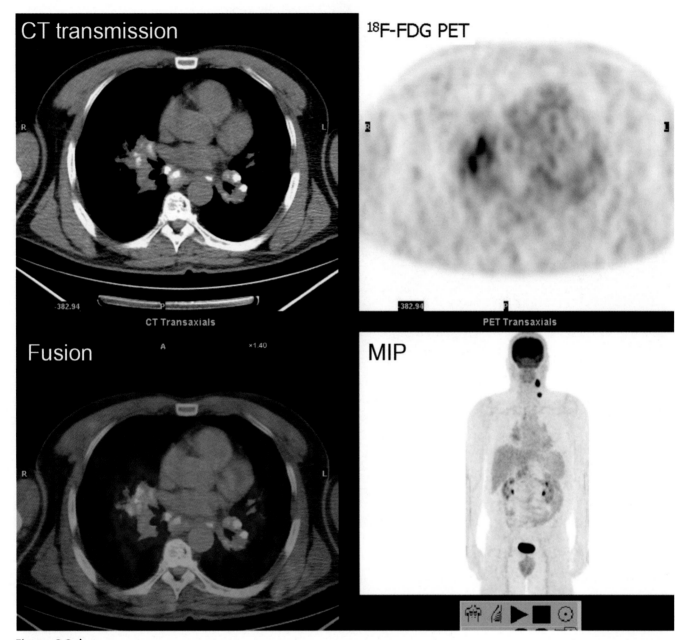

Figure 8.2 A

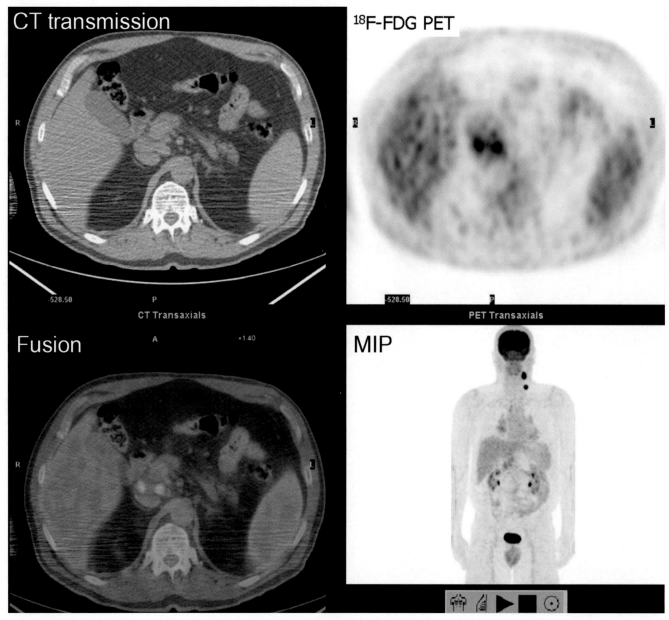

CT transmission

18F-FDG PET

-528.50   P
CT Transaxials
A   x1.40

-528.50   P
PET Transaxials

Fusion

MIP

R

R

Figure 8.2 B

Findings: Two foci of markedly increased uptake are seen in the left neck (Figs. 8.2 A, and 8.2 B), a maximum intensity projection (MIP) image, corresponding on the CT to a 2-cm submandibular and a 2-cm level III lymph node (CT not shown). In addition, there is moderate ^{18}F-FDG uptake in the mediastinum and porta hepatis corresponding to conglomerates of mediastinal, bilateral hilar (Fig. 8.2 A), and porta hepatis (Fig. 8.2 B) lymphadenopathy. The mediastinal nodes are partially calcified on CT.

Discussion: The intense uptake in the two lymph nodes in the neck is consistent with melanoma metastases. The role of PET/CT in evaluation of patients with melanoma is further discussed with Cases 8.19 and 8.20. However, the pattern of

moderate uptake in the mediastinum and porta hepatis is not typical for the malignancy of this patient, being more consistent with the patient's history of sarcoidosis.

Sarcoidosis is a multisystem disorder of unknown etiology most commonly affecting young adults and typically presenting with hilar lymphadenopathy, pulmonary infiltrates, and ocular and cutaneous lesions. The diagnosis is established when typical clinicoradiographic findings are supported by histologic evidence of noncaseating granuloma formation in more than one system unaccompanied by evidence of infection. The sensitivity and specificity of ^{18}F-FDG PET for the detection of malignancy are both greater than 90%, but the false-positive findings have generally been of inflammatory origin, including granulomatous (tuberculosis, atypical myobacteria, fungus, sarcoidosis, and suture granulomas) and nongranulomatous (bacterial abscess, postradiation, etc.) processes. ^{18}F-FDG PET imaging has also been demonstrated to be highly sensitive for the detection of inflammatory processes related to the high density of activated macrophages associated with inflammation (13,14). There is preliminary evidence that ^{18}F-FDG PET may be useful in monitoring the response of sarcoidosis to therapy and therefore guiding therapeutic intervention.

Diagnosis: (a) Metastatic melanoma restricted to the left neck. (b) Sarcoidosis.

CASE 8.3

History: A 10-year-old male with previous history of Hodgkin's lymphoma, stage 3B diagnosed 11 months earlier was referred for ^{18}F-FDG PET/CT imaging 4 months following completion of chemotherapy and radiation therapy. Prior to the ^{18}F-FDG injection, the patient's serum glucose was 96 mg/dL. A MIP image is displayed in Figure 8.3.

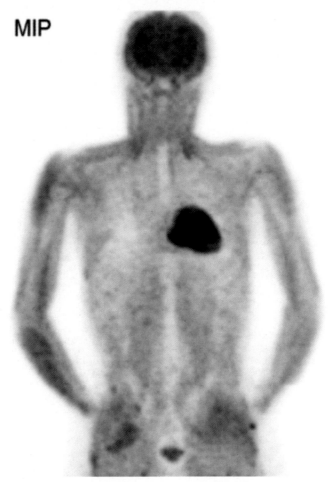

MIP

Figure 8.3

Findings: Intense diffuse symmetrical muscular uptake is seen. No abnormal focal ^{18}F-FDG metabolism is observed. Further history revealed that the patient had not complied with fasting instructions.

Discussion: The key to successful PET imaging is to prepare the patient properly so as to minimize the appearance of artifactual uptake patterns. All patients are instructed to fast for at least 6 hours and preferably 12 hours and to drink plenty of acaloric clear fluids. The serum glucose level should be measured just before ^{18}F-FDG administration to document euglycemia. Postprandial insulin secretion promotes ^{18}F-FDG uptake by skeletal muscle and myocardium, making ^{18}F-FDG less available for tumoral uptake (15). Therefore the sensitivity for detection of metastatic disease is decreased. The same considerations apply to diabetic patients after insulin administration, so administration of ^{18}F-FDG should be delayed for 2 or 3 hours after insulin injection.

Another consideration is ^{18}F-FDG uptake in activated musculature. At rest, skeletal muscle does not show significant accumulation of ^{18}F-FDG, but after exercise or if contraction takes place during the uptake period after the injection of the radiopharmaceutical, there can be marked uptake. Muscular uptake can usually be distinguished from malignant disease because it is often symmetrical and corresponds to the anatomy of muscular groups. Symmetrical uptake in the neck and thoracic paravertebral regions can be produced by patient anxiety alone. Occasionally, uptake can be focal and asymmetrical and very difficult to differentiate from malignant lesions. Therefore patients should be instructed to refrain from strenuous muscular activity for 24 hours prior to ^{18}F-FDG PET imaging. Abstention from talking and chewing during the distribution phase is of prime importance in patients evaluated for head and neck cancer.

Oral benzodiazepine administration should be considered before ^{18}F-FDG injection in patients considered at risk of showing muscle tension or brown fat uptake. Brown fat uptake is discussed in Case 8.25. Diazepam has anxiolytic and muscle-relaxant effects and may offer a simple solution to the diagnostic confusion that can arise between enhanced physiologic muscle uptake and malignant uptake.

Hyperglycemia represents a limitation for the sensitivity of ^{18}F-FDG PET imaging, because the excess of plasma glucose competes with ^{18}F-FDG and consequently reduces ^{18}F-FDG uptake in tumors by up to 50% (16). Therefore control of glycemia in diabetic patients and overnight fasting in normal patients are essential for high-quality ^{18}F-FDG images. The blood glucose level should always be measured before ^{18}F-FDG administration. Not uncommonly, patients with diabetes present with hyperglycemia because they have been instructed to fast overnight and have not appropriately adjusted their medications. Furthermore, unrecognized diabetes is not uncommon in elderly patients with malignancies.

Diagnosis: No evidence of gross recurrent disease; however, the sensitivity of this study for detection of malignant neoplasm is compromised because of diffuse skeletal muscle uptake.

CASE 8.4

History: ^{18}F-FDG PET/CT imaging was performed for initial staging of head and neck cancer (Figs. 8.4 A to 8.4 D) in a 76-year-old male recently found to have squamous cell carcinoma of the oral cavity extending to the left tonsillar region and submandibular region.

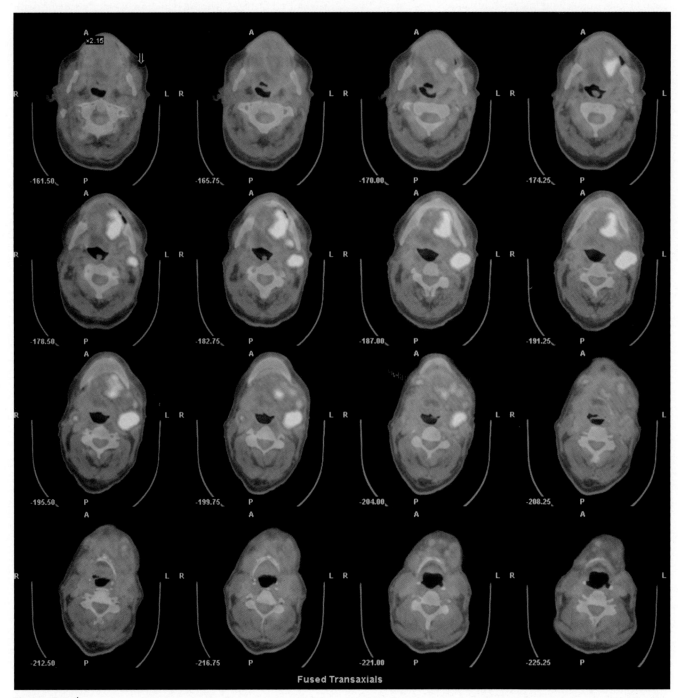

Figure 8.4 A

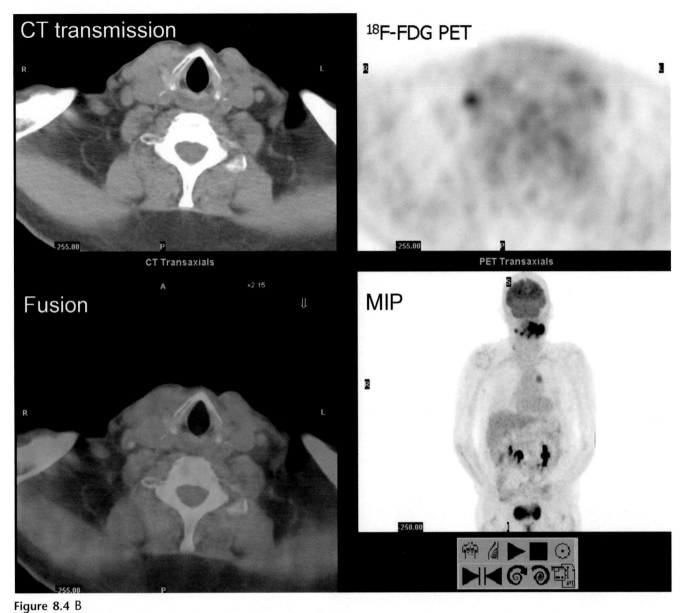

Figure 8.4 B

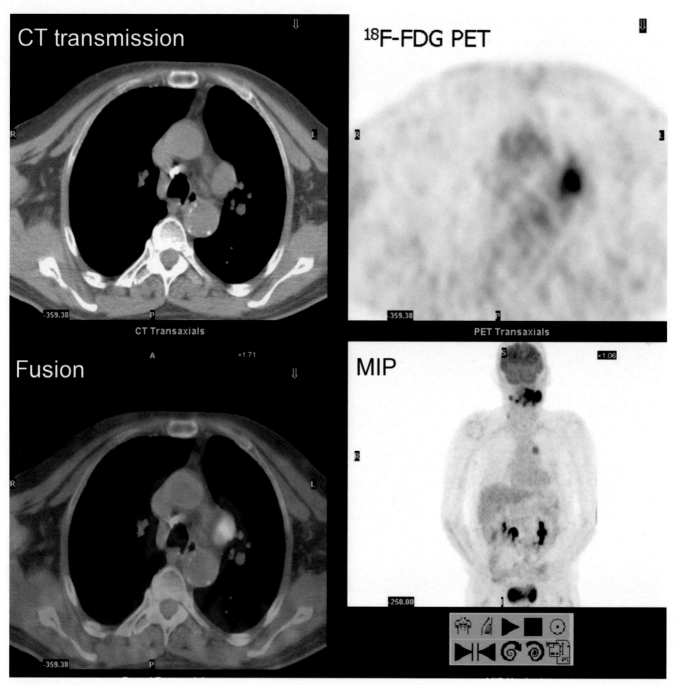

Figure 8.4 C

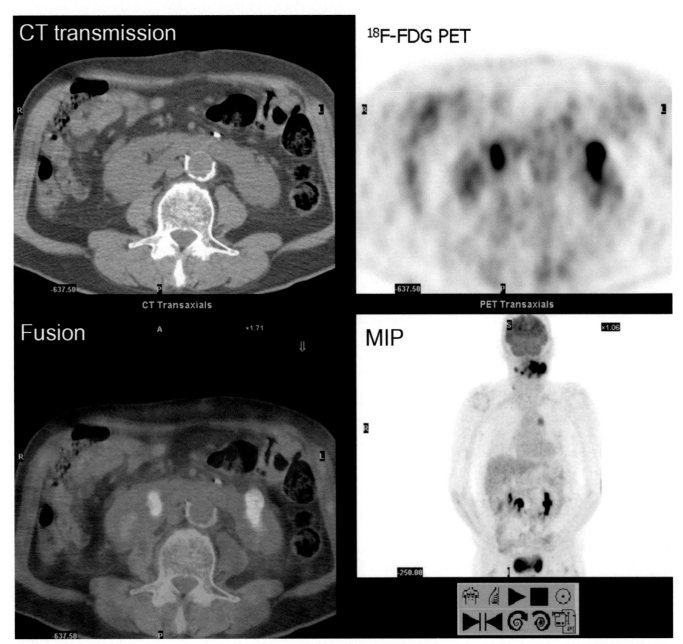

Figure 8.4 D

Findings: The fusion ^{18}F-FDG PET/CT images (Fig. 8.4 A) clearly show increased uptake in the floor of the mouth just to the left of midline extending posteriorly into the left parapharyngeal space, corresponding with a large soft tissue density mass on CT transmission images (CT not shown). There is also intense ^{18}F-FDG uptake corresponding to extensive lymphadenopathy in the left and right cervical region (levels I and II) on CT scan and to a right level III node (Fig. 8.4 B). There is also a focus of uptake in the mediastinum corresponding to a 2.3- by 3.2-cm lymph node in the aortopulmonary window (Fig. 8.4 C).

There is an incidental finding of horseshoe kidney (Fig. 8.4 D) and extensive vascular calcification.

Discussion: The findings are consistent with a large primary oropharyngeal tumor with extensive lymph node involvement and probable metastatic disease in the mediastinum, subsequently confirmed by mediastinoscopy and lymph node biopsy (stage IVC). He was treated with chemo- and radiation therapy.

For accurate staging of head and neck cancer, it is very important to be familiar with the TNM staging system recently updated by the American Joint Committee on Cancer (AJCC) (17). Although each primary site of tumor has a site-specific staging classification, typically primary tumors are staged according to size, from T1 to T4, with T4 indicating invasion of adjacent vessels, muscle, bone, or cartilage. For cervical nodes, N1 denotes a single ipsilateral node less than 3 cm, N2 indicates single or multiple nodes between 3 and 6 cm, and N3 refers to node(s) greater than 6 cm in greatest dimension. For all head and neck cancers regardless of the primary site, involvement of neck nodes has important therapeutic and prognostic implications. Therefore the knowledge of nodal anatomy and the standard system for describing the location of nodes is critical for proper communication with referring surgeons (18).

For initial staging of head and neck carcinoma, ^{18}F-FDG PET has a 10% advantage in sensitivity and specificity over CT, MRI, or ultrasound (US) (19,20). The reported change in management due to PET is in the range of 8% to 15% of the cases. As the accuracy of ^{18}F-FDG PET is superior to CT and MRI, ^{18}F-FDG PET/CT is recommended in the preoperative staging of patients with head and neck cancer. The high specificity (about 90%) and positive predictive value (PPV) (about 85%) of a positive PET scan indicates the need for neck dissection. The negative predictive value (NPV) is in the 90% range on a patient basis and there is still a debate regarding neck dissection in the N0 neck patient, since microscopic disease is below the resolution of any imaging modality and does occur in some 10% to 20% of patients (21,22).

In the post-therapy setting, there is a consensus that PET/CT has a clear advantage over CT or MR imaging in the evaluation of head and neck carcinoma. However, interpretation of ^{18}F-FDG PET images should be performed with the surgical and treatment history and correlation with CT and MRI for precise localization of the lesions (23,24).

^{18}F-FDG PET is also helpful for detection of the primary lesion of metastatic cancer of unknown primary (CUP). ^{18}F-FDG PET detects the primary in 43% (range 8% to 65%) of patients, which approximately doubles the rate of detection compared with conventional diagnostic procedures (25).

As for other primaries, the performance of PET/CT has been compared with that of PET alone. PET/CT aids in precisely localizing lesions and decreasing the number of equivocal lesions by 53%, resulting in a higher accuracy than PET alone (96% versus 90%) and a favorable impact on management in 18% of patients (26).

^{18}F-FDG is excreted by the kidneys, and transaxial and coronal images are usually most helpful in differentiating renal uptake from uptake in another anatomic structure. In this patient, the pattern of uptake clearly shows the shape of a horseshoe kidney. Unrecognized renal transplants can appear as malignant lesions. Although the absence of the native kidneys should be a warning sign, simultaneously acquired CT images delineate the anatomy and help avoid false-positive findings. Focal accumulation in the ureters is a common finding due to the pooling of radiotracer in the recumbent patient, although the intensity and location of uptake usually allow accurate identification of the ureters in patients with abdominal malignancies, especially on the coronal projections.

Diagnosis: (a) Carcinoma in the oral cavity. (b) Extensive bilateral metastatic cervical lymphadenopathy. (c) Metastatic focus in the aortopulmonary window, elevating the patient's disease to stage IV and changing management. (d) Horseshoe kidney.

CASE 8.5

History: This 43-year-old man was recently diagnosed with medullary carcinoma of the thyroid (MCT) on the basis of fine-needle aspiration (FNA) biopsy. The patient had not undergone any therapy. He was referred for ^{18}F-FDG PET/CT imaging (Fig. 8.5) for initial staging.

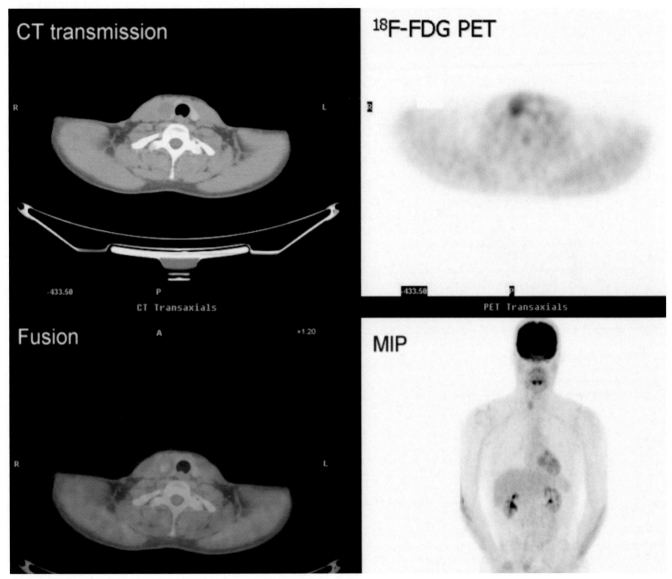

Figure 8.5

Findings: PET/CT imaging reveals a 2.1- by 2.0-cm solid nodule within the right lobe of the thyroid, which is moderately ^{18}F-FDG–avid, as is usually seen in MCT.

Discussion: ^{18}F-FDG PET is currently the most accurate technique for the detection of persistent/recurrent MCT and is more sensitive than CT or MRI (27). All imaging modalities are dependent on volume of disease and size of lesions for the detection of metastatic and recurrent MCT. While the overall sensitivity for detection of disease with ^{18}F-FDG PET/CT is only 63%, the sensitivity rises to 78% when the serum calcitonin is >1,000 pg/mL. With low-volume disease, sensitivity is quite low, 20% with serum calcitonin <1,000 pg/mL and

0% with calcitonin <500 pg/mL. When ^{18}F-FDG PET/CT is negative, conventional imaging and SSR imaging is also often negative (28).

Medullary carcinoma of the thyroid, representing approximately 3% to 5% of all thyroid cancers, is an intermediate-grade malignancy occurring in both sporadic (80%) and familial (20%) forms. There is an autosomal dominant inheritance in families with multiple endocrine neoplasia (MEN) 2A and 2B. Nearly 50% of patients have metastatic cervical adenopathy at presentation. With clinically palpable disease, surgical cure is rarely achieved, despite regional lymphadenectomy, but the 10-year survival rate is 86% even with persistent postoperative hypercalcitoninemia (29). Five-year survival is 94% in patients with metastatic lymphadenopathy but only 41% in those with extranodal disease (30). Only in the occasional patient with MCT is the tumor radioiodine-avid, so ^{131}I scintigraphy is not useful and ^{131}I treatment results in no improvement in survival or recurrence rate (31).

Surgery is currently the only potentially curative approach to the management of MCT. Persistent or recurrent disease is easily detected by elevated serum levels of tumor markers, calcitonin and carcinoembryonic antigen (CEA), but localization of persistent/recurrent disease remains a diagnostic problem. Most medullary tumors express SSRs, and the majority of patients with slow-growing or occult disease will have a positive localization with ^{111}In-octreotide scintigraphy, although the extent of disease may be underestimated (32). Like other neuroectodermal tumors, 40% to 50% of MCTs will take up ^{123}I/^{131}I-MIBG (33). Although less sensitive than

^{201}Tl, ^{99m}Tc-(V)-DMSA, and ^{99m}Tc-MIBI, ^{131}I-MIBG is poorly sensitive (about 30%) but highly specific and may thus be useful in conjunction with other localization modalities. Furthermore, the therapeutic efficacy of high-dose (100 to 300 mCi) ^{131}I-MIBG in patients with significant uptake appears promising (34,35). Although a complete response is uncommon, a partial response with significant symptom palliation and hormonal improvement has occurred in the majority of the cases.

In summary, ^{18}F-FDG PET appears to be the modality of choice for evaluation of patients with suspicion of recurrent MCT, especially in those with low-volume disease. There are few data regarding the role of scintigraphic imaging at initial staging.

Diagnosis: Primary medullary thyroid carcinoma without evidence of metastases.

CASE 8.6

History: A 78-year-old male with a history of papillary thyroid carcinoma treated by total thyroidectomy presented with a serum thyroglobulin elevated to 11.9 ng/mL. On three occasions, he had been treated with high-dose ^{131}I therapy. The most recent post-therapy ^{131}I whole-body scan revealed no evidence of cervical or distant radioiodine-avid metastases. ^{18}F-FDG PET/CT was requested for further assessment (Fig. 8.6). The patient received parenteral recombinant TSH 24 hours and 48 hours prior to administration of ^{18}F-FDG.

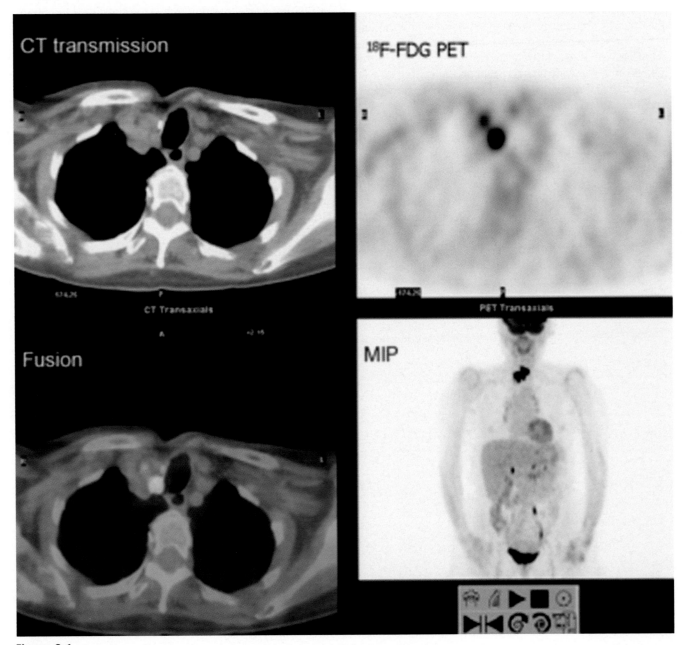

Figure 8.6

Findings: ^{18}F-FDG PET/CT images reveal a large conglomerate of intensely increased activity at the base of the neck in the midline extending into the right neck. The most inferior foci in the right neck shown on the transaxial images correspond to subcentimeter lymph nodes.

Discussion: These findings are consistent with metastatic thyroid carcinoma. A conglomerate of metastatic nodes was subsequently resected from the neck; 4 months postoperatively, serum thyroglobulin was undetectable and a repeat CT of the neck was unrevealing, indicative of a complete response to therapy.

Whole-body ^{131}I scintigraphy has a sensitivity of 60% to 70% for the detection of metastases, in part dependent upon the dose of radioiodine utilized. Metastases are more often seen with a 10-mCi diagnostic dose of ^{131}I than with a 2- to 5-mCi dose, and posttherapy scans obtained 5 to 8 days after a >100-mCi dose of ^{131}I reveal additional lesions or clarify equivocal abnormalities seen on a diagnostic scan in as many as 35% of patients. The visualization of ^{131}I-avid metastases is of utmost importance in view of the well-demonstrated efficacy of ^{131}I therapy in patients with such disease. However, as these differentiated neoplasms are subjected to various therapies, they may dedifferentiate, losing the iodine symporter and thus failing to accumulate radioiodine while retaining the ability to express thyroglobulin. Other differentiated thyroid neoplasms as well as less differentiated ones—including Hurthle cell, medullary, and anaplastic carcinomas—are not ^{131}I-avid. These thyroid neoplasms not detected by ^{131}I scintigraphy have been successfully imaged using ^{201}Tl, ^{99m}Tc-sestamibi, and ^{99m}Tc-tetrofosmin, but ^{18}F-FDG PET has demonstrated high sensitivity and specificity for the detection of these tumors and their metastases.

Although ^{18}F-FDG PET may demonstrate some ^{131}I-avid tumors, a heterogeneous population of ^{131}I-positive/^{18}F-FDG-negative and ^{131}I-negative/^{18}F-FDG-positive metastases may coexist in an individual patient. In an unselected population of patients with thyroid cancer, the sensitivity of ^{18}F-FDG PET is in the range of 50% to 75%. ^{18}F-FDG PET has proved most useful in the population of thyroid carcinoma patients who are suspected of harboring metastases due to elevated serum thyroglobulin but in whom conventional imaging and ^{131}I whole-body scintigraphy are negative, with a sensitivity in the range of 70% to 90%. PET has localized occult metastases in 50% to 82% of such patients and altered therapy in about 30% (36). High ^{18}F-FDG uptake indicates a poor prognosis, especially if there is high-volume disease (37). TSH stimulation enhances ^{18}F-FDG uptake by malignant thyroid tumors; therefore rhTSH or thyroid hormone withdrawal is recommended to improve the sensitivity for detection of recurrent and/or metastatic disease (38).

In summary, ^{131}I scintigraphy is the preferred modality for the detection of recurrent/metastatic differentiated thyroid carcinoma because of its ability to identify a tumor treatable with high-dose radioiodine administration. In patients suspected of metastatic disease but in whom ^{131}I imaging is unrevealing, ^{18}F-FDG PET offers high sensitivity and specificity for the detection of metastases, which may then be treated by surgical resection or external radiotherapy. TSH stimulation by thyroid hormone withdrawal or rhTSH administration enhances sensitivity. ^{18}F-FDG imaging is also helpful in patients with Hurthle cell carcinoma (39), medullary carcinoma, and probably anaplastic carcinoma.

Diagnosis: Radioiodine-negative, ^{18}F-FDG-positive metastatic thyroid cancer.

CASE 8.7

History: An 80-year-old male was referred for initial staging of esophageal carcinoma using ^{18}F-FDG PET/CT imaging (Figs. 8.7 A and 8.7 B).

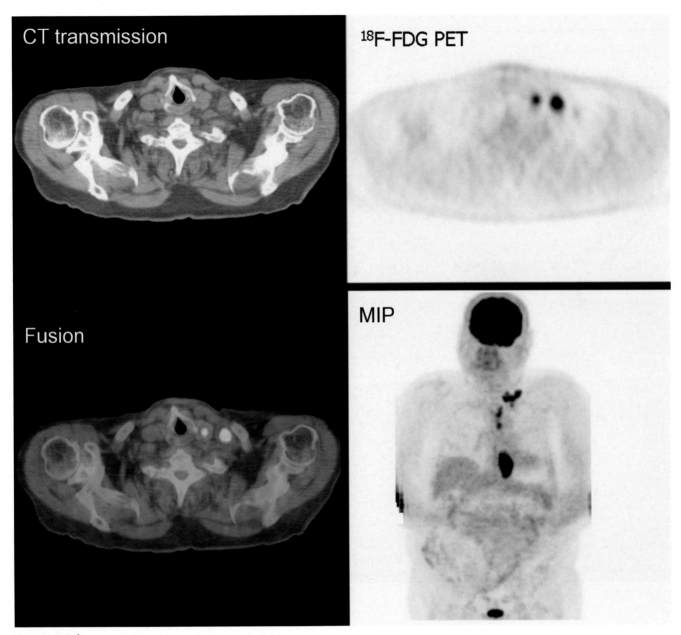

Figure 8.7 A

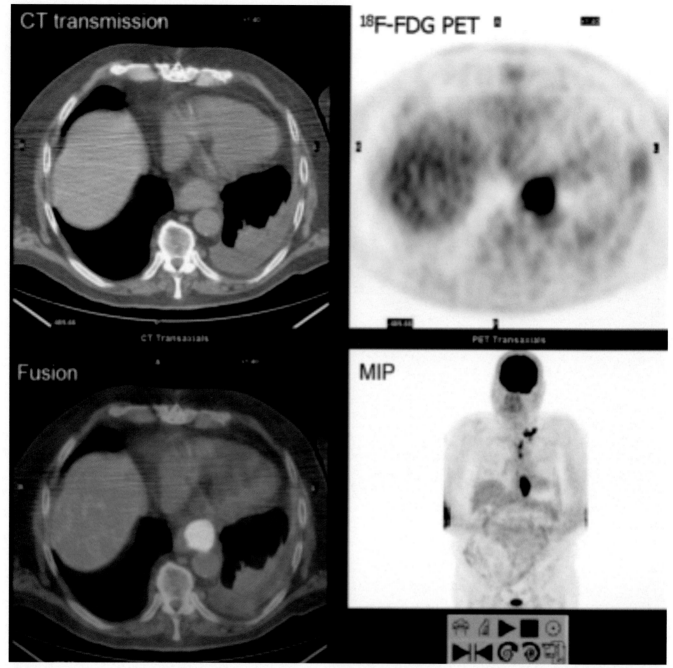

Figure 8.7 B

Findings: The images reveal marked ^{18}F-FDG uptake along the distal esophagus, corresponding to the portion of the esophagus with marked thickening on the CT scan (Fig. 8.7 B) and consistent with the patient's known primary esophageal carcinoma. In addition, multiple foci of ^{18}F-FDG uptake are seen in the mediastinum (paraesophageal and paratracheal) and left supraclavicular regions, corresponding to lymph nodes seen on the CT images (Fig. 8.7 B) and indicative of metastases.

Discussion: These findings are consistent with the patient's known primary esophageal carcinoma with involvement of mediastinal and left supraclavicular lymph nodes. This case demonstrates the value of preoperative ^{18}F-FDG PET imaging in the evaluation of esophageal carcinoma. ^{18}F-FDG PET is more sensitive than CT at detecting distant metastasis and at least as sensitive as CT in detecting regional metastasis. This is of critical importance, since approximately 20% of patients with esophageal cancer being considered for surgical therapy have distant metastases (40). ^{18}F-FDG PET also demonstrates the primary tumor in the vast majority of patients. Both CT and PET are limited by their inability to determine the depth of wall invasion; however, endoscopic ultrasound (EUS) is useful in this regard. When ^{18}F-FDG PET is performed in addition to CT, ill-advised surgery may be decreased by 90%. PET may play a role in differentiating responders from nonresponders after chemotherapy as well. Therefore PET imaging followed by EUS with FNA biopsy of abnormal lymph nodes or

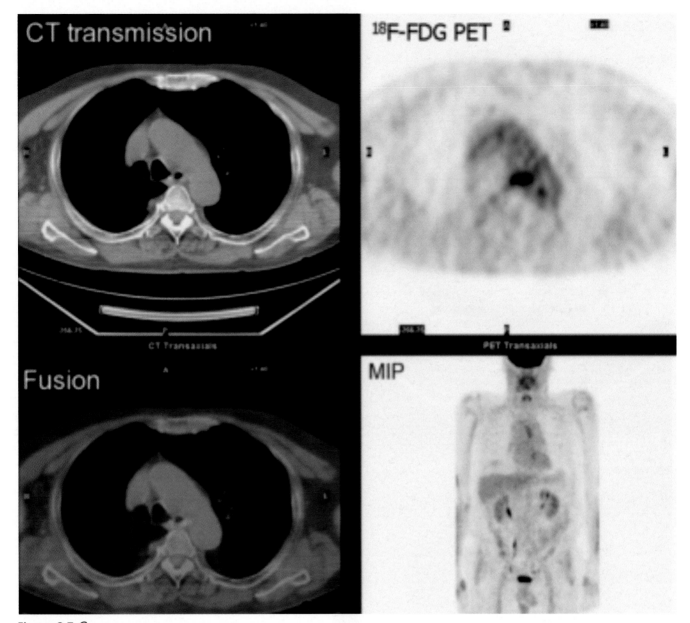

Figure 8.7 C

metastases provides the most cost-effective strategy for preoperative staging and management of patients with carcinoma of the esophagus (41).

Esophageal carcinoma is often treated preoperatively with neoadjuvant chemoradiation therapy, and ^{18}F-FDG PET is useful to assess the response to therapy prior to surgery. After radiation therapy, radiation-induced esophagitis occurs; these inflammatory changes should not be confused with residual tumor Fig. 8.6 C, as illustrated from a different patient with lung cancer who underwent PET/CT imaging 2 weeks following chemoradiation therapy. The uptake matches the radiation field and corresponds to a normal esophagus on the CT scan.

Diagnosis: Distal esophageal carcinoma with evidence of mediastinal and left supraclavicular metastases.

CASE 8.8

History: This 76-year-old female presented with a 1.5-cm pulmonary nodule in the right lower lobe. ^{18}F-FDG PET/CT imaging was performed to further characterize the lesion (Fig. 8.8)

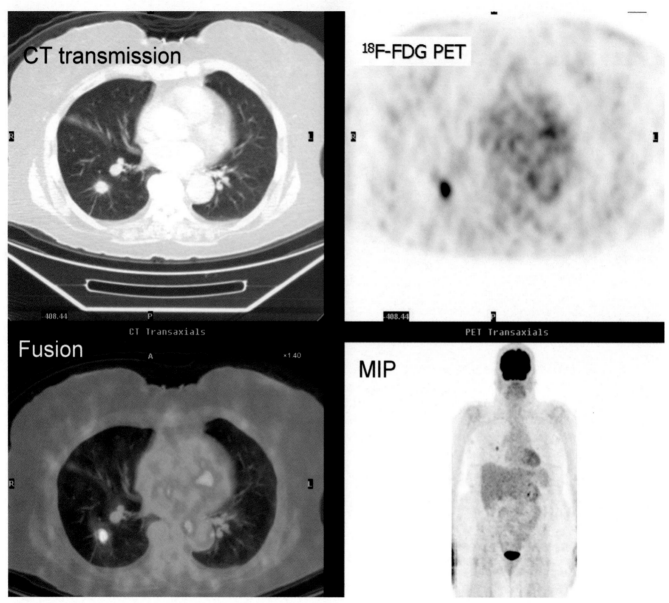

Figure 8.8

Findings: The pulmonary nodule in the right lower lobe demonstrates moderate ^{18}F-FDG avidity above that of normal liver parenchyma. No evidence of hypermetabolic foci is noted in the mediastinum.

Discussion: These findings indicate that the pulmonary nodule is likely malignant; a less likely explanation includes granulomatous infection. A biopsy demonstrated carcinoma.

In the United States, 130,000 new solitary pulmonary nodules (SPNs) are diagnosed annually, but only 30% to 50% are malignant. Chest radiography and CT have well-known limitations for differentiating benign from malignant nodules. This leads to a large number of invasive procedures. Transbronchial and percutaneous lung biopsy suffer from sampling error. In addition, percutaneous needle biopsy may be complicated by a pneumothorax, requiring chest tube placement in up to 5% to 10% of these patients (42). Functional imaging with ^{18}F-FDG can identify malignant lesions with a sensitivity ranging from 77% to 100% and an accuracy of 81% to 94%. In a meta-analysis including 40 studies and 1,474 focal pulmonary lesions, the maximum joint sensitivity and specificity of ROC curve was 91%; the authors concluded that to decrease the false-negative rate, ^{18}F-FDG PET must operate at sensitivity of 96% and specificity 78% (43). It has been suggested that some of these variations may be related to the regional prevalence of granulomatous diseases. False-negative exams are generally due to small-sized lesions relative to scanner resolution (partial volume effect), low cellularity of lesions (mucinous tumors) (44), or low metabolic activity of tumors—bronchioalveolar carcinoma (45) and carcinoid tumors (46). Lesions that are smaller than twice the size of the resolution of the imaging system at full width at half maximum suffer from partial volume averaging and may be falsely negative. The resolution of the newest state-of-the-art dedicated PET camera is 4 to 5 mm; therefore lesions greater than 1 cm in size can be evaluated without concern for partial volume averaging artifact.

Semiquantitative indices have been investigated to determine an optimal threshold of uptake to separate benign from malignant lesions. The most popular indices are the standardized uptake value (SUV) and the lesion to lung background ratio (L/B). However, SUV measurement requires rigorous quality control for accuracy as described in the introduction. Visual interpretation of the degree of uptake relative to normal liver parenchyma (average SUV about 2.0) is often adequate for clinical purposes. An SUV of 2.5 is accepted by most centers as the best threshold to differentiate benign from malignant lesions in the lungs. If a lesion greater than 1 cm in diameter has an SUV less than 2.5, malignancy can be excluded with a high degree of certainty. However, patients should always be managed by clinical and periodic imaging follow-up for 24 months. On the other hand, a positive study is not specific and requires further testing.

An analysis of potential cost benefits projects that appropriate utilization of ^{18}F-FDG PET in the evaluation of SPNs would save approximately $180 million in annual health-care costs in the United States by decreasing the number of thoracotomies and percutaneous needle biopsies performed (47).

Diagnosis: Malignant solitary pulmonary nodule.

CASE 8.9

History: A biopsy of a right hilar mass in a 66-year-old male revealed non–small cell carcinoma (NSCLC). ^{18}F-FDG PET/CT was performed for initial staging (Figs. 8.9 A and 8.9 B).

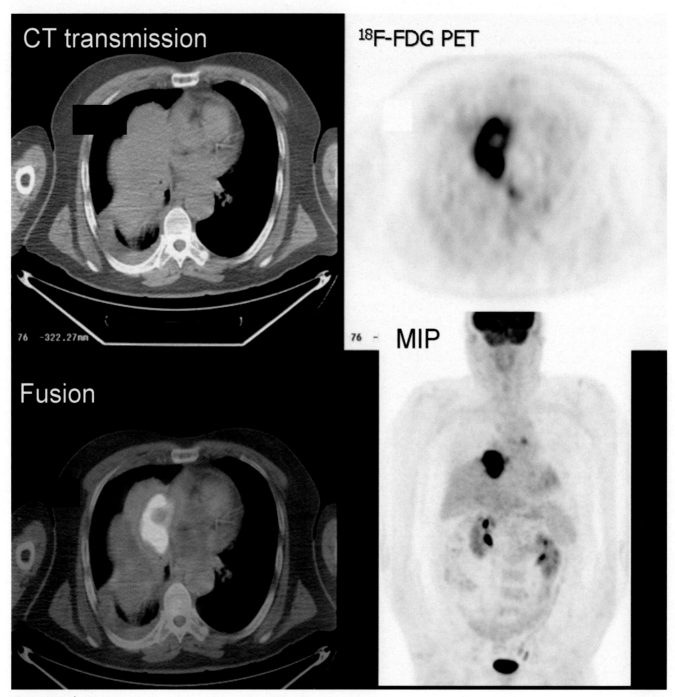

Figure 8.9 A

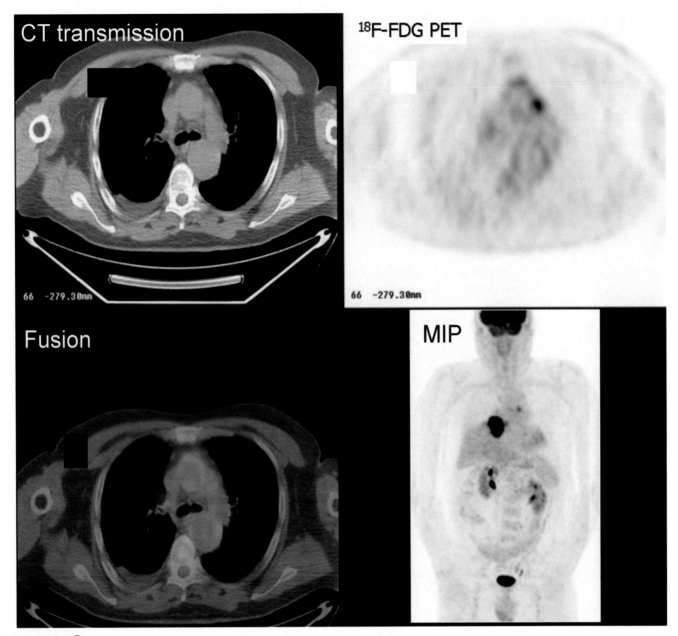

CT transmission

^{18}F-FDG PET

66 -279.30nn

66 -279.30nn

Fusion

MIP

Figure 8.9 B

Findings: There is increased ^{18}F-FDG uptake in the large right hilar mass with central photopenia, but the mass is much larger than the extent of uptake. There is also uptake in a subcentimeter paraesophageal node and a subcentimeter aortopulmonary lymph node. In addition there is a small right pleural effusion with partial consolidation. There is an aneurysm of the ascending and descending aorta.

Discussion: The image findings represent a stage IIIB NSCLC which is not curable by surgery. The landmark of stage IIIB is the presence of metastatic contralateral lymph nodes (N3). In this case, the lymph nodes do not meet size criteria for malignant involvement by CT, so PET was critical for optimal management. In addition the tumor is surrounded by a large area of atelectasism which has implications for determining the field of radiation therapy, as discussed in the introduction to this chapter (9). Using PET/CT, the gross target volume

(GTV) is altered (increased or decreased by 25%) in up to 56% of cases. The GTV variability between two independent oncologists is decreased and the treatment is changed from curative to palliative in some 15% of patients.

For accurate staging, it is very important to be familiar with the TNM staging system for NSCLC, recently updated by the AJCC (48). It is also very important to be familiar with the 1996 AJCC–Union Internationale Contre le Cancer (UICC) regional lymph node classification for lung cancer staging (49). Surgical resection is the treatment of choice for patients who have unilateral disease, including ipsilateral lymph nodes (stage N2). Involvement of contralateral lymph nodes (stage N3) is, however, a contraindication to surgery. The criteria for determining lymph node involvement on anatomic imaging studies (CT and MRI) are based on shape and size only. These criteria have obvious limitations, as small lymph nodes may be involved by tumor and benign inflammatory nodes may be enlarged. In a 1997 report, sensitivity and specificity of CT and MRI for detecting mediastinal involvement was 48% to 52% and 64% to 69% respectively (50). Twenty percent of patients with a negative CT have positive mediastinoscopy (51), and 15% of patients with a negative mediastinoscopy have N2 disease at surgery (52). Therefore CT cannot replace mediastinoscopy for accurate staging of the mediastinum, but mediastinoscopy is limited to the anterior mediastinum in addition to sampling error do underestimate mediastinal involvement.

^{18}F-FDG imaging detects mediastinal involvement with a sensitivity of 76% to 89% and specificity of 81% to 99%; however, ^{18}F-FDG PET does not permit evaluation of bronchial, vascular, and pleural involvement and therefore should be performed in addition to (not in place of) CT (53). In a meta-analysis including 14 studies (514 patients) for ^{18}F-FDG PET and 29 studies (2,226 patients) for CT, both the sensitivity and specificity of ^{18}F-FDG PET were superior to CT (79% versus 60% for sensitivity and 91% versus 77% for specificity) for staging the mediastinum (54). In a prospective study of 102 patients, the sensitivity of PET was 91% compared to 75% for CT, the specificity of PET was 86% compared to 77% for CT, and PET detected distant metastases in 10% of patients (55). The addition of PET to the conventional workup is cost-effective (56). PET/CT has proven to be more effective than the simple concomitant analysis of PET and CT alone (57).

If a PET/CT does not demonstrate mediastinal or distant metastases, surgery may proceed without mediastinoscopy. A positive PET showing the primary site and evidence of mediastinal involvement requires mediastinoscopy, not only to exclude false positive findings but also to separate patients with minimal N2 disease (that may be treated with neoadjuvant chemotherapy with subsequent surgery) from patients with more extensive N2 or N3 disease (58).

The effectiveness of PET in the staging of patients with NSCLC has been shown to change patient management in 19% to 41% of cases. Of particular importance is the exclusion of surgery by demonstration of unsuspected distant metastases. The multicenter PLUS trial included 188 patients from 9 hospitals who were randomized to conventional workup (CWU) and CWU plus PET. The endpoint was futile thoracotomy. This trial demonstrated that PET decreased futile thoracotomies in 50% of patients. There were 41% futile thoracotomies with CWU and only 21% with CWU plus PET.

Cerebral, skeletal, and adrenal metastases are common in patients with lung cancer and indicative of incurable stage IV disease. ^{18}F-FDG has limited sensitivity (about 60%) for detection of cerebral metastases because of the high physiologic uptake in the gray matter; MRI remains the standard of care. However, if the brain is in the field of view, careful examination will reveal unexpected metastases in some 0.5% of cases (59). For detection of skeletal metastases, ^{18}F-FDG PET has a sensitivity in the same range as skeletal scintigraphy but is much more specific (60). The topic of detection of skeletal metastases is further discussed in Case 8.11.

Incidental adrenal masses are identified in approximately 2% of patients undergoing CT imaging for reasons other than an adrenal mass. In patients without a known malignancy, the likelihood of an incidental (<5 cm) adrenal mass representing a malignant neoplasm is very low. After an appropriate endocrinologic evaluation to exclude a functioning adrenal neoplasm, a follow-up CT without biopsy is generally recommended. In patients with a known malignancy, an incidental adrenal mass may represent metastasis in 27% to 36% of patients; in such patients, accurate diagnosis is important for treatment planning. Many of these patients undergo percutaneous needle biopsy, which has an accuracy of 80% to 100%. On noncontrasted CT, most metastases are over 20 Hounsfield units (HU), and 85% of adenomas are <18 HU. All masses with <2 HU are benign. Metastases enhance more intensely than do benign lesions. Looking at attenuation with contrast enhancement and delayed contrast washout is also helpful to the extent that >60% enhancement washout at 15 minutes is indicative of benignity.

MRI is also emerging as a useful modality in differentiating benign from malignant adrenal and bone lesions. In a series of 20 patients with 24 incidental adrenal masses and a known malignancy, ^{18}F-FDG PET was able to separate benign (10) from malignant (14) lesions in all cases (61). Benign adrenal adenomas have ^{18}F-FDG activity less than or similar to that of normal liver parenchyma. ^{18}F-FDG PET is the modality of choice for masses indeterminate on CT and is a preferable technique in patients with known malignancy for staging the whole body.

PET has an important role in the evaluation of patients with small cell lung cancer. Patients are staged in a binary distinction between limited disease, with tumor confined to one hemithorax, and with extensive disease. Therefore accurate staging is important, since this determines subsequent therapy and prognosis. Several studies have demonstrated the potential usefulness of ^{18}F-FDG PET as a simplified staging tool in these patients (62). In treated patients, survival is lower in patients with PET-positive findings than in patients with PET-negative results; SUV max has a significant negative correlation with survival (63).

Diagnosis: (a) NSCLC, stage IIIB. (b) Large area of postobstructive atelectasis.

History: A 62-year-old woman was found to have carcinoma upon FNA biopsy of a left breast mass. After the intradermal injection of 240 μCi of filtered ^{99m}Tc–sulfur colloid in a circumferential pattern around the breast mass, delayed static images were acquired prior to lumpectomy and excisional biopsy of the axillary sentinel node (Fig. 8.10 A).

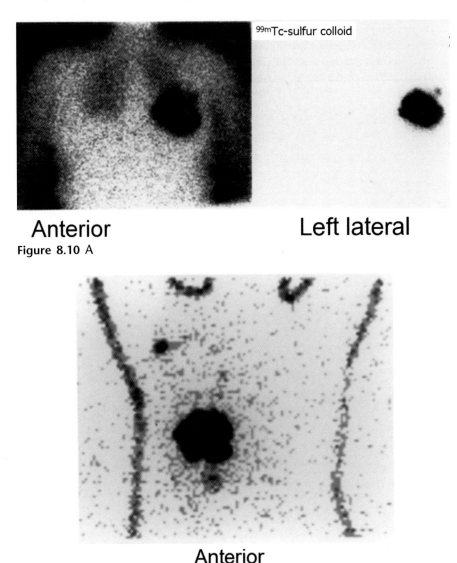

Anterior

Figure 8.10 A

Left lateral

^{99m}Tc-sulfur colloid

Anterior

Figure 8.10 B

Findings: A solitary focus of increased activity is identified in the left axilla on the left lateral view (Fig. 8.10 A). Because of the large amount of activity in the breast, the lesion is more difficult to visualize on the anterior views; the skin was tattooed to aid localization of the sentinel node at surgery performed later that morning.

Discussion: The accumulation of radiolabeled colloid merely identifies the first lymph node to which the breast mass drains; it does not indicate pathology. Following lumpectomy, a hand-held gamma probe was used intraoperatively to identify the axillary sentinel node for excisional biopsy.

A good review of this topic is available (64). There is strong evidence that the histopathology of the sentinel node does predict involvement of the other nodes in the region. The sentinel node(s) can be localized at minimally invasive surgery in 92% to 100% of patients using an intraoperative probe. False-negative sentinel nodes have been reported in <3% of patients, but many of these have occurred in patients with multicentric tumors. In fact, one investigator has reported a higher incidence (43%) of tumor when only the sentinel node was examined than when all the nodes within the axilla (29%) were examined, indicative of more accurate staging. The routine use of lymphoscintigraphy in patients with clinically negative axillary nodes results in the avoidance of axillary lymphadenectomy in the patients who do not have lymphatic tumor and reduces morbidity and costs considerably.

Furthermore, lymphoscintigraphy has documented drainage occurring across the breast to internal mammary or axillary nodes in 32% of patients with outer- or inner-quadrant lesions; drainage of an upper outer-quadrant mass may cross to the internal mammary chain in as many as 56% of patients (65). This is illustrated in another patient with a biopsy-proven breast carcinoma in the inferomedial quadrant of her right breast who underwent lymphoscintigraphy (Fig. 8.10 B). In addition to the right axillary sentinel node easily seen on the outlined body profile, there is faint activity in an internal mammary node superior to the medial border of the breast.

From the technical point of view, multiple routes including intradermal, intraparenchymal, periareolar, and subareolar have been used for ^{99m}Tc–sulfur colloid administration. A recent prospective randomized study of 400 patients demonstrated that the intradermal route demonstrated a greater frequency of localization, decreased time to first localization on preoperative lymphoscintigraphy, and decreased time to harvest the first sentinel lymph node (66).

Diagnosis: Breast cancer with localization of axillary sentinel node.

History: A 28-year-old female presented with recently diagnosed carcinoma of the left breast with previous history of mammoplasty. She was referred to ^{18}F-FDG PET/CT for initial staging (Figs. 8.11 A–D).

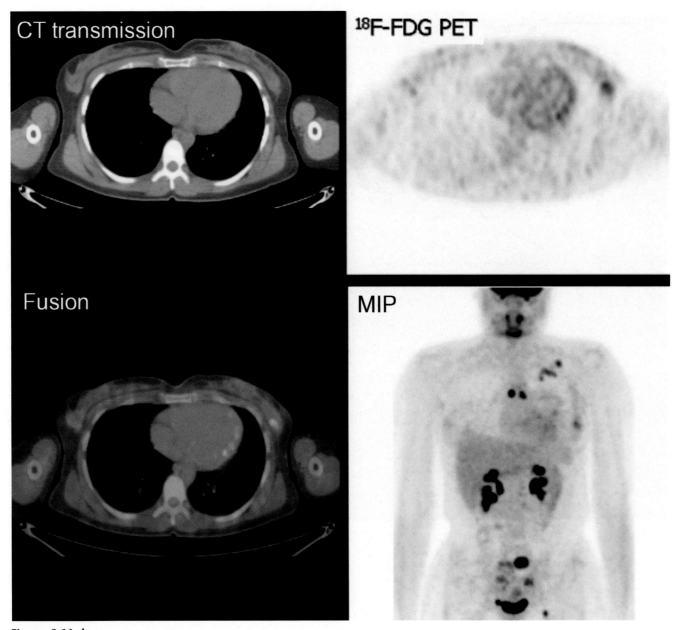

Figure 8.11 A

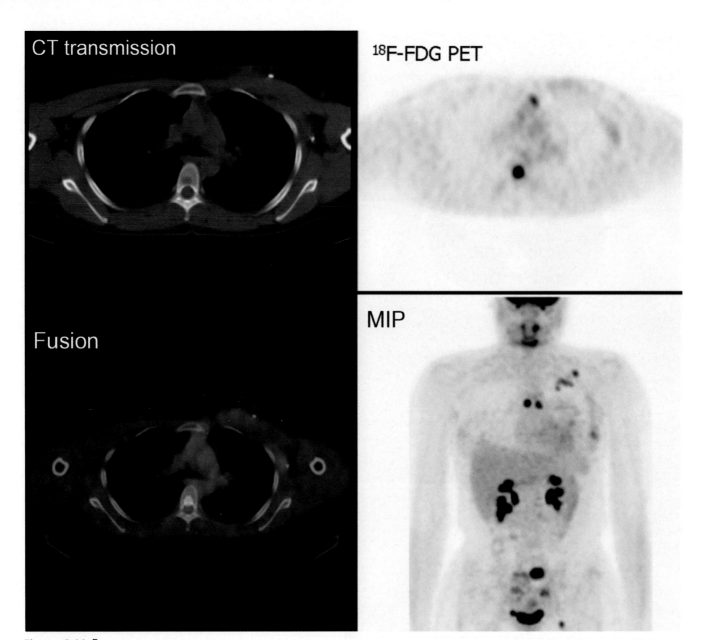

CT transmission

¹⁸F-FDG PET

Fusion

MIP

Figure 8.11 B

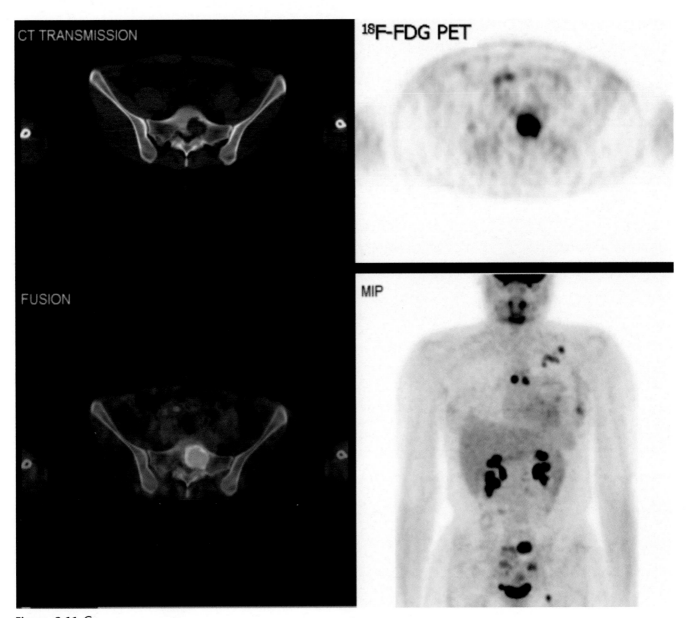

CT TRANSMISSION

¹⁸F-FDG PET

FUSION

MIP

Figure 8.11 C

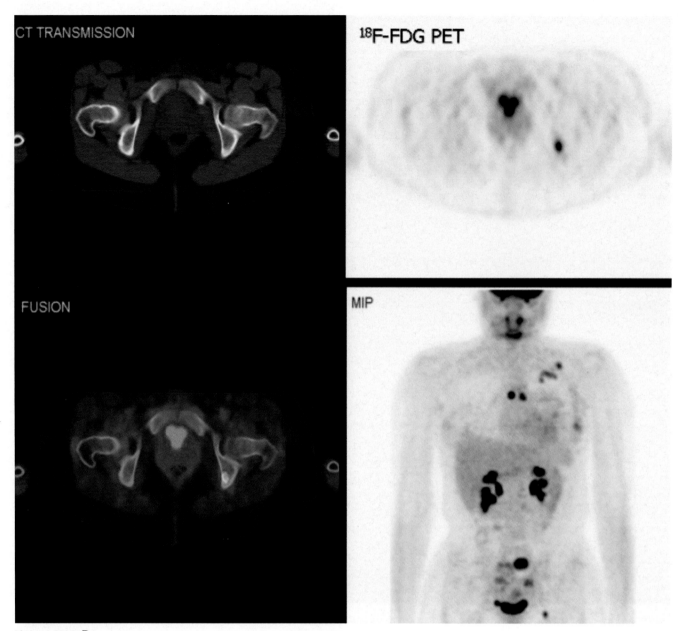

Figure 8.11 D

Findings: A focus of increased ^{18}F-FDG activity is noted in the region of the left breast and axilla. These areas are associated with postsurgical change and stranding on the transmission CT scan (Fig. 8.11 A). An additional focus of intense hypermetabolic activity is seen within a left internal mammary nodule (Fig. 8.11 B). Multiple hypermetabolic areas are seen in the spine congruent with lytic lesions within the vertebral bodies of T6, T10, T11 (MIP) as well as a lytic lesion within the left sacrum (Fig. 8.11 C). One other focus of activity is noted in the left posterior acetabulum without associated lytic change on the CT scan (Fig. 8.11 D).

Discussion: The foci of increased activity in the bones are consistent with metastatic skeletal lesions confirmed in most but not all by lytic lesions seen on CT. The skeleton is the most common site of distant metastases in breast cancer. Most patients with breast cancer have skeletal metastases

that are lytic, but 15% to 20% of patients have osteoblastic lesions.

Both ^{18}F-FDG PET and conventional diphosphonate bone scintigraphy are used to detect skeletal metastases in cancer patients. ^{99m}Tc-diphosphonate used in conventional bone scintigraphy is chemically adsorbed onto the bone surface; its uptake is dependent on local blood flow, osteoblastic activity, and capillary permeability. Since most metastatic skeletal lesions are associated with an osteoblastic reaction in the surrounding bone as well as increased vascularity, there is focal accumulation of the radiopharmaceutical in and around the metastasis. Purely lytic lesions, unaccompanied by osteoblastic activity, may demonstrate poor or absent activity.

^{18}F-FDG, on the other hand, accumulates in viable neoplastic tissues, including skeletal metastases, which have a higher glycolytic rate than the surrounding tissues and are not dependent upon other factors such as a surrounding osteoblastic reaction to the predominantly medullary tumor. Whole-body ^{18}F-FDG PET imaging can demonstrate not only skeletal metastases but also any other metastatic lesions as well as local recurrences. Furthermore, owing to its mechanism of uptake, the specificity of ^{18}F-FDG for malignant neoplasm is much higher than that of the diphosphonates. Because of their different mechanism of uptake, bone scintigraphy is more sensitive for detection of blastic metastases that are poorly detected with ^{18}F-FDG PET because of the low cellularity of these lesions and ^{18}F-FDG PET is more sensitive for the detection of lytic lesions. The hybrid PET/CT technology permits evaluation of both ^{18}F-FDG avidity and anatomic characterization on CT, which helps in detecting blastic metastases and differentiating benign from malignant lesions. Following treatment, ^{18}F-FDG–negative/CT-positive (usually sclerotic/blastic) lesions are more prevalent and probably reflect the efficacy of treatment.

The PET tracer ^{18}F-fluoride is also available for evaluation of the skeleton, and its mechanism of uptake, like that of diphosphonates, depends on bone mineralization. However, the first-pass extraction is higher than for the disphosphonates and the resolution of PET is better than that of planar or SPECT imaging. ^{18}F-fluoride PET/CT is more sensitive and specific than planar and SPECT diphosphonate scintigraphy and than ^{18}F-fluoride PET alone in prostate cancer and a variety of other neoplasms (67).

An excellent review of the role of ^{18}F-FDG PET imaging in breast cancer is available (68). For accurate TNM staging, it is important to be familiar with the TNM staging system as recently updated by the AJCC (69).

A large prospective study has demonstrated limited sensitivity of PET (61%) for detection of lymph node metastases (70). The sensitivity of PET is also limited in early-stage breast cancer compared to sentinel node biopsy (71). Microscopic lymph node metastases not detected by PET leads to the understaging of these patients. Therefore for staging early breast carcinoma, identification and sampling of the sentinel lymph node is the standard of care (see Case 8.10). If the sentinel lymph node is positive, axillary lymph adenectomy is usually performed as a diagnostic procedure for staging purposes since the presence of nodal metastases is the most important prognostic factor in patients with breast carcinoma (72).

For advanced local disease, the advantages of ^{18}F-FDG PET imaging include the detection of unsuspected distant metastases (73) and the ability to detect internal mammary and mediastinal lymph node metastases that are not routinely sampled with the current standard of care (74). ^{18}F-FDG PET imaging is the modality of choice for detecting recurrent disease and restaging. In a meta-analysis, the sensitivity and specificity were 93% and 82% respectively (75). The impact of PET on the management of patients with breast cancer, ranging from 22% to 36%, has been demonstrated in several studies (76,77). The incremental value of PET/CT has also been demonstrated (78).

Diagnosis: (a) Breast carcinoma. (b) Multiple metastatic lymph nodes within the left axilla, left supraclavicular region, and left mammary chain. (c) Widespread skeletal metastasis.

CASE 8.12

History: A 66-year-old female recently diagnosed with colon adenocarcinoma has a CT scan of the abdomen and pelvis demonstrating a suspected metastatic lesion in segment IV of the liver. The patient had not received treatment and is referred for initial staging with ^{18}F-FDG PET/CT imaging (Figs. 8.12 A and 8.12 B).

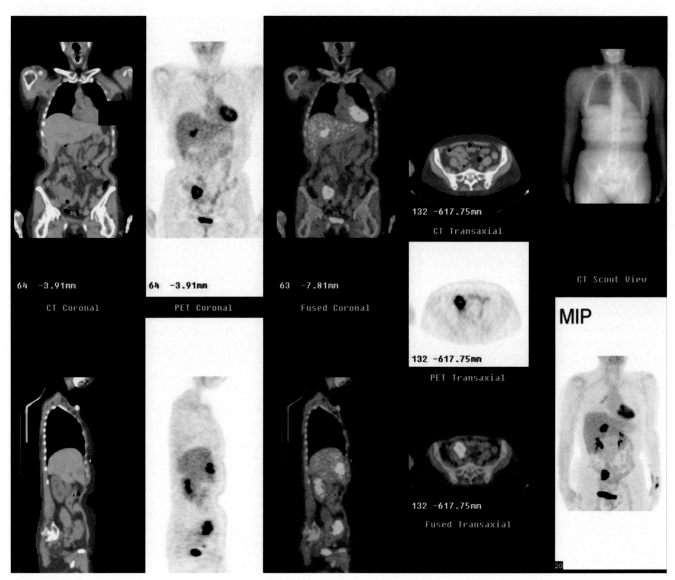

Figure 8.12 A

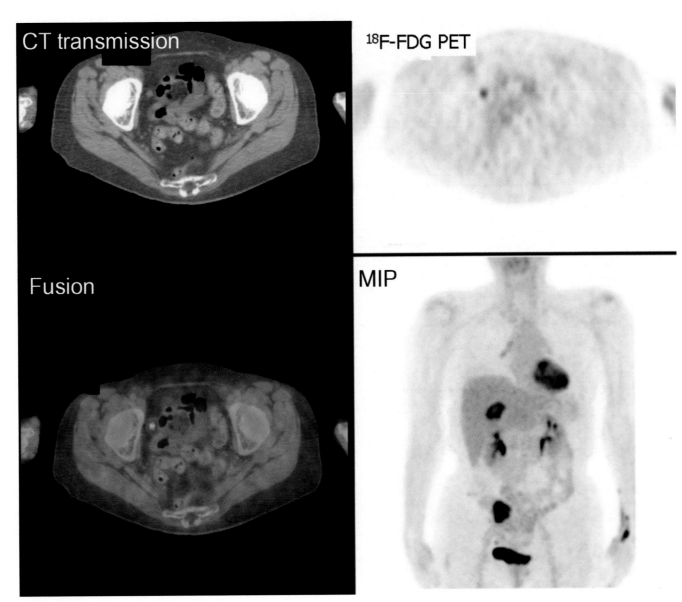

CT transmission

¹⁸F-FDG PET

Fusion

MIP

Figure 8.12 B

Findings: There is intense uptake in the primary cecal carcinoma which extends into adjacent loops of bowel as well as into the liver mass (Fig. 8.12 A). Activity within a right pelvic lymph node is also identified (Fig. 8.12 B).

Discussion: The large foci of uptake in the cecum and liver are consistent with the known primary tumor in the cecum and suspected hepatic metastasis.

A comprehensive review article discussing the role of PET in the evaluation of colorectal carcinoma is available (79). Approximately 135,000 new cases of colorectal carcinoma per year are diagnosed in the United States, and about 55,000 of these patients die of their disease annually.

Preoperative staging with imaging modalities is usually limited because most patients will benefit from colectomy to prevent intestinal obstruction and bleeding. The extent of the disease can be evaluated during surgery with excision of pericolonic and mesenteric lymph nodes along with peritoneal exploration. The performance of ¹⁸F-FDG PET preoperatively

may be helpful if the detection of distant metastases would result in cancellation of surgery in patients with increased surgical risk or in the performance of a less extensive surgical procedure. It may also be helpful as a baseline evaluation prior to chemotherapy in patients with advanced-stage disease. In the initial staging of colorectal cancer (80), ¹⁸F-FDG PET imaging identified most lesions and was superior to CT for the detection of hepatic metastases; however, it was as poor as CT for detecting local lymph node involvement. In one study, ¹⁸F-FDG PET imaging changed the management in 8% of patients and the extent of surgery in 13%.

¹⁸F-FDG PET imaging is better established in patients with suspected recurrent or metastatic colorectal carcinoma. About 14,000 patients per year present with isolated liver metastases as their first recurrence, and about 20% of these die with metastases exclusively to the liver. Hepatic resection is the only curative therapy in these patients, but it is associated with a mortality of 2% to 7% and significant morbidity. Early detection

and prompt treatment of recurrences may lead to a cure in up to 25% of patients. However, the size and number of hepatic metastases and the presence of extrahepatic disease affect the prognosis. The poor prognosis of extrahepatic metastases is believed to be a contraindication to hepatic resection. Therefore accurate noninvasive detection of inoperable disease with imaging modalities plays a pivotal role in selecting patients who would benefit from surgery.

In a meta-analysis, the sensitivity and specificity of ^{18}F-FDG PET for detecting recurrent colorectal cancer were 97% and 76% respectively (81). However, false-negative ^{18}F-FDG PET findings have been reported with mucinous adenocarcinoma. Other studies have compared the accuracy of ^{18}F-FDG PET and CT for the detection of hepatic metastases. A meta-analysis performed to compare noninvasive imaging methods (US, CT, MRI, and ^{18}F-FDG PET) for the differentiation of hepatic metastases from colorectal, gastric, and esophageal cancers demonstrated that at an equivalent specificity of 85%, ^{18}F-FDG PET had the highest sensitivity of 90% compared to 76% for MRI, 72% for CT, and 55% for US (82). A more recent meta-analysis confirmed these data (83). Valk et al. (84) compared the sensitivity and specificity of ^{18}F-FDG PET and CT for specific anatomic locations and found that ^{18}F-FDG PET was more sensitive than CT in all locations except the lung, where the two modalities were equivalent. The largest difference between PET and CT was found in the abdomen, pelvis, and retroperitoneum, where over one-third of PET-positive lesions were negative by CT.

In a meta-analysis of the literature, ^{18}F-FDG PET imaging changed the management in 29% (102 of 349) of patients (81). In a recent prospective study of 51 patients evaluated for resection of hepatic metastases, clinical management decisions based on conventional diagnostic methods were changed in 20% of patients based on the findings on ^{18}F-FDG PET imaging, especially by detecting unsuspected extrahepatic disease (85). The same group of investigators recently reported on patients' survival after resection of metastasis from colorectal carcinoma. The 5-year survival rate of patients evaluated with conventional diagnostic imaging is in the 30% range and does not appear to have changed over time (86). With the addition of ^{18}F-FDG PET imaging for preoperative restaging of patients with hepatic metastases, the 5-year survival rate improves to 58%. The main contribution is in detecting occult disease, leading to a reduction of futile surgeries. The incremental value of integrated PET/CT over PET alone has also been demonstrated (87).

In summary, the established indications for ^{18}F-FDG PET/CT in the evaluation of patients with colorectal carcinoma are as follows: (a) when there is a rising serum CEA level in the absence of a known source, (b) to increase the specificity of structural imaging when an equivocal lesion is detected, and (c) as a screening method for the entire body in the preoperative staging before curative resection of recurrent disease.

Diagnosis: (a) Adenocarcinoma of the cecum. (b) Hepatic and pelvic lymph node metastasis.

CASE 8.13

History: A 60-year-old male presented with metastatic colon carcinoma to the liver. ^{18}F-FDG PET/CT imaging was performed at the time of recurrence (Fig. 8.13, baseline) and 4 months following therapy with 50 mCi of ^{90}Y-labeled microspheres (SIRSpheres, Sirtex Medical, Inc.) infused in the right hepatic artery (Fig. 8.13). For each study, a MIP image and a transverse slice through the liver are displayed.

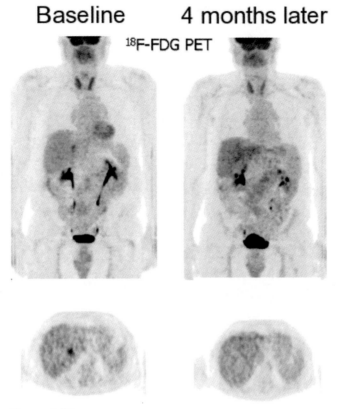

Figure 8.13

Findings: On the baseline study, there is a focus of uptake in the right lobe of the liver consistent with a metastasis. On the 4-month follow-up study, the uptake is no longer present, indicating a good response to therapy. Diffuse thyroid activity related to incidental autoimmune disease is present.

Discussion: Hepatic metastases can be treated with systemic chemotherapy or regional therapy to the liver. A variety of procedures to administer regional therapy to hepatic metastases have been investigated, including chemotherapy administered through the hepatic artery using infusion pumps, selective chemoembolization, radiofrequency ablation, cryoablation, alcohol ablation, and radiolabeled ^{90}Y-labeled microspheres (88,89). There are two types of ^{90}Y-labeled microspheres: ^{90}Y is either integrated into a glass matrix (TheraSpheres, manufactured by MDS Nordion) or attached to resin beads with diameters from 15 to 35 μm (SIRSpheres). Regional therapy with ^{90}Y-labeled microspheres is a palliative treatment for patients with unresectable hepatic metastases. Wong et al. (90) have compared ^{18}F-FDG PET imaging, CT, and MRI

with serum levels of CEA to monitor the therapeutic response of hepatic metastases to ^{90}Y-labeled glass microspheres. They found a significant difference between the ^{18}F-FDG PET changes and the changes on CT or MRI; the changes in ^{18}F-FDG uptake correlated better with the changes in serum levels of CEA. ^{18}F-FDG PET imaging also accurately monitors the efficacy of radiofrequency ablation for treatment of hepatic metastases, and it detects incomplete tumor ablation not detectable on CT. ^{18}F-FDG uptake decreases in responding lesions, and the presence of residual uptake in some lesions can help in guiding further regional therapy (91).

In summary, preliminary data suggest that ^{18}F-FDG PET imaging may be able to effectively monitor the efficacy of regional therapy to hepatic metastases, but these data need to be confirmed.

Diagnosis: Successful palliative regional therapy to hepatic metastases with ^{90}Y-labeled microspheres documented using ^{18}F-FDG PET.

History: A 61-year-old male with a 19-year history of prior hepatitis B infection was diagnosed with hepatocellular carcinoma; he had been treated with chemoembolization 3 months earlier. A recent CT suggested disease progression. He was referred to PET/CT for restaging (Fig. 8.14).

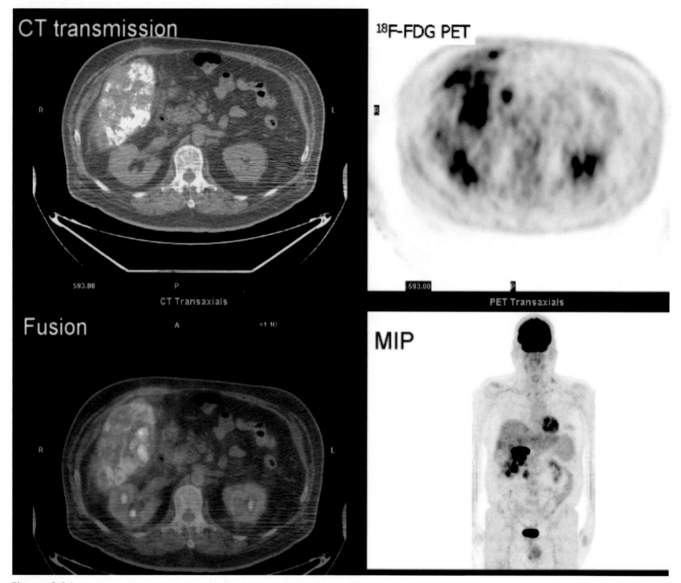

Figure 8.14

Findings: The ^{18}F-FDG PET images reveal intense uptake within the 6-cm heterogenous mass in the liver, corresponding on CT to an area of treatment with ethiodol (transaxial slice of Fig. 8.14). In addition, there is uptake corresponding to a lesion in the abdominal wall, retrospectively seen on CT, and in peripancreatic and pericaval lymph nodes (transaxial slice of Fig. 8.14).

Discussion: These findings are consistent with the known recurrent hepatocellular carcinoma in the liver and extrahepatic metastases.

The accumulation of ^{18}F-FDG in hepatocellular carcinoma is variable owing to the differing amounts of glucose-6-phosphatase present. It has been demonstrated that these tumors have increased levels of hexokinase activity and increased glucose metabolism; however, ^{18}F-FDG-6-phosphate does not accumulate intracellularly when significant levels of glucose-6-phosphatase activity are present. ^{18}F-FDG accumulation in hepatocellular carcinomas is greater than in normal liver parenchyma in approximately 50% to 70% of patients with the remaining patients having uptake equal to (30% of patients) or less than (15% of patients) background liver activity (92). ^{18}F-FDG uptake has been associated with high levels of alpha-fetoprotein and poorly differentiated tumors. Benign lesions such as regenerating nodules (which can represent significant diagnostic dilemmas on conventional imaging), focal nodular hyperplasia, adenomas, cysts, and cavernous hemangiomas do not result in increased uptake of ^{18}F-FDG (except in rare cases of abscesses with granulomatous inflammation). Therefore in this case the increased uptake of ^{18}F-FDG is consistent with the diagnosis of hepatocellular carcinoma in a patient with elevated serum alpha-fetoprotein.

^{11}C-acetate is complementary to ^{18}F-FDG imaging and accumulates in well-differentiated hepatocellular carcinoma. The combination of both tracers has a sensitivity greater than 95% for detection of hepatocellular carcinoma (93).

Diagnosis: Metastatic hepatocellular carcinoma accumulating ^{18}F-FDG.

CASE 8.15

History: A 34-year-old male with a history of cholangiocarcinoma, for which he had undergone a right hepatectomy 4 years earlier, presented with recurrent pain and jaundice. A CT scan of the abdomen revealed a low-attenuation lesion at the margin of resection. The patient was referred to ^{18}F-FDG PET/CT imaging for restaging. (Figs. 8.15 A and 8.15 B).

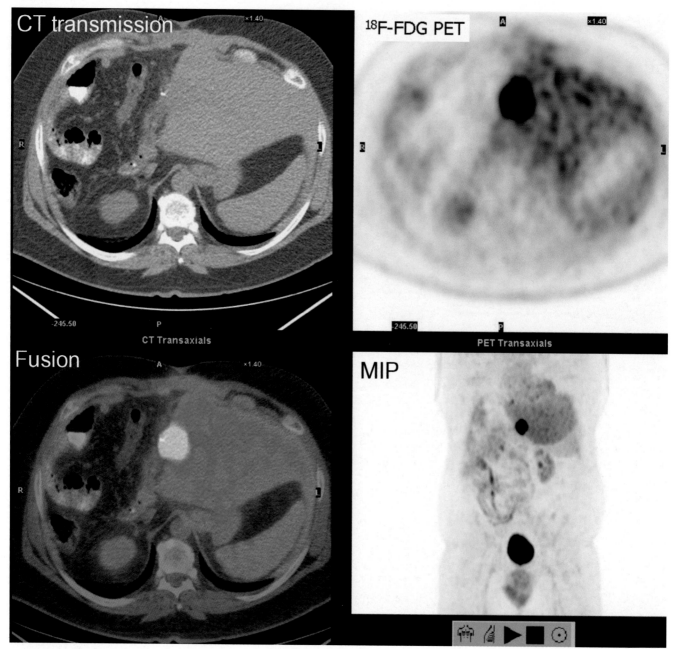

Figure 8.15 A

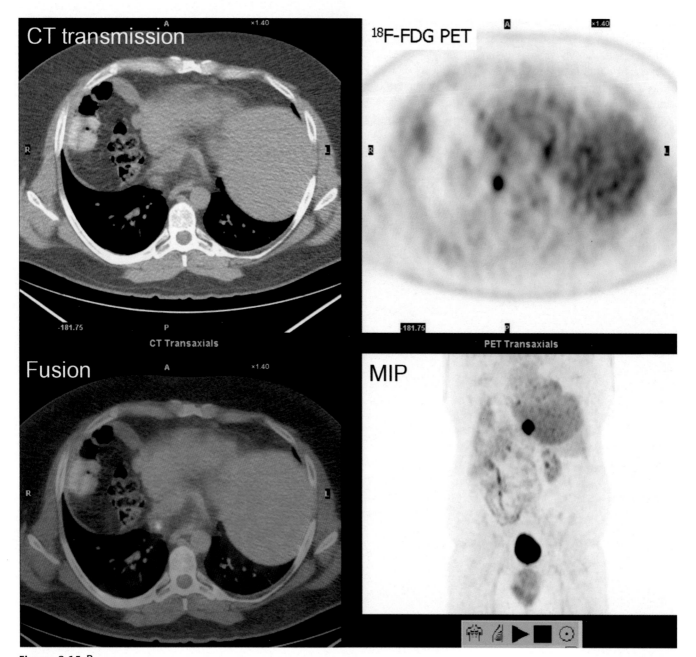

CT transmission

¹⁸F-FDG PET

CT Transaxials

PET Transaxials

Fusion

MIP

Figure 8.15 B

Findings: The images revealed a large area of uptake at the margin of resection indicating recurrent cholangiocarcinoma. In addition, there is a focus of uptake corresponding to a 1.2-cm retrocrural lymph node, indicating extrahepatic metastatic disease. The patient has had a right hepatectomy.

Discussion: Cholangiocarcinomas are relatively rare tumors, with 17,000 cases reported annually in the United States. Tumors that arise at the junction of the right and left hepatic ducts represent approximately 3,000 of these. Primary cholangiocarcinomas arising at this location are known as Klatskin's tumors (Klatskin reported a large series of these patients in 1965). Risk factors for cholangiocarcinoma include sclerosing cholangitis, alpha-1 antitrypsin deficiency, ulcerative colitis, Caroli's disease, choledochal cyst, infestation by the fluke *Clonorchis sinensis*, cholelithiasis, and exposure to Thorotrast. One of five

patients with cholangiocarcinoma has a predisposing factor. The majority of these tumors are unresectable at the time of presentation, although patients may survive for years, as these tumors tend to be slow-growing. Distant metastasis is relatively rare, although 50% of patients will have local lymph node metastases.

The diagnosis of cholangiocarcinomas using CT can be difficult, as the majority of these lesions are isodense to liver. The point at which intrahepatic ductal dilatation begins or where hepatic atrophy can be identified can suggest the extent of the tumor. MRI can be helpful in some cases, with a hypointense central scar identified on T2-weighted images in approximately 25% to 30% of cases (94).

¹⁸F-FDG PET imaging may be useful in the diagnosis and management of patients with suspected cholangiocarcinomas

and sclerosing cholangitis (95). Unlike hepatocellular carcinoma, which may have a variable degree of glucose-6-phosphatase activity and may not accumulate ^{18}F-FDG, cholangiocarcinomas do accumulate ^{18}F-FDG. However, false-negative results are not uncommon because of the frequent diffuse infiltrating pattern of this tumor (96). The sensitivity for the nodular morphology is 85%, but only 18% for infiltrating morphology. Carcinomatosis can be falsely negative and cholangitis falsely positive. Inflammatory changes along the tract of a biliary stent can lead to a false-positive interpretation also. Despite these limitations, ^{18}F-FDG PET can lead to a change in surgical management in up to 30% of patients because of the detection of unsuspected metastases.

Unsuspected gallbladder carcinoma is discovered incidentally in 1% of routine cholecystectomies. At present, the majority of cholecystectomies are performed laparoscopically, and occult gallbladder carcinoma found after laparoscopic cholecystectomy has been associated with reports of gallbladder carcinoma seeding of laparoscopic trocar sites. Increased ^{18}F-FDG uptake has been demonstrated in gallbladder carcinoma (97) and has been helpful in identifying recurrence in the area of the incision when CT could not differentiate scar tissue from malignant recurrence. In a study reviewing 14 patients with gallbladder carcinoma, the sensitivity for detection of residual gallbladder carcinoma was 78%. Sensitivity for extrahepatic metastases was 50% in 8 patients; 6 of these had carcinomatosis (96).

Diagnosis: Recurrent cholangiocarcinoma with local nodal metastasis.

CASE 8.16

History: A 55-year-old male presented with jaundice and epigastric pain. The CT scan revealed intra- and extrahepatic ductal dilatation and a 3.5-cm pancreatic mass. In addition, there were mildly enlarged retroperitoneal lymph nodes. The patient was referred to ^{18}F-FDG PET/CT imaging for initial staging (Figs. 8.16 A and 8.16 B).

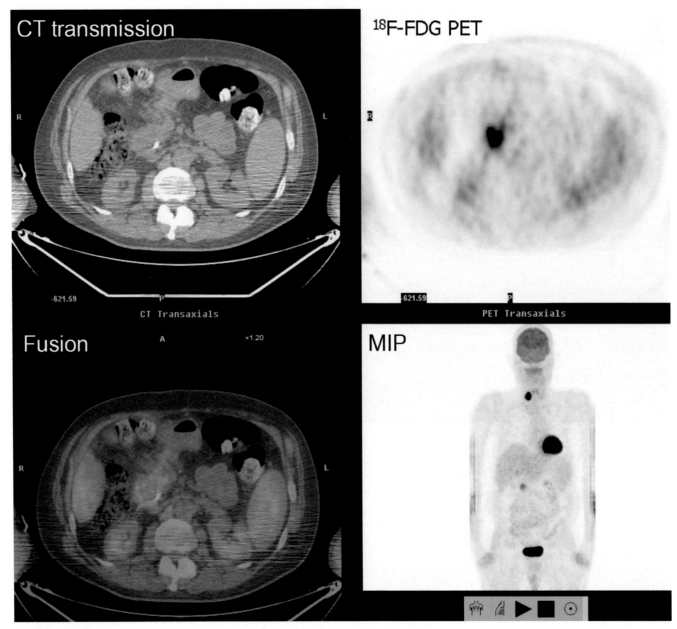

Figure 8.16 A

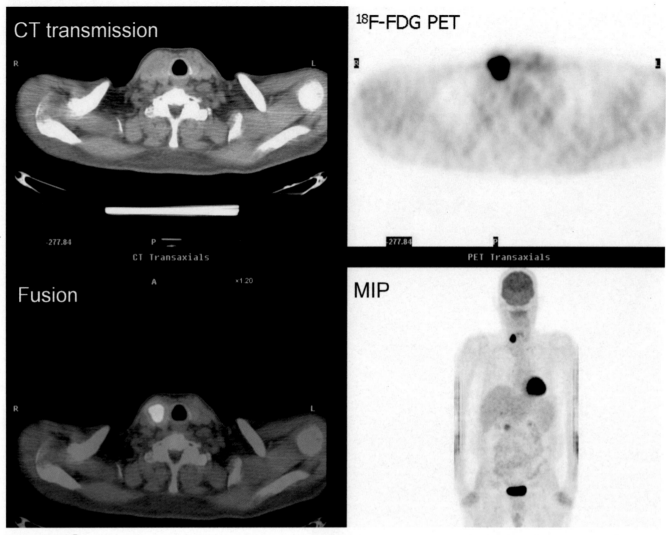

CT transmission

^{18}F-FDG PET

R — L

CT Transaxials

-277.84   P

A   ×1.20

Fusion

R — L

PET Transaxials

-277.84   P

MIP

Figure 8.16 B

Findings: The images revealed intense uptake corresponding to the mass in the head of the pancreas, consistent with malignancy. There is a stent in the common duct seen on the CT transmission image. In addition, there is intense uptake in the right lobe of the thyroid, which is also worrisome for malignancy. No ^{18}F-FDG uptake was seen in the mildly enlarged retroperitoneal lymph nodes on the CT (not shown).

Discussion: These findings are consistent with a carcinoma of the head of the pancreas. In this case, PET demonstrated the absence of distant metastases, as confirmed at surgery. The patient underwent a Whipple procedure and tissue obtained at surgery confirmed well-differentiated adenocarcinoma. A biopsy of the thyroid lesion revealed papillary thyroid carcinoma.

The role of imaging modalities in the staging of pancreatic carcinoma has been discussed in a review article (98). The typical initial evaluation of a pancreatic neoplasm includes CT and EUS with biopsy. CT has been to shown to have an accuracy of 70% in the diagnosis of pancreatic cancer and a positive predictive value of nonresectability of 90%. Endoscopic retrograde cholangiopancreatography (ERCP) is the other means of evaluating the pancreas and has an accuracy of 80% to 90% in

differentiating benign from malignant masses. There is an approximately 10% technical failure rate and up to 8% morbidity (iatrogenic pancreatitis, primarily) associated with ERCP. EUS allows FNA biopsy but is nondiagnostic in up to 30% of cases because of sampling error. PET is most helpful for the diagnosis of pancreatic cancer for these indeterminate patients. The diagnosis can also be difficult in mass-forming pancreatitis and in cases of enlargement of the pancreatic head without definite signs of malignancy. ^{18}F-FDG PET imaging has a sensitivity of 85% to 100%, a specificity of 67% to 99%, and an accuracy of 85% to 93% for the preoperative diagnosis of pancreatic carcinoma. ^{18}F-FDG imaging is particularly useful in determining the presence of metastatic disease, which can significantly alter surgical management. In one study, surgical management was altered in up to 41% of patients who underwent ^{18}F-FDG PET imaging in addition to CT scanning, in two-thirds of this group by identifying pancreatic carcinoma preoperatively and in one-third by identifying unsuspected metastasis or by confirming the benign nature of lesions that were equivocal on CT. Patients with high SUV values within the tumor have also been shown to have a significantly shorter survival time. It may be possible to exclude neoplasm in patients with chronic pancreatitis in up to 84% to 100% of those that present with a pancreatic mass.

Limitations of ^{18}F-FDG PET imaging are seen with respect to false-negative findings in patients with glucose intolerance and tumors smaller in size than twice the resolution of the PET system used for acquiring the images (less than 1 cm). False-positive findings can be seen in patients with acute pancreatitis. Therefore ^{18}F-FDG PET scans in patients with elevated serum levels of C-reactive protein should be interpreted with caution.

Incidental uptake in the thyroid gland is seen in approximately 2% of patients referred for ^{18}F-FDG PET/CT imaging. Diffuse uptake is seen in about 0.5% of patients and has been associated with Graves' disease and autoimmune thyroiditis. Focal uptake is seen in some 1.5% of patients and malignancy was found in one-third of the cases that were biopsied (99). Therefore, if there is intense focal uptake in the thyroid gland, an US should be recommended and biopsy if indicated.

Diagnosis: (a) Pancreatic carcinoma. (b) Papillary thyroid carcinoma.

CASE 8.17

History: This 41-year-old male presented with a history of diffuse large B-cell (DLBCL) non-Hodgkin's lymphoma (NHL) diagnosed with a biopsy of a right inguinal lymph node 1 year earlier. A recent CT scan showed extensive mediastinal adenopathy. He was referred to ^{18}F-FDG PET/CT imaging for restaging (Figs. 8.17 A and 8.17 C).

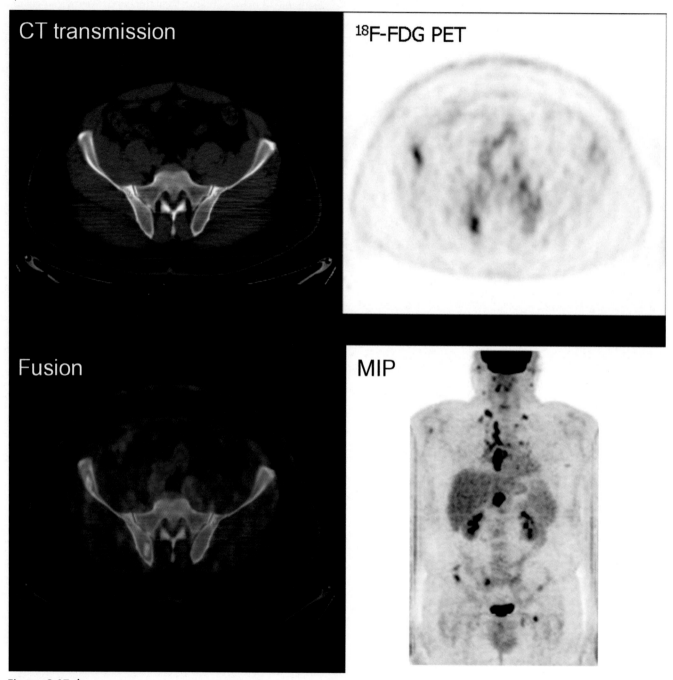

Figure 8.17 A

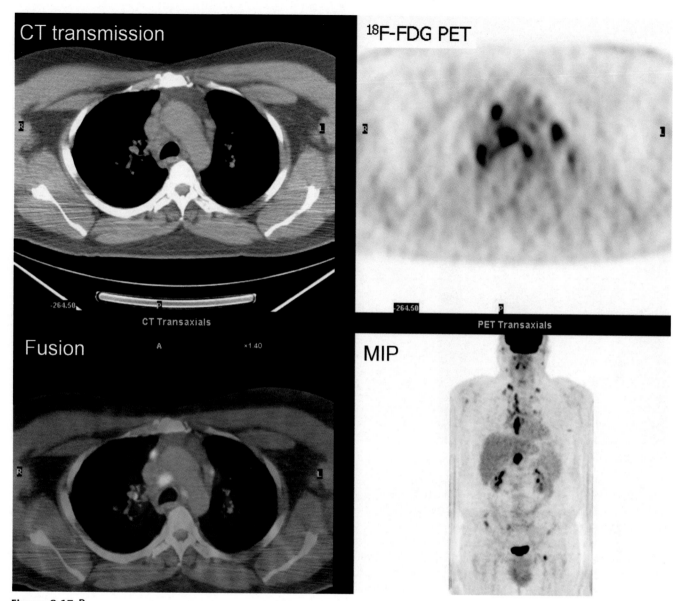

Figure 8.17 B

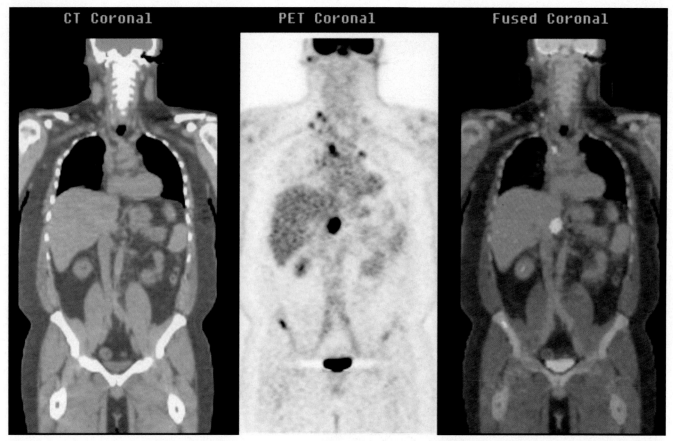

| CT Coronal | PET Coronal | Fused Coronal |

Figure 8.17 C

Findings: The ^{18}F-FDG images demonstrate multiple foci of intense ^{18}F-FDG uptake in the bilateral cervical, supraclavicular, and mediastinal nodes as well as in left inguinal node (Fig. 8.17 A MIP). These foci correspond to enlarged nodes on the CT transmission images (Figs. 8.17 B and 8.17 C). Additionally, there is large focus of uptake in a 4-cm retroperitoneal mass abutting the caudate lobe of the liver (Fig. 8.17 C). Multiple foci of intense uptake are seen in the skeletal pelvis (Fig. 8.17 A) and one in the right proximal humerus (MIP). There are no corresponding findings on the CT scan (Fig. 8.17 A).

Discussion: These findings are consistent with extensive involvement of lymph nodes and bone marrow with NHL. Because of the findings of PET, the right iliac crest should be preferentially selected for biopsy.

There are three major categories of lymphoma according to the World Health Organization (WHO) (100): (a) Hodgkin's lymphoma (HL), (b) B-cell neoplasms, and (c) T-cell/natural killer (NK)-cell neoplasms. HL is virtually always intensely ^{18}F-FDG–avid. Diffuse large B-cell lymphoma represents 30% of NHLs; they are aggressive and intensively ^{18}F-FDG-avid (101). Other relatively common aggressive lymphomas that are intensely ^{18}F-FDG–avid include mantle cell lymphoma (representing 6% of NHLs), adult T-cell leukemia/lymphoma, and Burkitt's lymphoma. Follicular lymphomas represent 22% of NHLs and are more indolent and only moderately ^{18}F-FDG–avid. Chronic lymphocytic leukemia/small cell lymphocytic lymphoma (CLL) and extranodal marginal zone B-cell lymphoma (MALT), each representing 7% of NHLs, are low-grade

and often poorly ^{18}F-FDG–avid unless they undergo transformation.

Stages I and II (lymph node involvement only on one side of the diaphragm) have a high cure rate (about 70% to 80%), whereas stages III (lymph node involvement on both sides of the diaphragm) and IV (systemic involvement) have a lower cure rate (about 40%).

^{18}F-FDG PET has both a higher sensitivity and specificity than CT for staging and restaging nodal and extranodal lymphoma (102,103). Many studies have shown the superiority of PET compared with CT for the detection of extranodal involvement because organomegaly is not always associated with disease involvement. For NHL and HL, the frequency of involvement of the spleen is about 22%; liver, 15% and 3% respectively; and bone marrow, 25% and 10% respectively. The ^{18}F-FDG PET criterion for diffuse involvement of the spleen or bone marrow is uptake more intense than in normal liver parenchyma, which has an average SUV of about 2.0. For the detection of bone marrow involvement, ^{18}F-FDG PET is more accurate than CT and equal to bone marrow biopsy (103). Bone marrow biopsy suffers from sampling error, and ^{18}F-FDG PET can guide the biopsy, as in this case. However, ^{18}F-FDG PET is poorly sensitive for the detection of bone marrow involvement of low-grade lymphoma owing to physiologic uptake in normal marrow. The diffuse pattern of uptake of reactive bone marrow hyperplasia after chemotherapy, and especially after concurrent administration of bone marrow stimulants, can mimic or mask diffuse bone marrow involvement. Therefore appropriate history is critical. A delay of 3 to 4 weeks after completion of therapy permits the physiologic marrow activity to abate.

The change of stage I/II to III/IV has major therapeutic implications. A change of stage and management has been reported in various studies summarized in a review article (104). Although a change in stage due to ^{18}F-FDG PET has been reported in 20% to 40% of patients, a major change in management involves only 10% to 35% because it occurs when patients are staged upward from stage I/II to III/IV.

Diagnosis: Stage IV diffuse large B-cell lymphoma involving lymph nodes on both sides of the diaphragm and bone marrow.

CASE 8.18

History: A 16-year-old male presented with dyspnea on exertion. A chest x-ray revealed a mediastinal mass that was confirmed by CT (Fig. 8.18 A). A biopsy demonstrated lymphoblastic lymphoma. He was referred for both ^{67}Ga and ^{18}F-FDG PET/CT imaging for initial staging (Fig. 8.18 A). He was treated with aggressive chemotherapy and referred for ^{18}F-FDG PET/CT imaging after two cycles of chemotherapy (May 2002), 2 months after completion of treatment (August 2002), and 6 months later (February 2003) (Fig. 8.18 B).

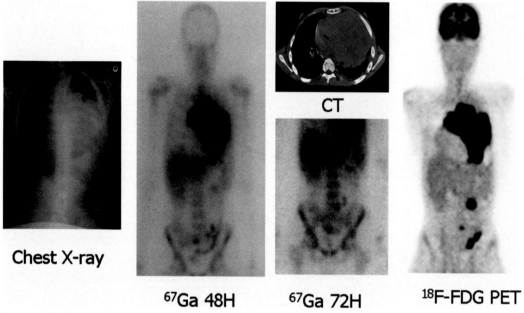

Figure 8.18 A

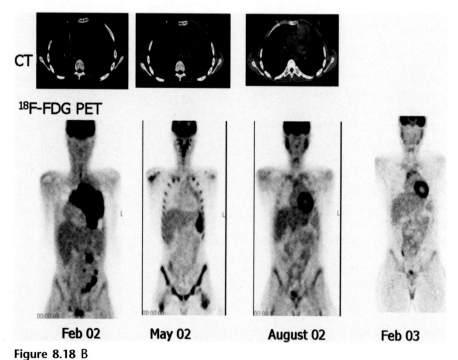

Figure 8.18 B

Findings: On the initial staging images (Fig. 8.18 A), there is intense ^{67}Ga and ^{18}F-FDG uptake corresponding to the large mediastinal mass seen on chest x-ray and CT. However, on the ^{18}F-FDG images, there are also three foci of intense uptake in the abdomen corresponding to bowel on the CT scan (not shown) and not seen on the ^{67}Ga images. On the follow-up CT images, the residual mass has decreased in size but is still present. On the follow-up ^{18}F-FDG PET images (Fig. 8.18 B), there is no longer uptake even after two cycles of chemotherapy (May 2002) indicating a good response to therapy. There is however diffuse uptake in the bone marrow and spleen due to reactive bone marrow hyperplasia and extramedullary hematopoiesis. Two months after completion of chemotherapy (August 2002), bone marrow hyperplasia and splenic uptake are resolving. Mild uptake is now seen in the mediastinum owing to thymic hyperplasia, which is becoming moderately intense after 6 months (February 2003).

Discussion: The patient had a GI bleed related to therapy-induced tumor lysis, and bowel involvement was confirmed at surgery. The ^{18}F-FDG PET images were more accurate than the ^{67}Ga images for staging, indicating stage IV disease, whereas the ^{67}Ga images indicated stage II.

The follow-up ^{18}F-FDG PET images indicated a good response to therapy despite a persistent large thoracic mass with the typical physiologic changes of reactive bone marrow hyperplasia and thymic rebound.

The sensitivity and specificity of ^{18}F-FDG PET for the detection of lymphoma is superior to that of ^{67}Ga (105). Therefore ^{18}F-FDG PET has supplanted ^{67}Ga imaging of patients with lymphoma.

Physiologic uptake in response to therapy can occasionally confuse interpretation. Reactive diffuse bone marrow hyperplasia and splenic uptake occur typically for 2 to 4 weeks after chemotherapy and can be intense after administration of marrow-stimulating factors such as filgrastim. Thymic hyperplasia is common in children and young adults, with an incidence of 16% (106). It typically occurs 2 to 6 months after completion of therapy and may persist for 12 to 24 months. The pattern of moderate ^{18}F-FDG uptake and the inverted V-shape are typical for thymic hyperplasia.

Data regarding monitoring therapy of lymphoma with ^{18}F-FDG PET have been summarized in a review article by Jerusalem et al. (107). Consensus recommendations regarding the use of ^{18}F-FDG PET/CT in monitoring therapy of lymphoma have been published (4): (a) Pretherapy ^{18}F-FDG PET imaging is strongly encouraged but not mandatory for aggressive lymphoma (HL, DLBCL, mantle cell lymphoma, and follicular lymphoma) because they are routinely ^{18}F-FDG–avid. However, pretherapy ^{18}F-FDG PET imaging is mandatory for lymphomas that are not typically ^{18}F-FDG–avid. (b) The timing of ^{18}F-FDG PET is critical to avoid equivocal interpretations. ^{18}F-FDG PET should be performed at least 3 weeks and preferably 6 to 8 weeks after completion of chemotherapy and 8 to 12 weeks after radiation therapy. For evaluation during therapy, ^{18}F-FDG PET imaging should be performed as close as possible before the subsequent cycle of therapy. (c) Visual assessment alone is adequate for interpreting PET findings as positive or negative. Mediastinal blood pool activity is used as a reference for assessment of residual masses greater than 2 cm. (d) Specific criteria for defining PET positivity in liver, spleen, lung, and bone marrow are described in the review article (4). (e) Treatment monitoring during the course of therapy should be done only in the setting of clinical trials.

The Society of Nuclear Medicine (SNM) procedure guidelines for tumor imaging using ^{18}F-FDG PET (3) recommend a comparison of extent and intensity of uptake between the pre- and posttherapy images. The comparison may be summarized as metabolic progressive disease, metabolic stable disease, metabolic partial response, or metabolic complete response, using the criteria published by the European Organization for Research and Treatment of Cancer (EORTC) (108), although these criteria have not yet been validated in outcome studies. A mixed response is considered progressive disease because the outcome of the patient depends on the behavior of the most aggressive part of the tumor. These criteria are as follows:

1. Progressive metabolic disease (PMD) would be classified as an increase in ^{18}F-FDG tumor SUV of greater than 25% within the tumor region defined on the baseline scan, visible increase in the extent of ^{18}F-FDG tumor uptake (>20% in the longest dimension), or the appearance of new ^{18}F-FDG uptake in metastatic lesions.

2. Stable metabolic disease (SMD) would be classified as an increase in tumor ^{18}F-FDG SUV of less than 25% or a decrease of less than 15% and no visible increase in extent of ^{18}F-FDG tumor uptake (>20% in the longest dimension).

3. Partial metabolic response (PMR) would be classified as a reduction of a minimum of 15% to 25% in tumor ^{18}F-FDG SUV after one cycle of chemotherapy, and greater than 25% after more than one treatment cycle. Reporting would need to be accompanied by adequate and disclosed reproducibility measurements from each center. An empirical 25% was found to be a useful cutoff point, but there is a need for a reproducibility analysis to determine the appropriate cutoffs for statistical significance. A reduction in the extent of the tumor ^{18}F-FDG uptake is not a requirement for PMR.

4. Complete metabolic response (CMR) would be complete resolution of ^{18}F-FDG uptake within the tumor volume so that it was indistinguishable from surrounding normal tissue.

A change of intensity of uptake with semiquantitative measurements, expressed in absolute values and percent change, may be appropriate in some clinical scenarios. However, the technical protocol and analysis of images must be consistent in the two sets of images.

Diagnosis: Initial staging of lymphoblastic lymphoma: stage II disease by ^{67}Ga and stage IV disease by ^{18}F-FDG PET, confirmed at surgery. Complete response to therapy.

CASE 8.19

History: A 34-year-old man was referred for sentinel node localization (SNL) (Fig. 8.19 A) following the excisional biopsy of an intermediate-level melanoma from the midposterior thorax. Six intradermal injections of 40 μCi of filtered (22 μm filter) ^{99m}Tc–sulfur colloid were performed surrounding the primary lesion. A series of 1-minute images was started immediately following injection for 5 minutes; then static images were obtained including trunk, axillary, cervical, and inguinal regions. A static 10 minute image over the upper chest (posterior projection) is displayed in Figure 8.19 A.

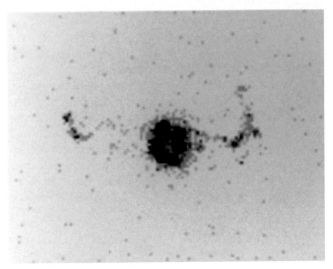

Figure 8.19 A

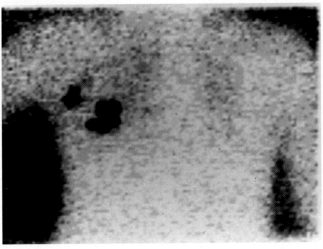

Figure 8.19 B

Findings: Sequential imaging (not shown) revealed lymphatic channels leading to two separate sentinel nodes, one in each axilla (Fig. 8.19 A). Orthogonal views and a hot marker were used to further localize the sentinel nodes, and the skin overlying these foci was marked and covered with an adhesive plastic covering to allow subsequent intraoperative localization and excision.

For improved anatomic landmarks in localization of sentinel lymph nodes, a cobalt-57 (^{57}Co) sheet source may be placed under the patient to create a transmission image, as illustrated in another patient (Fig. 8.19 B). In this patient, the sentinel node is easily identified in the left axilla superior and lateral to the injection site.

An alternative method of providing the surgeons with as much anatomic information as possible is to use a point source of ^{99m}Tc to "draw" an outline around the body after the sentinel node has been localized (Fig. 8.10 B).

Discussion: In the case presented in Figure 8.19 A, the skin surrounding the melanoma site drained to both axillae; if a lymphadenectomy had been performed on only one axilla or the other, a critical metastasis would have been missed. The sentinel node concept states that the first node(s) to receive lymphatic drainage from a tumor (the "sentinel node") will always contain tumor cells if lymphatic spread of the tumor has occurred, so that the histopathology of the sentinel node will reflect the histopathology of the entire nodal bed. This has been well validated in patients with melanoma, with a false-negative occurrence of <1%; the sentinel lymph node histology can predict over 99% of all recurrent lymph node metastases. In intermediate-level (stages I and II) melanoma, skip-nodal metastases have not been reported.

Staging of melanoma is based on the depth of invasion according to the anatomic level of invasion in the Clark classification (level I, intraepithelial or *in situ*; levels II and III, papillary dermis; level IV, reticular dermis; level V, subcutaneous tissue) and in millimeters in the Breslow classification, which more accurately predicts prognosis (109,110).

- 0.75 mm (comparable to Clark level II)
- > 0.75 to 1.5 mm (comparable to Clark level III)
- >1.5 to 4.0 mm (comparable to Clark level IV)
- >4.0 mm (comparable to Clark level V)

The staging system for melanoma was revised in 2002 (111). Patients with stages I and II disease have no lymph node involvement. Patients with stages III and IV disease have regional lymph node involvement and distant metastases, respectively.

Malignant melanoma appears to be increasing in incidence and mortality. As with most cancers, cure is dependent on early recognition and effective surgery. If melanoma lesions are <0.75 mm thick, survival is high, but if thickness is >3 mm, survival is only 50% at 5 years.

For stages I and II disease, in which there is no clinical evidence of spread and tumor thickness is <4 mm, elective regional lymph node dissection is usually recommended because of evidence that it reduces both the recurrence rate and mortality. However, approximately 75% to 80% of these patients do not have nodal metastases at the time of exploration and therefore could be spared the expense and morbidity of lymphadenectomy. Lymphoscintigraphy is therefore useful in detecting those who are most likely to benefit from lymphadenectomy. Furthermore, nodal basins identified by lymphoscintigraphy are discordant with the expected drainage pattern in over 60% of patients with head and neck melanoma and one-third of patients with truncal lesions, as in this case. If elective lymph node dissection is based on clinical experience or classic anatomic patterns, the procedure will be misdirected in approximately 50% of cases. The entire head, neck, and shoulder regions and the area within 10 cm of the midline have totally unpredictable lymphatic drainage, making lymphoscintigraphy even more important in these patients. Trunk lesions can drain to multiple sites including cervical, supraclavicular, and inguinal lymph nodes. Upper extremity lesions drain to the axillary and epitrochlear lymph nodes, and lower extremity lesions drain to inguinal and popliteal lymph nodes.

Using minimally invasive surgery, the sentinel node is identified via a small handheld gamma probe and excised. It is important for the node to be localized with orthogonal views or by using the probe and then marked so that the incision may be placed in the proper site. Including as much anatomic information on the images for the surgeon is critical, as illustrated in

Figure 8.19 B. Wide excision of the primary site is performed at the same operation. If the sentinel node is subsequently proven to be positive for melanoma by conventional hematoxylin and eosin (H&E) staining or by reverse transcription–polymerase chain reaction (RT-PCR) analysis, the patient subsequently undergoes regional lymphadenectomy.

The results of the Multicenter Selective Lymphadenectomy Trial (MSLT) suggest that there is a significantly better 5-year disease-free survival rate for patients staged with a sentinel node localization (SNL) procedure compared with those staged without such a procedure (112). The SNM has published a procedure guideline for SNL in the management of patients with melanoma (113). The radiopharmaceutical procedure is usually used in conjunction with methylene blue dye injected in the operating room. Blue and radioactive nodes are excised and extensively assessed histopathologically.

Lymphoscintigraphy allows localization of the sentinel node(s) without the expense and morbidity associated with complete lymphadenectomy, thus sparing the 75% to 80% of patients who do not have metastatic adenopathy yet identifying the group of patients likely to benefit from elective lymph node dissection.

Diagnosis: Intermediate-thickness melanoma; sentinel node localization.

CASE 8.20

History: This 76-year-old male underwent excision of a left facial melanoma 3 years earlier. Two years later, a right-lower-lobe metastatic lung nodule was resected. He was subsequently treated with investigational vaccine therapy and was referred to PET/CT imaging for restaging (Figs. 8.20 A to 8.20 D).

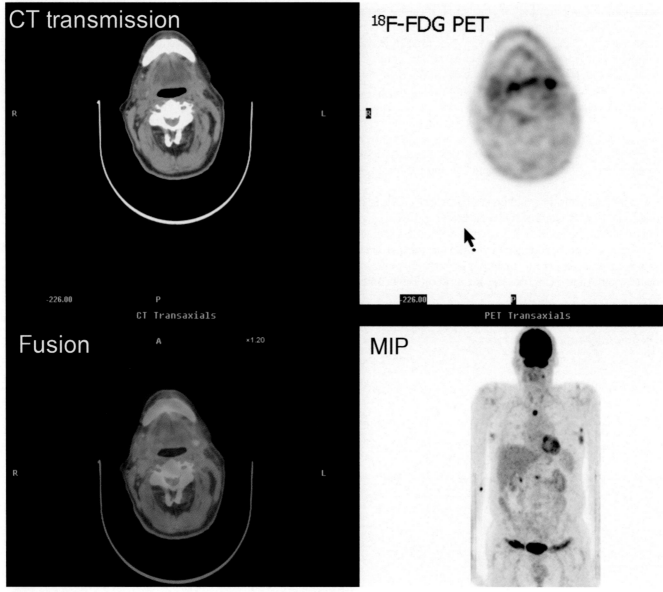

Figure 8.20 A

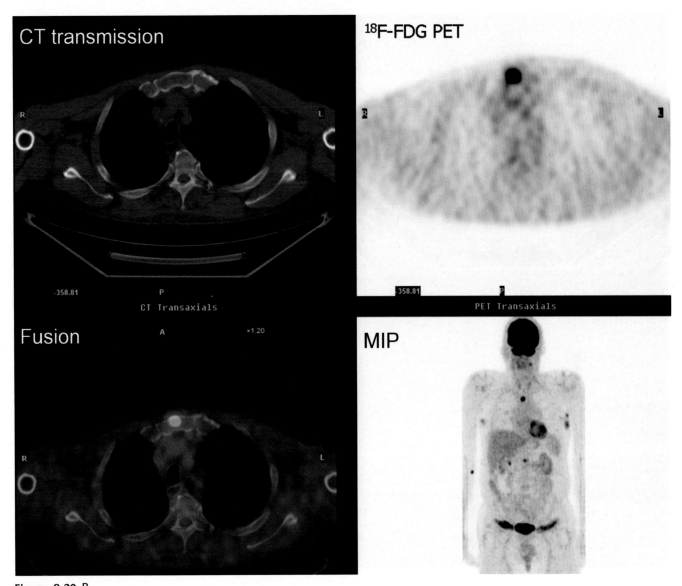

CT transmission

¹⁸F-FDG PET

Fusion

MIP

CT Transaxials

PET Transaxials

-358.81

-358.81

Figure 8.20 B

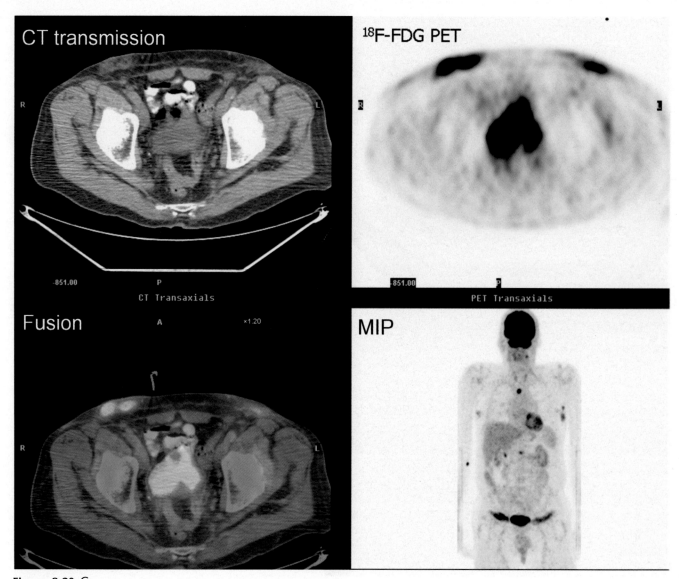

Figure 8.20 C

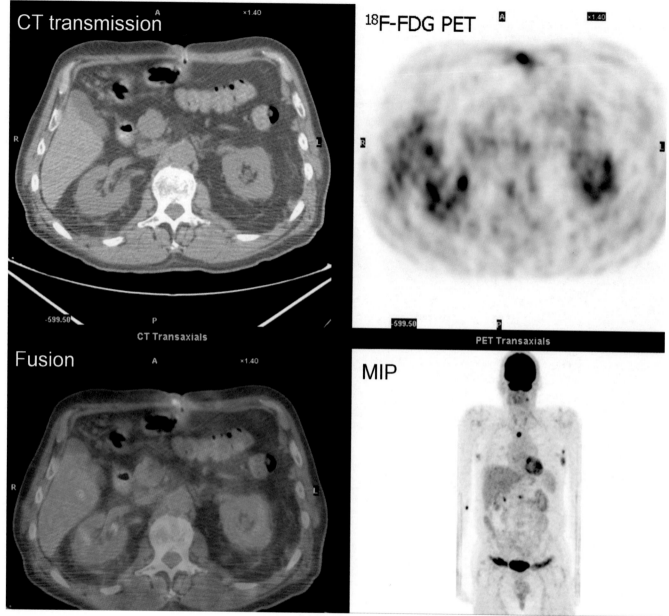

Figure 8.20 D

Findings: A small focus of uptake is seen in the left neck corresponding to a 1-cm lymph node in the lateral floor of the mouth (Fig. 8.20 A). A focus of intense uptake is also seen in the proximal sternum with no corresponding finding on the CT scan (Fig. 8.20 B). Multiple foci of moderate uptake are seen in the both axillae (MIP) and inguinal regions (Fig. 8.20 C). On the CT scan, there is corresponding stranding in the subcutaneous tissues. There is also a focus of uptake projecting in the upper midabdomen on the MIP image. This corresponds to soft tissue surrounding a feeding tube on the CT scan (Fig. 8.20 D).

Discussion: ^{18}F-FDG uptake in the left cervical lymph node and sternum are consistent with metastases, illustrating that ^{18}F-FDG PET can detect metastasis in normal-size lymph nodes and before anatomic changes occur in the skeleton. The uptake in the axillae and inguinal regions corresponds to stranding on the CT scan and is characteristic for an inflammatory reaction associated with subcutaneous injection of investigational treatments given to patients with metastatic melanoma. The uptake around the feeding tube is also typical of the inflammatory reaction around percutaneous stomas.

An excellent review article discusses the role of ^{18}F-FDG PET in the evaluation of patients with melanoma (114). The staging system for melanoma is described in Case 8.19. The incidence of metastases and therefore the prognosis are related to the depth of invasion.

For low-risk melanoma (Breslow thickness <1 mm), only 2% to 3% of patients have lymph node involvement, and there is no difference in survival (>95% at 10 years) whether observation or elective lymph node dissection is performed.

For intermediate-risk melanoma (Breslow thickness 1 to 3 mm), 20% to 50% of patients have lymph node involvement, so sentinel node biopsy is recommended and has largely replaced elective lymph node dissection (see Case 8.19); the 5-year survival is 75%. The sensitivity of ^{18}F-FDG PET for detection of metastases in this group of patients ist extremely low compared to sentinel node biopsy if there is no clinically palpable lymphadenopathy, because ^{18}F-FDG PET cannot detect micrometastases. The sensitivity of ^{18}F-FDG PET is 14% for detection of nodal metastases when the tumor volume is <78 mm^3 and 90% when the tumor volume is >78 mm^3 (115).

For high-risk melanoma (Breslow thickness >3 mm), 50% to 70% of patients have nodal metastases and more than 10% have distant metastases; the 5-year survival is less than 50%. ^{18}F-FDG PET is recommended for these patients, and multiple studies report a range of sensitivity of 84% to 97% for lesion detection.

For detection of melanoma recurrence, ^{18}F-FDG PET replaces multiple imaging modalities, and PET/CT offers the advantages of both modalities. For example, CT is more sensitive for detection of small pulmonary metastases that are below PET resolution. For patients with known recurrence, ^{18}F-FDG PET/CT is indicated for restaging and evaluation of the extent of disease prior to surgery.

In a meta-analysis, the sensitivity was 92% and specificity 90%; a change in management occurred in 22% of patients (116).

Diagnosis: (a) Metastatic melanoma to left cervical lymph node and sternum. (b) Inflammatory changes in bilateral axillae, inguinal region, and abdominal wall due to vaccine injections and feeding tube insertion site.

CASE 8.21

History: A 51-year-old woman recently diagnosed with invasive carcinoma of the cervix was referred to ^{18}F-FDG PET/CT imaging for initial staging (Figs. 8.21 A to 8.21 C).

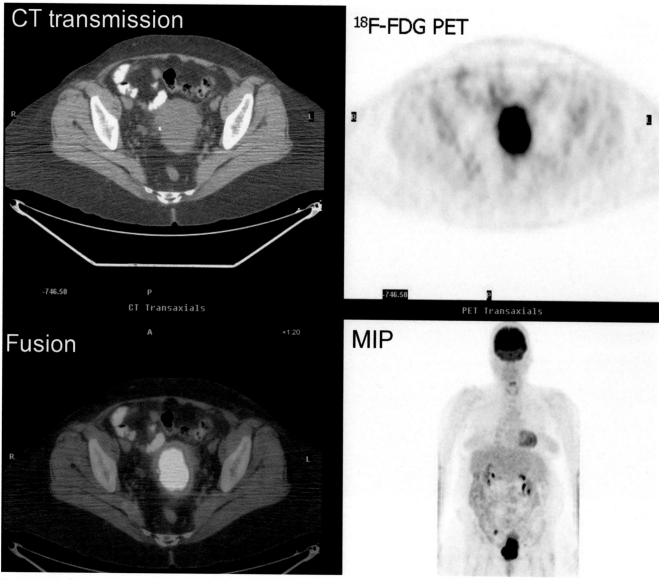

Figure 8.21 A

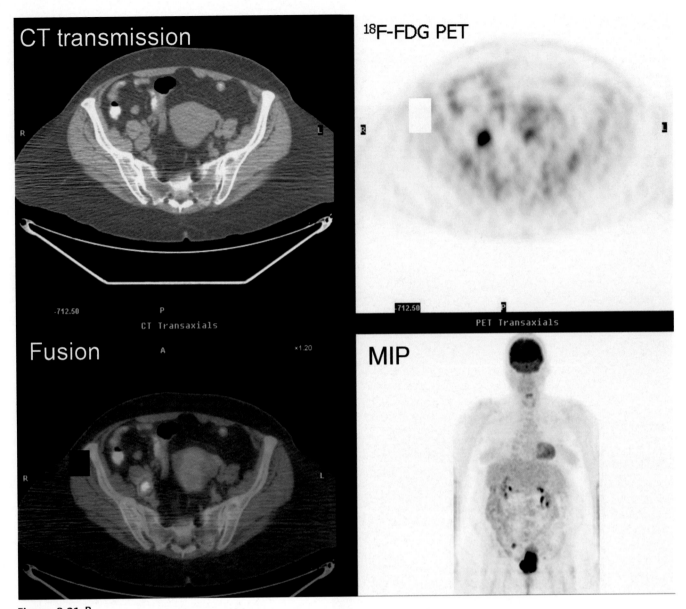

Figure 8.21 B

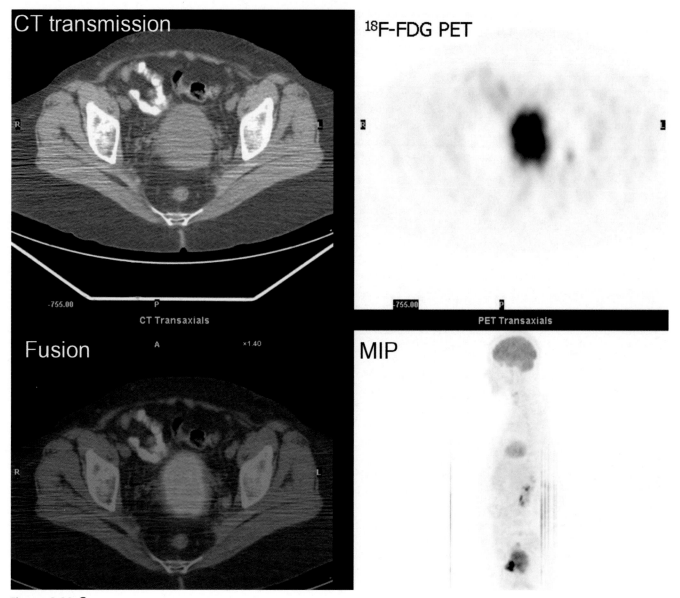

Figure 8.21 C

Findings: There is intense ^{18}F-FDG uptake in the cervix extending into the entire uterus, corresponding to a fungating mass on the CT scan (Figs. 8.21 A and 8.21 C). Fig. 8.21 C is displayed with the window level open compared to Fig. 8.21 A, which allows delineation of the tumor posterior to the bladder (lateral view of MIP). The urine-filled bladder is usually the organ with most intense ^{18}F-FDG uptake; ^{18}F-FDG uptake in tumors is usually less intense, as in this case. In addition, there is intense uptake corresponding to a 2.5-cm right iliac lymph node.

Discussion: These findings are consistent with the known primary cervical carcinoma and right iliac nodal involvement. Altering the window settings on the workstation is valuable in detecting bladder and rectal pathology as well as gynecologic disease.

Cervical cancer is the sixth most common solid malignancy in women and the third most common gynecological cancer, with almost 13,000 new cases of invasive disease annually.

With early detection, the prognosis of preinvasive disease has improved, but the overall 5-year survival of 70% for invasive cervical cancer has not changed over 20 years. The Fédération Internationale de Gynécologie Obstétrique (FIGO) staging system relies primarily on physical exam and basic tests and does not include cross-sectioning imaging. The pathologic status of pelvic and para-aortic lymph nodes is not included in the FIGO stage. However, in a series of 626 patients, the status of para-aortic nodes, determined by surgical staging, was the most significant prognostic factor in patients with cervical cancer (117). The detection of nodal involvement and distant metastases affects not only therapeutic decisions (surgery versus radiotherapy as well as radiotherapy treatment planning) but also prognosis. Survival decreases from 75% with negative nodes to 45% with positive nodes; when para-aortic nodes are involved, 5-year survival drops to 15%. Thirteen percent of patients present with advanced disease, experiencing a 50% to 62% five-year survival for stage III and 20% for stage IV disease. In this patient, the treatment was changed from surgery to radiation therapy based on the presence of metastatic iliac adenopathy. Retroperitoneal metastases appeared several months later. PET is more accurate than CT and MRI for the detection of metastatic lymph nodes (118). The positive predictive value for nodal metastases is 90% for PET and only 64% for MRI (119). Supraclavicular lymph nodes are detected by PET in 8% of patients (120). A meta-analysis showed that ^{18}F-FDG PET pooled sensitivity and specificity were 79% and 99%; they were 84% and 95% for pelvic and para-aortic lymph node detection respectively (121).

For detection of recurrence, the meta-analysis concluded that ^{18}F-FDG PET detected cervical cancer recurrence with a 96% pooled sensitivity and an 81% pooled specificity. ^{18}F-FDG PET can prevent unnecessary therapy by detecting unsuspected metastases and can modify therapy with a curative intent.

Diagnosis: (a) Carcinoma of the cervix. (b) Right iliac nodal metastases.

CASE 8.22

History: A 56-year-old female with a history of ovarian cancer who had been treated with hysterectomy, bilateral salpingo-oophorectomy, and adjuvant chemotherapy presented with rising serum levels of CA-125. She was referred for ^{18}F-FDG PET/CT imaging (Fig. 8.22).

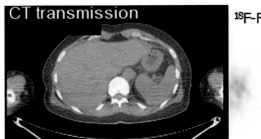 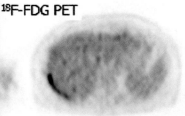 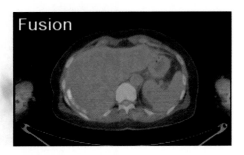

Figure 8.22

Findings: There is ^{18}F-FDG uptake along the posterolateral surface of the liver associated with free fluid. There was also mottled uptake superior to the bladder, also associated with some free fluid (not shown).

Discussion: These findings are diagnostic of peritoneal metastases. Ovarian cancer is the second most common gynecologic malignancy and the leading cause of gynecologic cancer deaths. Seventy percent of patients present with advanced disease (stages III or IV). Ovarian cancer spreads initially to local organs, then the retroperitoneum with dropped metastases into the pouch of Douglas, the omentum, and subphrenic space. Lymphatic spread occurs via inguinal, pelvic, and para-aortic lymph nodes while the patient is still asymptomatic.

Initial evaluation usually includes ultrasonography, tumor markers, peritoneal cytology and CT. The most accurate diagnosis and staging is performed at the time of surgery (FIGO staging system).

The performance of ^{18}F-FDG PET for characterization of adnexal masses was studied in a group of 101 asymptomatic women with adnexal masses scheduled to undergo laparoscopy, transvaginal US, and MRI. There were 12 ovarian cancers, 76 benign ovarian lesions, and 13 nonovarian lesions. ^{18}F-FDG PET had a sensitivity of only 58% (compared with 92% for US and 83% for MRI); specificity of 80% (compared with 60% for US and 84% for MRI); positive predictive value of 93% (compared with 23% for US and 42% for MRI); and accuracy of 77% (compared with 63% for US and 84% for MRI). The combination of US, MRI, and PET improved accuracy for characterizing adnexal masses, but negative MRI or PET did not exclude early-stage ovarian cancer (122).

The performance of ^{18}F-FDG PET for detection of residual disease has been compared with second-look laparoscopy in a series of 22 patients with advanced-stage ovarian cancer in terms of complete clinical (normalized CA-125) and radiologic response following therapy. Thirteen patients had persistent disease at second-look laparotomy. The sensitivity and specificity of ^{18}F-FDG PET was only 10% and 42% respectively (123).

For the diagnosis of recurrent ovarian cancer after completion of therapy, the performance of ^{18}F-FDG PET has an overall sensitivity of 83% and specificity of 83%. In a subgroup of patients with elevated levels of tumor markers or abnormal CT or US, the sensitivity of ^{18}F-FDG PET was greater than 90% (124). A meta-analysis (121) showed that PET had a pooled sensitivity and specificity of 90% and 86% in patients with clinical suspicion of recurrence.

Various patterns of carcinomatosis have been described: omental caking, macroscopic peritoneal implants, sheet-like spread in the peritoneum, and miliary spread. The macroscopic patterns of spread demonstrate ^{18}F-FDG uptake, but miliary carcinomatosis can be falsely negative.

^{18}F-FDG PET is mostly useful in detecting and restaging recurrent ovarian cancer, particularly in patients with rising CA-125 and negative or equivocal conventional imaging. There are known limitations in patients with small volumes of disease, and it is not recommended as a replacement for second-look laparoscopy.

Diagnosis: Metastatic ovarian cancer.

CASE 8.23

History: A 16-year-old male presented with anemia; bone marrow biopsy unexpectedly revealed metastatic rhabdomyosarcoma. Extensive workup failed to demonstrate a primary. He was referred to ^{18}F-FDG PET/CT imaging (Fig. 8.23)

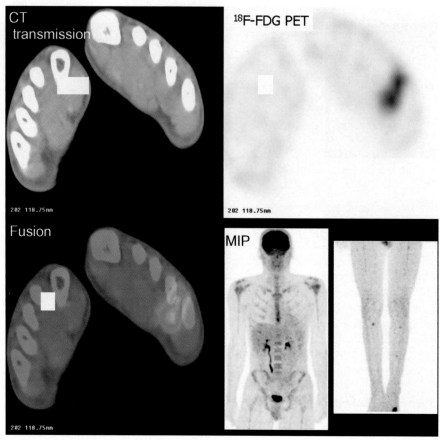

Figure 8.23

Findings: On the MIP images, there is diffuse uptake in the bone marrow of the axial and appendicular skeleton consistent with the known metastatic involvement. There is no focal abnormal uptake in the body. However, there is a focus of intense uptake in the lateral aspect of the left foot at the edge of the field of view. On the noncontrasted CT transmission images, there is a subtle corresponding lesion in the plantar aspect of the musculature in between the fourth and fifth metatarsals.

Discussion: The lesion was confirmed and better seen on a follow-up MRI of the left foot, and a biopsy revealed a rhabdomyosarcoma. Always look at the edges!

Approximately 8,640 new cases of soft tissue sarcoma occur in the United States annually, thus constituting only 1% of all cancers. Fifty percent occur in the extremities, 50% occur in children (usually Ewing's and rhabdomyosarcoma), and 50% will ultimately die of their disease. Although most of the extremity sarcomas exhibit local invasion, they usually spread hematogenously, with 88% of the metastases occurring in the lungs; nodal metastases are relatively unusual.

As with lymphoma, ^{18}F-FDG PET has been shown to be as useful as or more useful than CT for demonstrating the extent of disease in patients with intermediate- to high-grade soft tissue sarcomas, although experience is limited (125). All high-grade soft tissue sarcomas and most low-grade and intermediate-grade sarcomas are ^{18}F-FDG–avid and easily visualized, but many aggressive benign soft tissue lesions may also exhibit increased ^{18}F-FDG accumulation. As expected, benign lesions such as lipomas and leiomyomas do not accumulate ^{18}F-FDG, but inflammatory lesions may cause false-positive findings. The degree of ^{18}F-FDG activity as determined by tumor-to-background (TBR) ratios of >3 or SUVs of >2 tend to correlate with the grade (but not the histologic type) of tumor. Metastatic lesions have an SUV more than twice that of primary sarcomas, indicative of a more aggressive lesion (126).

Limb salvage is now possible in over 80% of patients with soft tissue sarcoma, and the presence of local or distant metastases does not necessarily contraindicate aggressive resection of the primary lesion; even resection of a pulmonary metastasis may be beneficial. In the treatment of soft tissue sarcoma of the extremities, control of the primary site with optimal functional outcome is the goal. Virtually all tumors are resected before or after chemotherapy or radiotherapy. Once metastases have occurred, median survival is only 9 to 12 months. As with other tumors, ^{18}F-FDG PET imaging may be useful for the assessment of response to therapy and the detection of distant metastases (127). False-positive findings can occur as a result of recent surgical intervention, so PET imaging should be delayed for at least 3 weeks after biopsy or other surgical procedures.

In summary, ^{18}F-FDG PET is useful for staging and monitoring therapy of high-grade sarcomas. At initial staging, it can guide biopsy at the site of more intense ^{18}F-FDG uptake, indicating the site of higher-grade tumor.

Diagnosis: (a) Diffuse involvement of the bone marrow by sarcoma. (b) The primary in the left foot detected by PET.

CASE 8.24

History: A 66-year-old man with a history of NSCLC presented with a new renal mass seen on a follow-up CT scan. He was referred to ^{18}F-FDG PET/CT imaging for restaging (Fig. 8.24).

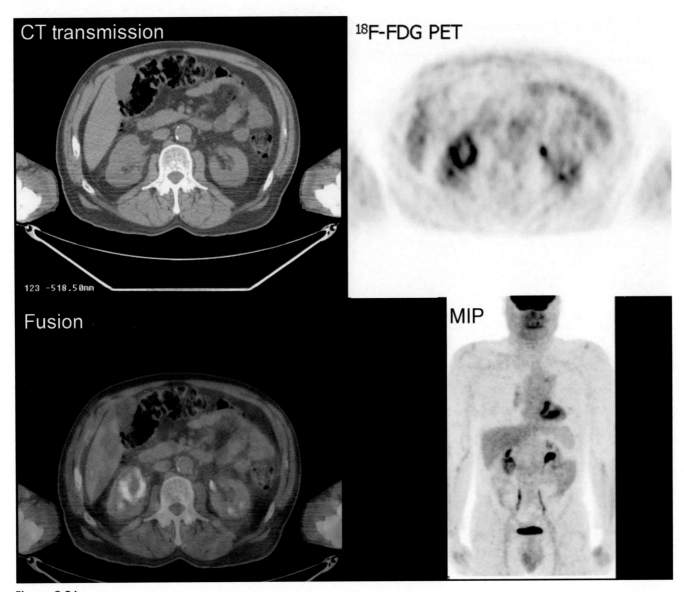

Figure 8.24

Findings: There is intense uptake corresponding to a 4-cm exophytic right renal mass with central photopenia characteristic of central necrosis (Fig. 8.24). There is also moderate uptake in the right pulmonary hilum and aortopulmonary window in the mediastinum (Fig. 8.24 MIP) corresponding to lymph nodes on the CT scan (not shown).

Discussion: Although there is physiologic uptake within the intrarenal collecting system, abnormal uptake is clearly seen in the right cortical mass, indicating a malignancy. As it is unusual for lung cancer to metastasize to the kidneys, this likely represents a primary, as renal cell carcinoma was subsequently proven by biopsy. Uptake in mediastinal lymph nodes is concerning for metastases in a patient with lung cancer, so

biopsy would be warranted to differentiate metastatic adenopathy from an inflammatory etiology.

Sometimes ^{18}F-FDG accumulation in the renal collecting system may interfere with the visualization of structures adjacent to the renal collecting system and the bladder and obscure visualization of urothelial tumors. However, anatomic information provided by CT allows proper assessment and characterization of renal masses. With good hydration, the administration of diuretics, and placement of a urinary catheter, visualization of perineal and paravesicular lesions can be improved.

The AJCC TNM classification is commonly used for staging renal cell carcinoma (128). Contrast-enhanced CT has become the procedure of choice for the diagnosis and staging of renal cell carcinoma. CT can characterize renal masses as cystic, solid or mixed, classifying them according to the Bosniak classification (129), and provide evaluation of lymph node and vascular involvement (130). The reported experience of ^{18}F-FDG PET imaging in patients with genitourinary neoplasms is limited to studies with small numbers of patients and has been summarized in a review article (131). The reported sensitivity of 60% for detection of the primary is relatively low, compared with 92% for CT (132). The sensitivity of PET was also lower (at about 75%) than that of CT or bone scintigraphy (at about 90%) for the detection of lymph node, lung, and skeletal metastases. This has an important implication for interpretation of PET/CT images; if a complex renal lesion is identified on PET/CT images, relatively low ^{18}F-FDG avidity does not exclude a renal cell carcinoma.

Malignancies other than renal cell carcinoma which may be falsely negative by ^{18}F-FDG PET owing to low ^{18}F-FDG avidity include neuroendocrine tumors, hepatocellular carcinomas, mucin-containing neoplasms, necrotic tumors, relatively well differentiated or low-grade adenocarcinomas, lymphomas and sarcomas, and some genitourinary tumors such as prostate carcinomas.

Diagnosis: ^{18}F-FDG–avid renal cell carcinoma.

CASE 8.25

History: A 26-year-old male diagnosed with testicular seminoma who had recently undergone surgery for resection was referred for ^{18}F-FDG PET/CT imaging (Figs. 8.25 A and 8.25 B).

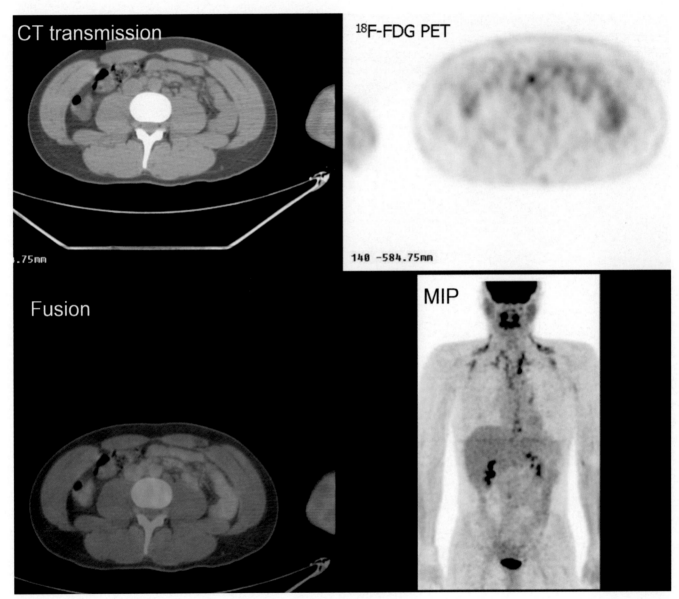

Figure 8.25 A

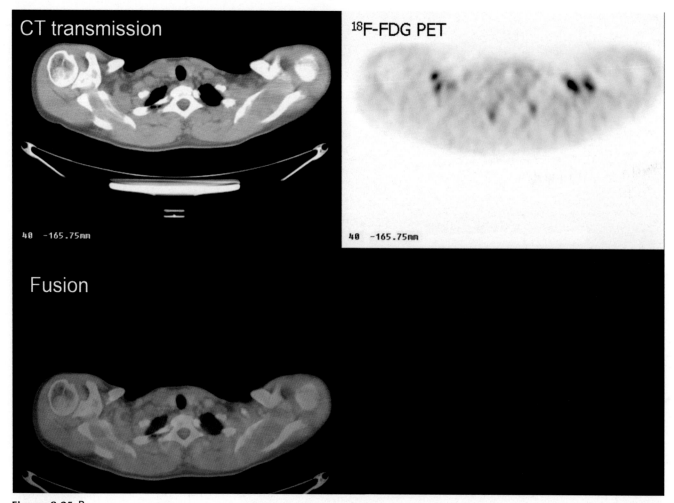

CT transmission

40 -165.75mm

18F-FDG PET

40 -165.75mm

Fusion

Figure 8.25 B

Findings: There is 18F-FDG uptake bilaterally in the supra-claviclar regions, mediastinum, and paravertebral region (MIP) in a pattern consistent with the uptake of brown fat. Examination of the PET/CT images confirmed that the uptake projected over a fatty region (Fig. 8.25 B). In addition there is a small focus of uptake in the aortocaval region below the level of the kidneys, corresponding to a subcentimeter lymph node on the CT scan (Fig. 8.25 A).

Discussion: This finding indicates a metastatic retroperitoneal lymph node despite its subcentimeter size, nondiagnostic by CT.

Seminoma represents 40% of germ cell tumors and nonseminomatous germ cell tumors (NSGCTs) 60%. NSGCTs include embryonal carcinomas, choriocarcinomas, mature and immature teratomas, and tumors with mixed histologies. Germ cell tumors affect young patients, and the prognosis of these tumors has improved with advances in chemotherapy.

As for other malignancies, accurate initial staging has prognostic significance and implications for treatment. At the time of diagnosis, approximately two-thirds of NSGCTs and one-third of seminomas have nodal involvement. Distant metastases commonly involve the lungs, liver, and brain. For nodal staging, the sensitivity of 18F-FDG PET ranges from 70% to 87% and is superior to that of CT (about 60%), which is lim-

ited by size criteria for lymph node involvement, as illustrated in this case. The specificity of PET ranges from 94% to 100%, also superior to that of CT. An impact on management has been demonstrated in 15% to 20% of patients (133).

18F-FDG PET also has a role in the evaluation of a residual mass after completion of therapy and in the evaluation of patients presenting with elevated tumor markers and a normal conventional workup. For patients with seminomas, a residual mass greater than 3 cm suggests viable tumor in 27% to 41% of the cases, and surgery is indicated. 18F-FDG PET has a good positive and negative predictive value to predict viable tumor in the residual mass and for the detection of recurrence when tumor markers are elevated (134).

For NSGCTs, 60% to 85% of patients with advanced disease have a residual mass after therapy. 18F-FDG PET has a good positive predictive value but a poor negative predictive value because there is overlap of uptake between mature teratoma and malignant tumors (135).

The uptake of brown fat is common in patients with a low body-mass index and in cold climates. Brown fat is a vestigial organ of thermogenesis; it is innervated by the sympathetic nervous system. Administration of benzodiazepines and beta blockers prior to 18F-FDG helps decrease uptake in brown fat. The pattern of uptake in brown fat is usually symmetrical

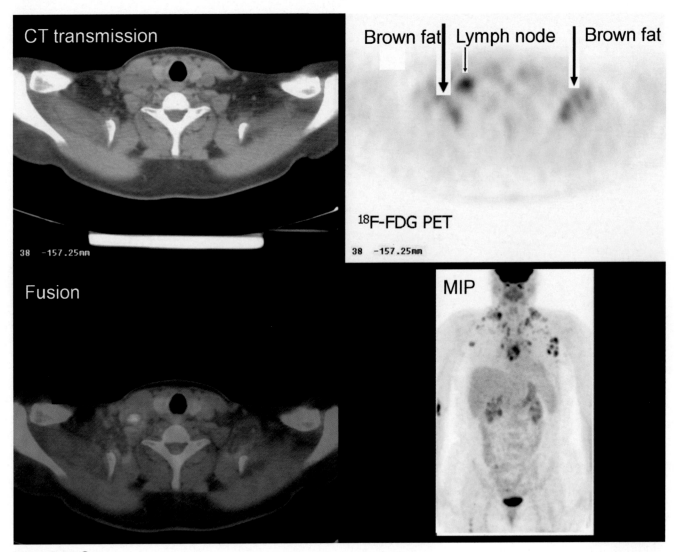

Figure 8.25 C

in the neck, supraclavicular, and paravertebral regions. It can also be present in the mediastinum and suprarenal fossa. With PET/CT, it is critical to inspect the CT images carefully to exclude the presence of ^{18}F-FDG–avid lymph nodes; these can be obscured on the PET images by adjacent brown fat uptake, as illustrated in Figure 8.25 C. This is a patient with lymphoma who has extensive brown fat uptake but also lymph nodes involved by lymphoma. The transaxial slice illustrates ^{18}F-FDG uptake corresponding to brown fat in both supraclavicular regions and a focus corresponding to a lymph node in the right supraclavicular region.

Diagnosis: Testicular cancer.

CASE 8.26

History: A 51-year-old woman presented with flushing, nausea, and early satiety. A CT scan (not shown) demonstrated multiple low-density hepatic lesions consistent with metastases. The largest mass involved the left lobe and appeared to be compressing the stomach, thus perhaps contributing to her symptoms. A percutaneous biopsy was positive for neuroendocrine tumor. She was referred for possible tumor resection and debulking. ^{18}F-FDG PET/CT (Fig. 8.26 A) and ^{111}In-octreotide (Fig. 8.26 B) imaging were performed for staging.

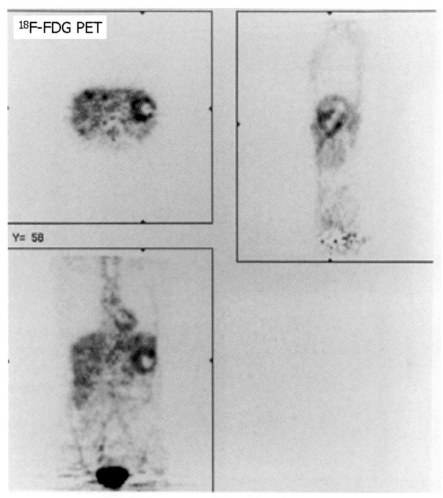

Figure 8.26 A

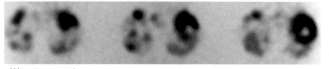

^{111}In-Octreotide

Figure 8.26 B

Findings: The axial, sagittal, and coronal PET images (Fig. 8.26 A) show a large hypermetabolic lesion within the left lateral lobe of the liver with a necrotic hypometabolic center, congruent with the large lesion seen on CT. In addition, there are several additional hypermetabolic lesions throughout the right and left lobes of the liver. The transaxial ^{111}In-octreotide SPECT images (Fig. 8.26 B) reveal somatostatin-positive activity within the large left-lobe lesion, again demonstrating the central necrosis and multiple additional hepatic lesions. No distant or regional extrahepatic metastases were identified with either modality. The primary, presumably a small bowel lesion, was not localized.

Discussion: The ^{18}F-FDG images are consistent with numerous hypermetabolic hepatic metastases with no evidence of extrahepatic disease. The ^{111}In-octreotide findings indicate that the tumor deposits are SSR-positive. At laparotomy, the large

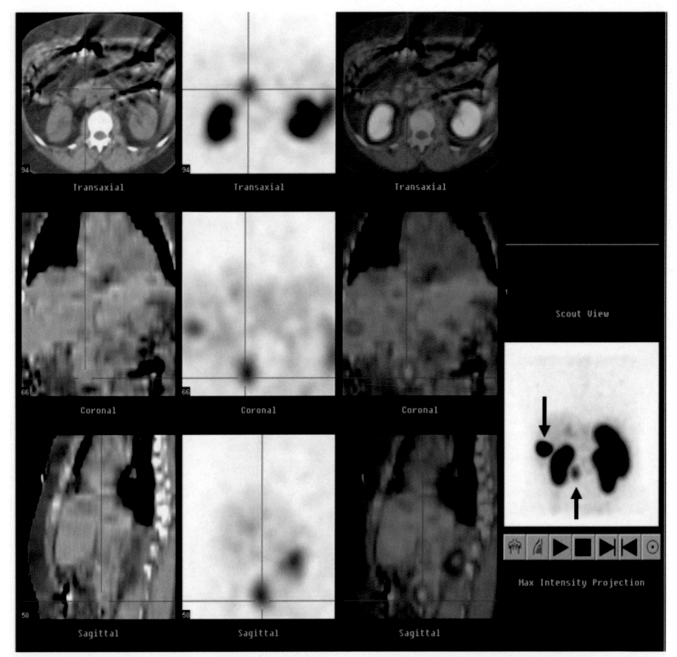

Integrated CT ¹¹¹In-Octreotide SPECT Fusion integrated SPECT-CT

Figure 8.26 C

left-lobe lesion was resected by segmentectomy, and multiple right-lobe lesions were enucleated. Histology was most consistent with metastatic carcinoid tumor.

Differentiated typical carcinoid expresses SSR with high density. In general, ¹¹¹In-octreotide scintigraphy is reported to be more sensitive than CT for the detection of metastatic carcinoid and other neuroendocrine tumors and may more accurately represent the extent of disease (136). This is especially true for extrahepatic and extra-abdominal disease. The therapeutic plan is altered in a substantial minority of patients owing to the superior sensitivity of scintigraphy for the detection of

extrahepatic disease. Furthermore, tumors that are somatostatin receptor–positive by scintigraphy have been found to be reliably responsive to systemic somatostatin analog therapy. Although ¹¹¹In-octreotide imaging may sometimes demonstrate a previously unknown primary tumor in patients with metastatic carcinoid, its clinical utility of this is uncertain. Carcinoid metastases may be heterogeneous for SSR, some being positive and some negative in the same patient. As these tumors dedifferentiate, they may lose their SSR expression and become ¹⁸F-FDG-positive. As in the case of other tumors, SPECT/CT has an incremental value compared with planar imaging or

SPECT alone by better characterization and localization of the lesions. The incremental value of SPECT/CT in patients with neuroendocrine tumors has been demonstrated in approximately 40% of patients, with an impact on therapy in 15% to 30% (137,138). This is illustrated in Figure 8.26 C from a patient with a history of carcinoid. The ^{111}In-octreotide projection image (MIP) demonstrates two lesions (arrows): one in the liver and one extrahepatic. The SPECT/CT images helped to localize the extrahepatic lesion in the head of the pancreas.

There are limited data comparing ^{18}F-FDG to SSR scintigraphy for the detection of carcinoid tumors, but these and other neuroendocrine tumors tend to be less hypermetabolic than the more common carcinomas and may be falsely negative with ^{18}F-FDG PET (139,140). Therefore ^{18}F-FDG PET should be reserved for patients who have negative SSR scintigraphy or additional lesions on CT or MRI that are not SSR-avid. Both techniques may be useful for following the response to therapy, whether it be resection or chemoembolization. An additional advantage of somatostatin-receptor scintigraphy is the potential for use of an intraoperative handheld gamma probe to aid in the resection of small tumor foci. Another important point: metastatic carcinoid patients with negative SSR imaging will not be effectively blocked by administration of somatostatin analogs at the time of ablation procedures and would be at increased risk for carcinoid crisis.

Diagnosis: Metastatic carcinoid tumor.

History: A 41-year-old man with a prior history of bronchial carcinoid resection presented with recurrent ACTH-dependent Cushing's syndrome. Chest x-ray and chest CT were interpreted as normal. ^{111}In-octreotide imaging (Figs. 8.27 A to 8.27 D) was performed.

^{111}In-Octreotide

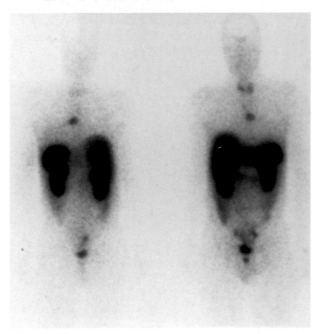

Figure 8.27 A

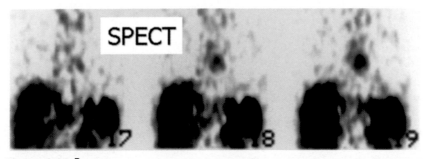

Figure 8.27 B

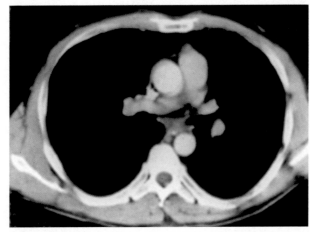

Figure 8.27 C

Figure 8.27 D

Findings: Anterior (right) and posterior (left) whole-body ^{111}In-octreotide images (Fig. 8.27 A) reveal two foci of increased uptake within the thorax, one near the left hilum and a smaller one in the mediastinum. Coronal SPECT images (Fig. 8.27 B) demonstrate both lesions clearly. Six months later, the ^{111}In-octreotide findings were unchanged, and close correlation with a repeat CT scan (Figs. 8.27 C and 8.27 D) resulted in confirmation of the scintigraphic findings.

Discussion: Despite the "normal" CT scan, ^{111}In-octreotide scintigraphy easily detected two metastatic SSR-positive metastases. Without knowledge of the scintigraphic findings, the subtle CT abnormalities could easily have been misinterpreted. Following resection of these deposits of carcinoid tumor, the patient's hypercortisolemia resolved.

The sensitivity for the detection of carcinoid metastases by ^{111}In-octreotide imaging is 85% to 90%, and GI primary tumors are detected in some of these patients. The sensitivity for the detection of bronchial and thymic carcinoids is also high. Adrenocorticotropic hormone (ACTH)-dependent Cushing's syndrome is due to a pituitary adenoma in 85% of patients and ectopic ACTH secretion in the remainder (141). Most of these with ectopic ACTH secretion are due to clinically obvious small cell lung carcinomas, but most of the remaining patients with chronic ACTH-dependent Cushing's syndrome not due to a pituitary adenoma are in fact found to be related to an ACTH-secreting carcinoid tumor of the lung or thymus. Petrosal sinus sampling for ACTH—an expensive, invasive, and complication-prone procedure—has been the standard technique for differentiating pituitary-dependent Cushing's from ectopic Cushing's syndrome. However, ^{111}In-octreotide imaging is now recommended as the procedure of choice for localizing an ectopic source of ACTH secretion in patients with Cushing's syndrome when conventional imaging is nondiagnostic. There are numerous case reports documenting the utility of somatostatin-receptor imaging in this population. In a series of 10 patients with ectopic ACTH syndrome, 8 were localized with ^{111}In-octreotide imaging, including two occult tumors. As in this patient, occult metastatic lesions may also be demonstrated.

In the Cushing's patient whose hypercortisolemia cannot be suppressed with dexamethasone, chest CT/MRI and ^{111}In-octreotide imaging with SPECT/CT of the chest should be performed prior to petrosal sinus sampling.

Diagnosis: Ectopic ACTH syndrome due to metastatic bronchial carcinoid.

CASE 8.28

History: A 10-year-old boy with a 3-year history of neuroblastoma had experienced marked progression of his tumor over the previous year despite chemotherapy. He was referred for ^{99m}Tc-HDP bone scintigraphy, ^{123}I-MIBG scintigraphy, and 18F-FDG PET/CT imaging (Fig. 8.28).

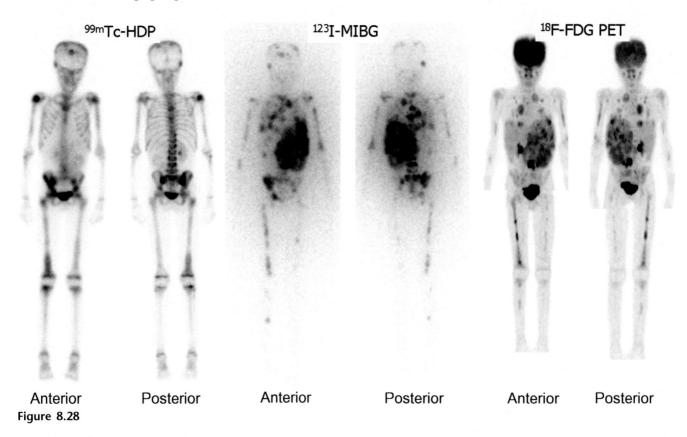

^{99m}Tc-HDP ^{123}I-MIBG ^{18}F-FDG PET

Anterior   Posterior   Anterior   Posterior   Anterior   Posterior

Figure 8.28

Findings: On the bone scan, there are a multiple foci of uptake in the calvarium; left proximal humerus; cervical, thoracic, and lumbar spine; right iliac wing; bilateral sacroiliac joints; right femur; and right proximal tibia. Mild uptake is also seen in the known left abdominal mass. The MIBG images show uptake in the large abdominal mass, metastases in the lungs, and additional skeletal lesions in the skull, right tibia, left humerus, and left femur. On the ^{18}F-FDG images, there is uptake in the abdominal mass, pulmonary metastases, and skeletal lesions seen on the MIBG images, but they are better delineated on the ^{18}F-FDG images. The skull lesions are not as well seen because of the physiologic uptake in the cerebral cortex.

Discussion: The soft tissue activity seen on the initial bone scan serves to illustrate the fact that neuroblastoma is one of the tumors more often detected on conventional bone scintigraphy, likely related to the virtually universal occurrence of microcalcification within this tumor; as many as 91% of primary tumors may be identified by bone scintigraphy. With MIBG imaging, the skeleton is visualized only if involved by tumor. ^{18}F-FDG PET has a better resolution than SPECT and therefore is more sensitive for detection of metastases except those in the calvarium (142,143).

Neuroblastoma is the third most common malignant tumor of childhood and the most common solid tumor occurring in infants under 1 year of age. Although most of the primary tumors arise in the adrenal gland, they may occur at any site along the sympathetic chain; 20% arise within the thorax. Prognosis is in general dismal, with a 10% to 20% two-year survival rate; but early detection and aggressive management can improve survival significantly.

Approximately 90% of neuroblastomas concentrate ^{131}I- or ^{123}I-MIBG. The usefulness of MIBG scintigraphy in the diagnosis, staging, and follow-up of neuroblastoma has been demonstrated in numerous reports. By convention, patients are initially staged with CT/MRI, bilateral iliac crest biopsies, and bone scintigraphy with ^{99m}Tc-labeled diphosphonates. Because of the physiologic activity at the epiphyseal growth plates and the tendency of neuroblastomas to metastasize to the distal femurs and proximal tibias, sometimes in a symmetrical pattern, ^{99m}Tc-diphosphonate bone scintigraphy is often difficult to interpret in these patients. The sensitivity of MRI for the detection of bone marrow metastasis is well established, but the specificity, particularly following chemotherapy, is much lower; MRI marrow signal may remain abnormal for up to 2 years following chemotherapy in the absence of viable tumor, and there is virtually always a delay as compared with MIBG scintigraphy. Since normal bone and bone marrow do not accumulate MIBG, the presence or absence of bone metastases is easily discerned; false-positive MIBG bone marrow findings have not been reported, although false-negative results do occur (144). MIBG scintigraphy is more sensitive than bone scintigraphy for staging neuroblastoma, and bone scintigraphy can be omitted if MIBG imaging is performed. Both MIBG and MRI are recommended and considered complementary in the staging and follow-up of patients with neuroblastoma. It has been recommended by some that ^{18}F-FDG PET/CT combined with marrow biopsies may be sufficient for follow-up and restaging.

MIBG scintigraphy may be useful in the detection, staging, and follow-up of patients with other neuroendocrine tumors. Approximately 80% to 90% of paragangliomas, 60% of carcinoid tumors, and <50% of medullary carcinomas of the thyroid concentrate MIBG (136). For neuroendocrine tumors demonstrated to be MIBG-avid, high-dose ^{131}I-MIBG treatment may provide palliation.

Diagnosis: Metastatic neuroblastoma.

CASE 8.29

History: A 37-year-old woman presented with an enlarging left neck mass. MRI and subsequently ^{111}In-octreotide scintigraphy and carotid arteriography (Fig. 8.29) were performed. Catecholamine excretion was normal.

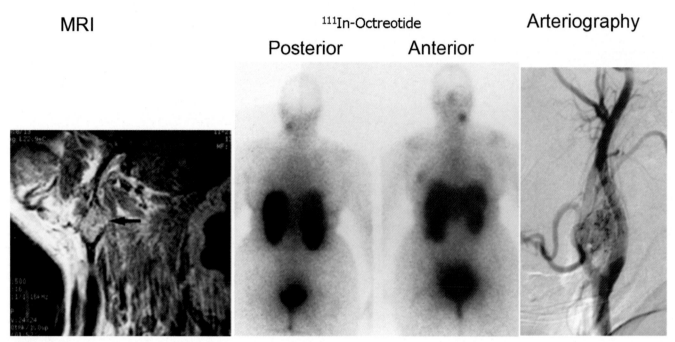

MRI   ^{111}In-Octreotide   Arteriography

Posterior   Anterior

Figure 8.29

Findings: The sagittal MRI image demonstrates a 2.5-cm vascular mass at the left carotid bifurcation (arrow). A CT scan (not shown) performed at an outside institution revealed a similar mass with mild contrast enhancement inseparable from the jugular vein, internal carotid artery, and external carotid. The posterior and anterior (right) whole-body ^{111}In-octreotide images demonstrate a solitary focus of abnormal activity in the left neck congruent with the mass seen on MR and CT. In addition to the usual physiologic activity at the liver, spleen, kidneys, and bowel, faint symmetrical activity in the thyroid and pituitary is identified; and this too is physiologic. The arteriogram shows a markedly vascular 2.4-cm mass at the left carotid bifurcation with splaying of the internal and external carotid arteries (the "lyre sign").

Discussion: The MR and CT are consistent with a paraganglioma or a schwannoma; lymphadenopathy is a less likely explanation. The scintigraphic finding of an SSR-positive mass narrows the diagnosis to a carotid body paraganglioma (or chemodectoma or glomus jugulare tumor). No additional paraganglioma tumors are identified in the neck, thorax, or abdomen. The carotid arteriogram is used principally for surgical planning but also for preoperative embolization, as in this case. At surgery, a 2- by 1.5-cm partially necrotic paraganglioma was resected; adjacent lymph nodes were negative for tumor.

[111]In-octreotide imaging has been reported to detect 33 of 33 paragangliomas and is preferable to the use of radioiodinated MIBG (sensitivity 52%), although the two may sometimes be complementary (136). In the proper clinical context, the specificity of SSR scintigraphy is excellent. With the high sensitivity of CT/MRI for the detection of localized paraganglioma, the advantage of whole-body ^{111}In-octreotide imaging lies in the detection of multiple tumors or metastases preoperatively.

Paragangliomas are neuroectodermal neoplasms arising from paraganglia of the autonomic nervous system and may occur anywhere along the autonomic chain, from the base of the brain to the urinary bladder. Paragangliomas of the head and neck occur most often in the jugular fossa and involve the carotid body or the vagal ganglia; they only rarely secrete catecholamines. Although paragangliomas are usually solitary, benign, and sporadic, approximately 10% of patients have a family history of paraganglioma. Those with a family history have a 26% incidence of multiple tumors and should be screened periodically.

Patients with suspected paraganglioma of the head and neck preoperatively undergo CT or MRI as well as carotid arteriography. The use of ^{111}In-octreotide permits the avoidance of bilateral carotid arteriography and is highly accurate for the detection of multiple tumors, metastases, and coexisting pheochromocytomas (136). For detection of benign pheochromocytoma, ^{123}I-MIBG is more sensitive than ^{111}In-octreotide, 90% compared with 25% (145). For malignant pheochromocytoma, the sensitivity is similar, but some MIBG-negative lesions may be octreotide-positive.

There is also evidence that ^{18}F-FDG PET may be the most sensitive imaging modality for the detection of malignant pheochromocytomas—more sensitive than MIBG (146,147). ^{18}F-FDG uptake is found in many pheochromocytomas, but in a greater percentage of malignant than benign tumors. ^{18}F-FDG PET is especially useful in defining the distribution of those pheochromocytomas that fail to concentrate MIBG.

Diagnosis: Solitary carotid paraganglioma.

CASE 8.30

History: A 64-year-old man with recurrent peptic ulcer disease was found to have an elevated fasting serum gastrin level. There was no family history of endocrinopathy. A contrast-enhanced CT scan was normal. An ^{111}In-octreotide scan was performed (Fig. 8.30 A) and repeated 4 months postoperatively (Fig. 8.30 B).

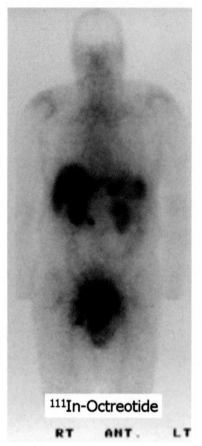

Figure 8.30 A

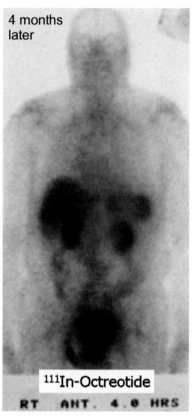

Figure 8.30 B

Findings: On the anterior planar images (Fig. 8.30 A), there is a solitary focus of abnormally increased activity in the midabdomen just medial to the inferior pole of the right kidney. The scintigraphic findings are most compatible with a SSR-positive tumor in the head of the pancreas despite the negative CT exam. At laparotomy, a solitary gastrinoma was enucleated from the head of the pancreas. Several small periportal malignant nodes were resected as well. Using intraoperative US and palpation, no additional tumor sites were detected. A repeat ^{111}In-octreotide scan performed 4 months (Fig. 8.30 B) postoperatively revealed no pathologic foci, and the patient was clinically improved.

Discussion: Functioning islet cell tumors of the pancreas tend to be small and are difficult to detect using conventional radiographic techniques. The diagnosis of these tumors is made clinically and confirmed biochemically, but accurate localization is necessary for surgical resection. Nonfunctioning islet-cell tumors are also typically SSR-positive, and SSR scintigraphy may be helpful to differentiate adenocarcinoma of the pancreas from nonfunctioning islet cell tumors.

The majority of gastrinomas are sporadic rather than familial. They are usually solitary and malignant and tend to occur in the pancreatic head and the surrounding peripancreatic regions. Metastatic adenopathy is often seen. Familial gastrinomas occurring in patients with MEN1, on the other hand, tend to be small and multifocal but less often malignant.

In the detection of gastrinomas, ^{111}In-octreotide SPECT is more sensitive than conventional radiographic imaging and possesses a very high specificity. Furthermore, SPECT is more accurate than CT in the determination of the extent of disease. In a series of 122 consecutive patients with gastrinoma, investigators at the National Institutes of Health (NIH) found that ^{111}In-octreotide scintigraphy was more sensitive (61%) than CT (48%) and MRI (50%) and equal in sensitivity to the results of a combination of all conventional radiographic studies (62%), including angiography (148). In patients with metastatic liver disease, ^{111}In-octreotide imaging was more sensitive (100%) than CT (64%) and MRI (80%). Preoperatively, management is altered in approximately half the patients. Although metastases are often detected with

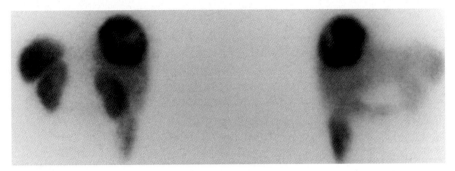

Figure 8.30 C

SPECT, the primary lesion is not always located. Figure 8.30 C is an example of posterior (left) and anterior whole-body ^{111}In-octreotide scintigraphy in a 34-year-old man with Zollinger-Ellison syndrome who was found to have a large 10-cm cystic lesion within the right lobe of the liver. The rim of SSR positivity surrounding the photopenic center was consistent with an islet cell tumor, and the serum gastrin of 3,800 pg/dL was indicative of a gastrinoma.

Resection of the right lobe of the liver revealed a partially necrotic gastrinoma, but a primary lesion could not be detected intraoperatively by palpation, US, or duodenal transillumination. While it is most likely that this lesion is metastatic, primary neuroendocrine tumors have rarely been reported in the liver. Postoperatively, the patient's postbulbar ulcerations healed and his serum gastrin decreased to normal at 80 pg/dL.

The intraoperative use of a handheld gamma probe after the preoperative injection of ^{111}In-octreotide has been reported to be more accurate than SPECT in detecting small (<1 cm) deposits of neuroendocrine tumors.

In summary, the overall sensitivity of ^{111}In-octreotide scintigraphy for the detection of gastrinoma is approximately 65% to 75%, with a relatively high positive predictive value, but a negative scan is less useful (149). In the patient with no evidence of metastases, the use of CT, MRI, and/or angiography may reveal a primary tumor in an additional 10% to 15% of SSR-negative patients. However, in view of the high accuracy of ^{111}In-octreotide imaging of hepatic metastases, additional imaging techniques are unlikely to reveal liver metastases in SSR-negative patients. The sensitivity of ^{111}In-octreotide scintigraphy remains high for the detection of other islet cell tumors, such as nonfunctioning tumors, glucagonomas, somatostatinomas, and VIPomas, but it is of little use in the detection of insulinomas.

Diagnosis: Gastrinoma, somatostatin receptor–positive.

REFERENCES AND SUGGESTED READING

1. Cook GJR, Fogelman I, Maisey MN. Normal physiological and benign pathological variants of 18-fluoro-2-deoxyglucose positron emission tomography scanning: potential for error in interpretation. *Semin Nucl Med* 1996;26:308–314.

2. Engel H, Steinert H, Buck A, et al. Whole body PET: physiological and artifactual fluorodeoxyglucose accumulations. *J Nucl Med* 1996;37:441–446.

3. Delbeke D (Chair), Coleman RE, Guiberteau MJ, et al. Society of Nuclear Medicine procedure guidelines for tumor imaging using FDG PET/CT. *J Nucl Med* 2006;47(5):885–895.

4. Juweid ME, Stroobants S, Hoekstra OS, et al. Use of positron emission tomography for response assessment of lymphoma: consensus of the Imaging Subcommittee of International Harmonization Project in Lymphoma. *J Clin Oncol* 2007;25(5):571–578.

5. Krenning EP, Kwekkeboom DJ, Reubi JC, et al. Somatostatin receptor scintigraphy. In: Sandler MP et al, eds. *Diagnostic Nuclear Medicine,* 3rd ed. Baltimore: Lippincott Williams & Wilkins, 1997;1047–1066.

6. Gelfand MJ. Metaiodobenzylguanidine in children. *Semin Nucl Med* 1993;23:231–242.

7. Zucker LS, DeNardo GL. Trials and tribulations: oncological antibody imaging comes to the fore. *Semin Nucl Med* 1997;27:10–29.

8. Gambhir SS, Czernin J, Schimmer J, et al. A tabulated summary of the FDG PET literature. *J Nucl Med* 2001;42(Suppl):1S–93S.

9. Ciernik IF, Dizendorf E, Ciernik IF, et al. Radiation treatment planning with an integrated positron emission and computer tomography (PET/CT): a feasibility study. *Int J Radiation Biol Phys* 2003;57:853–863.

10. Coleman RE, Delbeke D, Guiberteau MJ, et al. Intersociety dialogue on concurrent PET-CT with an integrated imaging system: from the Joint ACR/SNM/SCBT-MR PET-CT Working Group. *J Nucl Med* 2005;46:1225–1239.

11. Delbeke D (Chair), Coleman RE, Guiberteau MJ, et al. Society of Nuclear Medicine procedure guidelines for SPECT/CT imaging. *J Nucl Med* 2006;47:1227–1228.

12. Lerman H, Metser U, Grisaru D, et al. Normal and abnormal 18F-FDG endometrial and ovarian uptake in pre- and postmenopausal patients: assessment by PET/CT. *J Nucl Med* 2004;45:266–271.

13. Zhuang H, Alavi A. 18-Fluorodeoxyglucose positron emission tomographic imaging in the detection and monitoring of infection and inflammation. *Semin Nucl Med* 2002;32(1):47–59.

14. Lewis P, Salama A. Uptake of fluorine-18-fluorodeoxyglucose in sarcoidosis. *J Nucl Med* 1994; 35:1647–1649.

15. Huitink JM, Visser FC, van Leeuwen GR, et al. Influence of high and low plasma insulin levels on the uptake of fluorine-18 fluorodeoxyglucose in myocardium and femoral muscle, assessed by planar imaging. *Eur J Nucl Med* 1995;22(10):1141–1148.

16. Lindholm P, Minn H, Leskinen-Kallio S, et al. Influence of the blood glucose concentration on FDG uptake in cancer—a PET study. *J Nucl Med* 1993; 34(1):1–6

17. http://www.cancer.gov/cancertopics/pdq/treatment/laryngeal/HealthProfessional/page3#Section_48

18. http://www.bcm.edu/oto/studs/anat/neck.html

19. Adams S, Baum RP, Stuckensen T, et al. Prospective comparison of 18F-FDG PET with conventional imaging modalities (CT, MRI, US) in lymph node staging of head and neck cancer. *Eur J Nucl Med* 1998;25:1255–1260.

20. Hannah A, Scott AM, Tochon-Danguy H, et al. Evaluation of 18 F-fluorodeoxyglucose positron emission tomography and computed tomography with histopathologic correlation in the initial staging of head and neck cancer. *Ann Surg* 2002;236:208–217.

21. Myers LL, Wax MK, Nabi H, et al. Positron emission tomography in the evaluation of the N0 neck. *Laryngoscope* 1998;108:232–236.

22. Stoeckli SJ, Steinert H, Pfaltz M, et al. Is there a role for positron emission tomography with 18-F fluorodeoxyglucose in the initial staging of nodal negative oral and oropharyngeal squamous cell carcinoma. *Head Neck* 2002;24(4):345–349.

23. Anzai Y, Carroll WR, Quint DJ, et al. Recurrence of head and neck cancer after surgery or irradiation: prospective comparison of 2-deoxy-2-[F-18]fluoro-D-glucose PET and MR imaging diagnoses. *Radiology* 1996;200:135–141.

24. Kunkel M, Forster GJ, Reichert TE, et al. Detection of recurrent oral squamous cell carcinoma by [18F]-2-fluorodeoxyglucose-positron emission tomography: implications for prognosis and patient management. *Cancer* 2003;98:2257–2265

25. Delgado-Bolton RC, Fernandez-Perez C, Gonzalez-Mate A, et al. Meta-analysis of the performance of 18F-FDG PET in primary tumor detection in unknown primary tumors. *J Nucl Med* 2003;44:1301–1314.

26. Schoder H, Yeung HW, Gonen M, et al. Head and neck cancer: clinical usefulness and accuracy of PET/CT image fusion. *Radiology* 2004;231(1):65–72.

27. Diehl M, Risse JH, Brandt-Mainz K, et al., Fluorine-18 fluorodeoxyglucose positron emission tomography in medullary thyroid cancer: results of a multicentre study. *Eur J Nucl Med* 2001;28(11):1671–1676.

28. Ong SC, Schöder H, Patel SG, et al. Diagnostic accuracy of 18F-FDG PET in restaging patients with medullary thyroid carcinoma and elevated calcitonin levels. *J Nucl Med* 2007;48(4):501–507.

29. van Heerden JA, Grant CS, Gharib H, et al. Long term course of patients with persistent hypercalcitoninemia after apparent curative primary surgery for medullary thyroid carcinoma. *Ann Surg* 1990;212:395–400.

30. Ellenhorn JDI, Shah JP, Brennan MF. Impact of therapeutic regional lymph node dissection for medullary carcinoma of the thyroid gland. *Surgery* 1993;114:1078–1081.

31. Saad MF, Guido JJ, Samaan NA. Radioacive iodine in the treatment of medullary carcinoma of the thyroid. *J Clin Endocrinol Metab* 1983;57:124–128.

32. Kwekkeboom DJ, Reubi JC, Lamberts SW, et al. The potential value of somatostatin receptor scintigraphy in medullary thyroid carcinoma. *J Clin Endocrinol Metab* 1993;76:1413–1417.

33. Troncone L, Rufini V, Montemaggi P, et al. The diagnostic and therapeutic utility of radioiodinated metaiodobenzylguanidine (MIBG): 5 years of experience. *Eur J Nucl Med* 1990;16:325–335.

34. Skowsky WR, Wilf LH. Iodine-131 metaiodobenzylguanidine scintigraphy of medullary carcinoma of the thyroid. *South Med J* 1991;84:636–641.

35. Clarke SE. [131I]metaiodobenzylguanidine therapy in medullary thyroid cancer: Guy's hospital experience. *J Nucl Biol Med* 1991;35:323–326.

36. Wang W, Macapinlac H, Finn RD, et al. PET scanning with [18F] 2-fluoro-2 deoxy-D-glucose (FDG) can localize residual differentiated thyroid cancer in patients with negative [131I]-iodine whole-body scans. *J Clin Endocrinol Metab* 1999;84:2291–2302.

37. Wang W, Larson SM, Fazzari M, et al. Prognostic value of [18F]fluorodeoxyglucose positron emission tomographic scanning in patients with thyroid cancer. *J Clin Endocrinol Metab* 2000;85(3):1107–1113.

38. Chin BB, Patel P, Cohade C, et al. Recombinant human thyrotropin stimulation of fluoro-D-glucose positron emission tomography uptake in well-differentiated thyroid carcinoma. *J Clin Endocrinol Metab* 2004;89(1):91–95.

39. Lowe VJ, Mullan BP, Hay ID, et al. 18F-FDG PET of patients with Hurthle cell carcinoma. *J Nucl Med* 2003:44(9):1402–1406.

40. Flamen P, Lerut A, Van Cutsem E, et al. Utility of positron emission tomography for the staging of patients with potentially operable esophageal carcinoma. *J Clin Oncol* 2000;18(18):3202–3210.

41. Wallace MB, Nietert PJ, Earle C, et al. An analysis of multiple staging management strategies for carcinoma of the esophagus: computed tomography, endoscopic ultrasound, positron emission tomography, and thoracoscopy/laparoscopy. *Ann Thorac Surg* 2002;74(4):1026–1032.

42. Stambroglio L, Nosotti M, Bellaviti N, et al. CT-guided fine-needle aspiration cytology of solitary pulmonary nodules: a prospective, randomized study of immediate cytologic evaluation. *Chest* 1997;112(2):423–425.

43. Gould MK, Maclean CC, Kuschner WG, et al. Accuracy of positron emission tomography for diagnosis of pulmonary nodules and mass lesions: a meta-analysis. *JAMA* 2001;285(7):914–924.

44. Berger KL, Nicholson SA, Dehdashti F, et al. FDG PET evaluation of mucinous neoplasms: correlation of FDG uptake with histopathologic features. *Am J Roentgenol* 2000;174(4):1005–1008.

45. Higashi K, Ueda Y, Seki H, et al. Fluorine-18-FDG PET imaging is negative in bronchioloalveolar lung carcinoma. *J Nucl Med* 1998;39(6):1016–1020.

46. Erasmus JJ, McAdams HP, Patz EF Jr, et al. Evaluation of primary pulmonary carcinoid tumors using FDG PET. *Am J Roentgenol* 1998;170(5):1369–1373.

47. Gambhir SS, Shepherd JE, Shah BD, et al. Analytical decision model for the cost-effective management of solitary pulmonary nodules. *J Clin Oncol* 1998;16(6):2113–2125.

48. http://www.cancer.gov/cancertopics/pdq/treatment/non-small-cell-lung/HealthProfessional/page3

49. Cymbalista M, Waysberg A, Zacharias C, et al. CT demonstration of the 1996 AJCC-UICC regional lymph node classification for lung cancer staging. *Radiographics* 1999;4:899–900 (poster).

50. Steinert HC, Hauser M, Alleman F, et al. Non-small cell lung cancer: Nodal staging with FDG-PET versus CT with correlative lymph node mapping and sampling. *Radiology* 1997;202:441–446.

51. De Leyn P, Vansteenkiste J, Cuypers P, et al. Role of cervical mediastinoscopy in staging of non-small cell lung cancer without enlarged mediastinal lymph nodes on CT scan. *Eur J Cardiothorac Surg* 1997; 12:706–712.

52. De Leyn P, Schoonooghe P, Deneffe G, et al. Surgery for non-small cell lung cancer with unsuspected metastasis to ipsilateral mediastinal or subcarinal nodes (N2 disease). *Eur J Cardiothorac Surg* 1996;10: 649–654.

53. Scott WJ, Gobar LS, Terry JD, et al. Mediastinal lymph node staging of non-small-cell lung cancer: a prospective comparison of computed tomography and positron emission tomography. *J Thorac Cardiovascul Surg* 1996;111:642–648.

54. Dwamena BA, Sonnad SS, Angobaldo JO, et al. Metastases from non-small cell lung cancer: mediastinal staging in the 1990s – meta-analytic comparison of PET and CT. *Radiology* 1999;213(2):530–536.

55. Pieterman RM, van Putten JW, Meuzelaar JJ, et al. Preoperative staging of non-small cell lung cancer with positron emission tomography. *N Engl J Med* 2000;343(4):254–261.

56. Gambhir SS, Hoh CK, Phelps ME, et al. Decision tree sensitivity analysis for cost-effectiveness of FDG-PET in the staging and management of non-small-cell lung carcinoma. *J Nucl Med* 1996;37:1428–1436.

57. Lardinois D, Weder W, Hany TF, et al. Staging of non-small cell lung cancer with integrated positron-emission tomography and computed tomography. *N Engl J Med* 2003;348:2500–2507.

58. Andre F, Grunenwald D, Pignon J-P, et al. Survival of patients with resected N2 non-small cell lung cancer: Evidence for a subclassification and implications. *J Clin Oncol* 2000;18(16):2981–2989.

59. Ludwig, V, Komori T, Kolb DC, et al. Cerebral lesions incidentally detected on FDG PET images of patients evaluated for body malignancies. *Mol Imaging Biol* 2002;4(5):359–362.

60. Bury T, Barreto A, Daenen F, et al. Fluorine-18 deoxyglucose positron emission tomography for the detection of bone metastases in patients with non-small cell lung cancer. *Eur J Nucl Med* 1998;25:1244–1247.

61. Boland GW et al. Indeterminate adrenal masses in patients with cancer. Evaluation at PET with 2-(F-18)-fluoro-2-deoxy-D-glucose. *Radiology* 1995;194:131–134.

62. Kamle EM, Zwahlen D, Wyss MT, Stumpe KD, von Schulthess GK, Steinert HC. Whole-body 18-FDG PET improves management of patients with small-cell-lung-cancer. *J Nucl Med* 2003;44:1911–1917.

63. Pandit N, Gonen M, Krug L, et al. Prognostic value of 18-FDG-PET imaging in small cell lung cancer. *Eur Nucl Med Mol Imaging* 2003;30: 78–84.

64. Aarsvold JN, Alzaraki NP. Update on detection of sentinel lymph nodes in patients with breast cancer. *Semin Nucl Med* 2005;35(2):116–128.

65. Paganelli G. Sentinel node biopsy: role of nuclear medicine in conservative surgery of breast cancer. *Eur J Nucl Med* 1998;25:99–100.

66. Povoski SP, Olsen JO, Young DC, et al. Prospective randomized clinical trial comparing intradermal, intraparenchymal and subareolar injection routes for sentinel lymph node mapping and biopsy in breast cancer. *Ann Surg Oncol* 2006;13(11):1412–1421.

67. Even-Sapir E, Metser U, Mishani E, et al. The detection of bone metastases in patients with high-risk prostate cancer: 99mTc-MDP Planar bone scintigraphy, single- and multi-field-of-view SPECT, 18F-fluoride PET, and 18F-fluoride PET/CT. *J Nucl Med* 2006;47(2):287–297.

68. Eubank WB, Mankoff DA. Evolving role of positron emission tomography in breast cancer imaging. *Semin Nucl Med* 2005;35(2):84–99.

69. http://www.cancer.gov/cancertopics/pdq/treatment/breast/HealthProfessional/page3

70. Wahl RL, Siegel BA, Coleman RE, et al. Prospective multicenter study of axillary nodal staging by positron emission tomography in breast cancer: a report of the staging breast cancer with PET Study Group. *J Clin Oncol* 2004;22(2):277–285.

71. van der Hoeven JJ, Hoekstra OS, Comans EF, et al. Determinants of diagnostic performance of [F-18]fluorodeoxyglucose positron emission tomography for axillary staging in breast cancer. *Ann Surg* 2002;236(5):619–624.

72. Wilking N, Rutqvist LE, Cartensen J, et al. Prognostic significance of axillary nodal status in primary breast cancer in relation to the number of resected nodes. *Acta Oncol* 1992;31:29–35.

73. Avril N, Dose J, Janicke F, et al. Assessment of axillary lymph node involvement in breast cancer patients with positron emission tomography using radiolabeled 2-(fluorine-18)-fluoro-2-deoxy-D-glucose. *J Natl Cancer Inst* 1996;88(17):1204–1209.

74. Bellon JR, Livingston RB, Eubank WB, et al. Evaluation of the internal mammary lymph nodes by FDG-PET in locally advanced breast cancer (LABC). *Am J Clin Oncol* 2004;27(4):407–410.

75. Isasi CR, Moadel RM, Blaufox MD. A meta-analysis of FDG-PET for the evaluation of breast cancer recurrence and metastases. *Breast Cancer Res Treat* 2005;90(2):105–112.

76. Eubank WB, Mankoff D, Bhattacharya M, et al. Impact of FDG PET on defining the extent of disease and on the treatment of patients with recurrent or metastatic breast cancer. *AJR Am J Roentgenol* 2004;183(2):479–486.

77. Yap CS, Seltzer MA, Schiepers C, et al. Impact of whole-body 18F-FDG PET on staging and managing patients with breast cancer: the referring physician's perspective. *J Nucl Med* 2001;42(9):1334–1337.

78. Pelosi E, Messa C, Sironi S, et al. Value of integrated PET/CT for lesion localisation in cancer patients: a comparative study. *Eur J Nucl Med Mol Imaging* 2004;31(7):932–939.

79. Delbeke D. FDG PET and PET-CT for evaluation of colorectal carcinoma. *Semin Nucl Med* 2004;34:209–223.

80. Kantorova I, Lipska L, Belohlavek O, et al. Routine 18F-FDG PET preoperative staging of colorectal cancer: comparison with conventional staging and its impact on treatment decision making. *J Nucl Med* 2003;44:1784–1788.

81. Huebner RH, Park KC, Shepherd JE, et al. A meta-analysis of the literature for whole-body FDG PET detection of colorectal cancer. *J Nucl Med* 2000;41:1177–1189.

82. Kinkel K, Lu Y, Both M, et al. Detection of hepatic metastases from cancers of the gastrointestinal tract by using noninvasive imaging methods (US, CT, MR imaging, PET): a meta-analysis. *Radiology* 2002;224(3): 748–756.

83. Bipat S, vanLeeuwen MS, Comans EF, et al. Colorectal liver metastases: CT, MR imaging, and PET for diagnosis—meta analysis. *Radiology* 2005;237:123–131.

84. Valk PE, Abella-Columna E, Haseman MK, et al. Whole-body PET imaging with F-18-fluorodeoxyglucose in management of recurrent colorectal cancer. *Arch Surg* 1999;134:503–511.

85. Ruers TJ, Langenhoff BS, Neeleman N, et al. Value of positron emission tomography with [F-18] fluorodeoxyglucose in patients with colorectal liver metastases: a prospective study. *J Clin Oncol* 2002;20(2): 388–395.

86. Fernandez FG, Drebin JA, Linehan DC, et al. Five-year survival after resection of hepatic metastases from colorectal cancer in patients screened by positron emission tomography with F-18 fluorodeoxyglucose (FDG-PET). *Ann Surg* 2004;240(3):438–447; discussion 447–450.

87. Cohade C, Osman M, Leal J, et al. Direct comparison of FDG PET and PET-CT imaging in colorectal carcinoma. *J Nucl Med* 2003;44:1797–1803.

88. Liu LX, Zhang WH, Jiang HC. Current treatment for liver metastases from colorectal cancer. *World J Gastroenterol* 2003;9(2):193–200.

89. Gray B, Van Hazel G, Hope M, et al. Randomized trial of Sir-spheres plus chemotherapy vs chemotherapy alone for treating patients with liver metastases from primary large bowel cancer. *Ann Oncol* 2001;12 (12):1711–1720.

90. Wong CY, Salem R, Qing F, et al. Metabolic response after intra-arterial 90Y-glass microsphere treatment for colorectal liver metastases: comparison of quantitative and visual analysis by 18F-FDG PET. *J Nucl Med* 2004;45(11):1892–1897.

91. Langenhoff BS, Oyen WJ, Jager GJ, et al. Efficacy of fluorine-18-deoxyglucose positron emission tomography in detecting tumor recurrence after local ablative therapy for liver metastases: a prospective study. *J Clin Oncol* 2002;20:4453–4458.

92. Rose AT, Rose DM, Pinson CW, et al. Hepatocellular carcinoma outcome based on indicated treatment strategy. *Am Surg* 1998;64:1122–1135.

93. Ho CL, Chen S, Yeung DW, Cheng TK. Dual-tracer PET/CT imaging in evaluation of metastatic hepatocellular carcinoma. *J Nucl Med* 2007; 48(6):902–909.

94. Guthrie JA, Ward J, Robinson PJ. Hilar cholangiocarcinomas: T2-weighted spin-echo and gadolinium-enhanced FLASH MR imaging. *Radiology* 1996;201(2):347–351.

95. Keiding S, Hansen SB, Rasmussen HH, et al. Detection of cholangiocarcinoma in primary sclerosing cholangitis by positron emission tomography. *Hepatology* 1998;28:700–706.

96. Anderson CA, Rice MH, Pinson CW, et al. FDG PET imaging in the evaluation of gallbladder carcinoma and cholangiocarcinoma. *J Gastrointest Surg* 2004;8(1):90–97.

97. Hoh CK, Hawkins RA, Glaspy JA, et al. Cancer detection with whole-body PET using 2-[18F]fluoro-2-deoxy-D-glucose. *J Comput Assist Tomogr* 1993;17:582–589.

98. Delbeke D. Pancreatic tumors: role of imaging in the diagnosis, staging, decision making and treatment. *J Hepatobiliary Pancreat Surg* 2004; 11(1):4–10.

99. Kang KW, Kim SK, Kang HS, et al. Prevalence and risk of cancer of focal thyroid incidentaloma identified by 18F-fluorodeoxyglucose positron emission tomography for metastasis evaluation and cancer screening in healthy subjects. *Clin Endocrinol Metab* 2003;88:4100–4104.

100. National Cancer Institute: http://www.cancer.gov/cancertopics/

101. Ping Lu. Staging and classification of lymphoma. *Semin Nucl Med* 2005;35:160–164.

102. Israel O, Keidar Z, Bar-Shalom R. Positron emission tomography in the evaluation of lymphoma. *Semin Nucl Med* 2004;34:166–179.

103. Buchmann I, Reinhardt M, Elsner K, et al. 2-(fluorine-18)fluoro-2-deoxy-D-glucose positron emission tomography in the detection and staging of malignant lymphoma. A bicenter trial. *Cancer* 2001;91(5):889–899.

104. Hicks RJ, Mac Manus MP, Seymour JF. Initial staging of lymphoma with positron emission tomography and computed tomography. *Semin Nucl Med* 2005;35:165–175.

105. Bar-Shalom R, Mor M, Yefremov N, et al. The value of Ga-67 scintigraphy and F-18 fluorodeoxyglucose positron emission tomography in staging and monitoring the response of lymphoma to treatment. *Semin Nucl Med* 2001;31:177–190.

106. Ferdinand B, Gupta P, Kramer EL. Spectrum of thymic uptake at 18F-FDG PET. *Radiographics* 2004;24:1611–1616.

107. Jerusalem G, Hustinx R, Beguin Y, et al. Evaluation of therapy for lymphoma. *Semin Nucl Med* 2005;35:186–196.

108. Young H, Baum R, Cremerius U, et al. Measurement of clinical and subclinical tumour response using [18F]-fluorodeoxyglucose and positron emission tomography: review and 1999 EORTC recommendations. European Organization for Research and Treatment of Cancer (EORTC) PET Study Group. *Eur J Cancer* 1999;35(13):1773–1782.

109. www.cancer.gov/cancertopics/pdq/treatment/melanoma/healthprofessional/page1

110. Owen SA, Sanders LL, Edwards LJ, et al. Identification of higher risk thin melanomas should be based on Breslow depth not Clark level IV. *Cancer* 2001;91(5):983–991.

111. www.cancer.gov/cancertopics/pdq/treatment/melanoma/healthprofessional/page3

112. Morton DL, Thompson JF, Cochran AJ, et al. Sentinel-node biopsy or nodal observation in melanoma. *N Engl J Med* 355(13):1307–1317, 2006. Erratum in: *N Engl J Med* 355(18):1944, 2006.

113. Alazraki N, Glass EC, Castronovo F, et al. Society of Nuclear Medicine procedure guideline for lymphoscintigraphy and the use of intraoperative gamma probe for sentinel lymph node localization in melanoma of intermediate thickness, version 1.0, 2002. http://interactive.snm.org/docs/pg_ch24_0403.pdf)

114. Friedman KP, Wahl RL. Clinical use of positron emission tomography in the management of cutaneous melanoma. *Semin Nucl Med* 2004;34(4):242–253.

115. Wagner JD, Schauwecker DS, Davidson D, et al. FDG-PET sensitivity for melanoma lymph node metastases is dependent on tumor volume. *J Surg Oncol* 2001;77:237–242.

116. Schwimmer J, Essner R, Patel A, et al. A review of the literature for whole-body FDG PET in the management of patients with melanoma. *Q J Nucl Med* 2000;44(2):153–167.

117. Stehman FB, Bundy BN, DiSaia PJ, et al. Carcinoma of the cervix treated with radiation therapy. I. A multi-variate analysis of prognostic variables in the Gynecologic Oncology Group. *Cancer* 1991;67:2776–2785.

118. Grigsby PW, Siegel BA, Dehdashti F. Lymph node staging by positron emission tomography in patients with carcinoma of the cervix. *J Clin Oncol* 2001;19:3745–3749.

119. Reinhardt MJ, Ehritt-Braun C, Vogelgesang D, et al. Metastatic lymph nodes in patients with cervical cancer: detection with MR imaging and FDG PET. *Radiology* 2001;218:776–782.

120. Tran BN, Grigsby PW, Dehdashti F, et al. Occult supraclavicular lymph node metastasis identified by FDG-PET in patients with carcinoma of the uterine cervix. *Gynecol Oncol* 2003;90:572–576.

121. Havrilesky LJ, Kulasingam SL, Matchar DB, et al. FDG-PET for management of cervical and ovarian cancer. *Gynecol Oncol* 2005;97:183–191.

122. Grab D, Flock F, Stohr I, et al. Classification of asymptomatic adnexal masses by ultrasound, magnetic resonance imaging, and positron emission tomography. *Gynecol Oncol* 2000;77(3):454–459.

123. Rose PG, Faulhaber P, Miraldi F, et al. Positive emission tomography for evaluating a complete clinical response in patients with ovarian or peritoneal carcinoma: correlation with second-look laparotomy. *Gynecol Oncol* 2001;82:17–21.

124. Zimny M, Siggelkow W, Schroder W, et al. 2-[Fluorine-18]-fluoro-2-deoxy-d-glucose positron emission tomography in the diagnosis of recurrent ovarian cancer. *Gynecol Oncol* 2001;83:310–315.

125. Schwarzbach MH, Dimitrakopoulou-Strauss A, Willeke F, et al. Clinical value of 18-F fluorodeoxyglucose positron emission tomography imaging in soft tissue sarcomas. *Ann Surg* 2000;23:380–386.

126. Folpe AI, Lyles RH, Sprouse JT, et al. F-18 fluorodeoxyglucose positron emission tomography as a predictor of pathologic grade and other prognostic variables in bone and soft tissue sarcoma. *Clin Cancer Res* 2000;6:1279–1287.

127. Schuetze SM, Rubin BP, Vernon C, et al. Use of positron emission tomography in localized extremity soft tissue sarcoma treated with neoadjuvant chemotherapy. *Cancer* 2005;103(2):339–348.

128. http://www.cancer.gov/cancertopics/pdq/treatment/renalcell/healthprofessional

129. Bosniak MA. The current radiographic approaches to renal cysts. *Radiology* 1986;158:1–10.

130. Russo P. Renal cell carcinoma: presentation, staging, and surgical treatment. *Semin Oncol* 2000;27:160–176.

131. Schoder H, Larson SM. Positron emission tomography for prostate, bladder, and renal cancer. *Semin Nucl Med* 2004;34:274–292.

132. Kang DE, White RL, Jr, Zuger JH, et al. Clinical use of fluorodeoxyglucose F 18 positron emission tomography for detection of renal cell carcinoma. *J Urol* 2004;171:1806–1809.

133. Hain SF, O'Doherty MJ, Timothy AR, et al. Fluorodeoxyglucose PET in the initial staging of germ cell tumours. *Eur J Nucl Med* 2000;27:590–594.

134. De Santis M, Becherer A, Bokemeyer C, et al. 2-18fluoro-2-deoxy-D-glucose positron emission tomography is a reliable predictor for viable tumor in postchemotherapy seminoma: an update of the prospective multicentric SEMPET trial. *J Clin Oncol* 2004;22:1034–1039.

135. Stephens AW, Gonin R, Hutchins GD et al. Positron emission tomography of residual radiological abnormalities in postchemotherapy germ cell tumour patients. *J Clin Oncol* 1996;14:1637–1641.

136. Krenning EP. Somatostatin receptor scintigraphy. In: Sandler MP et al, eds. *Diagnostic Nuclear Medicine,* 3rd ed. Baltimore: Lippincott Williams & Wilkins, 1996.

137. Even-Sapir E, Keidar Z, Sachs J, et al. The new technology of combined transmission and emission tomography in evaluation of endocrine neoplasms. *J Nucl Med* 2001;42(7):998–1004.

138. Krausz Y, Israel O. Single-photon emission computed tomography/computed tomography in endocrinology. *Semin Nucl Med* 2006;36(4):267–274.

139. Scanga DR, Martin WH, Delbeke D. Value of FDG PET imaging in the management of patients with thyroid, neuroendocrine, and neural crest tumors. *Clin Nucl Med* 2004;29(2):86–90.

140. Belhocine T, Foidart J, Rigo P, et al. Fluorodeoxyglucose positron emission tomography and somatostatin receptor scintigraphy for diagnosing and staging carcinoid tumours: correlations with the pathological indexes p53 and Ki-67. *Nucl Med Commun* 2002;23(8):727–734.

141. Orth DN. Cushing's syndrome. *N Engl J Med* 1995;332:791–803.

142. Kushner BH, Yeung HW, Larson SM, et al. Extending positron emission tomography scan utility to high-risk neuroblastoma: fluorine-18 fluorodeoxyglucose positron emission tomography as sole imaging modality in follow-up of patients. *J Clin Oncol* 2001;19(14):3397–3405.

143. Shulkin BL, Hutchinson RJ, Castle VP, et al. Neuroblastoma: positron emission tomography with 2-[fluorine-18]-fluoro-2-deoxy-D-glucose compared with metaiodobenzylguanidine scintigraphy. *Radiology* 1996;199(3):743–750.

144. Lebtahi N et al. Evaluating bone marrow metastasis of neuroblastoma with iodine-123-MIBG scintigraphy and MRI. *J Nucl Med* 1997;38: 1389–1392.

145. van der Harst E, de Herder WW, Bruining HA, et al. [(123)I]metaiodo-benzylguanidine and [(111)In]octreotide uptake in benign and malignant pheochromocytomas. *J Clin Endocrinol Metab* 2001;86(2):685–693.

146. Shulkin BL, Thompson NW, Shapiro B, et al. Pheochromocytomas: imaging with 2-[fluorine-18]fluoro-2-deoxy-D-glucose PET. *Radiology* 1999;212(1):35–41.

147. Timmers HJ, Kozupa A, Chen CC, et al. Superiority of fluorodeoxyglucose positron emission tomography to other functional imaging techniques in the evaluation of metastatic SDHB-associated pheochromocytoma and paraganglioma. *J Clin Oncol* 2007;25(16):2262–2269.

148. Termanini B, Gibril F, Reynolds JC, Doppman JL, et al. Value of somatostatin receptor scintigraphy: a prospective study in gastrinoma of its effect on clinical management. *Gastroenterology* 1997;112:335–347.

CHAPTER NINE

ARTIFACTS

James A. Patton

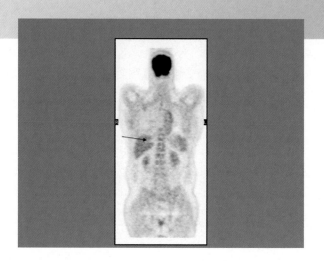

The performance of routine quality assurance procedures on nuclear medicine equipment is necessary to ensure that the equipment is functioning properly prior to its use in nuclear medicine procedures. A daily routine of checking the isotope peak calibration and performing either an intrinsic flood (point source without the collimator) or an extrinsic flood (plane source with the collimator on) can identify many problems. An acceptable intrinsic flood is shown in Figure 9 A. Examples of unacceptable intrinsic flood are window off photopeak (Fig. 9 B), a photomultiplier tube not functioning (Fig. 9 C), failure of the uniformity correction circuitry (Fig. 9 D), and a broken crystal (Fig. 9 E). Performing a flood extrinsically using a plane source with the collimator in place permits an evaluation of the entire detector system in its imaging configuration and can be used to identify collimator damage that might interfere with the proper acquisition of a nuclear medicine study

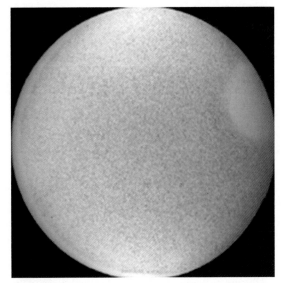

Figure 9 C

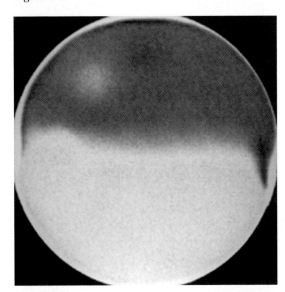

Figure 9 D

Figure 9 A

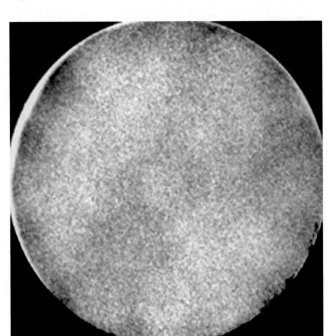

Figure 9 B

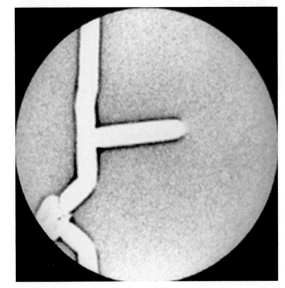

Figure 9 E

Figure 9 F

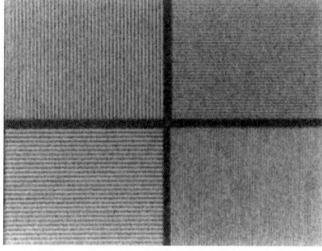

Figure 9 H

(Fig. 9 F). The use of computer-based scintillation cameras permits the implementation of automated protocols to check window and peak positioning and the evaluation of uniformity correction circuitry both visually and quantitatively by calculating the value of integral uniformity in the corrected image (Fig. 9 G). When they are obtained daily, these quantitative values can be used to track trends and maintenance can be scheduled before problems become significant. Weekly monitoring of linearity and spatial resolution with a bar pattern that tests the spatial resolution of the camera (Fig. 9 H) permits the identification of problems that would otherwise go undetected.

The use of single photon emission computed tomography (SPECT) requires the implementation of additional quality control procedures. The center of rotation should be evaluated monthly to ensure that the center of the acquired image at every location corresponds to the center of rotation of the scanning system. Discrepancies in these values will result in circular or ring artifacts in the reconstructed images (Fig. 9 I). The use of a high-count flood for uniformity correction of the acquired planar images prior to image reconstruction is also recommended. Otherwise the presence of a nonuniformity (either hot or cold) in the response of the scintillation camera will result in the amplification of this nonuniformity into a hot or cold ring in the reconstructed images.

However, even with the most diligent approach to routine quality assurance, there are many instances where unusual findings are noted in the images acquired in routine

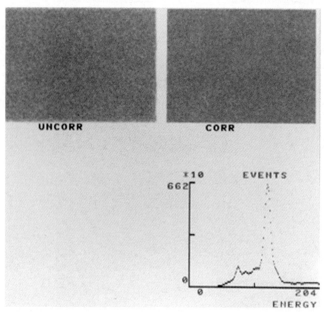

Figure 9 G

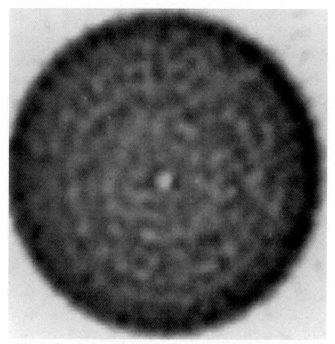

Figure 9 I

nuclear medicine procedures. The following cases describe examples of these abnormalities. Some are due to improper calibration of equipment or equipment failures. Others are due to improper techniques. And finally, others are simply due to patients being studied with clinical conditions that al- ter the routine course of the radiotracers being used for the studies. It is the goal of this chapter to make the reader aware of the many circumstances that may produce apparent arti- facts that warrant further investigation in order to identify their causes.

History/Procedure: A patient presented for a gastroesophageal reflux study. The study was performed with 500 μCi of ^{99m}Tc–sulfur colloid administered orally followed by dynamic acquisition of 15 sequential anterior images, each 1 minute in length, using a large field-of-view camera (Fig. 9.1).

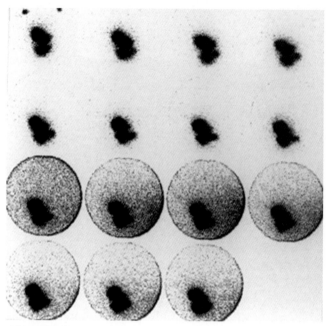

Figure 9.1

Artifact: Nine minutes into the study, the background suddenly increased and remained constant and nonuniform, increasing in intensity from the patient's left to right.

Discussion: When the background suddenly changes in an image, the technologist immediately suspects an equipment malfunction. However, it is useful to first investigate the possibility of a source of high-energy photons that may have entered the vicinity of the procedure currently being performed. In this case, a patient injected with 10 mCi of ^{18}FDG had entered an adjacent room for a stress perfusion/rest metabolism cardiac study. The shielding of the mobile camera was not sufficient to completely absorb the primary and scattered radiation resulting from the 511-keV annihilation radiation from ^{18}F; thus the camera detected the scatter background from the cardiac patient. This is a relatively new problem in nuclear medicine owing to the recent implementation of ^{18}FDG in laboratories that perform a majority of their studies using low-energy photon emitters. It is always important to be certain that injected patients are situated so that their presence will not interfere with ongoing procedures.

Conclusion/Diagnosis: Artifact due to interference from a high-energy source in close proximity to the scintillation camera during part of the imaging procedure.

CASE 9.2

History/Procedure: A patient presented for a bone scan. The study was performed with 20 mCi of ^{99m}Tc-oxidronate (HDP) administered intravenously, followed 2 hours later by static imaging of the whole body using a rectangular field-of-view scintillation camera.

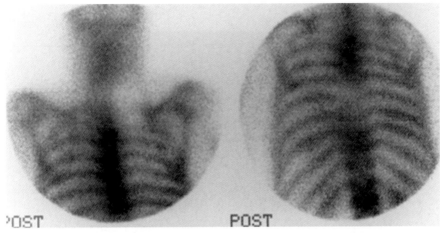

Figure 9.2 A

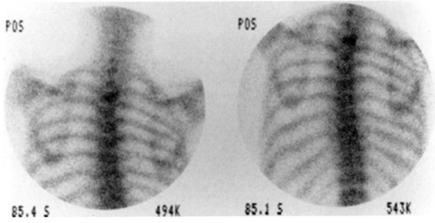

Figure 9.2 B

Artifact: An area of decreased uptake was noted in each of the images, as demonstrated in the neck region and the spine (Fig. 9.2 A). It was noted that artifacts occurred in exactly the same area of the camera in each of the images. When the study was repeated on a different scintillation camera, the areas of decreased uptake were not seen (Fig. 9.2 B).

Discussion: When an area of decreased uptake is noted in multiple images from the same area of the camera, a photomultiplier tube/preamplifier drift or failure is immediately suspected. This problem can be easily verified by performing a flood, as shown earlier in Figure 9 C (not the same camera as used for the study described here). Usually, systems failures of this type are easily identified. However, occasionally they are very subtle and the technologists and physicians should carefully review abnormal findings of this type to be sure that they represent true abnormal uptake of the radiopharmaceutical and not equipment malfunctions.

Conclusion/Diagnosis: Artifact due to photomultiplier tube drift.

History/Procedure: A patient presented for a bone scan to evaluate for metastatic disease. The patient was administered 20 mCi of ^{99m}Tc-oxidronate (HDP), and whole-body images were obtained 2 hours later using a rectangular field-of-view digital scintillation camera. Multiple areas of increased uptake were identified that were consistent with metastatic disease (Fig. 9.3 A). However, it was observed that the overall quality of the images was poor, and there appeared to have been a degradation in spatial resolution.

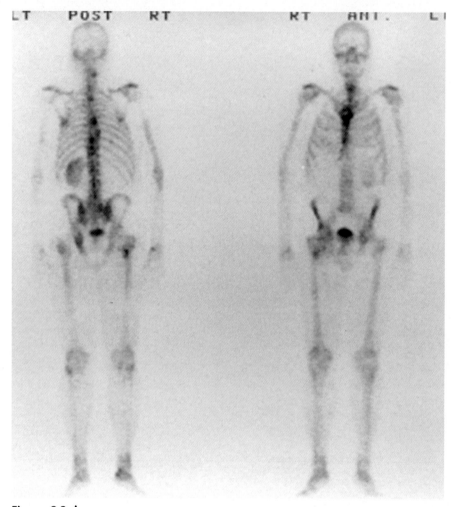

Figure 9.3 A

Artifact: An intrinsic flood (without collimation) was performed with a ^{99m}Tc point source to evaluate peaking and uniformity before and after automated uniformity correction (Fig. 9.3 B). Both floods were very nonuniform, with an integral uniformity of 24% on the corrected flood. The automatic peaking circuitry had set the peak at 107 keV (33 keV below the actual value for ^{99m}Tc at 140 keV). This failure of the autopeaking circuitry resulted in the patient being imaged in the scatter region of ^{99m}Tc, where the camera provides a nonuniform response with a degradation in spatial resolution and contrast.

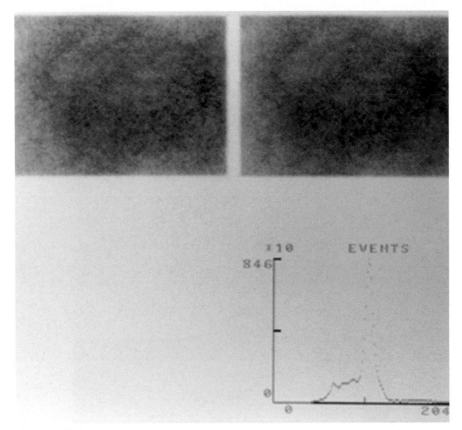

Figure 9.3 B

Discussion: The use of digital scintillation camera technology with preset acquisition protocols and automated peaking procedures has significantly improved and simplified the procedure for performing a diagnostic nuclear medicine study. However, technologists and physicians must be alert to failure of these automated systems and be able to identify potential causes for abnormalities that may appear.

Conclusion/Diagnosis: Poor image quality because the pulse-height analyzer window was off peak.

History/Procedure: A patient presented for a bone scan and was administered 20 mCi of ^{99m}Tc-oxidronate (HDP); static images of the whole body were obtained 2 hours later.

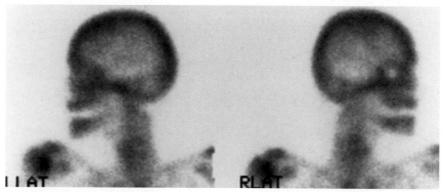

Figure 9.4 A

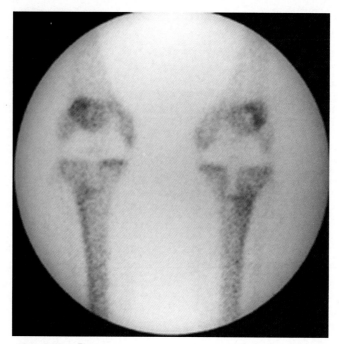

Figure 9.4 B

Artifact: In comparing the right and left lateral views (Fig. 9.4 A) of the head, it was noted that the patient had a "cold" area in the region of the right eye. In discussion with the patient, it was noted that the patient had an artificial right eye that was attenuating photons from the skull.

Discussion: It is known that any article of clothing that contains metal can potentially interfere with the acquisition of a nuclear medicine study. This is also true of prosthetic devices.

The patient should be screened before the study for such devices, and although it may not be possible to remove them, they should be identified and labeled on the images in order to assist the nuclear medicine physicians in image interpretation. Some prosthetic devices may be very obvious, such as the bilateral knee replacements in another patient shown in Figure 9.4 B.

Conclusion/Diagnosis: Prosthetic device artifact.

CASE 9.5

History/Procedure: A 51-year-old male presented with chronic right groin pain. The patient had a history of right total hip replacement, and the symptoms caused suspicion of infection. The patient was administered 570 μCi of ^{111}In labeled white blood cells and images of the pelvis were acquired 24 hours postinjection (Figs. 9.5 A and 9.5 B).

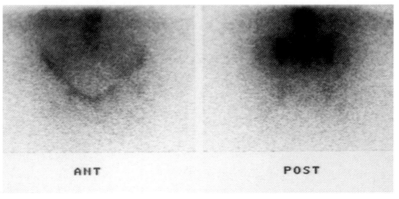

Figure 9.5 A   Figure 9.5 B

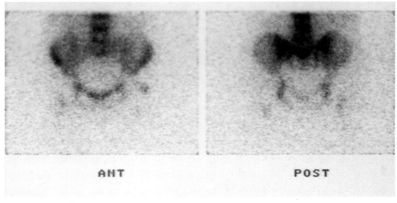

Figure 9.5 C   Figure 9.5 D

Artifact: When the images of the study were reviewed, it was observed that they were of poor quality. On further review with the technologist performing the study, it was discovered that the images were obtained with the scintillation camera peaked for ^{99m}Tc (140 keV) instead of ^{111}In (172 keV and 247 keV).

Discussion: Imaging of a photon-emitting radionuclide with a window positioned below the photopeak energy of the radionuclide results in the acquisition of a scatter image with very poor spatial information and therefore degraded spatial resolution and contrast. Using the appropriate window settings resulted in images of acceptable diagnostic quality (Figs. 9.5 C and 9.5 D), which were negative for infection.

Conclusion/Diagnosis: Pulse-height analyzer settings selected for incorrect radionuclide.

CASE 9.6

History/Procedure: A patient diagnosed with thyroid carcinoma was treated post-thyroidectomy with 100 mCi of ^{131}I administered orally. A whole-body scan was performed 72 hours after administration using a dual-head rectangular field-of-view scintillation camera with medium-energy collimators.

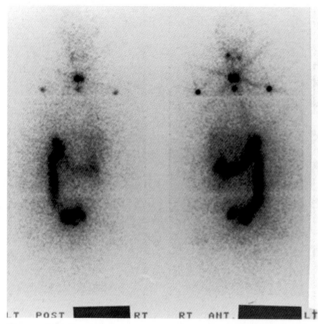

Figure 9.6 A

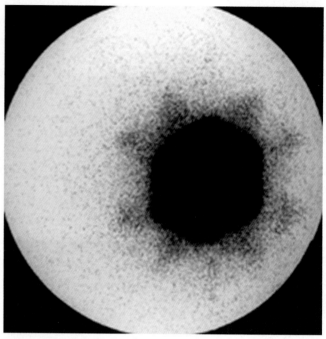

Figure 9.6 B

Artifact: The images (Fig. 9.6 A) demonstrate activity in the gastrointestinal tract as well as in residual thyroid tissue in the neck. The high background common in ^{131}I scanning is obvious, along with the "star effect" in the neck that is often seen in areas of increased activity such as the bladder, malignant lesions, and residual thyroid tissue. The star effect occasionally causes problems in image interpretation when an arm of the star passes through a suspicious region of increased activity.

Discussion: The high background and the star effect are due to septal penetration [i.e., photons passing through the walls (septa) of the holes of the collimator without being attenuated and being detected in the scintillation camera]. The star effect is a special case that is observed in the vicinity of small, discrete areas of increased uptake. The geometry of the star is determined by the geometry of the collimator, with the number of arms of the star typically equal to the number of sides

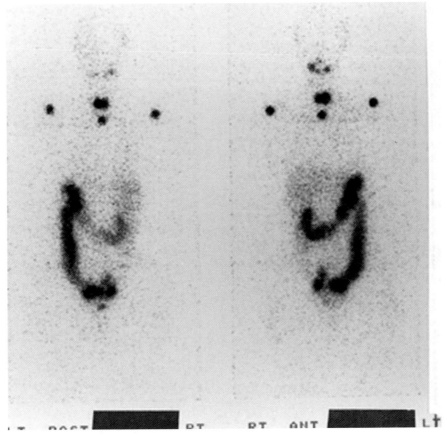

Figure 9.6 C

of a single hole. For example, the collimators used in this case had hexagon-shaped holes and were packed in a hexagonal pattern. Thus the star has six arms, since the holes are aligned such that the walls of the holes are parallel in six directions from the center of each hole, thereby presenting a smaller amount of lead for photon absorption than in the directions where the corners of the holes are aligned. Figure 9.6 B is an image of a 10-cm circular disk source of ^{131}I imaged with a medium-energy collimator. With the display intensity in-creased, the disk appears to be hexagonal in shape owing to the hexagonal pattern holes in the collimator. A collimator fabricated with square holes arranged in a square pattern would thus generate a star with four arms. The availability of high-energy collimators fabricated with thicker septa significantly reduces the background and often eliminates the star effect (Fig. 9.6 C)

Conclusion/Diagnosis: Septal penetration of collimator.

CASE 9.7

History/Procedure: A patient presented for a thyroid scan. The patient was administered 15 mCi of ^{99m}Tc-pertechnetate and routine imaging of the thyroid was performed using a pinhole collimator (Fig. 9.7).

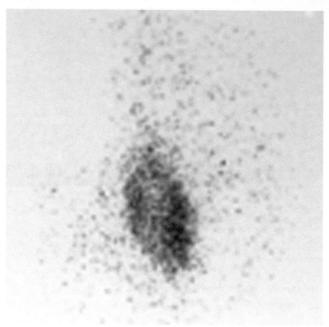

Figure 9.7

Artifact: The technologist performing the study immediately noticed that the measured count rate from the neck region was abnormally low. The technologist checked the camera for proper peak and window settings and evaluated the injection site for possible infiltrate of the administered dose. After no problems were identified, the label on the syringe used for administering the dose was examined, and it was determined that the patient was injected with 7.5 mCi of ^{99m}Tc-mercaptylacetyltriglycine (^{99m}Tc-MAG3). Although this was a recordable misadministration, there was enough free pertechnetate in the dose to obtain marginal images of the thyroid. This was true even though the dose of MAG3 had successfully passed radiopharmaceutical quality control testing.

Discussion: Extreme care must be exercised in the performance of any nuclear medicine procedure to verify that the proper patient is administered the correct radiopharmaceutical at the prescribed level of activity for the procedure. This involves checking the patient's identity (identification bracelet with medical record number for inpatients) and comparing it with the procedure request form and the dose syringe label.

Conclusion/Diagnosis: Radiopharmaceutical misadministration.

CASE 9.8

History/Procedure: A patient presented for a rest and stress cardiac perfusion study with ^{99m}Tc-sestamibi. SPECT imaging was performed with a dual-head, fixed 90-degree geometry scintillation camera using a 180-degree acquisition.

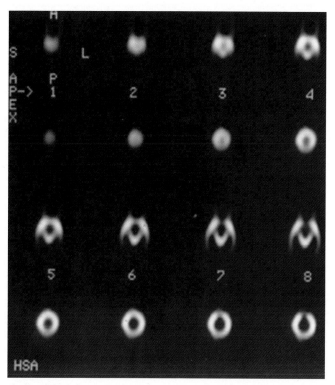

Figure 9.8

Artifact: When the images were reconstructed from the initial resting study, it was observed that there were gross errors in the geometric reconstruction of the data. A 180-degree SPECT acquisition of a cardiac phantom was performed using the suspect camera, and short-axis views of the phantom were reconstructed. These images (rows 1 and 3 of Fig. 9.8) clearly indicate a gross geometric error in the reconstruction. A center-of-rotation evaluation was performed, and it was determined that there had been a major shift in the center of rotation for one of the detector heads. After this detector was recalibrated, a new center of rotation was performed and found to be acceptable. The cardiac phantom was imaged again, and the short-axis views (rows 2 and 4 of Fig. 9.8) demonstrated that the geometric error had been eliminated.

Discussion: Routine monitoring of the center of rotation of SPECT is necessary to ensure the quality of SPECT image reconstruction. Small errors result in the generation of circular or ring artifacts; however, large errors can be catastrophic, as was the case in the example described here.

Conclusion/Diagnosis: SPECT center-of-rotation error.

CASE 9.9

History/Procedure: A patient was administered autologous white blood cells labeled with 473 μCi of ^{111}In-oxine for a whole-body survey to identify a site of infection and was imaged 24 hours later with a scintillation camera.

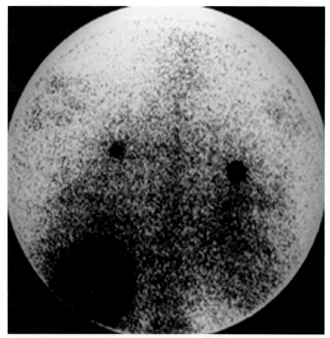

Figure 9.9

Artifact: In the image of the posterior chest (Fig. 9.9) there was diffuse uptake in the bases of both lungs, consistent with the bilateral basilar atelectasis process. In addition, two focal areas of increased uptake were noted in both the right and left lung apices.

Discussion: In the preparation of labeled white blood cells, the procedure protocol must be followed carefully not only to ensure proper labeling of the cells but also to prevent them from clumping together. In this case, it was determined that some clumping of cells occurred, resulting in the clumps being trapped in the capillaries of the lungs and producing the artifacts demonstrated in Figure 9.9.

Conclusion/Diagnosis: Artifact due to the clumping of white blood cells during the labeling procedure.

CASE 9.10

History/Procedure: A patient was administered 20 mCi of ^{99m}Tc-oxidronate (HDP) and a whole-body bone scan was performed 2 hours later to evaluate for metastatic disease.

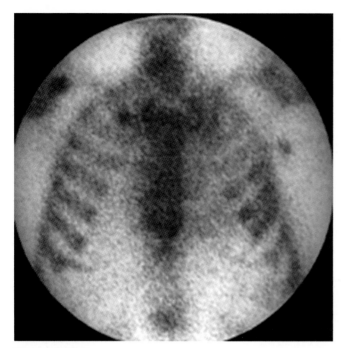

Figure 9.10 A

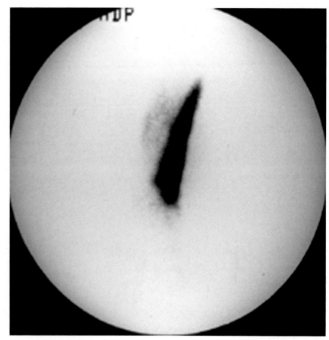

Figure 9.10 B

Artifact: In the anterior view of the chest (Fig. 9.10 A), an area of increased uptake was noted in a left axillary lymph node in addition to multiple areas of increased uptake in this image that were consistent with metastatic disease.

Discussion: The technologist noted that part of the dose was infiltrated during injection and an image of the injection site in the left arm was obtained to verify the infiltrate (Fig. 9.10 B). It was concluded that the uptake in the lymph node was due to the infiltrate and not related to the patient's disease. Whenever an infiltrate of the administered dose is suspected, it is important that the technologist verify that this has occurred and inform the nuclear medicine physician so that this situation may be considered when image interpretation is performed. This procedure may result in the prevention of an error in diagnosis, as was the situation in the case presented here.

Diagnosis/Conclusion: Infiltrate of ^{99m}Tc-oxidronate (HDP) appearing in lymph node.

CASE 9.11

History/Procedure: This 70-year-old female presented with progressive memory loss. A brain MRI showed diffuse cortical atropy appropriate to age. A ^{99m}Tc-HMPAO (hexamethylpropylene amine oxime or exametazime) SPECT scan of the brain was performed to evaluate for the presence of Alzheimer's disease.

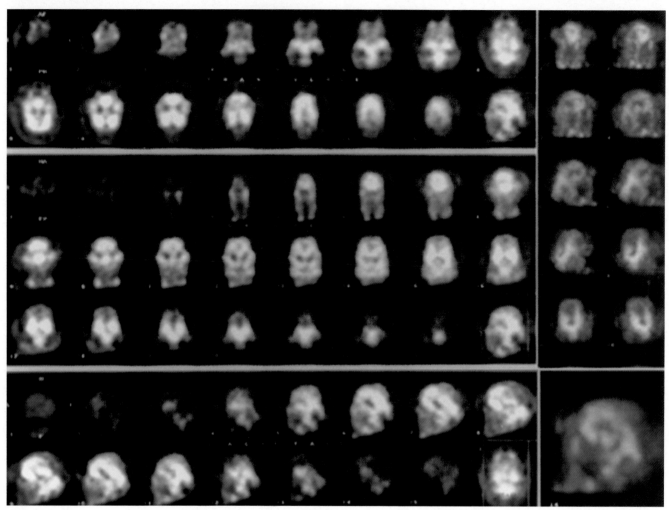

Figure 9.11

Findings: Figure 9.11 shows the entire set of images displayed in a standard report including transaxial slices from base to vertex of the brain on top left, coronal slices from anterior to posterior poles in the middle left, and sagittal slices from right to left on the bottom left of the image. Serial static views taken at different angles during the SPECT acquisition are shown on the top right and the cine loop display that has been stopped in a left lateral projection is shown at the bottom right of the image. There is virtually no uptake in the cortex and subcortical gray matter. The structures with most uptake are in a central location and have the shape of the ventricular system, which can best be recognized on the sagittal slices or the lateral view of the cine loop display.

Discussion: The pattern of ventricular uptake is most probably due to an excessive amount of free ^{99m}Tc-pertechnetate in the radiopharmaceutical preparation. Pertechnetate is ex-

creted by the choroid plexus into the cerebrospinal fluid and the ventricular system.

When ^{99m}Tc-pertechnetate is added to HMPAO in the presence of stannous reductant, a lipophilic technetium complex is formed that crosses the blood-brain barrier and fixes in the brain. Any oxidants present in the preparation may adversely affect the quality of the preparation. For example, the generator must be eluted within 24 hours for the eluate to be used to label HMPAO. Sodium chloride injection, USP, must be used as the diluent, not the bacteriostatic sodium chloride, which contains oxidants. The radiochemical purity of the radiopharmaceutical must be evaluated by chromatography and should be greater than 80%. Potential contaminants are free pertechnetate, reduced-hydrolyzed technetium, and a secondary ^{99m}Tc-HMPAO complex.

Conclusion/Diagnosis: Free pertechnetate in HPAO preparation for brain SPECT.

CASE 9.12

History/Procedure: A 79-year-old female presented to the emergency department with palpitations. SPECT images of the myocardium were acquired at rest after administration of 14 mCi of ^{99m}Tc-tetrofosmin (Figs. 9.12 C, 9.12 F and 9.12 I). The patient was unable to exercise; therefore a dobutamine infusion was administered, followed by the administration of 39 mCi of ^{99m}Tc-tetrofosmin at peak stress. SPECT images were obtained with attenuation correction using correction factors acquired from a low-output CT scanner (Figs. 9.12 A, 9.12 D and 9.12 G). Images without attenuation correction (Figs. 9.12 B, 9.12 E and 9.12 H) were also displayed for comparison purposes.

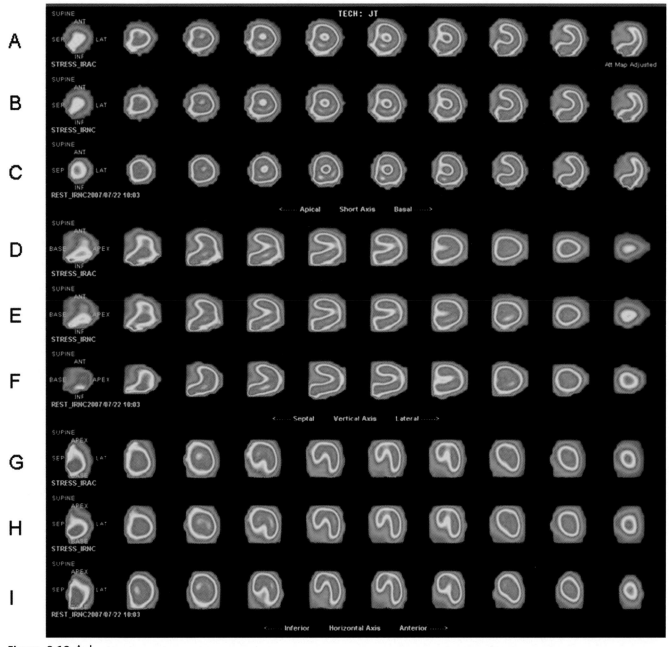

Figure 9.12 A–I

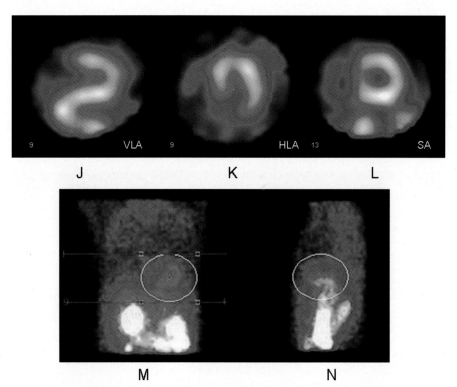

J   K   L

M   N

Figure 9.12 J–N

Artifact: The quality of the study was fair, with some noticeable thickening of the inferior wall. A review of the monitor images used to set limits prior to reconstruction (Figs. 9.12 J to 9.12 L) revealed a very unusual distribution in the vertical long-axis view (Fig. 9.12 J). Further inspection of the acquired data reviewed in cine mode (Figs. 9.12 M and 9.12 N) showed that this abnormality was due to gastrointestinal (GI) activity adjacent to the myocardium. The study was interpreted as negative for ischemia and infarct.

Discussion: The presence of GI activity after the administration of ^{99m}Tc-tetrofosmin is not an uncommon finding. Repeat imaging after having the patient drink water is often helpful. The GI activity is often reduced with time, and delayed imaging can also be performed. Therefore it is important to review the acquired data in order to identify any condition that may affect the quality of the study.

Conclusion/Diagnosis: GI activity interfering with myocardial perfusion imaging.

CASE 9.13

History/Procedure: A 50-year-old male diagnosed with thyroid carcinoma underwent thyroidectomy followed by ^{131}I therapy. Whole-body scans of the patient posttherapy are shown in Figures 9.13 A and 9.13 B. The patient returned after 6 months for posttherapy follow-up, and whole-body scans were acquired after the administration of 10 mCi of ^{123}I (Figs. 9.13 C and 9.13 D).

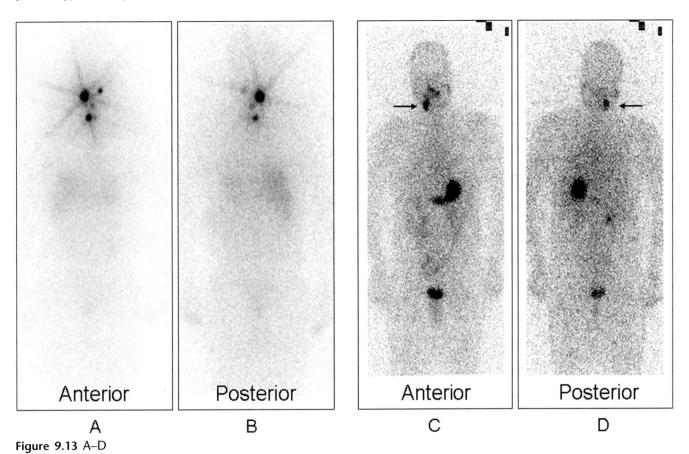

Figure 9.13 A–D

Findings: Some activity was noted in the thyroid bed (anterior view) along with a focal area of increased activity in the neck, visualized in both the anterior and posterior views. The initial impression was that this area was tumor, and additional ^{131}I treatment was contemplated. However it was decided to perform an image fusion study for anatomic correlation to determine the precise location of the focal area of increased activity. A SPECT study of the neck was acquired to image the ^{123}I distribution, along with a CT scan of the neck for anatomy, using a hybrid SPECT-CT system utilizing a low-output CT scanner. Coronal views reconstructed from the acquired data with the CT scanner (Fig. 9.13 E) and the scintillation camera (Fig. 9.13 F) were combined in registered format (Fig. 9.13 G) to correlate anatomy and function. The lesion identified on the ^{123}I study correlated precisely with a discrete opaque lesion on the CT scan. This lesion was better visualized on the transverse

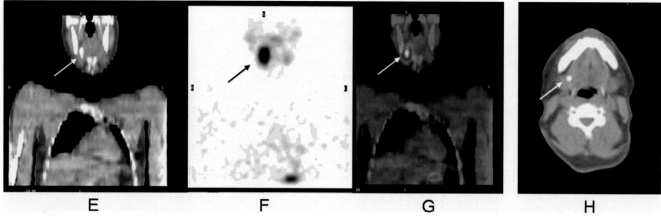

Figure 9.13 E–H

CT view (Fig. 9.13 H), and the density of the lesion was not consistent with tumor. The lesion proved to be a stone that was blocking a salivary gland and the study was read as negative for tumor.

Discussion: Combined SPECT-CT studies are extremely useful for correlating anatomy and function in order to identify anatomic locations of increased radiopharmaceutical uptake.

These combined images often increase the level of confidence of the interpreting physician and occasionally provide information that is not available independently from the separate modalities.

Conclusion/Diagnosis: Stone blocking drainage of salivary gland.

CASE 9.14

History/Procedure: A 68-year-old male with a history of adenocarcinoma of the left upper lobe of the lung who was treated with surgery and chemoradiation therapy in the past presented for follow-up evaluation. The patient was administered 10 mCi of ^{18}F-FDG and PET-CT imaging was performed at 75 minutes postinjection. A low-dose CT scan was performed as part of the study in order to correct for body attenuation and to provide anatomic correlation with the PET scan.

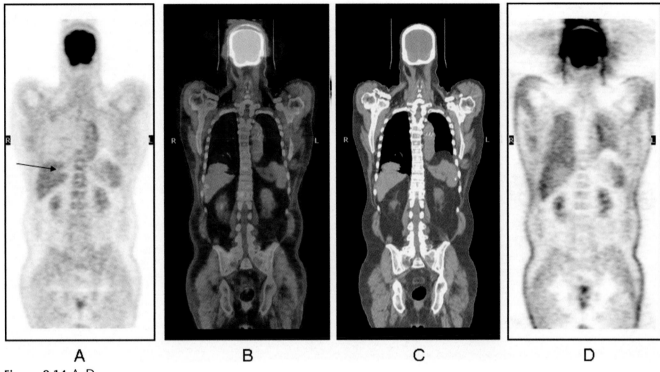

Figure 9.14 A–D

Artifact: Review of the coronal views of the attenuation-corrected PET scan (Fig. 9.14 A) indicated the presence of a wedge-shaped area of decreased activity in the liver (arrow). Further review of the corresponding view from the CT scan (Fig. 9.14 B) and the fused images of the two views (Fig. 9.14 C) demonstrated that this was an artifact in the CT scan data. The wedge-shaped defect was not present in the PET scan without attenuation correction (Fig. 9.14 D). It was determined that the defect was actually an attenuation correction artifact. The CT scan was acquired very rapidly at an acquisition rate of 8 slices per 0.5 seconds, resulting in stop-action viewing of physiologic motion of the diaphragm. Coronal views reconstructed from transverse data resulted in different components of the physiologic cycle being visualized at different times, yielding a poor representation of the actual anatomy of organs affected by diaphragm movement. On the other hand, the PET scan was acquired slowly, so that physiologic motion was aver-

aged over the acquisition time. Using very fast anatomic acquisitions to provide attenuation correction for very slow physiologic acquisitions in regions where motion is present often results in artifacts in the attenuation-corrected PET images.

The study was positive for recurring tumor in the upper left lobe in the region of prior surgery.

Discussion: In order to identify potential artifacts, it is important to view PET images without attenuation correction in regions where motion may give rise to poor registration of anatomy and physiology. Work is ongoing to develop alternative CT acquisitions (slow scanning or multiple scanning of the same region) in regions where motion may be a problem. An alternative method is the use of respiratory gating in both PET and CT to eliminate the effects of motion.

Conclusion/Diagnosis: Attenuation-correction artifact due to diaphragmatic motion.

INDEX

Page numbers followed by *f* and *t* denote figure and table, respectively.

Hibernated myocardium, 133, 139–140, 139f
HIDA. *See* Hydroxy iminodiacetic acid
High probability
  of acute pulmonary embolism, 46–47, 46f
  of CAD, 101, 102, 102f, 104
  of pulmonary embolism, 38–39, 38t, 43–45, 43f–44f
    false positive of, 50–51, 50f–51f
High-grade glioma, 172–173, 172f–173f
  low grade v., 159, 168–169, 168f–169f, 173
High-grade tumor, with adjacent ictal seizure focus, 184–185, 184f
Hilar lymphadenopathy, sarcoidosis with, 432
Hilar node enlargement, with pulmonary sarcoidosis, 83–84, 83f
Hip(s)
  osteoid osteoma of, 347
  osteonecrosis in, 311–312
  SPECT for, 308
Hip fracture, musculoskeletal scintigraphy of, 381, 381f
Hip prosthesis, bone scan of, 313
Histiocytosis X, normal bone scan and, 331f, 332
HIV
  brain infection in patients with, 167, 195
  dementia with, 167, 167f
  Pneumocystis carinii pneumonia with, 85–86, 85f
HIVAN. *See* HIV-associated nephropathy
HIV-associated nephropathy (HIVAN), 299
HMPAO. *See* Hexamethylpropylene amine oxime or exametazime
Hodgkin's disease, 474
  ^{18}F-FDG for, 434
  sclerotic metastasis with, 317
Hormone therapy, hepatic adenoma with, 205
Horseshoe kidney, 296, 296f, 439, 439f
HPO. *See* Hypertrophic osteoarthropathy
Human antimouse antibody (HAMA), formation of, 426
Humeral head, lesions in, 324f–325f, 325
Humerus
  bone island in, 354
  Paget's disease in, 401
Huntington's disease, 159, 182–183, 183f
Hydration
  for diuretic renography, 261
  for ^{18}F-FDG imaging, 424
Hydrocephalus. *See* Normal-pressure hydrocephalus (NPH)
Hydronephrosis, 261
Hydrothorax, hepatic, 243, 243f
Hydroxy iminodiacetic acid (HIDA), for hepatobiliary scintigraphy of
    chronic cholecystitis, 217, 217f
Hydroxyapatite crystal
  diphosphonate compound binding of, 307
  ^{18}F-fluoride ion and, 307
  osteogenic activity and, 308
Hydroxydiphosphonate (HDP), for bone scanning, 307
Hydroxyethylene diphosphonate (HEDP), for bone scanning, 307
Hyperacute rejection, renal allograft failure and, 286
Hypercalcemia, 28
  atherosclerotic heart disease and, 418
  muscle bone scan and, 342
Hypercalcitoninemia, MCT and, 441–442
Hypercortisolemia, with Cushing's syndrome, 501
Hyperemia
  avascular necrosis and, 412, 412f
  bone tumors and, 310
  three-phase bone scan and, 311
Hyperemia of synovitis, with reflex sympathetic dystrophy, 408
Hyperglycemia, ^{18}F-FDG uptake in patients with, 174, 174f, 435
Hyperinsulinemia euglycemic clamp, for promoting cardiac ^{18}F-FDG
    uptake, 138
Hyperparathyroidism
  musculoskeletal scintigraphy of, 313, 315–316, 331f, 332
  osteoporosis and, 387

with parathyroid adenoma, 28–30, 28f–30f
  postparathyroidectomy, 29f–30f, 30
  with renal osteodystrophy, 402
  superscan and, 309, 326
Hyperphosphatemia, with renal osteodystrophy, 403
Hypertension. *See* Portal hypertension; Pulmonary arterial hypertension;
    Renovascular hypertension
Hyperthermia, rhabdomyolysis with, 396
Hyperthyroidism
  classification of, 10t
  with Graves' disease, 10–12, 10f–11f, 10t
  with postpartum autoimmune thyroiditis, 13–14, 13f
  superscan and, 328
  toxic autonomously functioning follicular adenoma imaging, 6–7
  with toxic multinodular goiter, 10–12, 10f–11f, 10t
Hypertrophic osteoarthropathy (HPO), musculoskeletal scintigraphy of, 415,
    415f
Hypertrophic pulmonary osteoarthropathy, shin splints v., 378
Hypervitaminosis A, hypertrophic osteoarthropathy and, 415
Hypervitaminosis D, superscan and, 309, 326–327
Hypocalcemia
  with renal osteodystrophy, 403
  rhabdomyolysis with, 396
Hypokinesis
  with chemotherapy, 130, 130f
  with dilated cardiomyopathy, 131, 131f
Hypothalamic-pituitary-thyroid axis, 2–3, 2f
Hypothyroidism, neonatal, 24–25, 24f–25f
Hypoxia, alveolar, 71

^{123}I. *See* Iodine 123
^{125}I. *See* Iodine 125
^{131}I scintigraphy, for thyroid cancer, 443–444
^{131}I therapy
  for AFTNs, 7
  for follicular carcinoma of thyroid, 17–20
  for goiter, 16
  for Graves' disease, 12
  for multinodular goiter, 9, 12
  for toxic multinodular goiter, 12
Iatrogenic postoperative leaks, 177
IBD. *See* Irritable bowel disease
^{123}I-BMIPP, for viability evaluation, 134
Ictal SPECT
  of cortical dysplasia and closed-lip schizencephaly, 196–197, 196f
  for seizure localization, 162–163, 162f–163f
IDA. *See* Iminodiacetic acid
^{123}I-IMP, 156
^{125}I-iothalamate, 260
Imaging technique, for ventilation/perfusion (V/Q) scintigraphy, 37
^{123}I-MIBG, 206
  for adrenal medulla scintigraphy, 3
  for metastatic neuroblastoma, 502
  for oncologic imaging, 425–426
  for pheochromocytoma, 31–34, 31f–32f, 505
^{131}I-MIBG, 206
  for adrenal medulla scintigraphy, 3
  for oncologic imaging, 425–426
  for pheochromocytoma, 31–34, 31f–32f, 32
Iminodiacetic acid (IDA), 204
Immunocompromise, *Pneumocystis carinii* pneumonia with, 85–86, 85f
IMP. *See* Iodo-amphetamine
Impurity
  in HMPAO, 528, 528f
  in macroaggregated albumin, 80, 80f
^{111}In. *See* Indium 111
^{111}In radiolabeled monoclonal antibody, for OncoScint immunoscintigraphy,
    206
Indications, for neurologic imaging, 157–160